U. Heim K. M. Pfeiffer

Internal Fixation of Small Fractures

Technique Recommended by the AO-ASIF Group

Third Edition of Small Fragment Set Manual

In Collaboration with
J. Brennwald C. Geel R.P. Jakob T. Rüedi B. Simmen
H.U. Stäubli

Translated by T.C. Telger

With 258 Figures in more than 700 Separate Illustrations
Drawings by K. Oberli

Springer-Verlag Berlin Heidelberg New York
London Paris Tokyo

Priv. Doz. Dr. URS HEIM
Mattenstrasse 17a
CH-3073 Gümligen-Bern

Prof. Dr. KARL M. PFEIFFER
Chirurgisches Departement
Kantonsspital Basel
CH-4031 Basel

Translated from the German by
TERRY C. TELGER
6112 Waco Way
Ft. Worth, TX 76133/USA

ISBN-13: 978-3-642-72616-3 e-ISBN-13: 978-3-642-72614-9
DOI: 10.1007/978-3-642-72614-9

Library of Congress Cataloging-in-Publication Data. Heim, U., 1924–. [Periphere Osteosynthesen. English] Internal fixation of small fractures: technique recommanded by the AO-ASIF Group / U. Heim, K.M. Pfeiffer; in collaboration with J. Brennwald ... [et al.]; translated by T.C. Telger; drawings by K. Oberli. – 3rd ed. p. cm.
Rev. translation of: Periphere Osteosynthesen. First English edition published in 1974 under title: Small fragment set manual. Bibliography: p.
Includes index. 1. Internal fixation in fractures. I. Pfeiffer, K.M. (Karl Maria), 1927–. II. Brennwald, J. III. Arbeitsgemeinschaft für Osteosynthesefragen. IV. Title. RD103.I5H4413 1988 617'. 15–dc19 87-28711 CIP

Softcover reprint of the hardcover 3rd edition 1988

Reproduction of the figures: Gustav Dreher GmbH, Stuttgart

2124/3130-543210

Preface to the Third Edition

The second English-language edition of the *Small Fragment Set Manual* was enthusiastically received and quickly went into a second printing.

In preparing a third edition, we found it necessary to revise the text extensively and partly restructure it. The reasons for this are numerous.

Experience of recent years has brought technical refinements in the operative treatment of many types of small fracture. Many of these changes stem from the small-fragment-set training programs conducted in Switzerland since 1980, and also from courses and symposia that have been held in other European countries and the United States. These events were occasions for a fruitful exchange of experience with surgeons who were critical of our methods. As a result of this exchange, we perceived a need both to revise our indications and to give greater attention to alternative techniques.

We also felt it necessary to respond to criticisms of the first two editions concerning the catalog-like instrument lists and illustrations, and the attention given to fundamental techniques. Many surgeons who work or would like to work with small implants, especially those practicing abroad, are inexperienced in operations on the larger bones. It is imperative that these colleagues be given a basic introduction to the "biomechanical thinking" of the Swiss Association for the Study of Internal Fixation (ASIF).

We have tried to place greater emphasis on soft-tissue techniques (incisions, approaches, wound closure) and on potential dangers and errors that can occur in specific situations. Clinical examples were added where necessary in order to document new experiences. Also, previous descriptions were made more concise so that we could expand the contents of the book while maintaining its compact size.

The list of references, considered too general in the previous editions, has been broken down by chapters for the present edition, although its length had to be greatly curtailed. The dangers of this are well known. Also, some repetitions are unavoidable when this type of arrangement is used.

A major goal of the third edition is to present innovations in our armamentarium that have been developed in the last few years or are about to be introduced. We have tried to integrate and illustrate their practical use.

By consulting with qualified experts from the ASIF, we were able to add depth and detail to specific chapters in cases where developments appeared to warrant it. We are deeply indebted to these colleagues for their assistance.

Course organizers and authors of instructional materials are commonly blamed for the failures of participants and readers. No type of teaching is immune, whether it is given in courses, at the operating table, or in the literature. Yet ultimately, every surgeon is responsible for acquiring his own experience and expertise. Human inadequacies – including one's own – set painful limits to "progress", despite technical innovations.

As the age and situation of the authors make it unlikely that this material will be reworked again at a later time, we must look upon this third edition as the culmination of many years' work devoted to the study and description of a specialized area of traumatology.

As before, we are indebted to many friends and colleagues for their help, advice, and criticisms. We express special thanks to our illustrator, Mr. K. Oberli. His superb drawings document his wealth of knowledge and his ability to grasp this difficult material. We also thank Mr. U. Keller of the ASIF Documentation Center in Bern for the excellent X-ray reproductions. We once again acknowledge the tireless work of our secretaries, Mrs. M. Keller and Mrs. L. Gutzwiller, and the efforts of others who quietly gave their help and council in the disposition of many details. Finally, we thank the staff at Springer-Verlag for their thoughtful cooperation and outstanding production work.

Gümligen and Basel, October 1987

U. Heim
K.M. Pfeiffer

Contents

I. **History and Goals** 1

General Section

II. **Implants and Instruments** 5

1. Screws 5
2. Plates 8
3. Additional Implants 10
4. The Small External Fixator 10
5. Instruments 10
6. Instrument Cases 13
7. Mini Compressed Air Machine 13

III. **General Techniques for the Internal Fixation of Small Fractures** 31

1. Basic Principles 31
2. Interfragmental Compression with Lag Screws 32
3. Tension-Band Wires 34
4. Axial Interfragmental Compression with a Plate 35
5. Neutralization Plates 37
6. Buttress Plates 38
7. Combined Internal Fixation Using Small and Large Implants 38
8. Multiple Fractures 38
9. Operative Technique with Special Plates 39
10. Open Fractures 40
11. Small External Fixator – Technique and Indications 40

IV. **Preoperative, Operative, and Postoperative Guidelines** 69

V. **Removal of Implants** 73

VI. **Autogenous Bone Grafts** 75

VII. **Reconstructive Surgery** 77

Special Section

VIII. Introduction and Overview 83

IX. The Shoulder Girdle 85

1. Clavicle 85
2. Scapula 87
3. Proximal Humerus 89
4. Illustrative Clinical X-Rays 89

X. The Elbow 107

1. Distal Humerus 107
2. Radial Head 109
3. Olecranon 112
4. Illustrative Clinical X-Rays 113

XI. The Shafts of the Radius and Ulna 139

XII. The Wrist and Carpus 145

1. Distal Radius 145
2. Distal Ulna 149
3. Scaphoid (Navicular) 149
4. Other Carpal Bones 150
5. Arthrodesis of the Wrist 151
6. Illustrative Clinical X-Rays 151

XIII. The Hand 179

A. Introduction 179

B. Injuries of the First Ray 180

1. Fractures of the Base of the First Metacarpal 180
2. Distal Fractures of the First Ray 182
3. Secondary Operations on the First Ray 182
4. Illustrative Case Reports and X-Rays 183

C. Injuries of the Second through Fifth Rays 204

1. Approaches 204
2. Fractures of the Second through Fifth Metacarpals 206
3. Articular Fractures 207
4. Fractures of the Phalangeal Shafts 208
5. Secondary Operations on the Second through Fifth Rays . . . 209
6. Fixation Techniques for Complex Injuries and Amputations of the Hand 210
7. Illustrative Case Reports and X-Rays 211

XIV. The Knee 247

1. Patella 247
2. Tibia 248

3. Ligament Repairs 248
4. Lateral Avulsion Fractures (Femoral Condyle, Fibular Head) 249
5. Osteochondral Fractures 249
6. Secondary Operations 249
7. Illustrative Case Reports and X-Rays 249

XV. The Tibial Shaft 259

XVI. The Ankle Joint 261

A. Distal Intra-Articular Fractures of the Tibia 261

1. Split Fractures without a Cancellous Bone Defect 262
2. Simple Depressed Fracture 262
3. Complex Fractures with a Cancellous Bone Defect 263
4. Secondary Operations 265
5. Illustrative Case Reports and X-Rays 266

B. Malleolar Fractures 286

1. Classification and Patient Selection 286
2. Internal Fixations and Ligament Repairs on the Lateral Side . . 287
3. Internal Fixations on the Medial Side 295
4. Aftertreatment 296
5. Secondary Operations after Malleolar Fractures 297

C. Fractures of the Talus 297

D. Illustrative Case Reports and X-Rays 297

XVII. The Foot 337

1. Calcaneus 337
2. Tarsal Navicular 338
3. Cuneiforms and Cuboid 339
4. Dislocations and Fracture-Dislocations 339
5. Fractures of the Metatarsal Shaft and Neck 340
6. Fractures of the Fifth Metatarsal 341
7. Fractures of the Big Toe 342
8. Secondary Operations on the Forefoot 342
9. Illustrative Case Reports and X-Rays 343

XVIII. Special Indications 373

1. Internal Fixations in Children 373
2. Use of the SFS in Rheumatoid Surgery 373
3. Illustrative Case Reports and X-Rays 373

References 383

Subject Index 389

List of Collaborators

Authors

Urs Heim, Priv.-Doz. Dr., Specialist in Surgery, Mattenstrasse 17a, CH-3073 Gümligen-Bern

Karl M. Pfeiffer, Prof. Dr., Chief of Hand Surgery, Kantonsspital Basel, CH-4031 Basel

Collaborators

Jürg Brennwald, Priv.-Doz., Staff Physician, Division of Hand Surgery, Department of Surgery, Kantonsspital Basel, CH-4031 Basel and Lab. f. Experimental Surgery, Schweiz. Forschungsinstitut, CH-7270 Davos-Platz (Fixation Techniques for Complex Injuries and Amputations of the Hand)

Christof Geel, Dr., Staff Physician, Department of Orthopedic Surgery, Upstate Medical Center, 550 Harrison Street, Syracuse, New York 13202, USA (Scapula)

Roland P. Jakob, Priv.-Doz., Assistant Director, Clinic for Orthopedics and Surgery of the Musculoskeletal System, Inselspital Bern, CH-3010 Bern (Small External Fixator)

Thomas Rüedi, Prof., Chief of Surgery, Surgical Clinic, Kantonsspital Chur, CH-7000 Chur (Scapula)

Beat Simmen, Dr., Staff Physician, Department of Surgery, Kantonsspital Basel, CH-4031 Basel (The Foot)

Hans-Ulrich Stäubli, Dr., Chief of Surgery, Surgical Clinic, Tiefenauspital of the City of Berne, CH-3006 Bern (Distal Humerus)

Illustrator

Klaus Oberli, Technical Illustrator, Berchtoldstrasse 29, CH-3012 Bern

I. History and Goals

Practical experience in the operative treatment of fractures quickly demonstrated a need to supplement the standard instrument set of the ASIF with smaller implants. Certain situations pointed up obvious deficiencies in the instruments and appliances developed between 1958 and 1960.

This first became apparent during the fixation of thin, narrow fragments in large cylindrical bones. The large drill holes jeopardized the viability of the fragments, and the conical screw heads threatened to crack them. The prominent, dome-like screw heads also proved troublesome on diaphyseal borders and in certain other areas.

The relatively thick and inflexible plates of the standard set created unacceptably large foreign bodies on the metaphyses of the upper extremity and distal tibia. In these cases a gross disproportion existed between the bone and implant, and often this was detrimental to the soft tissues, especially the skin.

Comminuted fractures involving smaller joints such as the elbow and ankle, in which the long-term prognosis depends critically on an accurate reduction and fixation, were difficult to manage with bulky cancellous screws. It was usually necessary to resort to Kirschner wires in these situations, with a corresponding sacrifice of rigidity.

Clinical experience and experimental studies have repeatedly shown that loose, isolated fragments of cortex will become revascularized if they can be stably reintegrated into a living environment. This led to the use of small, individual implants as components of a "combined" internal fixation.

Finally, the standard-size implants were not at all appropriate for the short, thin, tubular bones of the hand and foot. In 1946 Kilbourne, prompted by functional considerations, became the first surgeon to perform internal fixations with small screws and plates. His results in 17 cases were published in 1958. Great hopes were placed in the stable internal fixation of hand fractures and the avoidance of postoperative casting, which can lead to joint stiffness if prolonged.

In 1959 the ASIF developed the "scaphoid screw" for cancellous bone. Later it was modified for more universal applications and was renamed the "small cancellous screw." In its new form, this implant is suitable for scaphoid fractures only in highly selected cases. But the problem of coping with the diverse shapes and dimensions of the peripheral bones could be solved only by the creation of a complete instrument set having the widest possible range of applications. The credit for developing this set belongs to Dr. Robert Mathys of Bettlach. The first prototypes of small cortex screws with unthreaded shanks produced excellent interfragmental compression, but they were extremely difficult to remove from the cortical bone. Then, in 1964, a standard set of small implants and instruments was assembled in rapid order and made available for clinical testing.

The small fragment set of the ASIF (hereafter abbreviated as SFS) was designed both in the realm and in the spirit of the Swiss watchmaking industry. All the instruments and implants of the SFS are delicate, and they are designed to be handled with skill rather than force. While the screws are remarkably strong and provide excellent stability, they have their limitations. It would be inappropriate to use them in areas where mechanical or anatomic factors demand the use of standard-size implants. The availability of small implants should never tempt the surgeon to compromise stability. In the past, many failures of operative fracture treatment resulted from the use of implants that were too short or too weak. The small screws and plates should never be used to obtain a feeble hold in an open reduction. Like the implants from the standard set, their purpose is to provide the degree of stability that is necessary for early postoperative mobilization. A major purpose of this book is to emphasize that goal.

Today, basic questions on the indications for internal fixation and operative techniques have been resolved for most fractures and nonunions by animal experiments and clinical results. The SFS makes skeletal injuries of the hand and foot, as well as small fractures of other bones, accessible to management by the same, basic principles of open reduction and rigid internal fixation.

Veterinarians and maxillofacial surgeons have developed specialized instrument sets from the SFS, and information on these sets is available in the literature.

To date we have had more than 20 years' clinical experience with the internal fixation of small fractures. Many of the small implants are described and illustrated in the *Manual of Internal Fixation* (2nd edition, Springer-Verlag).

As in the first two editions of the *Small Fragment Set Manual*, the material that follows represents a clinical study whose primary goal is the advancement of surgical practice.

General Section

II. Implants and Instruments

Experience has shown that the diversity of implants can be a source of confusion. Because a number of innovations are described, we have adhered to our previous format, although every implant is not drawn to scale so that its function can be more clearly demonstrated.

1. Screws (Fig. 1)

There are six different types of screw in the SFS:

a) The 4.0-mm Small Cancellous Screw with a Smooth Shank

Dimensions (Fig. 1): Outer diameter of thread 4.0 mm, core diameter 1.9 mm, pitch 1.75 mm, shank diameter between head and thread 2.3 mm. The threaded length increases from 5 to 15 mm in proportion to the overall screw length. Lengths: 10 mm to 30 mm in 2-mm increments, 30 mm to 50 mm in 5-mm increments.

Technique (Figs. 2, 22): For screw fixation: The hole is predrilled with the 2.5-mm bit through the corresponding double drill guide, then threaded with the 3.5-mm *cancellous* tap using the double drill guide as a tap sleeve.

Applications: The slightly undersized tap diameter is practically unnoticed when the screw is driven into the cancellous bone and causes no clinical problems. The wide thread of the screw ensures a solid hold. In exceptional cases the screw may be used with the one-third tubular plates or special plates. It has replaced the "malleolar screw" for many applications.

Disadvantages: A weak point exists at the junction of the smooth shank and thread, where the screw is liable to fracture on removal (Figs. 174, 247). Recently the back surface of the threads has been sloped toward the screw tip so that the screw will, in effect, cut a new thread as it is removed.

b) The 4.0-mm Fully Threaded Small Cancellous Screw (Fig. 1)

This screw supplements the partially threaded 4.0-mm cancellous screw and has the same diameter. It was designated in 1986 as the successor to the old 3.5-mm cortex screw having the same 1.75-mm pitch.

Production of the latter was discontinued because the operator might confuse it with the new 3.5-mm cortex screw and use the wrong implant, bit, or tap. The older screw had certain disadvantages and did not conform to international standards. Once the new 3.5-mm cortex screw with a larger core and reduced pitch had become established, it was possible to go to the 4.0-mm outer diameter exclusively for cancellous bone.

Technique (Fig. 2): For screw fixation: The hole is predrilled with the 2.5-mm bit through the 3.5/2.5-mm insert drill sleeve, then threaded with the 3.5-mm *cancellous* tap using the large end of the 3.5/2.5-mm double drill guide as a tap sleeve.

Applications: Plate fixation in loose cancellous bone; cancellous screw fixations that do not require a gliding hole (avulsions, chip fractures, fixation of washers, etc.).

c) The 3.5-mm Small Cortex Screw

This implant was introduced in 1983.

Dimensions (Fig. 1): Outer diameter of thread 3.5 mm, core diameter 2.4 mm, pitch 1.25 mm. Lengths: 10 mm to 28 mm in 2-mm increments, 28 mm to 50 mm in 4-mm increments.

Screw lengths up to 110 mm are available for special applications (pelvis).

The dimensions of this screw conform to international standards.

Technique (Figs. 2, 23): For screw fixation: The gliding hole is drilled with the 3.5-mm bit through the corresponding bronze-colored double drill guide. The thread hole is drilled with the bronze-colored 2.5-mm bit through a separate 3.5/2.5-mm insert drill sleeve or through the small end of the 3.5/2.5-mm double drill guide. The hole is tapped with the 3.5-mm *cortex* tap (bronze) using the large end of the double drill guide as a tap sleeve.

For plate fixation: The hole is drilled with the 2.5-mm bit (bronze) through the small end of the double drill guide or DCP drill guide and threaded with the 3.5-mm *cortex* tap (bronze) using the large end of the double drill guide as a tap sleeve.

Applications: The new 3.5-mm small cortex screw can be used in both cortical and cancellous bone. Despite the larger core, the smaller pitch provides a greater area of bony contact, and so this screw holds better than the older screw with the same outer diameter, renamed the *small cancellous screw*.The new 3.5-mm *cortex* tap may give better results in hard cortical bone. The screw is used in all plates of the 3.5-mm series, particularly the 3.5-mm dynamic compression plate (DCP). The thicker core keeps the screw from deforming when inserted, providing better axial displacement of the plate and better interfragmental compression than was possible with previous screws.

d) New Technique for Small Screws

- Today a 2.5-mm thread hole is used for all three screws described above, replacing the 2.0-mm hole formerly used. It has been shown clinically and experimentally that this does not weaken the hold of the cancellous screws.

The 2.5-mm drill bit is substantially stronger than the 2.0-mm bit and is less apt to bend on encountering an oblique cortical surface. Owing to this simplification and the systematic introduction of double drill guides for all screw sizes, it has been possible to standardize and simplify the instruments used.

- The drilling technique has been standardized for all the small screws. It now corresponds to the classic ASIF technique as originally recommended for the 4.5-mm cortex screw (see *Manual of Internal Fixation*, pp. 36ff.).

This was made possible by the introduction of double drill guides having a sleeve design.A single instrument can now perform the functions of a gliding-hole drill guide, insert drill sleeve, and tap sleeve. Each end of the instrument corresponds to the outer diameter or the core diameter of the screw being used (Figs. 11-13). The narrow sleeve enables the drill bit to be directed with greater precision, especially in plate holes, where a vertical, oblique, central, or eccentric drill placement can be accurately achieved.

Separate insert drill sleeves with a round handle are additionally available for the 3.5- and 2.7-mm cortex screws. They are intended for use in bones with wide medullary cavities. Separate insert sleeves of this type cannot be produced in smaller dimensions for technical reasons.

With a moderately wide or narrow medullary cavity, the small end of the double drill guide can be used as an insert drill sleeve in the predrilled gliding hole (Fig. 12).

The procedure formerly called the "small fragment technique" is still applicable: First a thread hole is drilled through both cortices, then both cortices are tapped, and finally the near hole is drilled out with a larger bit to make the gliding hole (Fig. 12). Potential problems with this technique are illustrated in Figs. 26 and 27.

e) The 2.7-mm Small Cortex Screw

Dimensions (Fig. 1): Outer diameter of thread 2.7 mm, core diameter 1.9 mm, pitch 1.0 mm, fully threaded. Lengths: 6 mm to 40 mm in 2-mm increments.

Technique (Figs. 2, 12): For screw fixation: The gliding hole is drilled with the 2.7-mm bit through the corresponding double drill guide. The thread hole is drilled with the 2.0-mm bit through a separate 2.7/2.0-mm insert sleeve or through the double drill guide used as an insert sleeve. The hole is threaded with the 2.7-mm tap using the appropriate double drill guide.

For plate fixation: The hole is drilled with the 2.0-mm bit through the corresponding double drill guide and threaded with the 2.7-mm tap using the appropriate double drill guide as a tap sleeve.

Applications: The 2.7-mm small cortex screw is suitable for use in the metacarpals and metatarsals, and for the fibula or distal forearm in selected cases. It is used to fix the 2.7-mm plates for hand and foot surgery, the quarter tubular plate, and the 2.7-mm DCP. It is also used with the spiked plastic washer to reattach avulsed ligaments (Figs. 1, 28).

f) The 2.0-mm Mini Cortex Screw

Dimensions (Fig. 1): Since 1984 the mini cortex screws have carried an hexagonal socket that measures 1.5 mm across the flats.This makes the head slightly taller than in the older Phillips head screw. Outer thread diameter 2.0 mm, core diameter 1.4 mm, pitch 0.6 mm, fully threaded. Lengths: 6 mm to 24 mm in 2-mm increments.

Technique (Figs. 2, 24): For screw fixation: The gliding hole is drilled with the 2.0-mm bit through the corresponding double drill guide. The thread hole is drilled with the 1.5-mm bit through the double drill guide used as an insert sleeve. The hole is threaded with the 2.0-mm tap using the appropriate double drill guide as a tap sleeve. The hole is countersunk.

For plate fixation: The hole is drilled with the 1.5-mm bit through the corresponding double drill guide, measured with the mini depth gauge, and threaded with the 2.0-mm tap using the corresponding double drill guide as a tap sleeve.

Applications: The 2.0-mm mini cortex screw is suitable for the peripheral bones of the hand (proximal and middle phalanx, small metacarpals). It is used to fix the "mini plates," the 2.0-mm DCP, the 2.0-mm mini condylar plate, and the 2.0-mm H plate.

g) The 1.5-mm Mini Cortex Screw

Dimensions (Fig. 1): The 1.5-mm mini cortex screws also come with an hexagonal socket, making the head slightly taller than in the pre-1984 design. Outer thread diameter 1.5 mm, core diameter 1.1 mm, pitch 0.5 mm, fully threaded.Lengths: 6 mm to 12 mm in 1-mm increments, 12 mm to 20 mm in 2-mm increments.

Technique (Figs. 2, 24): For screw fixation: The gliding hole is drilled with the 1.5-mm bit through the corresponding double drill guide. The thread hole is drilled with the 1.1-mm bit through the double drill guide used as an insert sleeve. The hole is measured with the mini depth gauge and threaded with the 1.5-mm tap using the appropriate double drill guide as a tap sleeve.

For plate fixation: The hole is drilled with the 1.1-mm bit through the corresponding double drill guide, measured with the mini depth gauge, and threaded with the 1.5-mm tap using the double drill guide as a tap sleeve.

Applications: The 1.5-mm mini cortex screw is suitable for use in the phalanges, radial head, and small butterfly fragments. It is used to fix the 1.5-mm mini plate, the 1.5-mm mini condylar plate, and the 1.5-mm H plate.

The hold of this smallest screw is excellent and is surprising considering the size of the implant.

h) Special Dimensions

Extra-long screws with diameters of 2.7 mm and 2.0 mm are available by special order for arthrodeses of the hand.

i) The Screw Heads (Fig. 3)

All the small screws now have a uniform head design. The surface of the head is vaulted but not too prominent. All the screw heads carry an hexagonal socket.

In 1984 the mini screw heads were redesigned to improve the hold of the screw and make it easier to drive and manipulate with the hexagonal screwdriver. Screw removal is also facilitated. This design change has proved successful in every respect, dispelling fears that the slightly taller head might jeopardize the soft tissues.

The undersurface of the head is spherical to ensure solid seating in plate holes.This also provides better axial compression than a conical head design when the screw is placed eccentrically.

If fixation is obtained with screws alone in thick cortical bone, countersinking is recommended. A washer is useful on thin cortex to prevent subsidence of the head (Figs. 1, 28).

A single screwdriver fits the 4.0-, 3.5-, and 2.7-mm screw sizes.A special, smaller screwdriver fits the hexagonal socket of the 2.0- and 1.5-mm screws. Although the screwdriver fits snugly into the screws, the holding sleeve was retained at the request of numerous surgeons (Fig. 4).

All of the drawings on operating technique show the new screw heads with hexagonal sockets, but many of the clinical examples show the older Phillips heads, since most of these cases date from several years ago.

k) Washers

Small metal washers were developed to keep the screw heads from sinking into thin cortical bone and to distribute the head pressure more evenly to prevent the splitting of narrow fragments. The larger washers are designed for the 4.0- to 2.7-mm screw sizes, and the smaller washers for the 2.0- and 1.5-mm mini screws (Figs. 1, 28).

Wide plastic washers with spikes are available for the fixation of avulsed ligaments to the bone and for the compression of very small avulsion fractures or small comminuted areas. A thin metal ring is incorporated into these washers to provide a radiographic marker. These claw-shaped implants are fixed with the 4.0- and 3.5-mm screws, and a smaller size is fixed with the 2.7-mm screw (Figs. 1, 28).

2. Plates

In response to demands, the assortment of plates has been expanded considerably in recent years, especially in the smaller dimensions. It has also undergone modifications.

All holes in the shaft portion of the plates are oval to provide the option for axial compression through eccentric screw placement. Oval holes also permit the screws to be inserted obliquely if required. All the flat plates are flexible so that they can be contoured with pliers or shortened with the cutting forceps for finger plates and Kirschner wires. The thicker DCPs are shaped with bending irons or the bending press.

a) The 3.5-mm Plates

Straight Plates

One-third Tubular Plate (Figs. 5, 31): This is the most commonly used plate in the SFS. It is trough-shaped, 10 mm wide, 1 mm thick, and comes in lengths of 25 mm (2-hole) to 145 mm (12-hole). Axial compression can be applied either by eccentric screw placement or by use of the tension device (Fig. 31). The plate is most commonly used on the lateral malleolus, metatarsus, distal ulna, and olecranon.

In the tubular plates for 3.5- and 2.7-mm screws (one-third and quarter tubular), the rims of the holes are raised on the concave side of the plate to prevent direct contact between the screw head and cortex (Fig. 5a). This contact is believed to lessen the stability of the plate fixation.

The 3.5-mm DCP (Figs. 5, 32): This plate is identical to the one-third tubular plate in length, width, and the number and spacing of the holes, but its 3-mm thickness gives it considerably greater strength.Its applications have been greatly expanded in recent years (forearm bones, clavicle, etc.).

Shaped Plates

Small T Plate (Fig. 6): This plate has an arched cross section and is slightly angled at the head.

The shaft is 10 mm wide. The plate comes in lengths of 50 and 57 mm, and the head comes with 3 holes. This implant, originally designed for the volar side of the distal radius, has proved useful on the olecranon, lateral clavicle, ankle joint, first metatarsal, and other areas.

Small Oblique T Plate (Fig. 6):The holes of this flat plate are beveled on both sides, and the oblique head is angled 120°. The plate is designed for use on the dorsal aspect of the distal radius, where it can grip the styloid process more securely than the 90° T plate. It is equally effective on the right and left sides.

Cloverleaf Plate (Fig. 6): This plate was specially designed for the medial aspect of the distal tibial epiphysis. It can be modified for use in other areas (e.g., the humeral head) by cutting off one of the cloverleaf tabs.

All the plate holes are compatible with 3.5- and 4.0-mm screws. The strong 3.5-mm cortex screw is used in the shaft. This eliminates the need for 4.5-mm cortex screws and simplifies the use of these plates (SFS implants and instruments are used exclusively).

Special Plates

Reconstruction Plate (Fig. 5): This plate comes in various lengths and is notched along the sides to facilitate 3-dimensional contouring with bending irons.

H Plate. This is specially designed for the cervical spine and is available in various lengths.

b) The 2.7-mm Plates

Straight Plates

Quarter Tubular Plate (Figs. 7, 35): The holes of this straight, trough-shaped plate have raised rims (Fig. 7c) that help to make the plate stronger than the older flat version. Lengths range from 23 mm (3-hole) to 63 mm (8-hole). The plate is used chiefly on the metacarpus and foot.

The 2.7-mm DCP (Fig. 7): This plate is most commonly used in veterinary and mandibular surgery. Because of its thickness, it is used only occasionally in secondary operations for delayed unions or nonunions of the hand. Lengths range from 20 mm (2-hole) to 100 mm (12-hole).

Shaped Plates

Small T Plate and Oblique L Plates for the Hand and Foot (Figs. 7, 34):These plates are 35 mm long and have 5 screw holes. The neck of the plate has been widened for increased strength. The right-angled L plates are no longer manufactured.

c) The 2.0- and 1.5-mm Mini Plates (Fig. 8)

A new line of small plates has been developed for use with 2.0- and 1.5-mm screws. They are extra-long and are cut to the desired length with plate cutting forceps. Mini plates with a T-shaped end are available. The T piece comes with 3 holes (central sequence) or 4 holes (eccentric sequence).

Mini Condylar Plates (Figs. 8, 36): These plates are specially designed for use about the joints of the hand and are patterned after the large condylar plates of the standard set (*Manual of Internal Fixation*, pp. 86 ff.).

They are produced in two sizes for 2.0- and 1.5-mm screws (respective lengths 28 mm and 26 mm). The shaft carries 4 screw holes and is notched between the holes, like the reconstruction plates, to make contouring easier.

The widened, reinforced distal end of the plate terminates in a flat, sharpened pin 14 mm long that is angled 90°. An extra plate hole, coaxial with the pin, is provided for the insertion of a parallel screw.The center of the pin is offset 4 mm from the center of the hole in the plate for 2-mm screws, and 3 mm in the plate for 1.5-mm screws.

The tab-like end of the plate around the distal screw hole projects 2.5 mm past the center of the pin in the 2-mm plate, and 2 mm in the 1.5-mm plate.

The pin length and plate shaft must be adapted to local anatomy and are shortened as needed with the plate cutting forceps.

Mini H Plate (Figs. 8, 37): The mini H plate is specially designed for the reïmplantation of transversely amputated fingers, where extensive exposure is not desired. Like the mini condylar plate, it comes in two sizes for 2.0- and 1.5-mm screws.

The 2.0-mm Mini DCP (Fig. 8): The strength of this plate makes it excellent for secondary operations on the distal bones of the hand.

3. Additional Implants (Fig. 7)

Some of these implants are used for provisional retention, others for constructing tension-band systems or transosseous wire fixation.

Kirschner Wires: These are available in diameters of 0.6, 0.8, 1.0, 1.25, 1.6, and 2.0 mm. The different diameters are supplied in different lengths to facilitate identification.

Cerclage Wires: Cerclage wires are supplied in precut lengths in diameters of 0.4, 0.6, 0.8, and 1.0 (1.25) mm. Again, the diameters come in different lengths to make identification easier. The earlier use of rolled wire had numerous disadvantages.

4. The Small External Fixator (Figs. 9, 42)

The instrument set for the small external fixator was developed in 1978 and described in detail in a 1982 ASIF Bulletin. All the parts are contained in one case.

The components include:
- Kirschner wires with thread, 2.5 mm diam., 150 mm long
- Connecting rods, 4.0 mm diam., 60-200 mm long
- Swivel clamps in two sizes:
- 4.0/2.5-mm clamp for use on Kirschner wires and

connecting rods
- 4.0/4.0-mm clamp for assembling the connecting rods

The clamps are provided with spring-loaded nuts that facilitate provisional tightening by hand.

The set also contains:
- 1 Tap sleeve (2.5 mm i.d.)
- 1 Combination wrench
- 1 Socket wrench for definitive tightening of the clamps

The large wire cutter or 2.5-mm bolt cutter is additionally recommended for shortening the Kirschner wires.

Recently this system has been augmented by Schanz screws 4.0 mm in diameter with a 2.7- and 3.5-mm diameter thread. They are more stable than the 2.5-mm Kirschner wires. The 4/4-mm clamps are used for assembly.

Applications: The small external fixator was originally designed as a transarticular stabilizer for complex fractures of the distal radius. Since then it has proved useful for numerous applications in the peripheral skeleton.

5. Instruments

A number of additions and changes have been made in the SFS. Some instruments that proved unsatisfactory in clinical use have been dropped from the set.The innovations make it necessary to describe the new instruments, calling particular attention to their function and applications.

a) Instruments for Reduction and Provisional Fixation (Figs. 14, 15)

Reduction Forceps with Points ("towel clip"): Traditional instrument with scissors handle, heavy-duty construction, flared jaws, and sharp points. Can reduce even markedly displaced fragments, but associated soft-tissue displacement can cause problems. The newest model is equipped with a fine ratchet lock to make handling easier and more precise.

This instrument is considered tóo bulky for the small bones of the hand, and so new, finer forceps have been developed:

"Termite" Forceps: A very small, short, and light-weight reduction forceps (about 15 g) with flared jaws, very fine points, and an extra-fine ratchet lock. Owing to its light weight, the forceps tends to stay in the selected position without displacing.

Applications: Phalanges or small metacarpal fragments.

"Stag-beetle" Forceps: A slightly longer forceps of similar design. The jaws resemble the antler-like mandibles of the male stag beetle.

Applications: Same as "termite" forceps, except that the instrument must be held in place by hand because of its greater weight.

The fine points of the "termite" and "stag-beetle" forceps make it possible to fix the bone on one side through the soft tissues or even percutaneously without having to strip them aside. This has great practical value in areas of limited access, such as the phalanges.

Forceps with Sliding Jaws: This forceps has two jaws that move parallel to each other, and an angulated handle. Either of two interchangeable carriages, one with a sharp point and the other with a small footplate, apposes against a stationary, pointed hook. The instrument is equipped with a fine thread lock.

Applications: Reduction and provisional fixation of the third and fourth metacarpals (where access is a problem). The wide footplate can also be used to hold small plates against the bone.

Small ASIF Reduction Forceps ("lobster"): Small traditional reduction forceps with curved, serrated jaws. The forceps has been refined and equipped with a thread lock that swings aside when not in use.

Applications: Reduction and retention of fragments, and provisional plate fixation on bones of moderate size (forearm, fibula, clavicle, metatarsus, metacarpus, etc.).

Self-Centering Bone-Holding Forceps for Small Fragments ("Verbrugge"): The smallest traditional instrument. The jaws have been refined, and a thread lock has been added.

Applications: Correspond to small ASIF reduction forceps.

Small Hohmann Retractors: Earlier models have been supplemented by fine instruments designed for use in the hand.

b) Drill Bits (Fig. 2)

All drill bits are available with adapters that snap into the quick coupling of the small air drill. They are easily distinguished from one another by their different lengths.

The 2.7-, 2.0-, 1.5-, and 1.1-mm drill bits are also available with adapters for the mini quick coupling, and they fit the corresponding drill heads of the mini compressed air machine.

c) Drill Guides and Tap Sleeves (Figs. 2, 11, 12, 13)

The drill bits and taps are fine, delicate instruments that may bend or break under oblique pressure. They can also cause severe trauma to the soft tissues. Consequently, they should never be used without a guide. The surgeon should hold the appropriate drill guide or sleeve with the nondominant hand while drilling or tapping the bone with the other. An assistant should never hold the drill guide for the surgeon, as this might lead to misdirection or breakage of the bit.

A double drill guide has been developed for each screw size. Two thin sleeves of different calibers are mounted at opposite ends of the guide, one corresponding to the core diameter of the screw, the other to the outside diameter. With their thin walls, the sleeves provide a less obstructed view of the operative field and permit optimum drilling accuracy.

Thus, a single guide can be used to drill both the gliding hole and the thread hole. The large end of the guide is used to make the gliding hole, whereupon the small end is introduced through the gliding hole for drilling the thread hole in the far cortex. The large sleeve then functions as a tap sleeve when the far hole is threaded.

The small sleeve is also used to guide the drill bit in the plate hole. The thin-walled construction of the sleeve makes it easy to position the drill bit centrally or eccentrically in the oval plate hole, as desired.

It is also easier to center an obliquely drilled hole with the thin-walled sleeves than with the older thick-walled drill guides.

The handle of the double drill guide carries an extra guide hole at the ends, close to each sleeve. A preliminary Kirschner wire can be inserted into the guide hole, enabling the surgeon to drill a parallel hole under vision. The distance of the guide hole from the center of the sleeve corresponds in the mini condylar plate to the distance from the pin center to the center of the hole for the condylar screw. The hole is also positioned such that a washer may be placed next to the Kirschner guide wire; this is done mainly in cancellous bone.

Double drill guide for 3.5- and 4.0-mm screws: inside diameters 3.5 and 2.5 mm.

Double DCP drill guide for drilling the thread hole in 3.5-mm DC plates (Fig. 5): inside diameter 2.5 mm. Analogous double drill guides are available for the 2.7- and 2.0-mm DC plates.

Double drill guide for 2.7-mm screws: inside diameters 2.7 mm and 2.0 mm.

Double drill guide for 2.0-mm screws: inside diameters 2.0 mm and 1.5 mm.

Double drill guide for 1.5-mm screws: inside diameters 1.5 mm and 1.1 mm.

Insert drill sleeve 3.5/2.5 mm (Fig. 23): outside diameter 3.5 mm, inside diameter 2.5 mm. For use in the 3.5-mm gliding hole in bones with wide medullary cavities.

Insert drill sleeve 2.7/2.0 mm:outside diameter 2.7 mm, inside diameter 2.0 mm. For use in the 2.7-mm gliding hole in bones with wide medullary cavities or in the gliding hole for arthrodesis with 2.7-mm screws.

d) Taps (Fig. 2)

The 3.5- and 2.7-mm taps fit the quick-coupling sockets of the straight handle and T-grip handle. A special handle with a mini quick coupling is used for the 2.0- and 1.5-mm taps.

The 3.5-mm cancellous tap for 4.0-mm cancellous screws is used in 2.5-mm drill holes.

The 3.5-mm cortex tap for 3.5-mm cortex screws is bronze colored to distinguish it from the cancellous tap; it is used in 2.5-mm drill holes.

The 2.7-mm tap for 2.7-mm cortex screws is used in 2.0-mm drill holes.

The 2.0-mm tap for 2.0-mm mini screws is used in 1.5-mm drill holes.

The 1.5-mm tap for 1.5-mm mini screws is used in 1.1-mm drill holes.

e) Screwdrivers

Small screwdriver (width across flats 2.5 mm) for 4.0-, 3.5-, and 2.7-mm screws. The holding sleeve (Fig. 4) has been retained.

Small screwdriver attachment: same size and use as the small screwdriver; fits handles with quick coupling.

Mini hexagonal screwdriver (width across flats 1.5 mm) for 2.0- and 1.5-mm mini screws with hexagonal sockets.

Mini hexagonal screwdriver attachment: fits handle with mini quick coupling.

Mini screwdriver for cross-slotted heads with holding sleeve: fits handle with mini quick coupling; for insertion and removal of all mini screws with cross-slotted heads.

f) Other Instruments

Small depth gauge: length measurement for 4.0-, 3.5-, and 2.7-mm screws (Fig. 23).

Mini depth gauge: length measurement for 2.0- and 1.5-mm mini screws (Figs. 24, 25).

Small countersink: fits handle with quick coupling; for 3.5- and 2.7-mm screws (Fig. 23).

Mini countersink: fits handle with mini quick coupling; for 2.0- and 1.5-mm mini screws (Fig. 24).

Handle with quick coupling: accepts 3.5- and 2.7-mm taps, small screwdriver attachment, and small countersink (Fig. 2).

Handle with mini quick coupling: accepts 2.0- and 1.5-mm taps, mini screwdriver attachment, and mini countersink (Fig. 2).

Bending pliers and bending irons: for bending and twisting of DC plates (3.5- and 2.7-mm) and reconstruction plates (Fig. 5).

g) Recommended Supplementary Instruments

- T-grip handle with quick coupling: has same functions as the straight handle. Permits more force to be exerted when tapping hard bone (Fig. 2).
- Small hand chuck: for inserting all sizes of Kirschner wires in cancellous bone (Fig. 7).
- Plate cutting forceps: specially designed for mini plates; can also be used on 2.7-mm plates except DCPs (Fig. 8).
- Small bending pliers: for bending and twisting quarter tubular plates, T plates, L plates, and mini plates (Fig. 8).
- Small bone spreader: useful for inspection of fracture surfaces and for distraction of osteotomies (Fig. 200 d).
- Articulated tension device: can be used on 3.5-mm plates. Useful for fine reduction in difficult situations, permits fine control of interfragmental compression with 3.5-mm DCPs and one-third tubular plates. Distraction can be applied by reversing the position of the hook (Fig. 33).
- Small compression forceps for bone fragments and for 2.7- and 2.0-mm plates. The angled points fit into a 2.0-mm drill hole and an adjacent plate hole for applying compression (Figs. 33, 34).
- Mini wire cutters: for cutting fine Kirschner wire and cerclage wire.
- Wire bending pliers: for grasping, bending, and cutting Kirschner and cerclage wires (Fig. 7).
- Mini bending iron for Kirschner wires: for bending Kirschner wires of 0.6- to 1.25-mm diam. close to the bone or skin surface (Fig. 7, 25b9, 116d).

6. Instrument Cases

Various combinations of the instruments and implants are supplied in special metal cases.The contents of the cases have been modified in recent years, and also they vary regionally according to the preferences of different surgical groups.For these reasons it was decided not to show illustrations of standard instrument cases in the present edition.

All the screw racks have a graduated scale at the edge for the convenient measurement of screw lengths (Fig. 4). Screw lengths should be checked as a matter of routine whenever a screw is taken from the rack.

7. Mini Compressed Air Machine (Fig. 10)

The mini compressed air machine, built by the R. Mathys Co. in 1973, is shaped like a large pencil and, unlike the machines with a pistol grip, can be operated with three fingers. This gives the operator a better "feel" for precision work. It was specially designed for hand surgery, mandibular surgery, and neurosurgery and is supplied in its own case along with instruments and attachments.

The machine consists of a motor, a double hose, and attachments for different functions (drilling, reaming, sawing).

The motor speed is variable and is controlled with a slide switch.

Several new attachments have been added, and some of the existing parts have been improved:

- Straight drill head: the torque has been increased and the speed reduced from 15,000 to 3,000 rpm, making the attachment slightly longer and heavier than before, and increasing its power.
- Right-angle (90°) drill head: for drilling in areas of restricted access.

Each of these drill heads has a mini quick coupling and accepts 2.7- to 1.1-mm drill bits and various types of reamer and bur.

- Oscillating saw: the new saw blades, only 0.3 mm thick, are used for osteotomies and for resecting the articular surfaces of small bones.

- Attachment for inserting Kirschner wires: this component has been redesigned. Its 45° angle was retained. The locking mechanism for the Kirschner wire is activated by pressure on a lever. This simplifies insertion, feeding, and removal of the wire in the instrument without the need for further manipulations.

Thread ⌀	4.0	3.5	2.7	2.0	1.5 mm
Core ⌀	2.0	2.4	2.0	1.3	1.0 mm
Shank ⌀	2.3 mm				

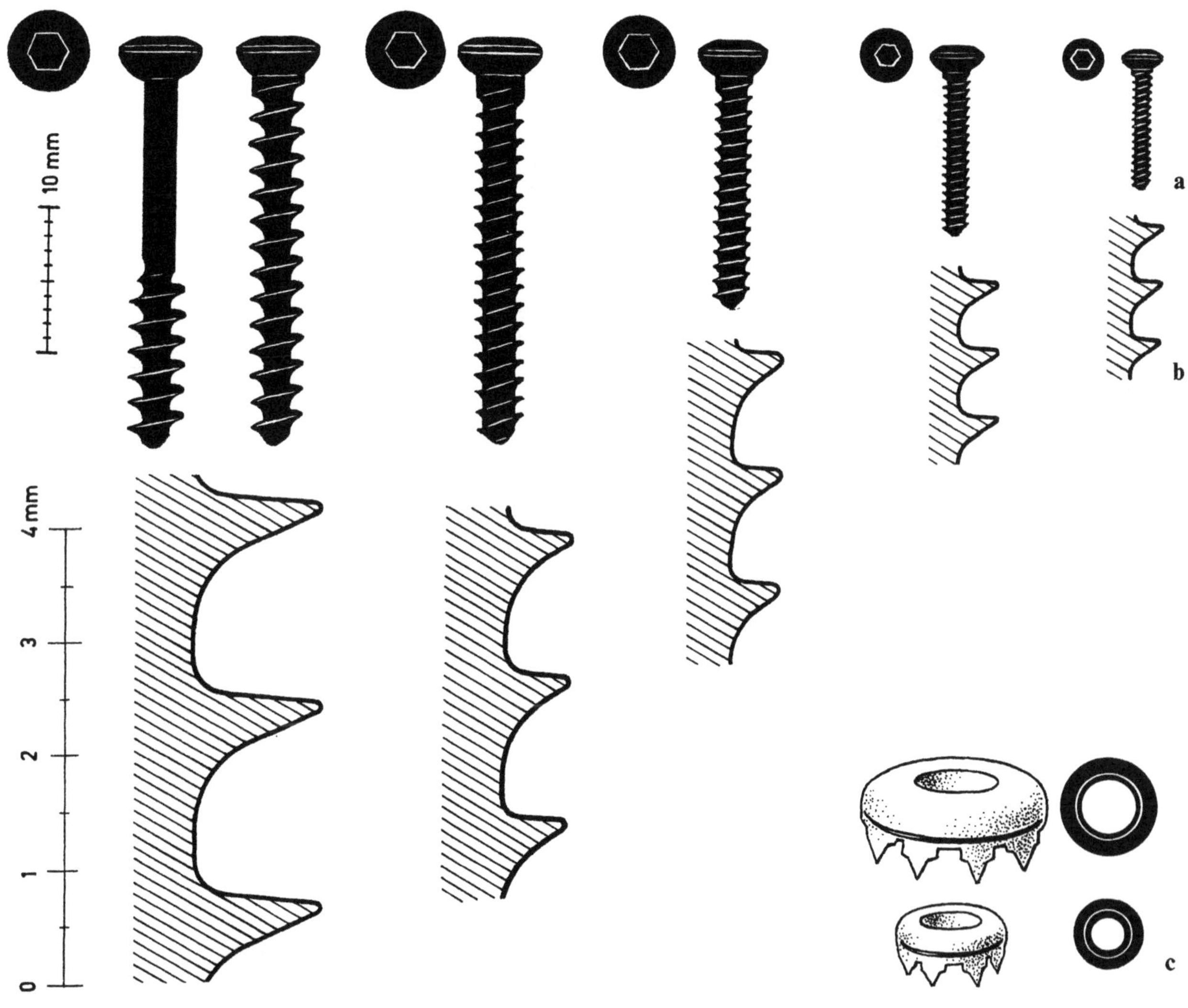

Fig. 1a–c. The small ASIF screws, enlarged (measurements in mm)

a Details of screw heads with hexagonal sockets (SW = width across flats), cores, and threads: 4.0-mm cancellous screw with unthreaded shank and with full-length thread; 3.5-, 2.7-, 2.0- and 1.5-mm cortex screws

b Close-up view of the threads (with scale)

c Metal washers: large model for 4.0-, 3.5- and 2.7-mm screws, small model for 2.0- and 1.5-mm screws. Spiked plastic washers incorporating a metallic ring: large model for 3.5- and 4.0-mm screws, small model for 2.7-mm screws

Thread ⌀	4.0	3.5	2.7
Core ⌀	2.0	2.4	2.0
Shank ⌀	2.3 mm		

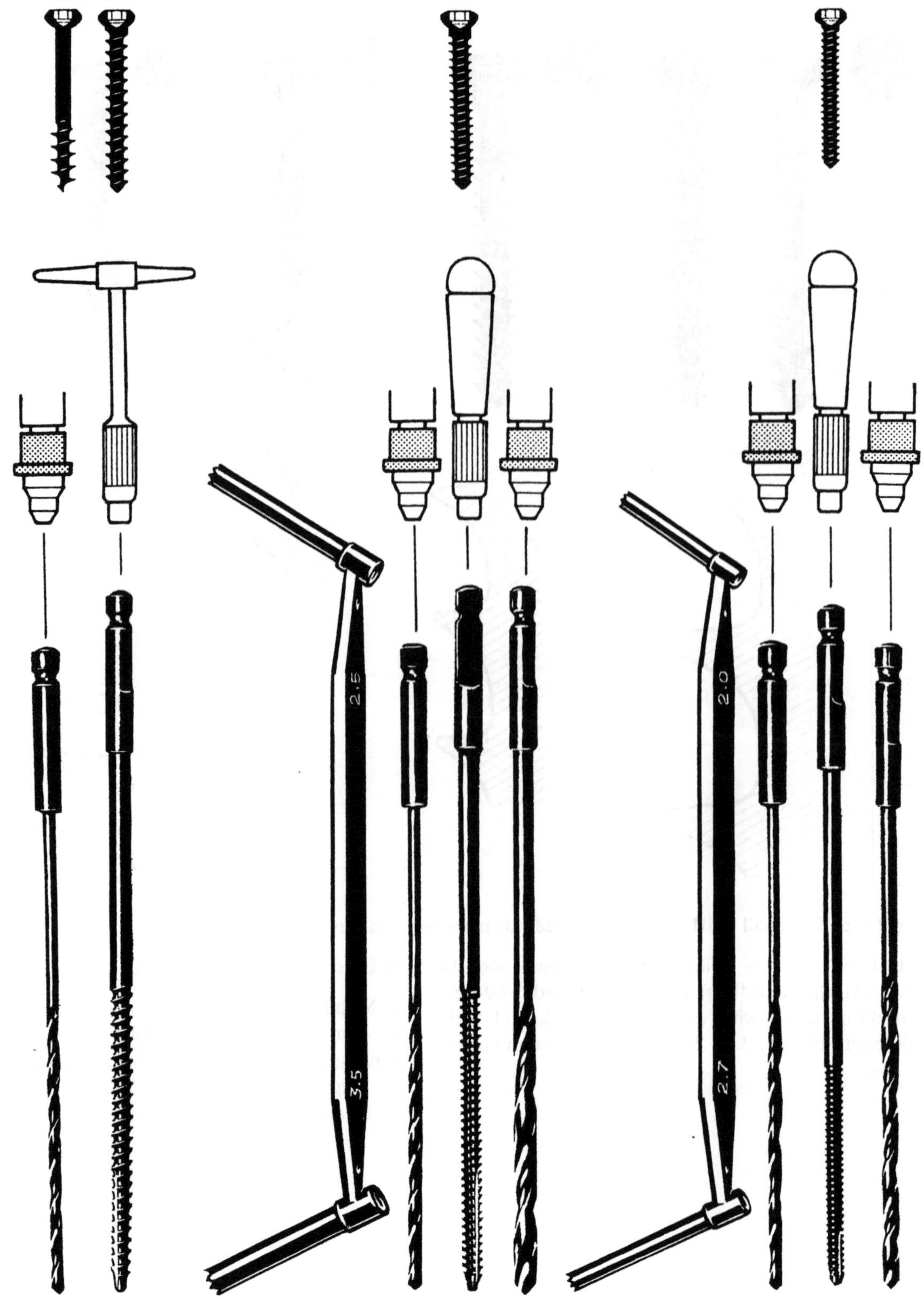

⌀	2.5	3.5	2.5	3.5	3.5	2.0	2.7	2.7

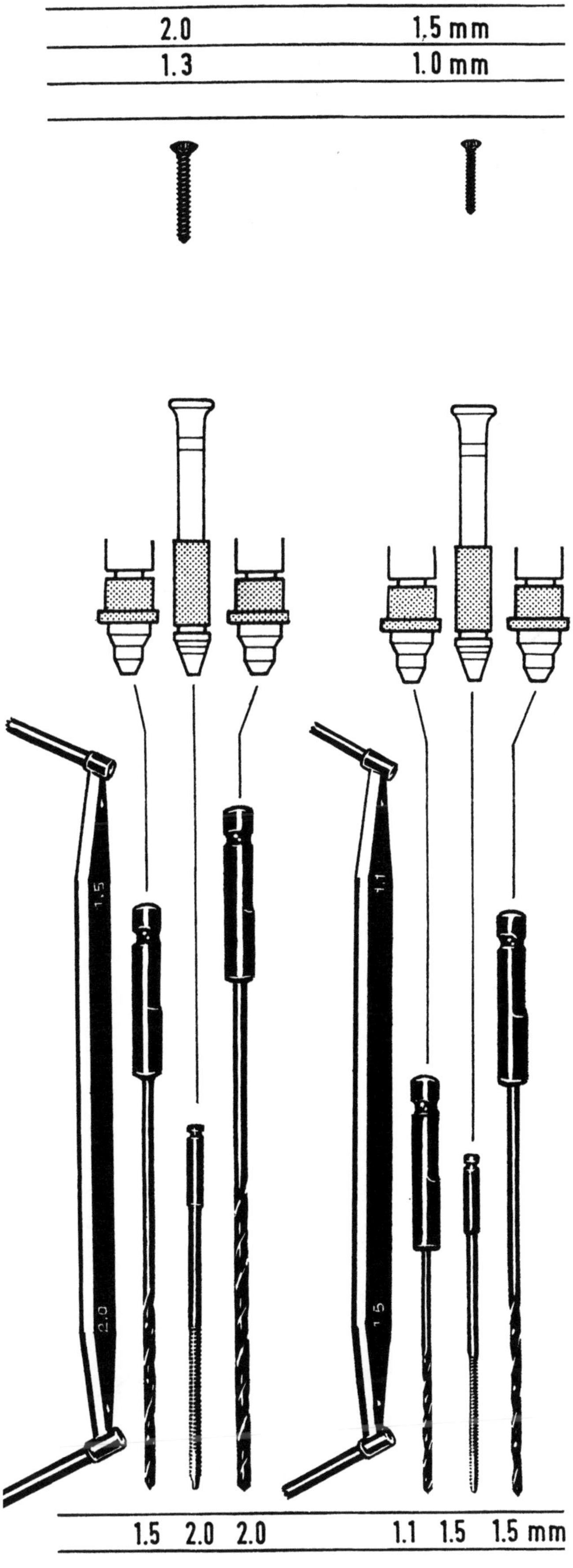

Fig. 2. The small ASIF screws and the instruments needed for their insertion

The five small ASIF screws (Fig. 1) are shown with their associated instruments (double drill guide, drill bit, tap). Size data are given in the top and bottom margins. The drill bits are shown with quick-coupling attachments. The 2.7-, 2.0-, 1.5- and 1.1-mm bits are also available with mini quick-couplings to fit the mini compressed air machine. The T-grip handle and straight handle with quick coupling (reduced) are pictured above the corresponding taps. The handle with mini quick coupling (reduced) is pictured above the corresponding mini taps

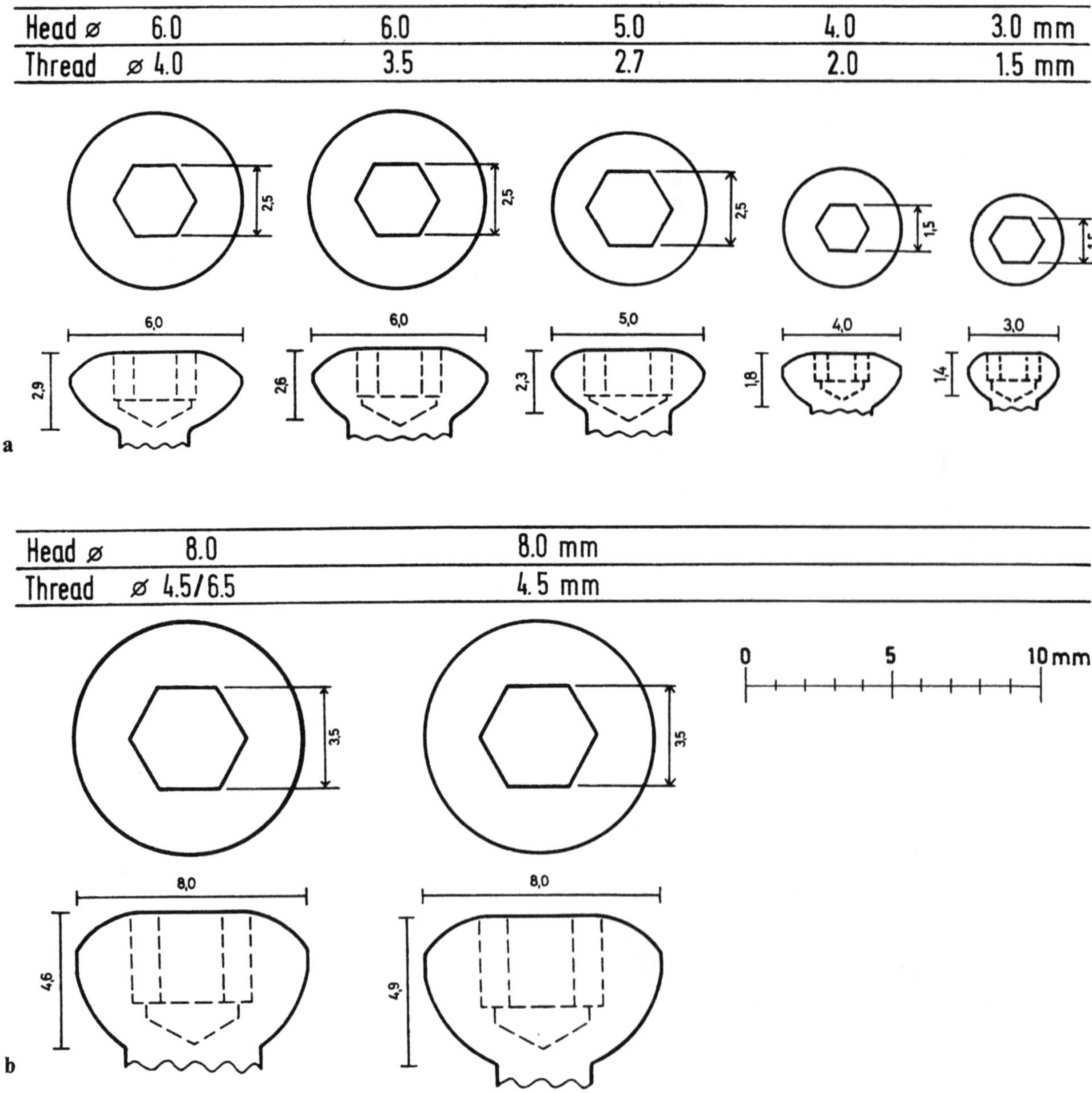

Fig. 3a, b. Close-up views of the ASIF screw heads (scale indicated)

a *Top half:* the heads of the small ASIF screws with hexagonal socket (width across flats 2.5 and 1.5 mm)

b *Bottom half:* The heads of the large screws are shown for comparison. *Left:* the standard screw head (4.5-mm cortex and 6.5-mm cancellous). *Right:* the "malleolar screw"

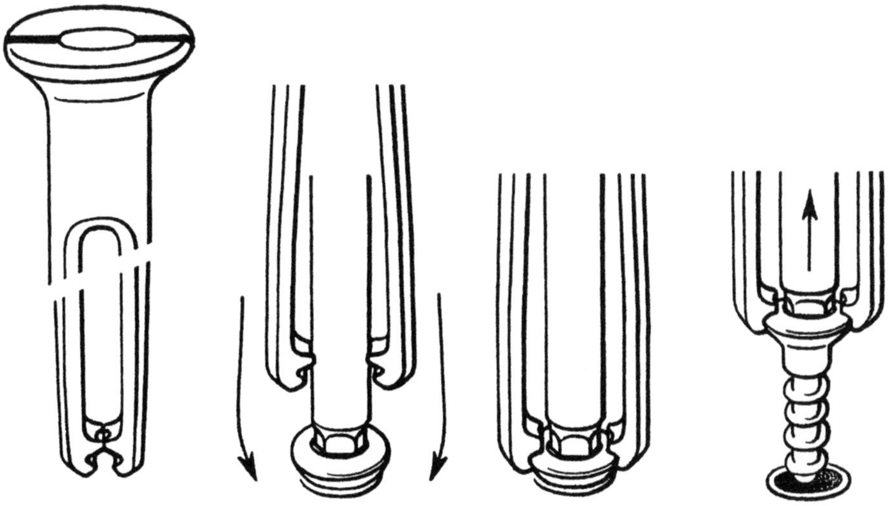

a

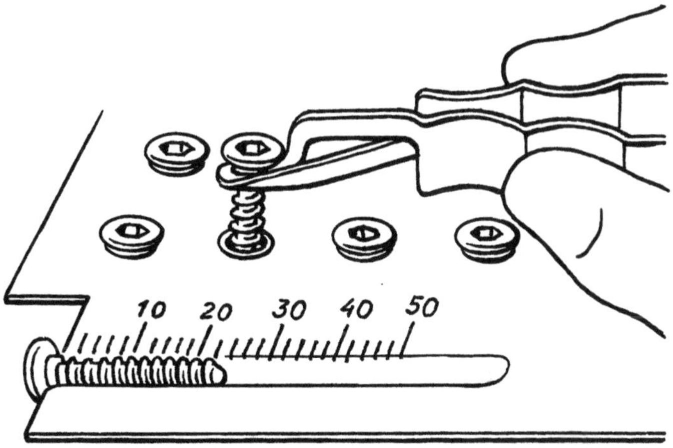

b

Fig. 4a, b. Taking the screws from the rack and measuring their length

a Use of the holding sleeve to remove a screw from the storage rack: The holding sleeve may be used to lift the screw directly from the rack, or the screwdriver may first be inserted into the screw socket and the sleeve slid down to engage the head

b Removing a screw with the screw forceps. The screw length is measured in the graduated slot at the edge of the rack

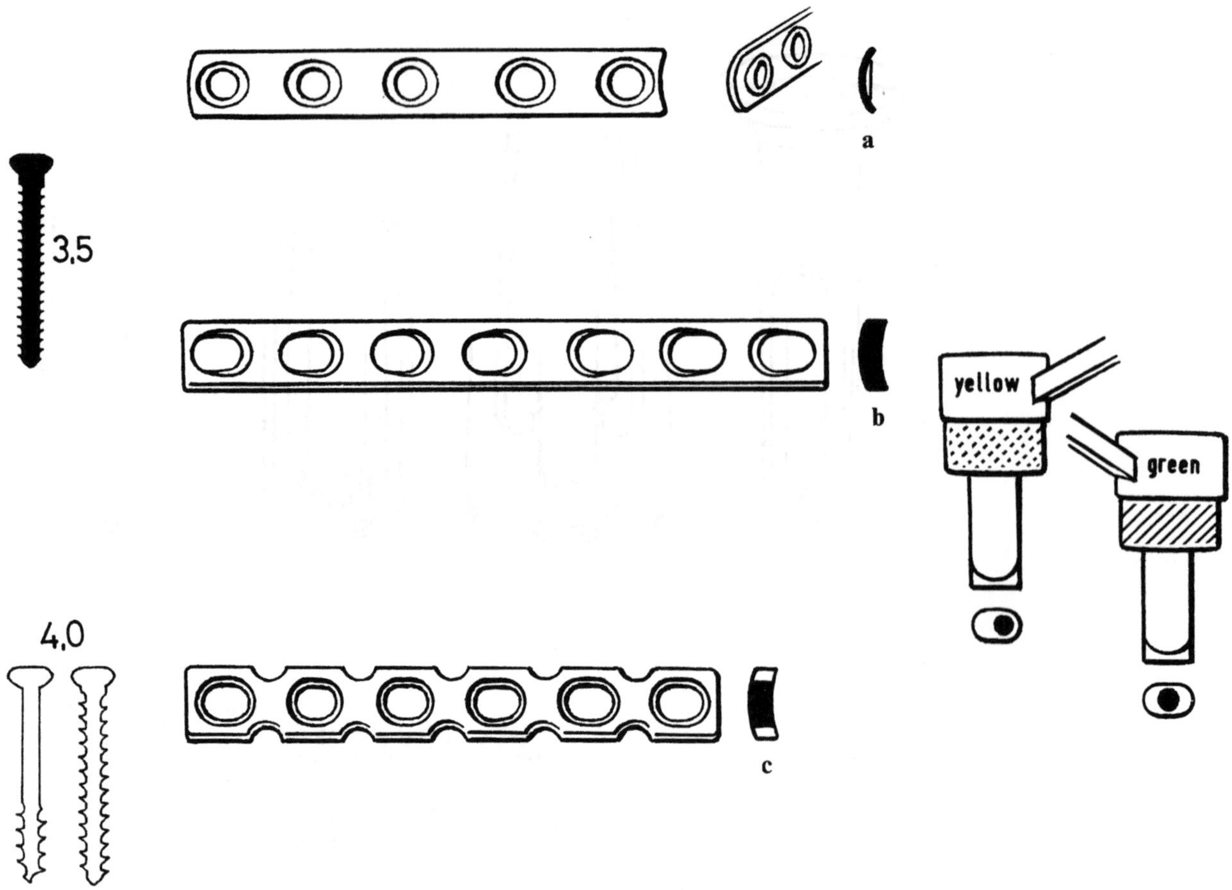

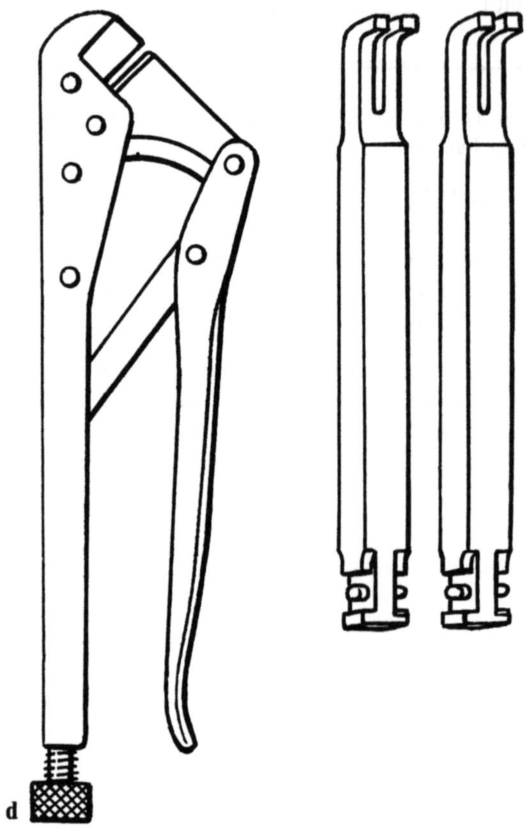

Fig. 5a–d. Straight standard plates of the 3.5-mm size (scale 1:1)

The size designation refers to the corresponding screw diameter: 3.5-mm cortex screws (or 4.0-mm cancellous screws in exceptional cases)

a One-third tubular plate with raised-rim holes

b The 3.5-mm dynamic compression plate (DCP) with corresponding drill guides (*yellow* for drilling an *eccentric* hole, *green* for drilling a *centered* hole)

c The 3.5-mm reconstruction plate

d Plate bending pliers and bending irons for contouring the above plates

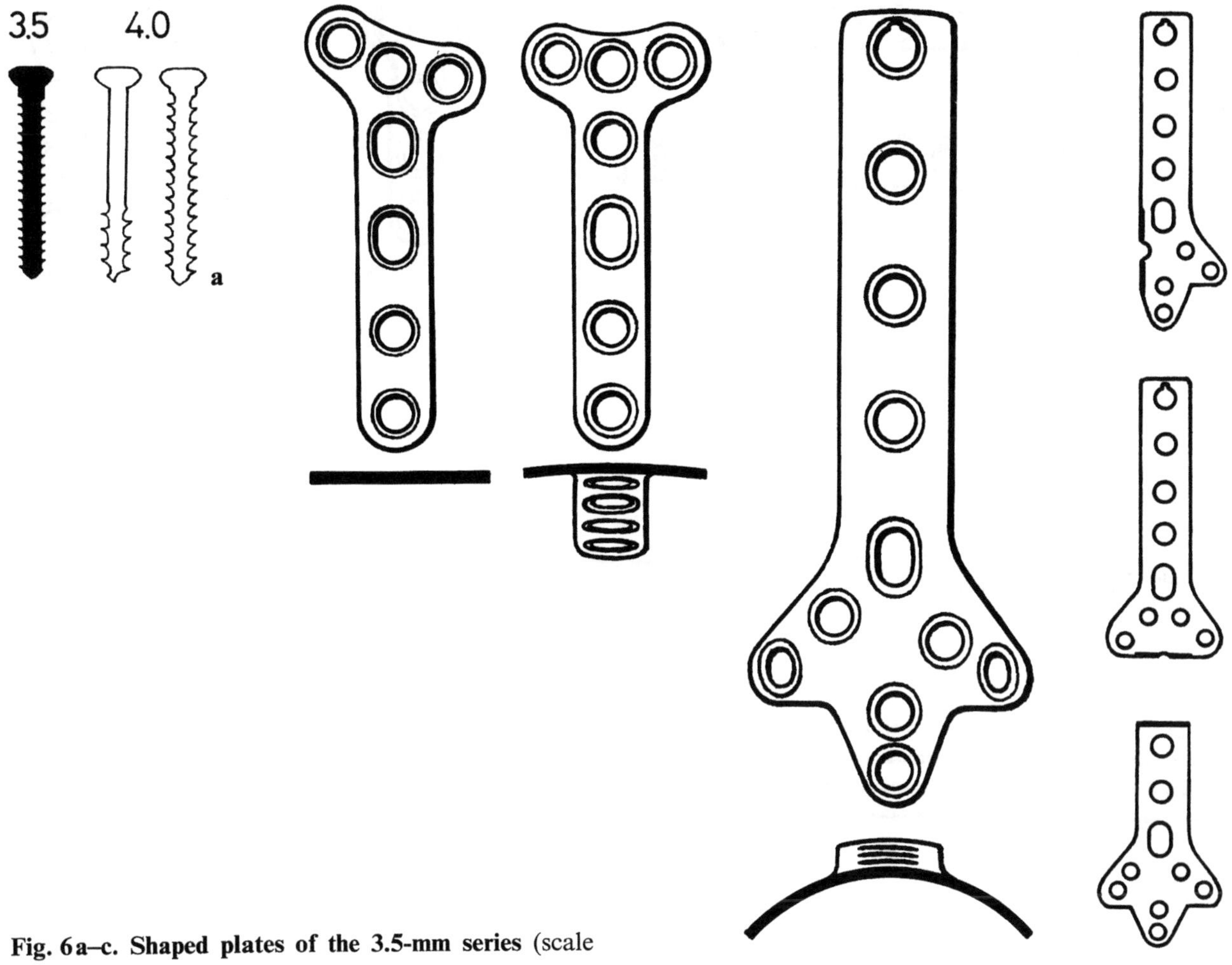

Fig. 6a–c. Shaped plates of the 3.5-mm series (scale 1:1)

The size designation refers to the corresponding screw diameter: 3.5-mm cortex screws (or 4.0-mm cancellous screws in exceptional cases)

a The straight and oblique T plate for the distal radius (top view and cross-section)

b The cloverleaf plate. The drawings show three ways the plate can be modified with cutting forceps: One of the side tabs may be removed, the distal tab may be removed, or the plate itself can be shortened

c Flat-nose parallel pliers and cutting forceps for bending and twisting the plates or for cutting off extensions

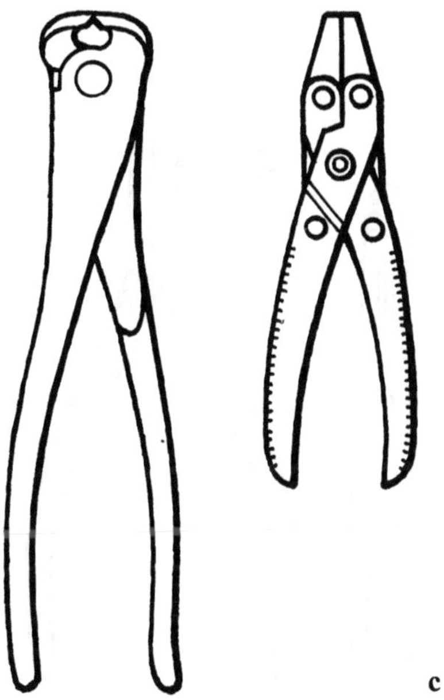

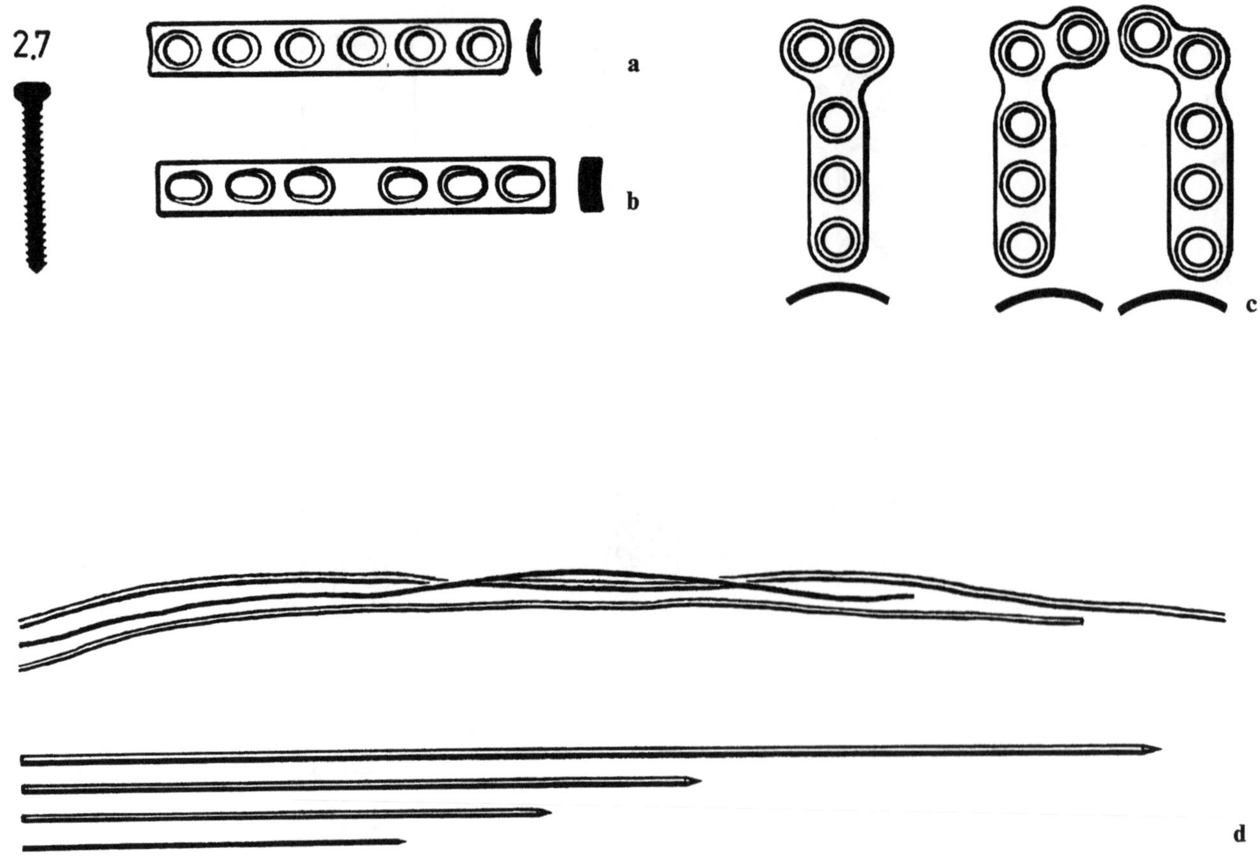

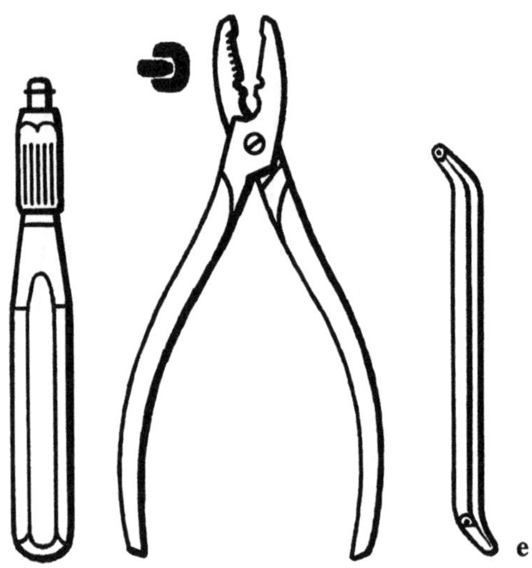

Fig. 7a–e. The plates of the 2.7-mm series, Kirschner wires, and cerclage wires.

The system is named for the corresponding 2.7-mm cortex screws.

a The quarter tubular plate with raised-rim holes

b The 2.7-mm dynamic compression plate (DCP)

c The T plate and oblique L plates

d Precut cerclage wires of various lengths (diam. 0.4, 0.6, 0.8, 1.0 and 1.25 mm) and Kirschner wires (diam. 0.6, 0.8, 1.0, 1.25, 1.6 and 2.0 mm)

e Hand chuck for inserting Kirschner wires. Wire bending pliers, which permits right-angle bending and cutting. Doubly angled bending iron for bending 0.6- to 1.25-mm Kirschner wires close to the bone or skin (see also Fig. 25/9 and 116 c)

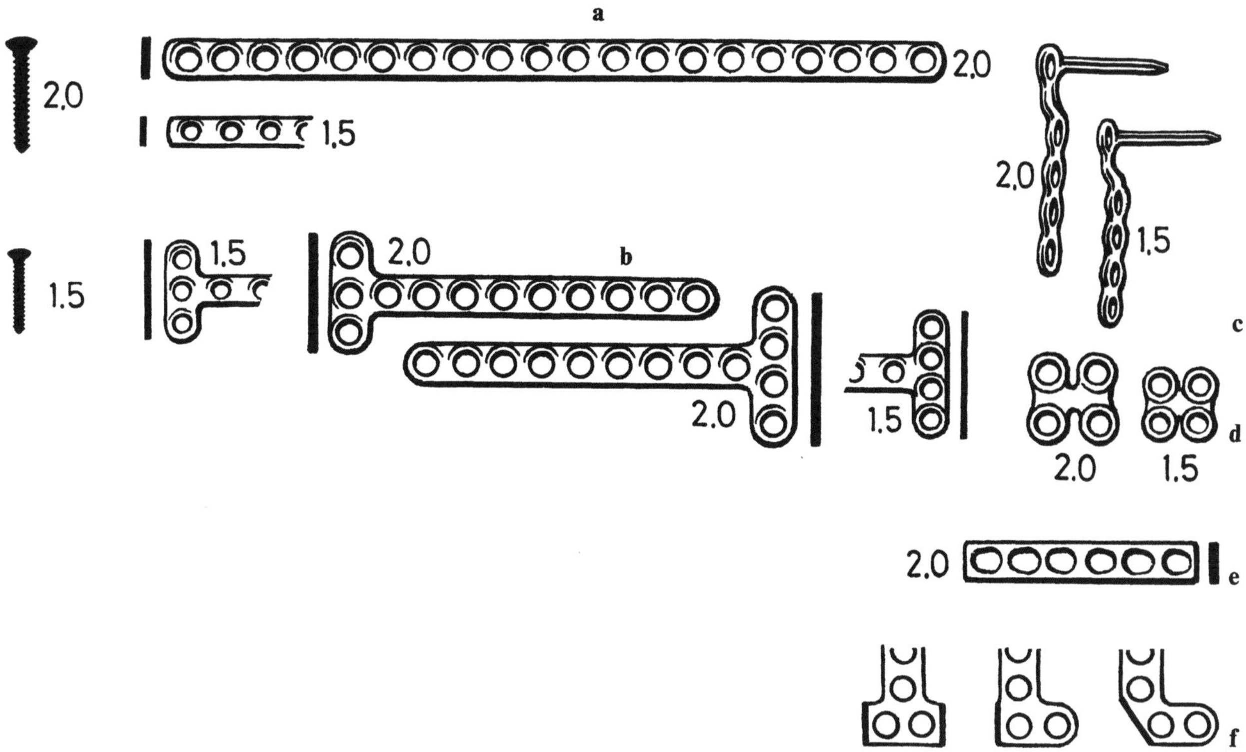

Fig. 8a–g. The mini implants of the 2.0- and 1.5-mm series

The system is named for the corresponding 2.0- and 1.5-mm cortex screws

a The straight 2.0- and 1.5-mm plates, which are cut to length by the user

b The 2.0- and 1.5-mm T plates with a variable hole sequence in the crosspiece; these plates also are cut to length by the user

c The 2.0- and 1.5-mm mini condylar plates

d The 2.0- and 1.5-mm mini H plates

e The 2.0-mm dynamic compression plate (DCP)

f Examples of how the crosspiece of the T plate can be modified for user requirements

g Plate cutting forceps and small forceps for bending and twisting mini plates and small quarter tubular plates

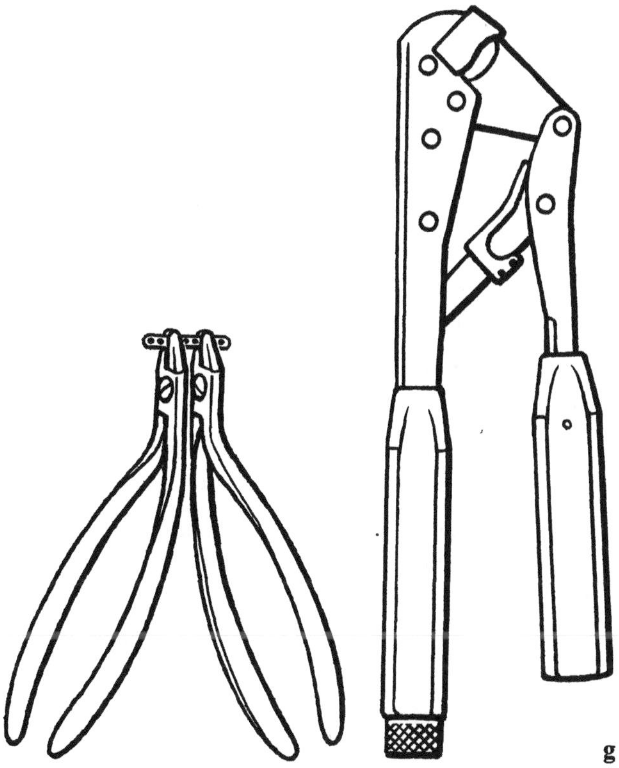

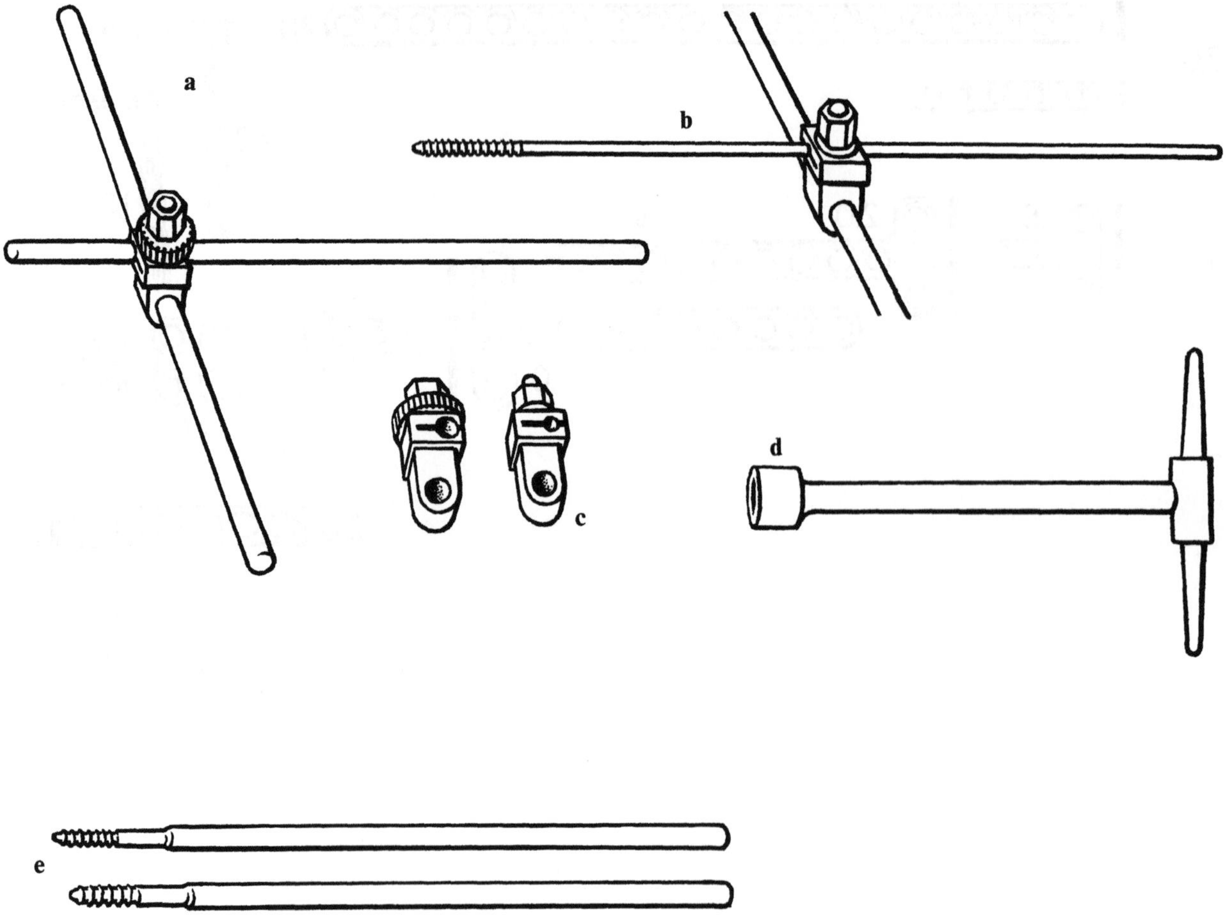

Fig. 9a–e. The components of the 2.5-mm mini external fixator

The system is designed for use with 2.5-mm threaded Kirschner wires and 4.0-mm connecting rods

a Connecting rods, interconnected with a 4/4-mm clamp

b Connecting rod and 2.5-mm threaded Kirschner wire, interconnected with a 2.5/4.0-mm clamp

c Close-up view the 4/4-mm and 4/2.5-mm clamps. The nuts have knurled edges for tentative hand tightening

d The socket wrench is used for definitive tightening of the nuts

e Schantz screws with 2.7-mm and 3.5-mm thread for use with the 4.0-mm rod

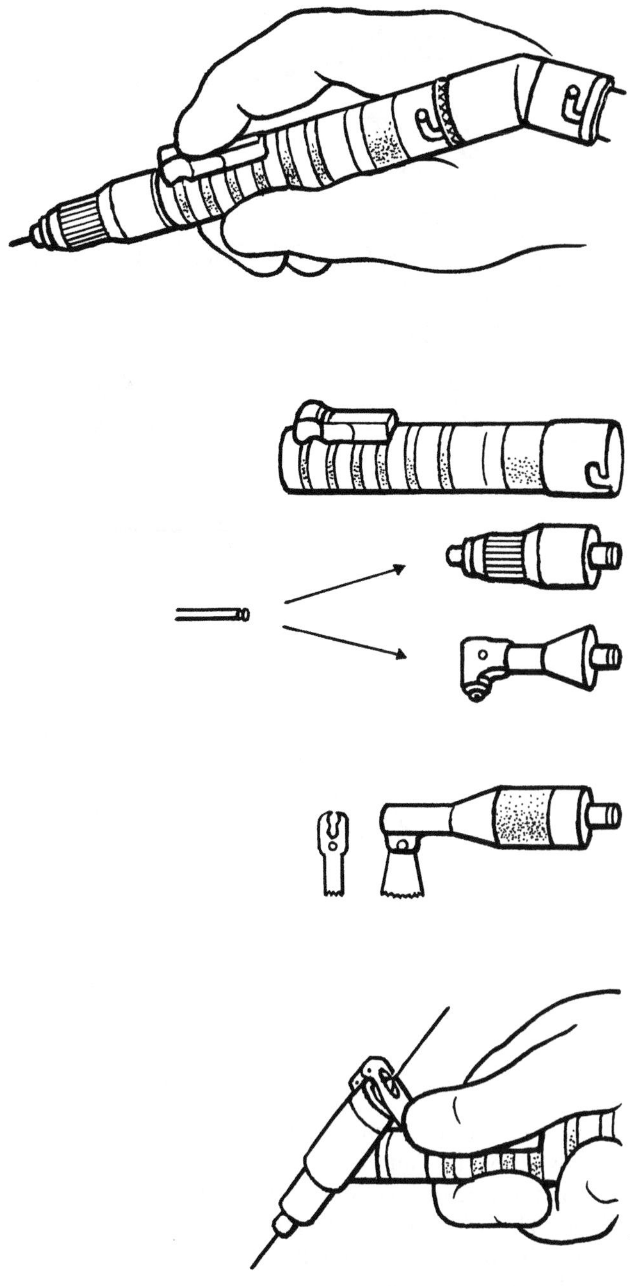

a

b

c

d

e

Fig. 10 a–e. The mini compressed air machine and principal accessories

a The mini compressed air machine is held in the hand like a pencil. Motor speed is controlled by moving a slide switch with the index finger

b The body of the machine, without attachments

c Straight and right-angled drill heads (with mini quick coupling) for drilling or reaming

d Oscillating saw with blades

e Attachment for Kirschner wires. Thumb pressure locks and releases the wire

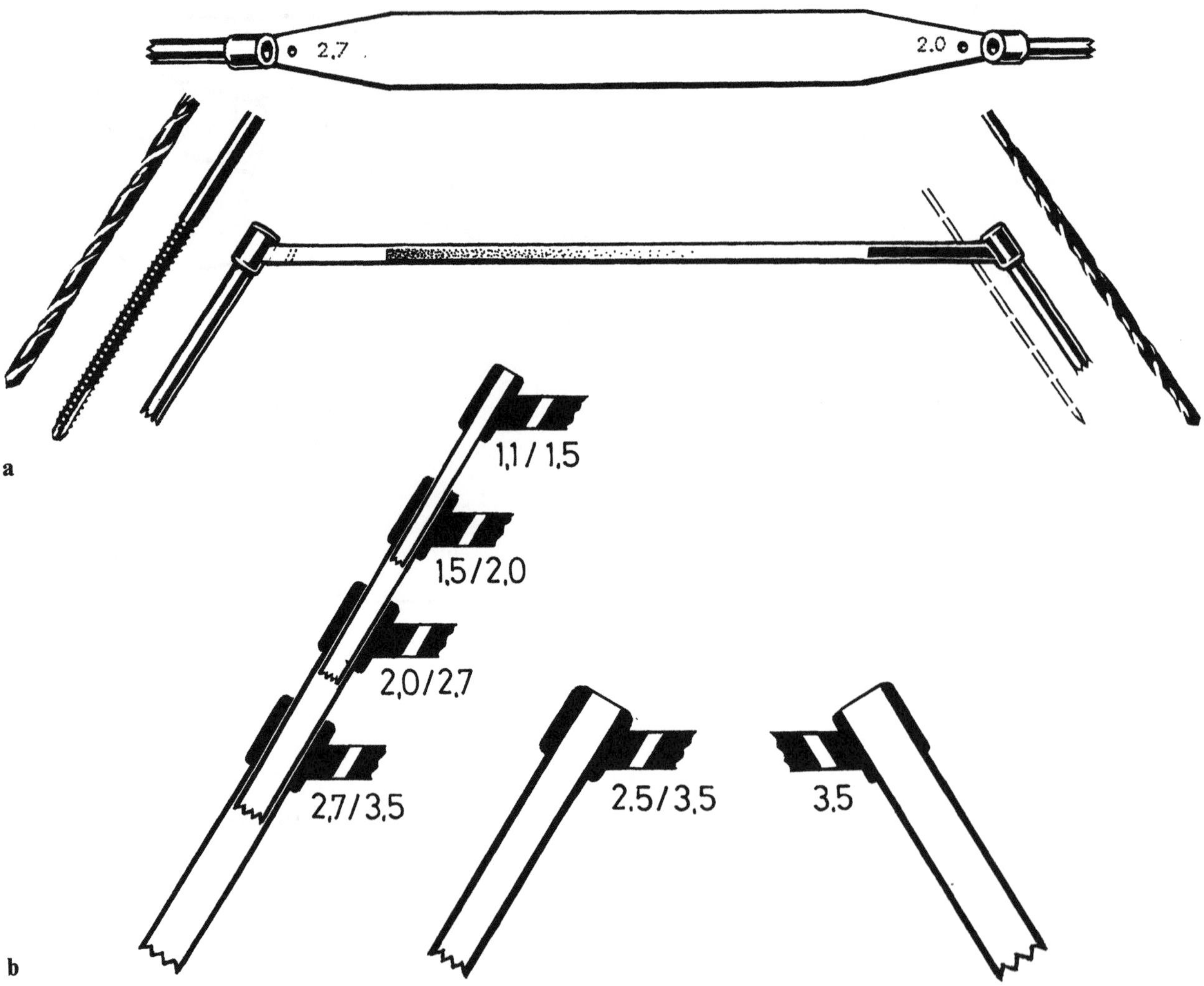

Fig. 11 a, b. A double drill guide is produced for each screw size (example: 2.7 mm)

a Top and side views of the double drill guide: The narrow sleeve (2.7 mm o.d., 2.0 mm i.d.) guides the bit for the thread hole and serves as an insert drill sleeve. The wide sleeve (3.5 mm o.d., 2.7 mm i.d.) guides the bit for the gliding hole and serves as a tap sleeve. The perforations near the ends of the handle permit holes to be drilled parallel to a previously placed Kirschner wire.The hole is larger than the outside diameter of the wire. The distance from the center of the hole to the center of the sleeve is sufficient to accommodate a washer; in the 2.0- and 1.5-mm system it equals the distance between the pin and condylar screw of the mini condylar plate

b Sleeve dimensions in longitudinal section (enlarged): The inside and outside diameters of the sleeves coincide, so it would be possible to telescope the sleeves into each other. An exception is the 3.5/2.5-mm drill guide

Fig. 12 a, b. Use of the double drill guide for lag screw insertion in cortical and cancellous bone

Left: wide sleeve *Right:* narrow sleeve
(Steps in the use of the drill guide are marked sequentially with numbers and arrows)

a The classic ASIF technique (insert drill sleeve)

b The "small fragment technique" (thread hole is cut through both fragments as an initial step)

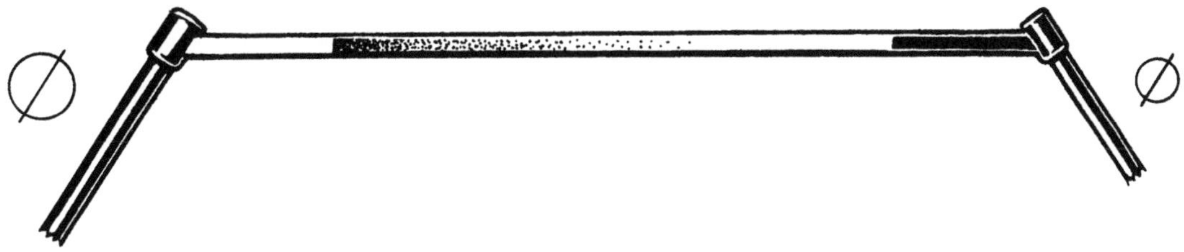

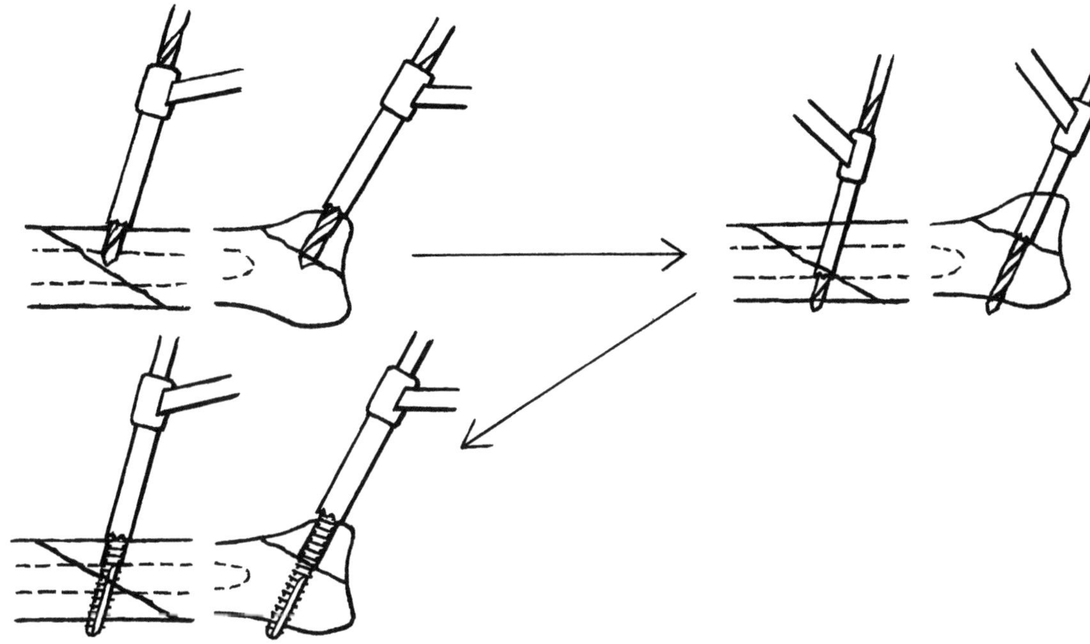

a

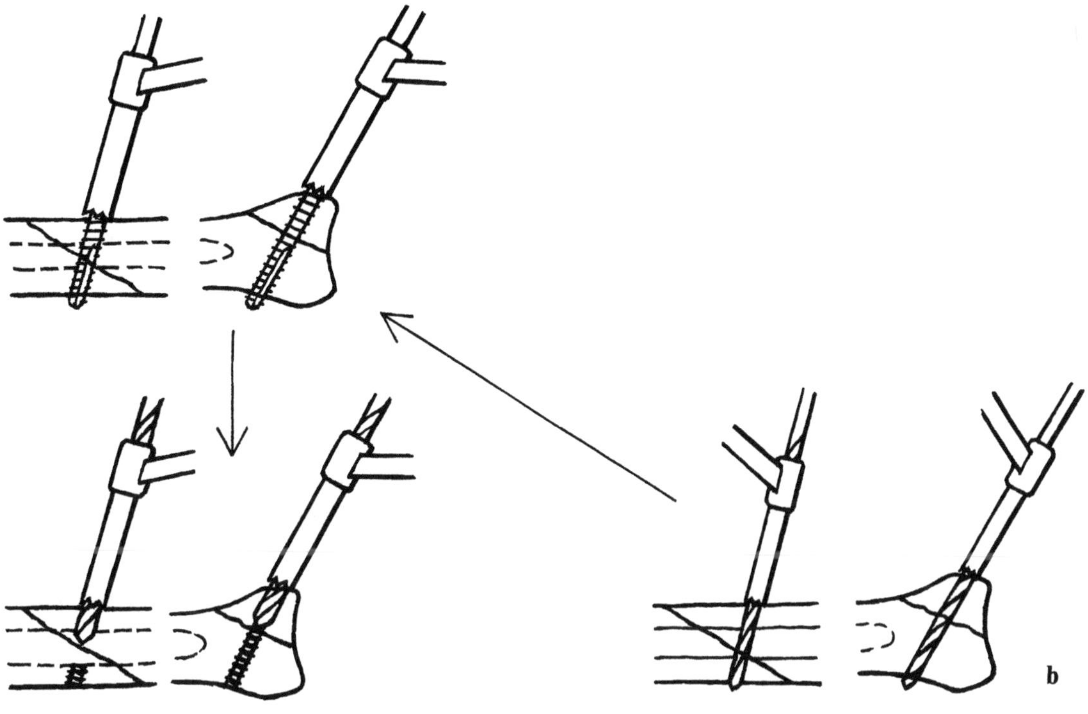

b

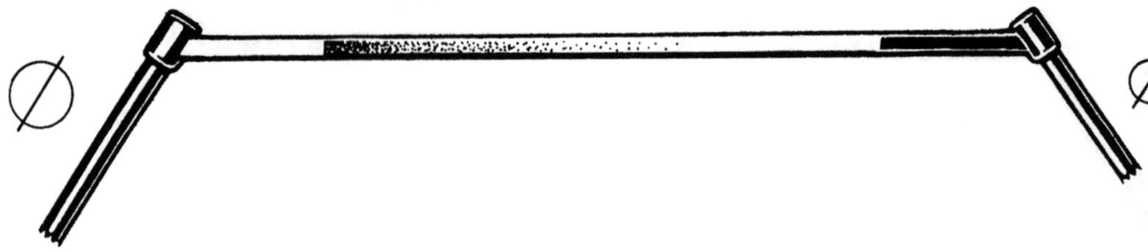

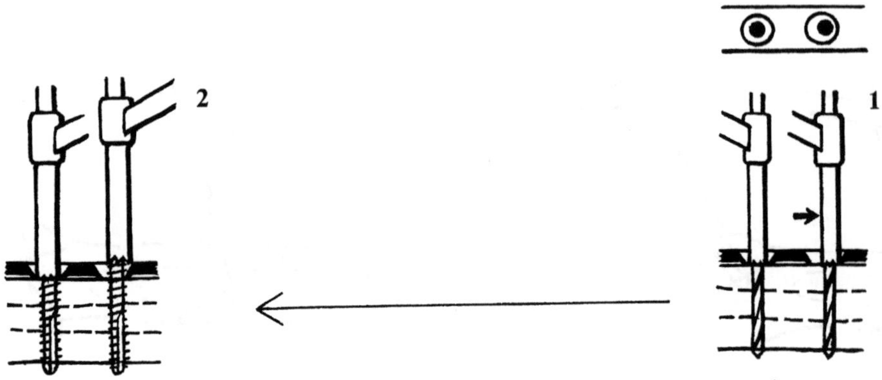

a

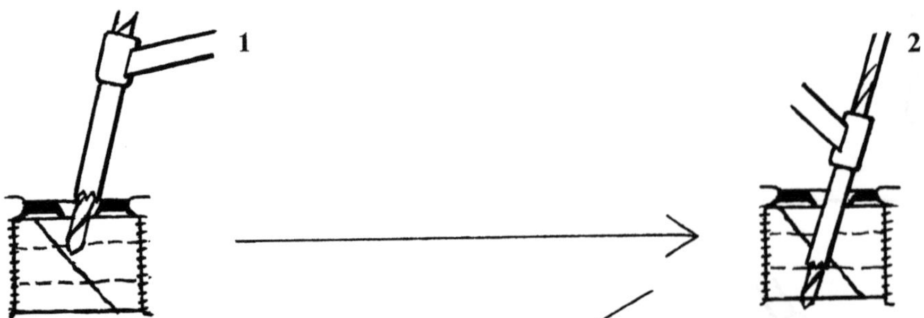

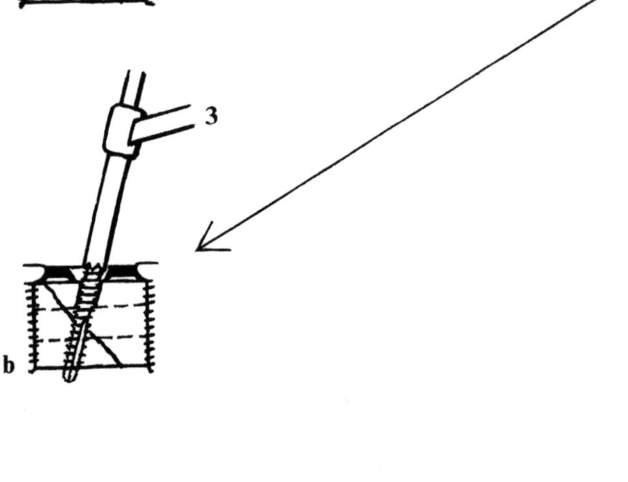

b

Fig. 13a, b. Use of the double drill guide for plating

Left: wide sleeve *Right:* narrow sleeve

a Standard technique for drilling plate holes: The thread hole may be placed centrally or eccentrically. In either case the narrow sleeve is held directly against the bone. Tapping is done through the wide sleeve, which is not in full contact with the bone. For tapping an eccentric drill hole, the wide sleeve rests on the edge of the plate opening

b Placing an oblique lag screw through the plate: The gliding hole is drilled first, through the center of the plate hole.The end of the wide sleeve has only partial contact with the bone. The thread hole is drilled through the narrow sleeve, which is inserted through the gliding hole. The tap does not touch the edge of the plate

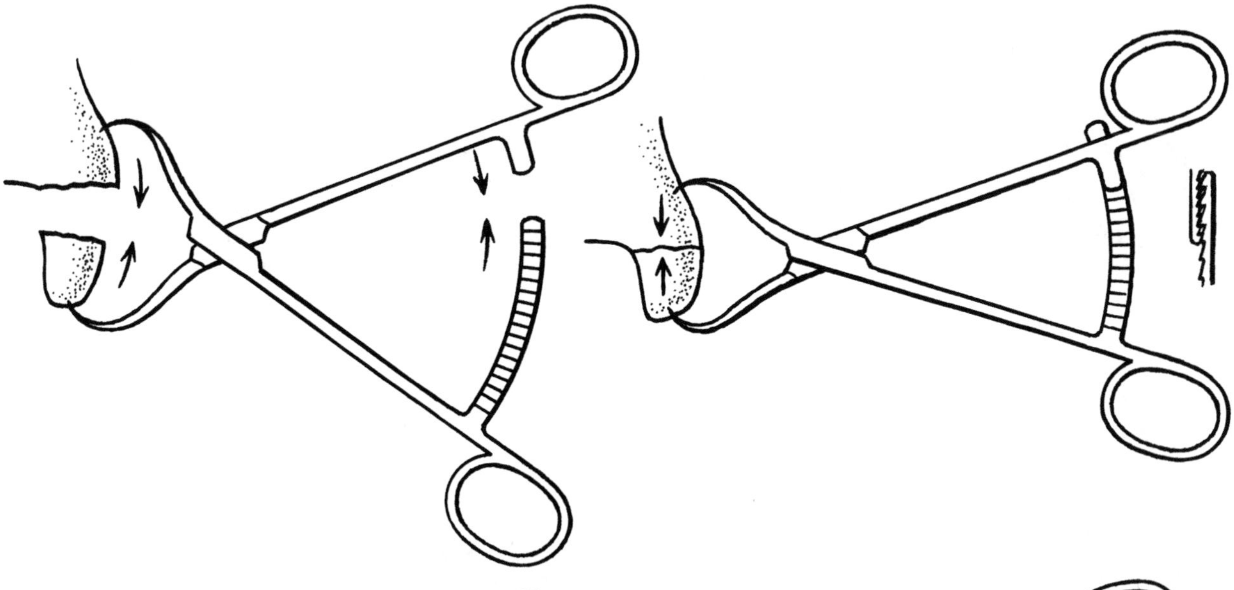

a

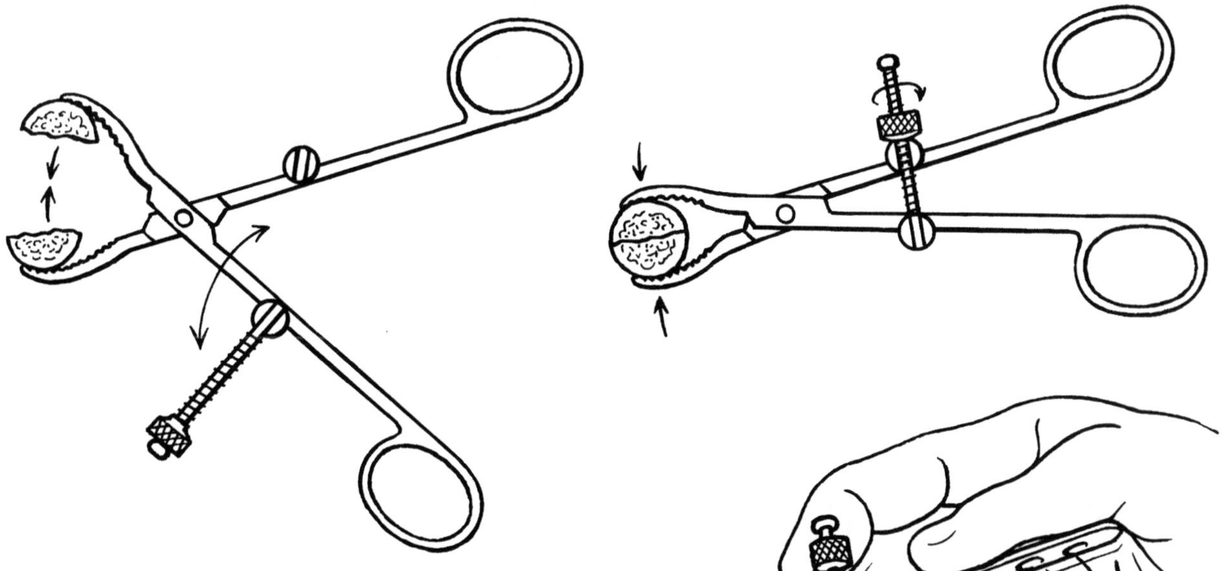

b

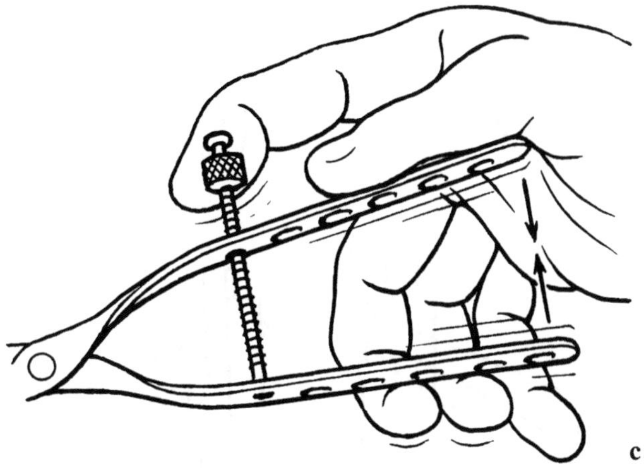

c

Fig. 14a–c. Reduction forceps: locking mechanisms

a The reduction forceps with points has a scissors handle and ratchet lock. Even markedly separated bone ends can be reduced with this instrument. The ratchet teeth were made smaller to permit finer control of compression and make the forceps easier to open with one hand

b Small "lobster" forceps with fine cross-serrations and a swiveling thread lock on the scissors handle. This forceps, too, can reduce markedly separated fragments. When reduction is accomplished, the threaded rod is swung into place, and the lock nut is tightened with the index finger

c The thread lock on the compression forceps is operated by rotating the lock nut with the index finger. The pliers-type handle is perforated and slightly elastic

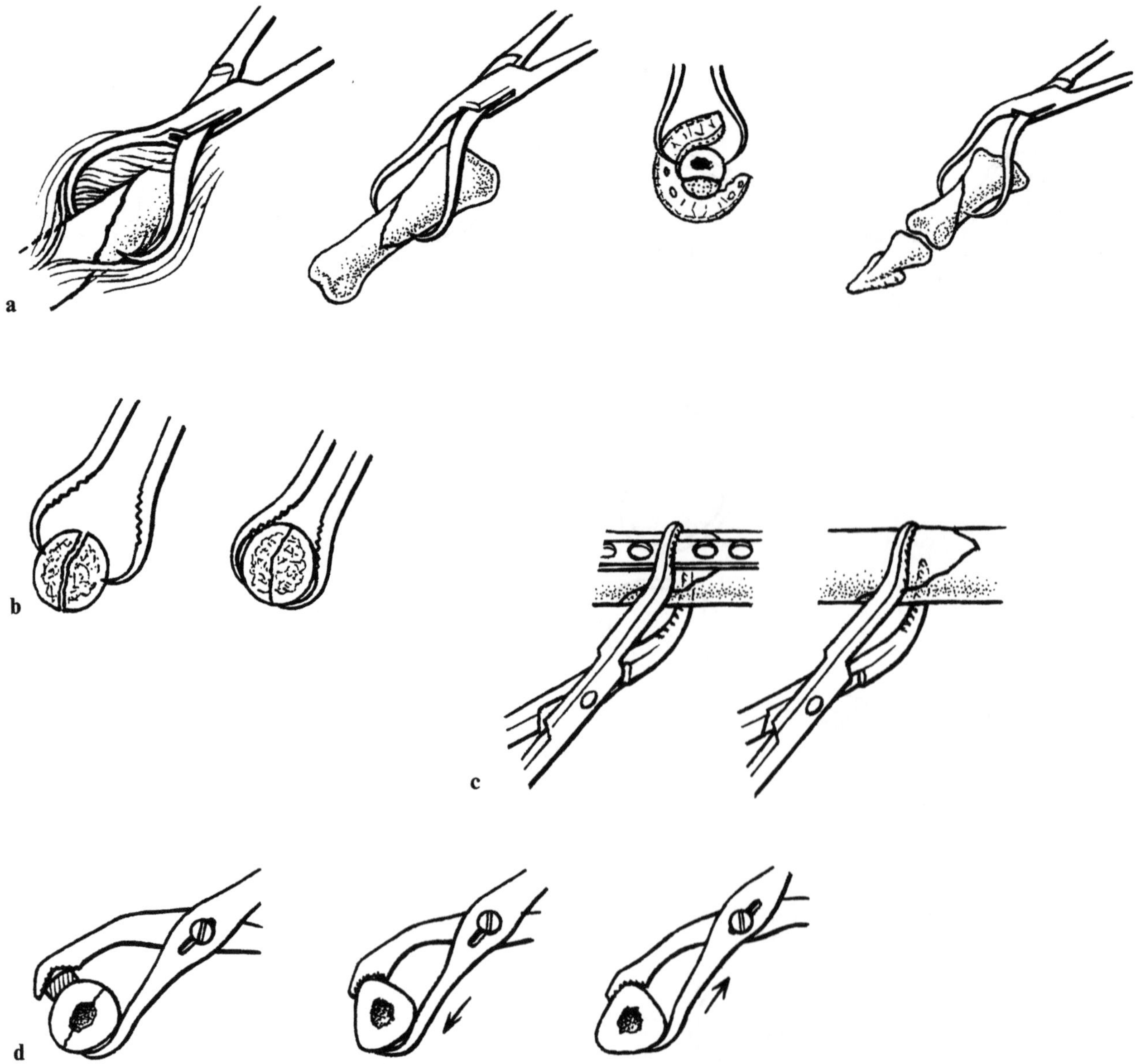

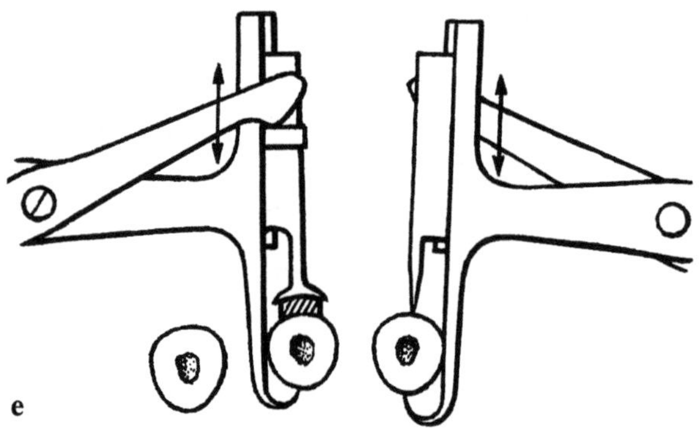

Fig. 15a–e. Reduction forceps: jaw design and holding function

a The previous wide jaw design caused displacement of the soft tissues. The new, fine points ("termite" and "stag beetle") allow percutaneous fixation of the bone on one side, resulting in less soft-tissue trauma

b Combination of sharp points and cross-serrations in a single forceps, for reduction and holding

c The finely serrated jaws of the "lobster" forceps are excellent for the temporary retention of plates and fragments

d The slip joint permits modification of the reduction and holding functions

e Forceps with sliding jaws (central metacarpals): interchangeable jaws with a sharp point or a footplate for reduction and retention

III. General Techniques for the Internal Fixation of Small Fractures

1. Basic Principles

The basic techniques of the ASIF are described in detail in the *Manual of Internal Fixation*. Because these techniques are essential for understanding rigid internal fixation, and because they may be unfamiliar to some surgeons, it is appropriate to review them briefly here (Figs. 16–21).

Rigid internal fixation is a necessary prerequisite for early postoperative function and rapid, economical fracture union. It can be achieved in various ways, depending on the nature of the fracture and the loading of the bone. The basic methods of rigid internal fixation are: splinting, interfragmental compression, neutralization, and buttressing. In practice, it usually is necessary to combine two or more of these methods to obtain optimum stability.

Splinting may be accomplished with an intramedullary implant or by simple approximation with Kirschner wires.

Interfragmental compression can be effected with a lag screw, dynamic compression plate (DCP), or compression device ("static" interfragmental compression), or it may be achieved with a tension band ("dynamic" interfragmental compression). When applied under sufficient primary tension, these devices convert potentially disruptive asymmetrical forces into symmetrical, compressive forces that enhance the stability of the fixation.

Simple fixation with cancellous lag screws is ideal for epiphyseal and metaphyseal fractures and avulsions that have a large area of interfragmental contact. In the diaphysis, fixation with cortex screws is suitable for very long spiral or oblique fractures in which optimum interfragmental compression can be achieved, and shearing and bending forces can be neutralized.

Careful attention should be given to a biomechanically correct placement of the screws in relation to the fracture line. The intent is to distribute the compression as evenly as possible across the fracture interface. This is why it is best to insert screws in "skewed" fashion wherever possible, rather than parallel (Fig. 16). Ideally each screw should bisect the angle formed by the perpendicular to the shaft axis and the perpendicular to the fracture plane.

The most frequent combination of internal fixation methods in use today is screw fixation combined with a neutralization plate. The purpose of the neutralization plate is to absorb bending and shear forces that might disrupt the fixation (Fig. 19a).

Pure axial compression across the fracture line can be achieved by use of the tension device or by the eccentric placement of a screw through the oval hole of a DCP. The DCP principle (DCP = "dynamic compression plate") has become universally established in fracture therapy and is an effective way of applying primary tension to neutralization plates and tension-band plates.

Besides plates, the tension-band effect can be produced with wire loops or by combining a wire loop with a Kirschner wire (splinting) (Fig. 18a, b). These techniques are gaining in popularity.

When the weight-bearing ability of a fracture site has been seriously compromised by comminution or bone loss, the site can be buttressed with a plate or with an external fixation device. The combination of a buttress plate and lag screws is most commonly used (Fig. 21).

In fractures with bone loss and devascularization, increasing use is made of autogenous cancellous bone grafts, which produce mainly a biological effect, and of corticocancellous grafts, whose effect is chiefly mechanical.

The general techniques of the ASIF apply fully to internal fixations of small fractures. This is not surprising when one considers that ASIF techniques are based on the application of fundamental biomechanical laws. However, the small implants call for specific additions and modifications made necessary by the topography of the peripheral skeleton and the smaller amount of bony stock. Special technical considerations apply to the stabilization of these cases.

2. Interfragmental Compression with Lag Screws

Whether screws are used by themselves for the fixation of a fracture or for the attachment of a plate, their use demands technical precision. Technical errors committed while working with wood or metal usually are immediately apparent; this is not the case in the biologic milieu.The soft-tissue envelope, which must be spared, limits exposure of the operative field. Stability may appear excellent at operation, even though the area of interfragmental contact is extremely small. Radiographs, in turn, give little information on fine details. It is our experience that many poor results of internal fixations are based on a too-liberal use of screws. This affects not only the unskilled novice but also the self-assured "expert" who works largely from habit.

The smaller the dimensions, the greater the importance of minor details. This is why we devote a greater amount of space to describing the lag screw technique (and its pitfalls) in words and especially in drawings (Figs. 26, 27, 29, 38).

a) Fixation with Small Cancellous Screws (4.0 mm)

The deep thread and wide head of this screw can produce substantial interfragmental compression. The thread should engage the "far fragment" only. The pilot hole is drilled with a 2.5-mm bit and tapped with the 3.5-mm *cancellous* tap. There is no need to tap the full depth of the hole, especially in osteoporotic bone, and the 4.0-mm diameter screw drives easily into the slightly undersized hole.

Example: Oblique fracture of the medial malleolus (Fig. 22).

(The technique of interfragmental compression in cancellous bone using small, fully threaded screws is described in Section **i** below.)

b) Cutting the Thread

Even with small screws, it is necessary to tap the drill hole (i.e., cut an internal thread) so that the screw can seat properly in the bone and function correctly. Without a precut threat, it may be impossible to insert the screw at all, or the bone may crack when this is attempted. Also, the frictional heat generated by driving a screw into an untapped hole can cause a thermal necrosis that predisposes to loosening. The ASIF has always been very skeptical toward the use of "self-tapping" screws in cortical bone.

It is standard practice to cut the thread by hand. The small bones of the peripheral human skeleton are covered by a delicate soft-tissue envelope whose preservation is essential, and these tissues would be jeopardized if tapping were done with a power instrument.Manual tapping enables the operator to feel the thickness of the cortex and to assess the screw hold that it will afford. This reduces the danger of stripping the thread when the screw is tightened.

c) Fixation with Small Cortex Screws in Cylindrical Bones with a Wide Medullary Cavity (Fig. 23)

The standard ASIF technique is used in this type of bone, but with implants of smaller caliber. The gliding hole is predrilled in the near cortex with a 3.5-mm bit. The 3.5/2.5-mm insert drill sleeve is introduced, and the thread hole is drilled in the far cortex with the 2.5-mm bit. This hole is tapped with the 3.5-mm *cortex* tap (bronze colored) (Fig. 2) using the larger end of the double drill guide as a tap sleeve.

Example: Use of individual small screws for mixed internal fixation of long cylindrical bones (Fig. 213).

d) Small Cortex Screws in Cylindrical Bones with a Narrow Medullary Cavity (Fig. 23)

In cylindrical bones with a narrow medullary cavity (radius, ulna, fibula, clavicle, tubular bones of hand and foot), the new double drill guide permits use of the classic ASIF technique: The gliding hole is drilled first, and the smaller sleeve of the drill guide is inserted until it abuts against the far cortex. This results in a thread hole that is precisely coaxial with the initial gliding hole. Afterward, the far drill hole is easily located with the tapered end of the tap. Note that in this technique the tap is twisted through *one cortex only*, resulting in better safety and precision. Diminishing resistance will tell the operator when the thread has been completely cut. This is especially critical in the hand and foot, where delicate soft tissues would be damaged if the tap were driven too far. This can be avoided by measuring the width of the predrilled cortex with the mini depth gauge (Fig. 29) to estimate the depth of tap insertion.

Example: Fixation of a spiral fracture of the lateral malleolus with a 3.5-mm cortex screw (Fig. 23) or a central metacarpal with a 2.7-mm cortex screw.

e) Previous "Small Fragment Technique"

In the technique formerly recommended by the ASIF for narrow cylindrical bones, the operator first uses the smaller bit to drill through both cortices at once. With this technique the operator can gauge the strength of the far cortex in advance and estimate the hold that it will afford a lag screw.

The screw length having been determined, the tap is twisted through both cortices, and the near hole is drilled out with a larger-gauge bit to make the gliding hole.

The disadvantage of this technique is that the far hole is made without benefit of an insert drill guide, and so the bit may skid when it encounters an oblique far cortex. In this case the far hole will not be coaxial with the near hole, and the gliding hole will be imperfectly centered. Another danger is that the threaded hole will become damaged when the gliding hole is cut (Fig. 26).

This technique, while not ideal, was the only option available before the development of small insert drill sleeves. Thus it has become standard practice for many surgeons, and certainly it will continue to be used. It is perfectly safe when the medullary cavity is narrow and a large-gauge bit is used.Especially in bones with a thin far cortex and in many cancellous fractures (see **f** and **i**), it continues to be a favorable alternative.

f) Primary Compression with Reduction Forceps

When the far cortex is thin (visible on X-rays and palpable when drilling and tapping by the "small fragment technique"), it is safer not to make the gliding hole in the near cortex as the initial step. Before the thread is cut, the reduction forceps is tightened to create some amount of interfragmental compression. The stability achieved with this method may be sufficient in small bones and especially in cancellous bone (Fig. 27).

g) Metal Washer

When the near cortex is thin or splintered, it is recommended that a washer be used to prevent subsidence of the screw head or cracking of the adjacent cortex (Fig. 28).

h) Countersink

Cutting a recess for the screw head is recommended only when the cortex is thick or there is a danger of soft-tissue injury by a projecting screw head. Experience has shown that this is rarely the case in the hand and foot (Figs. 23, 24).

i) Use of Small Screws in Cancellous Bone

The threads of the 2.7-, 2.0-, and 1.5-mm screws are basically designed for use in cortical bone. Special cancellous screws with a wider thread, steeper pitch, and unthreaded neck–as exist in the 6.5- and 4.0-mm sizes–are not necessary for very small-scale work.The hold of the small cortex screw is remarkably good, especially in the hard cancellous bone of the hand and foot.

On the other hand, because the cancellous bone lacks a medullary cavity, interfragmental compression can present problems. An ideal solution would be to drill the large gliding hole in the smaller fragment before reducing the fracture, i.e., with vision of the open fracture site. Then the thread hole in the far fragment could be drilled through a narrow sleeve passed through the first hole. This would correspond to the standard technique for cortical bone. There is a danger of tearout of small near fragments with this technique, so it should be reserved for exceptional cases (Fig. 27a).

Usually it is necessary for practical reasons to carry out the reduction and provisional fixation before drilling the bone. This makes the drilling depth for the gliding hole uncertain. If the gliding hole is too short, interfragmental compression will not be obtained when the screw is tightened. If the gliding hole is cut too deeply, the threaded hole will be shortened or weakened and may become stripped when the screw is tightened (Fig. 27b). This problem can be minimized by introducing the screw through the smaller fragment.

In certain cases, then, the technique of primary external compression with the reduction forceps (described above) should be used with the mini screws. This method is appropriate in cases where juxta-articular fragments fit together cleanly so that an anatomic reduction can be obtained (Fig. 27e).

Stabilization Rule 1: Screw Fixation (Fig. 39)

The resistance of screws to tearout forces depends chiefly on the screw diameter (and bone strength) and on the length of screw thread gripping the bone (cortical thickness).

The core diameter of the screw is not a significant factor in cortical bone.

As the thickness of the cortex decreases, so does the number of *active screw threads* (threads that grip the bone). At least three active screw threads are needed to maintain resistance to dislodgment.

Conclusion: With a thin cortex, use a finely threaded screw with more active threads (larger contact area). Example: 3.5-mm cortex screw (pitch 1.25 mm) instead of a fully threaded cancellous screw (pitch 1.75 mm).

Two smaller, staggered screws produce a more uniform and symmetrical compression of the fracture surfaces and resist bending and shear forces better than one centrally placed screw.

Basic rule: *Match the screw size to the size of the bone. A small, fine screw may be mechanically superior to a larger, coarse screw in thin cortical bone. Two are definitely superior.*

Exception: Cancellous fractures and avulsions with interdigitating fragments can be perfectly stabilized (even against rotation) with a single lag screw (Fig. 39c).

3. Tension-Band Wires (Fig. 30)

"The tension-band wire provides dynamic compression and is used in cases where it can absorb all the tensile forces acting on the fracture, while bending and shear forces are overcome by interfragmental friction alone or by supplementary splintage with Kirschner wires" (*Manual of Internal Fixation*, p. 42).

Tension-band wiring is indicated chiefly for avulsion fractures, for the fixation of arthrodeses, and occasionally for the attachment of corticocancellous grafts.

Kirschner wires aid in the reduction and, because they are inserted sequentially, facilitate provisional fixation. Parallel Kirschner wires enhance rotational stability and provide symmetric anchoring posts for a wire loop.

One end of the wire loop may pass through a strong tendinous structure close to the bone, or it may be brought through a channel drilled in the bone. On the other side of the fracture, the loop is usually passed around the projecting ends of the Kirschner wires.

Crossing the wire loop over the fracture line centers the compressive force on the midline. Asymmetric tension is avoided by stressing each limb of the wire loop independently. This places right-angle bends in the wire at the edges of the bony channel and at the Kirschner wires, thereby preventing stress transfer from one limb of the wire to the other. The wire is tightened by twisting it. Two shorter wires can be twisted together at their ends, or the ends of a longer wire can be twisted together and a small loop formed in the middle of the other side with a pliers.

The wires are twisted and tightened with a flat-nosed parallel pliers (or special pliers with flared jaws). The operator grasps the twisted wire segment at the base (Fig. 30b) so that he can feel the amount of tension being applied and avoid wire breakage. The twist is started by hand. Then the twisted segment is grasped with the pliers, raised vertically from the bone (Fig. 30a), and twisted further while vertical tension is slowly released. After each complete turn, the twisted segment is released and regrasped at its base, each time pulling the wire vertically before the twist is made. This maneuver is done alternately on both sides until the wire can no longer be raised from the bone. Generally each limb of the wire will have to be twisted several times, depending on the primary tension in the loop.

After the wire has been tightened, any excess is trimmed off with the wire cutter, and the twisted segment is turned to one side (while preserving wire tension) so that it does not directly underlie the skin incision and does not tent the skin, which often is traumatized and sensitive.

With very small avulsion fractures of the hand, absorbable suture material is used in place of a wire loop. Care is taken that the suture is made tense when the knots are tied. The advantage of this method is that it obviates the need for later wire removal.

4. Axial Interfragmental Compression with a Plate

A plate should be used according to the tension-band principle whenever the biomechanical configuration permits (asymmetric tensile forces). This means applying the plate to the tension side of the bone, such as the dorsal aspect of the metacarpus. Whenever possible, a supplementary lag screw should be placed on the second plane (Fig. 35b) or, with a short oblique fracture, one of the central plate screws should be driven across the fracture line in lag-screw fashion (Figs. 31–35). Stability is demonstrably improved by this technique.

Prebending the plate at its center (about 1 mm from the bone surface) is an excellent means of ensuring uniform compression of the fracture, even on the side opposite the plate. But this method is reliable only in a purely transverse, "osteotomy-like" fracture. It can hinder anatomic reduction and will cause axial displacement unless the opposite cortex is completely intact. In peripheral fractures, the presence of small marginal fragments often is not apparent on X-rays. Meanwhile, the danger of devascularization makes it advisable to limit the extent of the exposure as much as possible. For this reason we have decided not to describe the technique of plate prebending in this context, despite its ability to improve axial interfragmental compression when correctly performed. The interfragmental lag screw is more reliable, and we prefer to use it whenever possible.

With small plates, particular care must be taken to adapt the plate to the contour of the bone; otherwise displacements can occur when the screws are tightened (Fig. 33). Special pliers are used for this purpose. Generally the bending press and bending irons are used for contouring the thicker DCP plates. To make this easier, aluminum templates are available for the 3.5- and 2.7-mm sizes that are bent manually to the shape of the bone and then serve as a pattern for contouring the plate.

Axial Compression with the One-Third Tubular Plate (Fig. 31). After the fracture has been reduced and the plate contoured, eccentric drill holes (away from the fracture line) are made through the plate holes adjacent to the fracture. Tightening the spherical-head screws distracts the plate and presses the bone ends together. The articulated tension device (Fig. 33) also may be used to prestress the plate.

The 3.5-mm Dynamic Compression Plate (Fig. 32). Again, axial compression is obtained by drilling an eccentric hole through a plate hole adjoining the fracture. For this we use the special DCP double drill guide, which fits exactly into the deep holes of the DCP. The green end of the guide is used first to drill a centered hole (neutral position). The opposite end of the guide, colored yellow, produces a drill hole that is off-center by 1 mm. The arrow on the guide must point toward the fracture. Tightening the screws produces a compressive displacement of 1 mm; i.e., the fragments are pushed toward each other by a distance of 1 mm and are correspondingly compressed.

A compressive displacement of 2 mm is obtained by placing an eccentric drill hole on each side of the fracture (Fig. 32). The second hole is not drilled until the first screw has been inserted. The first screw creates friction between the plate and underlying bone, so that screw should be loosened slightly before the second screw is tightened. Since the small core of the 3.5-mm cortex screw has a relatively low bending strength, it is better to use the articulated tension device (Fig. 33) when there is a need for greater compressive displacement. This device is also useful for fine reduction.

The 3.5-mm DCP can also function as a neutralization plate. In this case all the screw holes are drilled centrally through the green, neutral drill guide.

The oval holes of the DCP permits screws to be inserted at an angle if required. This may be necessary to avoid a fracture line or a previously placed lag screw (Fig. 32d).

Oblique fracture lines should be compressed with a plate screw whenever possible, as this significantly augments the stability of the fixation (Fig. 32c).

For the *2.7- and 2.0-mm DCP*, the technique is the same, using correspondingly smaller instruments and a smaller compressive displacement.

Axial compression with the 2.7-mm plates is more difficult to obtain, especially when shaped plates are used. The main reason for this is that while a perfect reduction can be obtained under vision, provisional fixation of the fragments is quite difficult. Reduction forceps and thin, oblique Kirschner wires often cannot be used, or the fracture itself may be obscured by the implant in cases where soft-tissue factors contraindicate a wider exposure. In this situation, secondary displacements can occur unnoticed when the screws are inserted.

Our technique for applying shaped plates in difficult cases is as follows (Fig. 34):

- The fragments are reduced under vision and temporarily held in place by an assistant.
- The proper plate is selected and contoured to the bone (especially important on the metaphysis).
- The first drill hole is made on the long axis of the shorter fragment. Accurate placement of this hole is critical.
- The plate is fixed to the shorter fragment with this first screw.
- The plate is used as a handle to assist the reduction and is fixed to the larger fragment with a reduction forceps. At this time axial alignment is checked and adjusted as needed.
- The second screw is driven into the shorter fragment. Rotational alignment is checked and corrected either by bending the plate or by adjusting its position on the larger fragment.
- The eccentric (load) hole is now drilled in the larger fragment, and axial compression is applied by inserting and tightening the screw. The reduction forceps is removed.
- The remaining screws are inserted in the larger fragment.

Definitive tightening of the screws is done as a last step to avoid thread damage in the event the plate has to be loosened and repositioned. The original holes are reused after the plate has been properly adapted. It is virtually impossible to correct malalignment by drilling new holes.

This technique is designed to avoid the two most common errors in this type of internal fixation:

- Axial malalignment with use of the T plate. This results from eccentric tensile forces that arise when the fracture is compressed before both screws have been inserted in the T piece of the plate (Fig. 38b).
- Rotational malalignment with the oblique L plate. This occurs when the delayed insertion of a screw off the long axis of the plate alters the rotational alignment of the bone (Fig. 38c).

If malrotation occurs despite all precautions, this should be recognized after the third screw is inserted. The plate can then be loosened or removed, twisted with the bending pliers to counter the deformity, and reattached with the original screws. The final screws are not inserted into the larger fragment until correct alignment has been established.

Common errors of internal fixation with small plates are illustrated in Fig. 38. They tend to occur when the plates are not accurately contoured to the bone, or when screws are inserted obliquely.

5. Neutralization Plates

The neutralization principle is commonly applied in the peripheral skeleton, and virtually any plate can be used for this purpose.

Two different techniques are employed for oblique and spiral fractures:

- If the visible apex of the fragment is not on the plane of the plate, the fracture is first reduced and fixed with a separate lag screw in standard fashion. Then the plate is contoured to the bone and attached with screws on a different plane; the lag screw does not pass through the plate (Fig. 35b).
- If the apex of the fragments is directly beneath the plate, the latter will cover the fracture line. The following technique has proved useful in this situation (Fig. 35a):
- The fracture is reduced and held with forceps.
- The appropriate neutralization plate is selected and tentatively contoured.
- An interfragmental lag screw is inserted across the fracture at a site coinciding with the central plate hole. The screw tip should protrude from the bone slightly.
- The operator checks the quality of the reduction and the position of the peripheral joints in flexion.
- If reduction and alignment are satisfactory, the screw is removed and reinserted through the plate. The plate should fit snugly against the reduced fracture. Otherwise it is removed, recontoured, and reattached with the initial screw.
- Once the plate has been accurately fitted, the remaining screws are inserted.

This technique virtually eliminates the danger of secondary displacement and fully utilizes the protective effect of the plate in neutralizing shearing and bending forces.

Mini plates are applied according to the techniques used for the small plates for 2.7-mm screws.

Stabilization Rule 2: Plate Stability

The implant and bone should be correctly matched biomechanically. The plate must be matched to the fractured bone in such a way that, given its intrinsic mechanical properties, length, and position, it is able to resist bending and shear forces that might disrupt the fixation postoperatively. Interfragmental compression is particularly effective against rotational forces.

The number and type of screws pressing the plate against the bone, and their threads, are significant.

Because the lever arm forces and functional loads increase in the direction of the trunk, the number of cortices that must be gripped by the screw threads increases in a peripheral-to-central direction.

Generally it is sufficient to engage three cortices per main fragment in the phalanges, and four cortices in the metacarpals and metatarsals. In the more proximal skeleton, oblique fractures will require five cortices per main fragment, and transverse fractures, which are subject to greater shearing forces, will require six. This rule also may be adapted to special implants (e.g., the mini condylar plate).

Basic rule: *Three or four cortical threads in each main fragment distally, and five or six proximally.*

Exception: In transverse interdigitating fractures, interfragmental compression and plate length are more important than the number of cortical threads in terms of resistance to bending and shear. If the cortex is thick, it is sufficient to have a short, terminal screw that engages one cortex only.

6. Buttress Plates

Use of a buttress plate is frequently necessary in unstable diaphyseal or metaphyseal fractures. In multiple fractures, small irreducible or devitalized fragments must be replaced with cancellous bone graft if the reduction yields an assembly that is unstable or prone to secondary collapse.

A special type of buttress plate used on severely comminuted areas in the peripheral skeleton, and especially the hand, is called the "bridge plate" (Fig. 19b).Its only function is to create a mechanical linkage between the main fracture fragments. Small, viable fragments are not fixed, but are biologically optimized by the addition of cancellous bone. Nonviable fragments are removed and replaced with a corticocancellous block whose cortical side is placed opposite the plate (for optimum mechanical effect).

7. Combined Internal Fixation Using Small and Large Implants

Skeletal areas that are intermediate between "large" and "small" often call for the concurrent use of different techniques or different implants.Examples are the distal tibia, the malleoli, the elbow, the distal forearm, etc.. In these areas the SFS may form the core of the internal fixation, or it may serve only as an adjust. Small and large implants are most frequently combined in the tibia, where it may be necessary to fix small, pointed fragments to larger fracture elements or to fit partially or completely devitalized fragments accurately into place so that they can become revascularized from adjacent bone.

8. Multiple Fractures

Multiple fractures are relatively common in the peripheral skeleton. They may be mechanically independent of each other (we call these "autonomous fractures"), or they may show a mechanical interdependence. In the latter case one fracture will be predominant; we call it the *dominant fracture*. The other fracture, which is less conspicuous and whose position and stability are dependent on the dominant fracture, is called the *vassal fracture* or *subordinate fracture*.

This relationship is most commonly seen in fractures of the second through fifth metacarpals, the malleoli, and the distal forearm. It can also exist in certain segmental fractures. A classic example in the major skeleton is an oblique fracture of the distal fibula associated with a spiral fracture of the tibia (see Fig. 41 b). Therapeutic efforts should be concentrated on the dominant fracture.For practical reasons, this economy of effort is particularly valuable in the treatment of multiple fractures.The internal fixation of these cases is often technically demanding, and the time factor can be crucial in terms of maintaining blood supply, avoiding infection, and preserving the soft tissues. This brings us to our third rule of stabilization:

Stabilization Rule 3: The "Vassal Rule" or Rule of Fracture Dominance (Fig. 41)

When a mechanical interdependence exists between two fractures, the dominant fracture should be reduced first. Then the subordinate fracture either will be very easy to reduce or will reduce spontaneously.

The dominant fracture is stabilized with an (external) implant that is able to bear loads. This will eliminate the danger of secondary displacement of the subordinate fracture–although its fixation is often recommended in the interest of early mobilization. Fixation of the subordinate fracture can be accomplished by very simple means (e.g., a single lag screw or Kirschner wire), and even this is unnecessary in some cases.

Basic rule: *Plate only the dominant fracture.*

9. Operative Technique with Special Plates

a) Reconstruction Plates (Fig. 5)

The need to bend plates not just about a transverse axis but also about an axis perpendicular to the plane of the plate ("edgewise" bending) first became evident in surgery of the mandible. By adding the capability of bending the plate in a third dimension, it became possible to fix fractures at or near the angle of the mandible, and even to stabilize the entire mandibular arch (excluding the condylar processes) and reconstruct it with bone grafts.

Edgewise bending is made possible by notching the edges of the plate between the plate holes. Naturally this reduces the stability of the plate in comparison with a straight plate of the same size. Special pliers and bending irons are required for edgewise plate bending.The holes are oval in shape so that interfragmental compression by the DCP principle can be applied.

The reconstruction plate for 3.5-mm screws, with 5 to 8 holes spaced 12 mm apart, is designed for use on the distal humerus, acetabulum, clavicle, and scapula; other sites are also possible.

A special type of 3.5-mm plate is the Y plate for the distal humerus, which has the same features but is rarely used because of the difficulty of removing implants from the dorsal side of the forearm.

Straight and prebent reconstruction plates for 2.7-mm screws with 8 to 24 holes spaced 8 mm spart are used chiefly in mandibular surgery. They are rarely if ever indicated for other parts of the skeleton.

The same design principle is applied in the shaft of the mini condylar plates for 2.0- and 1.5-mm screws.

b) Mini Condylar Plate (Fig. 36)

The rigid internal fixation of juxta-articular fractures of the metacarpals and phalanges often cannot be satisfactorily accomplished with small, straight plates or even with L or T plates, especially when there is T- or Y-shaped fragmentation. The mini condylar plates are excellent for fractures of this type. Generally the 1.5-mm size is used on the phalanges and the 2.0-mm size on the metacarpals.

First the articular fragments are carefully reassembled and transfixed with a thin Kirschner wire inserted parallel to the joint plane. This may be done from within the fracture using the "inside-out" technique, inserting the wire first into one fragment and then drilling it back into the second, or the wire may be drilled directly through both fragments held in reduction with a sharp forceps. The placement of the wire should be carefully planned, for it marks the site where the definitive lag screw will be inserted. Depending on the position of the plate on the bone, this screw may come to lie dorsal or volar to the pin of the mini condylar plate, since the plates are not made in separate "right" and "left" designs.Next the wire is threaded through the barrel of the appropriate drill guide, and a parallel hole (1.5 or 2.0 mm) is drilled to accommodate the pin of the plate. The depth of the channel is measured, and the pin is trimmed to the required length with cutting pliers and sharpened. The remainder of the plate also must be cut to the proper length and contoured to the bone surface. The pin of the mini condylar plate is inserted by threading the adjacent plate hole over the Kirschner guide wire and seating the pin tentatively in its channel. Discrepancies of plate shape or pin angle are corrected by removing the plate and rebending it. When the fit is perfect, the pin is definitively driven in by hand or with an impactor. The wire is then replaced by a screw inserted parallel to the plate pin. With a Y-shaped fracture, the screw is introduced in lag fashion. It also may engage the shaft fragment as a lag screw in certain types of fracture. Finally the shaft fragment is reduced against the stabilized articular fragment, and axial compression is applied with a first, eccentric screw. The possibility of inserting an interfragmental lag screw should again be checked at this time.Then the remaining screws are inserted.

The mini condylar plate has also proved very useful for comminuted fractures that involve the joints or occur in proximity to them. Fixation of the fracture is carried out in the same way, starting from the joint and working toward the diaphysis. Separate lag screws placed away from the plate may be necessary for difficult fragments.

While the implants are basically designed for use on the lateral or medial aspect of the metacarpals and phalanges, experience has shown that they can be used on various surfaces, according to the requirements of the situation.

c) Mini H Plate (Fig. 37)

This mini plate was specifically designed for transverse fractures. Its use differs in some respects from a conventional plate and is described below:

- *Indications:* Internal fixations of the phalanges, especially transverse fractures of the shaft and metaphysis. Y fractures of the metaphysis. Comminuted fractures (in combination with lag screws).
- *Contraindications:* Comminution of the cortex opposite the plate. This would not allow early mobilization, even when combined with cancellous bone grafting, as it will tend to loosen before the fracture has consolidated.
- *Approach:* For reimplantations and in complex injuries, approach is made through existing soft-tissue injuries, and an effort is made to expose the bone sparingly.
- *Internal fixation*: The sequence of screw insertion is shown in Fig. 37. Some interfragmental compression can be produced by drilling the holes eccentrically.

In *thin* phalanges, the screws in one fragment should be inserted in different directions so that their points do not touch (Fig. 37b)

In *Y fractures* of the metaphysis (Fig. 37 c), the DCP principle of eccentric screw placement can be utilized to produce interfragmental compression and increase stability.

10. Open Fractures

Today it is recognized that osseous stability and wound rest are essential to the uncomplicated healing of an open fracture.

When selecting metallic implants, consideration must be given to existing wounds and defects as well as to contusions, degloving injuries, and the degree of contamination. The problem of venous drainage, especially on the dorsal sides of the hand and foot, limits the free extension of incisions.It is imperative that wound-closing sutures be placed without tension.In doubtful cases wounds should be left open and closed secondarily. Often, however, wounds on the hand and foot will require primary closure using flap techniques. For these reasons, standard procedures may not always be appropriate for open fractures.

An external fixator modified for use on small bones has proved useful in the management of these cases (see Chap. 11).

Kirschner wires are also commonly used. Despite their relatively poor stability, they are useful for the temporary immobilization of peripheral joints (e.g., during the treatment of tendon and ligamentous injuries).

The objective in all cases is an essentially open wound care followed if possible by postoperative treatment without a cast.

By adhering to these principles, we have seen a significant decline in the infection rate among our patients with peripheral fractures. The infection rate at present is approximately 10% for open fractures and 1.9% for closed fractures.

11. Small External Fixator–Technique and Indications

The small external fixator performs the same functions on the peripheral skeleton as the tubular external fixation system does on the larger bones: immobilization, distraction, and compression. However, the topography of the peripheral bones demands that more careful attention be given to the soft tissues. That is why the small external fixator is most commonly used in the unilateral or "half-frame" configuration.

In most cases the fracture is reduced and fixed with percutaneous Kirschner wires before the external rods are applied.In fractures with extensive comminution and in closed, irreducible fractures, the external fixator is applied first in the distracting mode in order to facilitate open reduction, screw or Kirschner wire fixation, and cancellous grafting.

The drill sites on the bone are exposed through longitudinal incisions held open with small retractors (Fig. 42a). We recommend pre-drilling both cortices with the 2.0-mm bit through the appropriate drill guide. This ensures correct placement of the implants and reduces heat generation and the danger of cracking. As the threaded end of the pin or Kirschner wire is twisted into the bone, the resistance felt in the far cortex will enable the operator to gauge the depth of insertion. The thread must grip both cortices solidly, making certain that the sharp point does not injure the soft tissues.

Kirschner wires of 2.5 mm diameter with a low thread pitch may be inserted with a low-speed power drill. In delicate areas it is best to work under image intensifier guidance. Schanz screws with a steep pitch should always be twisted in by hand (using the T-grip handle or universal chuck with handle).

Assembly as a Half Frame (Figs. 42, 43a). For the most frequent indication–a comminuted fracture of the distal radius–two pairs of threaded wires are inserted in converging ("V") fashion into the radius and second metacarpal. Angling the wires in this way increases the intraosseous distance and improves stability once the connecting rods are in place.

The two end wires are inserted first, making sure their axial and rotational alignment are correct, and they are provisionally attached to the connecting rod with the spring-loaded nuts. Then the central wires are inserted, using the two central clamps as guides (Fig. 42b). The rod should be relatively close to the skin surface.

The rotational stability of the assembly is reinforced with a a second connecting rod mounted 2-3 cm from the first with 4 additional clamps. Stability can be further increased by manually compressing the wires toward each other, as in the large tubular system.

After both rods are in place, distraction can still be applied by loosening the clamps.

The clamps are definitively tightened with the open-end wrench after first removing the spring-loaded nuts and replacing them with ordinary nuts.

The axial alignment of the frame can be secondarily adjusted by replacing the long 4-mm rods with two shorter rods connected at the center with 4/4-mm clamps (Fig. 43a).

Rotational alignment can be corrected by adding a third pair of rods at the center, though this is more difficult.

Assembly as a Quadrilateral Frame (Fig. 43b): Short rods anchored on two implants can be cross-connected to create a stable, quadrilateral assembly. It is unnecessary to mount additional rods above the frame.

When the assembly has been completed, any skin tension noted about the wires is released with transverse incisions. Loose approximating sutures are placed, and the sites are covered with petrolatum gauze and a protective dressing. The incisions are checked regularly.

Applications as a Half-Frame

- Immobilization of the wrist in unstable distal radial fractures
- Stabilization of the carpus in fracture-dislocations of the wrist, with connection of 3rd metacarpal and radius
- Infected nonunions and osteitis of the forearm (possibly supplemented by a plaster splint)
- Open fractures of the upper and lower extremity in small children

Applications as a Quadrilateral or Triangular Frame

- Intermetacarpal stabilization in complex comminuted fractures
- Fracture-dislocations of the metatarsus
- Temporary reduction aid (as a distractor) during the internal fixation of calcaneus fractures (Fig. 228)
- Open fractures of the tarsus, especially the calcaneus

Combined Applications

- Complex injuries with tissue loss about the wrist and distal forearm

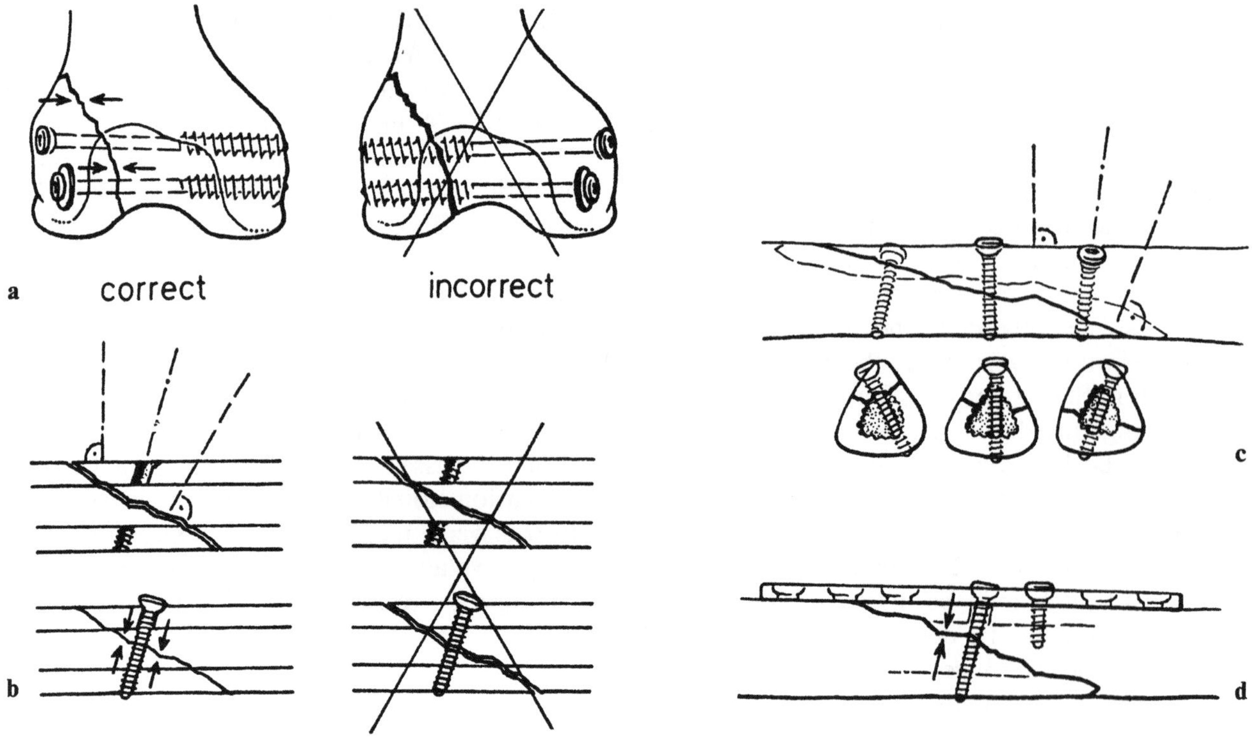

Fig. 16a–d. Technical fundamentals: interfragmental compression with lag screws (see also *Manual of Internal Fixation*)

a Internal fixation of a simple fracture of the lateral femoral condyle with cancellous screws. Principle: The screw shank is unthreaded, and all of the threaded portion is beyond the fracture line. One cancellous screw is placed over a washer to keep its head from perforating the thin cortex

b Fixation with cortex screws: The hole in the near cortex must be as wide as the outer diameter of the screw (gliding hole). The hole in the far cortex is smaller and is tapped (thread hole). Tightening the screw effects interfragmental compression

c Correct placement of the screws (in a long spiral fracture): Multiple screws placed in staggered fashion exert uniform compression over the length of the fracture. The optimum screw position is on a line bisecting the angle formed by the fracture line and shaft axis. In cross-section, the screws should be perpendicular to the fracture plane

d If the hole in the near cortex is large enough, a screw driven through a plate is able to function as a compressive lag screw

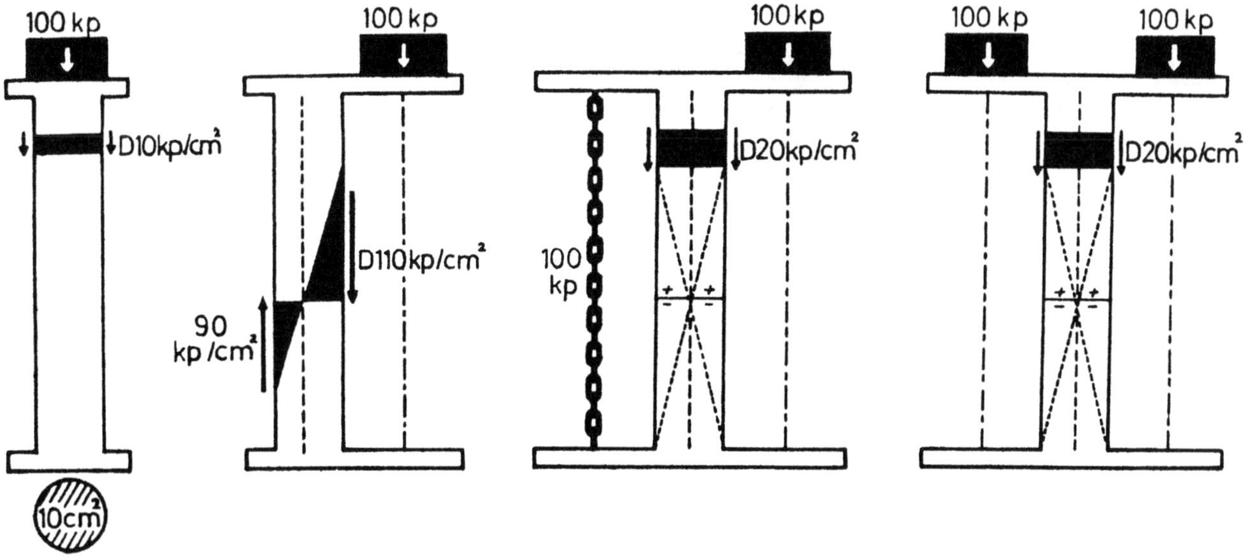

Fig. 17. Technical fundamentals: the tension-band principle (see also *Manual of Internal Fixation*)

Pauwels' model of a weight-bearing T beam: An eccentrically placed weight causes tensile and compressive stresses to develop in the interior of the column. These can be neutralized, and converted to uniform axial compression, by a chain or a weight applied to the opposite side of the beam

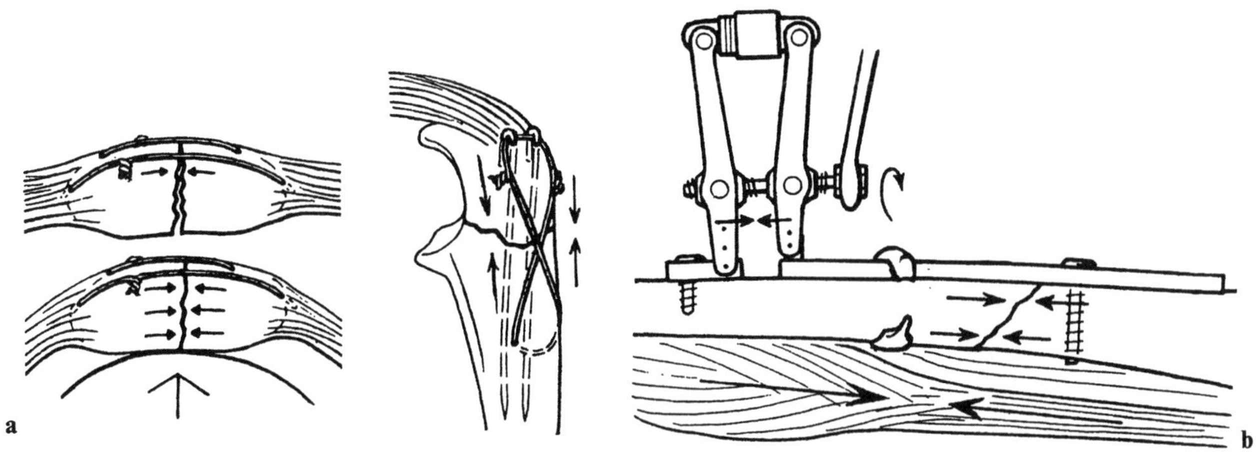

Fig. 18 a, b. Application of the tension-band principle: the wire tension band and the tension-band plate

a The wire loop must overcome the muscular tensile forces acting on the fracture. The skeletal pressure accompanying flexion of the joint leads to uniform compression of the fracture surfaces. Shear forces are neutralized by the parallel Kirschner wires

b Tension-band plate: The eccentrically applied plate provides uniform compression of the fracture owing to muscular tension exerted from the opposite side

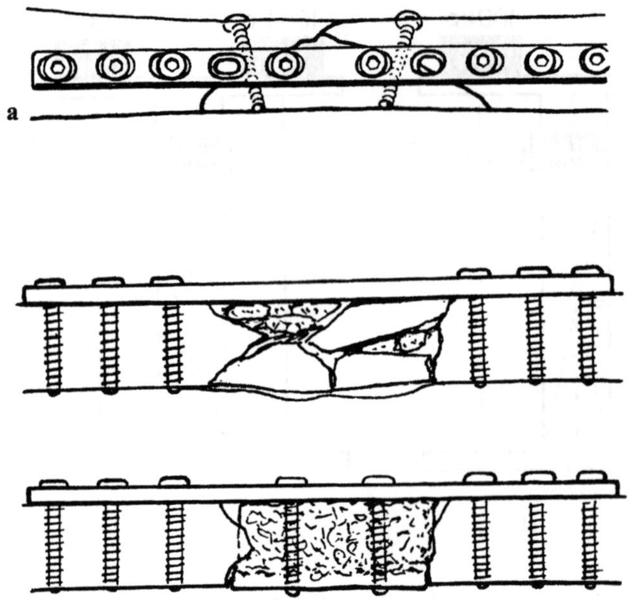

Fig. 19a, b. **Technical fundamentals: neutralization plate, bridge plate**

a Neutralization plate in a fracture with a butterfly fragment: Lag screws produce compression between the two main fragments and the butterfly. Bending and shear forces acting on the fracture are neutralized with a plate that bridges the butterfly and unites the main fragments

b Bridge plate for comminuted fractures: Blood-flow considerations prohibit the direct fixation of a central comminuted area with viable fragments. One solution is to bridge the site with a plate attached only to the main fragments. If the comminuted fragments are nonviable, they are removed and replaced with a cancellous or corticocancellous graft with its cortical side opposite the plate

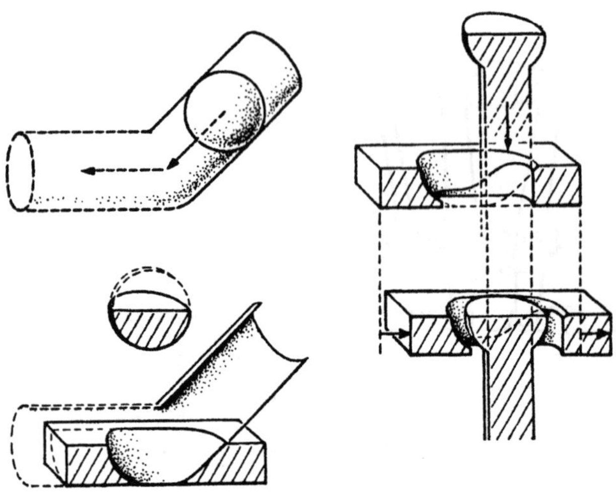

Fig. 20. Technical fundamentals: dynamic axial compression (DCP principle)

With an appropriate configuration of the oval plate hole and eccentric placement of the drill hole, the screw head will exert a pushing force on the plate as the screw is tightened. This principle is utilized to produce axial compression with the dynamic compression plate (DCP)–often without the need for a separate tension device

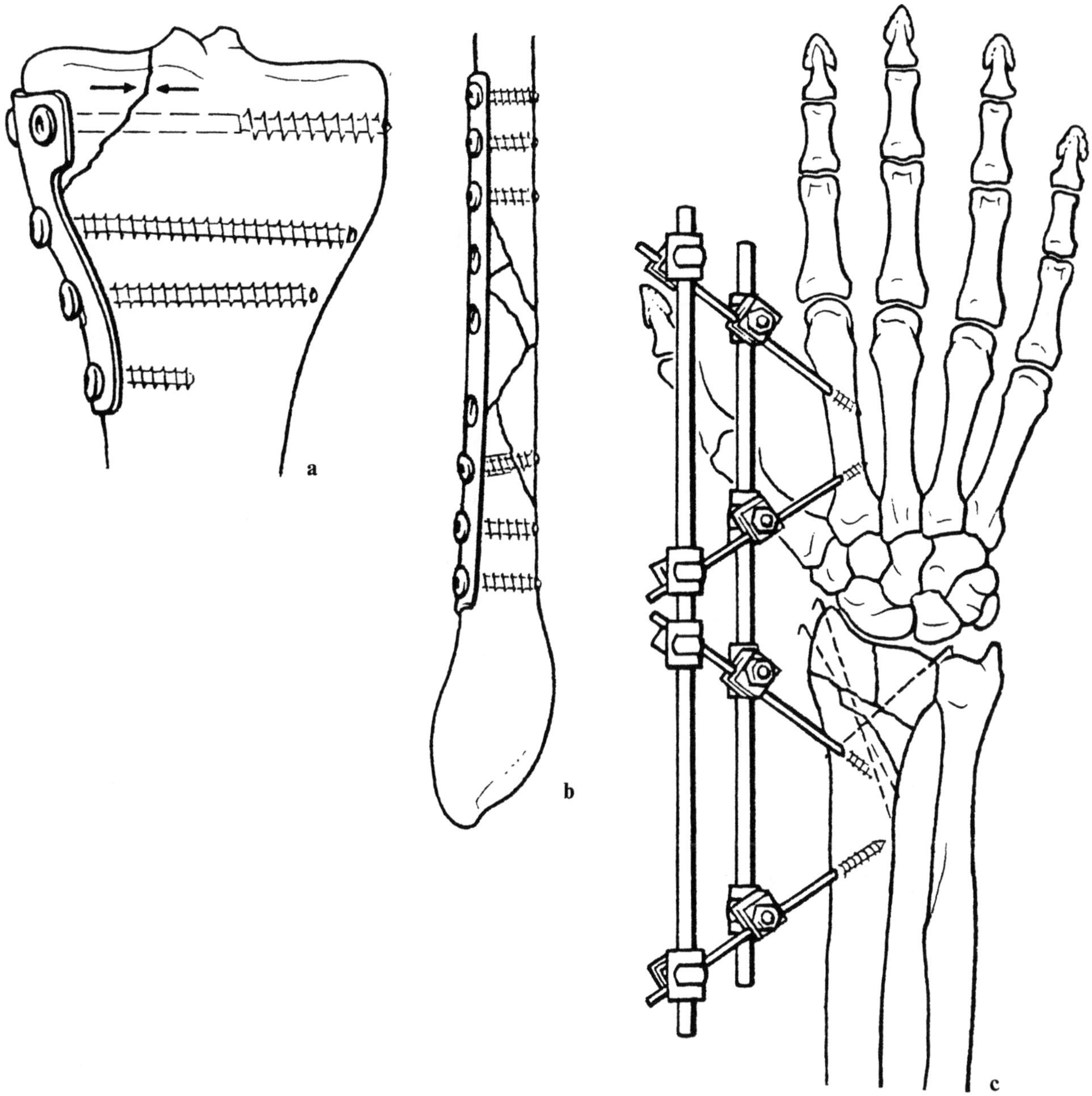

Fig. 21 a–c. Technical fundamentals: buttressing

The buttress plate protects an epiphyseal or metaphyseal fragment from secondary collapse and prevents shortening of a comminuted diaphysis. A similar function is performed by the external fixator

a Buttress plate on a tibial plateau fracture

b Bridge plate on a complex type C malleolar fracture

c Transarticular immobilization with the external fixator for a complex fracture of the distal radius

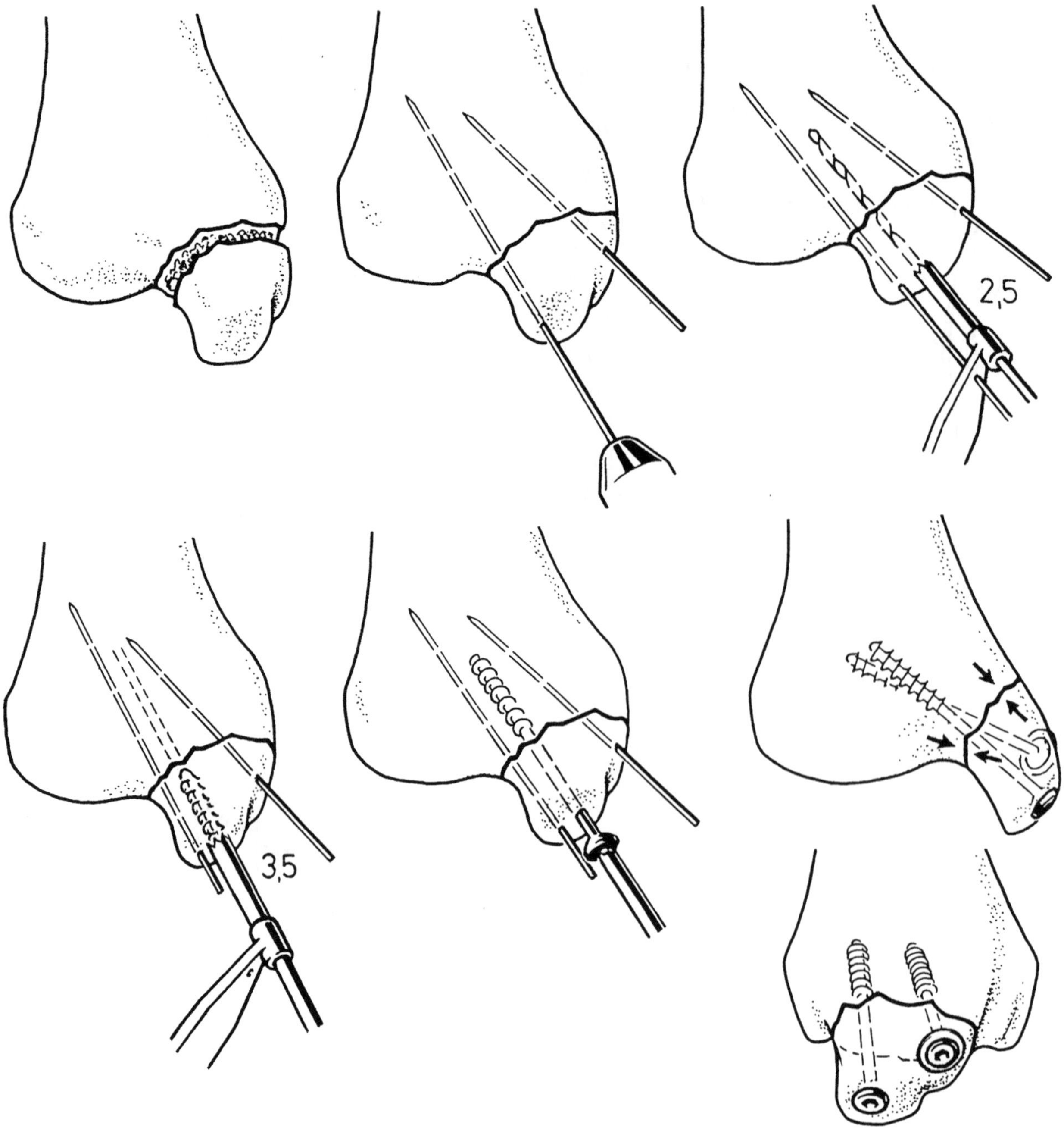

Fig. 22. Fixation with the 4.0-mm small cancellous screw

This oblique fracture of the medial malleolus is reduced and temporarily fixed with Kirschner wires. A parallel hole is drilled with the 2.5-mm bit and tapped using the 3.5-mm *cancellous* tap and tap sleeve. The first screw is inserted. The second Kirschner wire is removed and replaced with a second screw, which is placed over a washer. The screws are definitively tightened after the Kirschner wires are removed

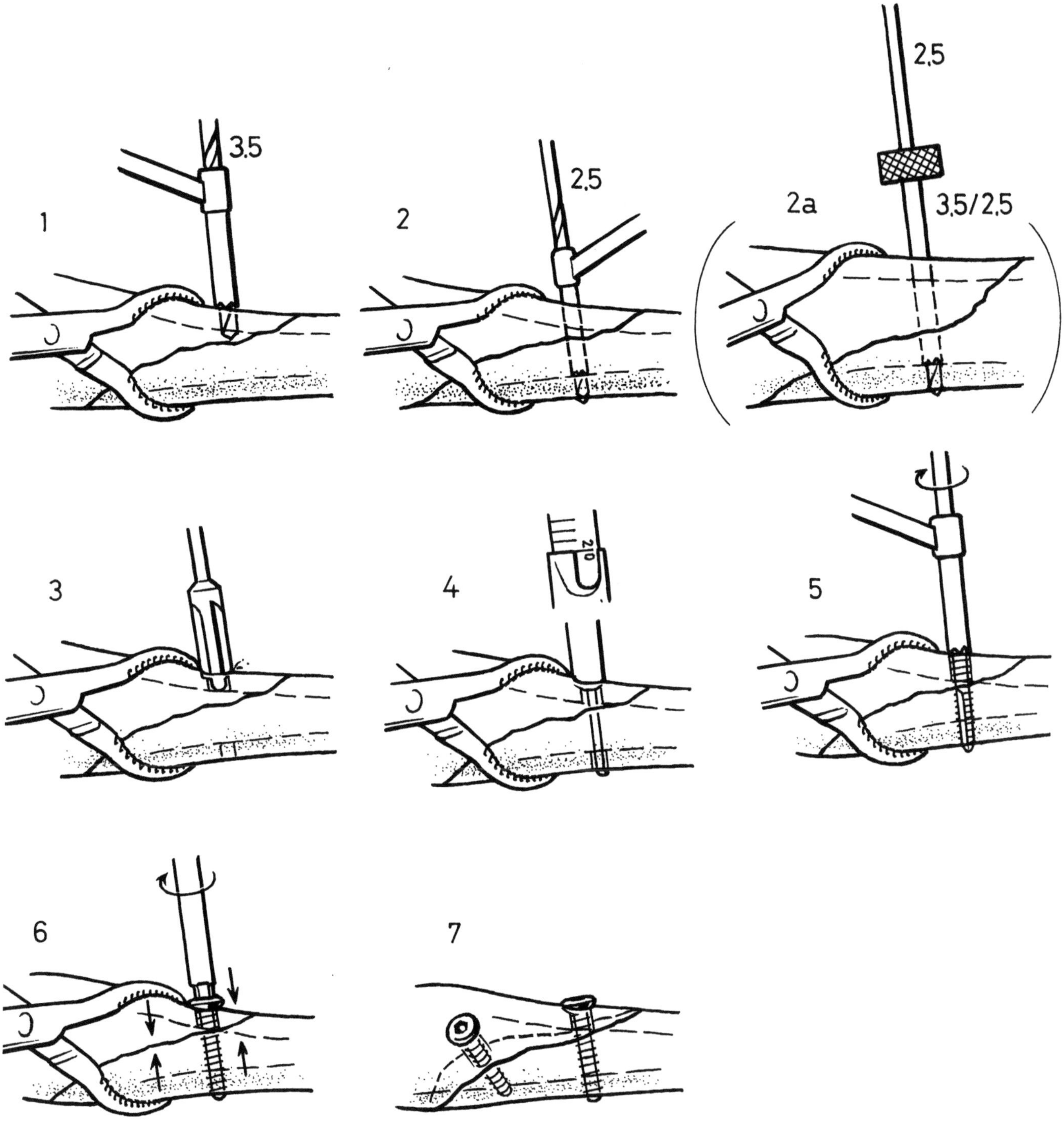

Fig. 23. Fixation with the 3.5-mm cortex screw on bone with a wide or moderately wide medullary cavity

This spiral fracture is reduced and held in place with forceps. The gliding hole is drilled in the near cortex with the 3.5-mm bit (1). The narrow end of the double drill guide is introduced as an insert sleeve (moderately wide medullary cavity), and the 2.5-mm thread hole is made in the far cortex (2). With a wide medullary cavity, the separate insert drill sleeve may be used to guide the 2.5-mm bit (2a). The gliding hole is countersunk for the screw head (3). Screw length is determined with the depth gauge (4). The hole is tapped with the 3.5-mm *cortex* tap using the double drill guide as a tap sleeve (5). The first screw is inserted, and the reduction forceps is replaced by a second screw using the same technique (6, 7)

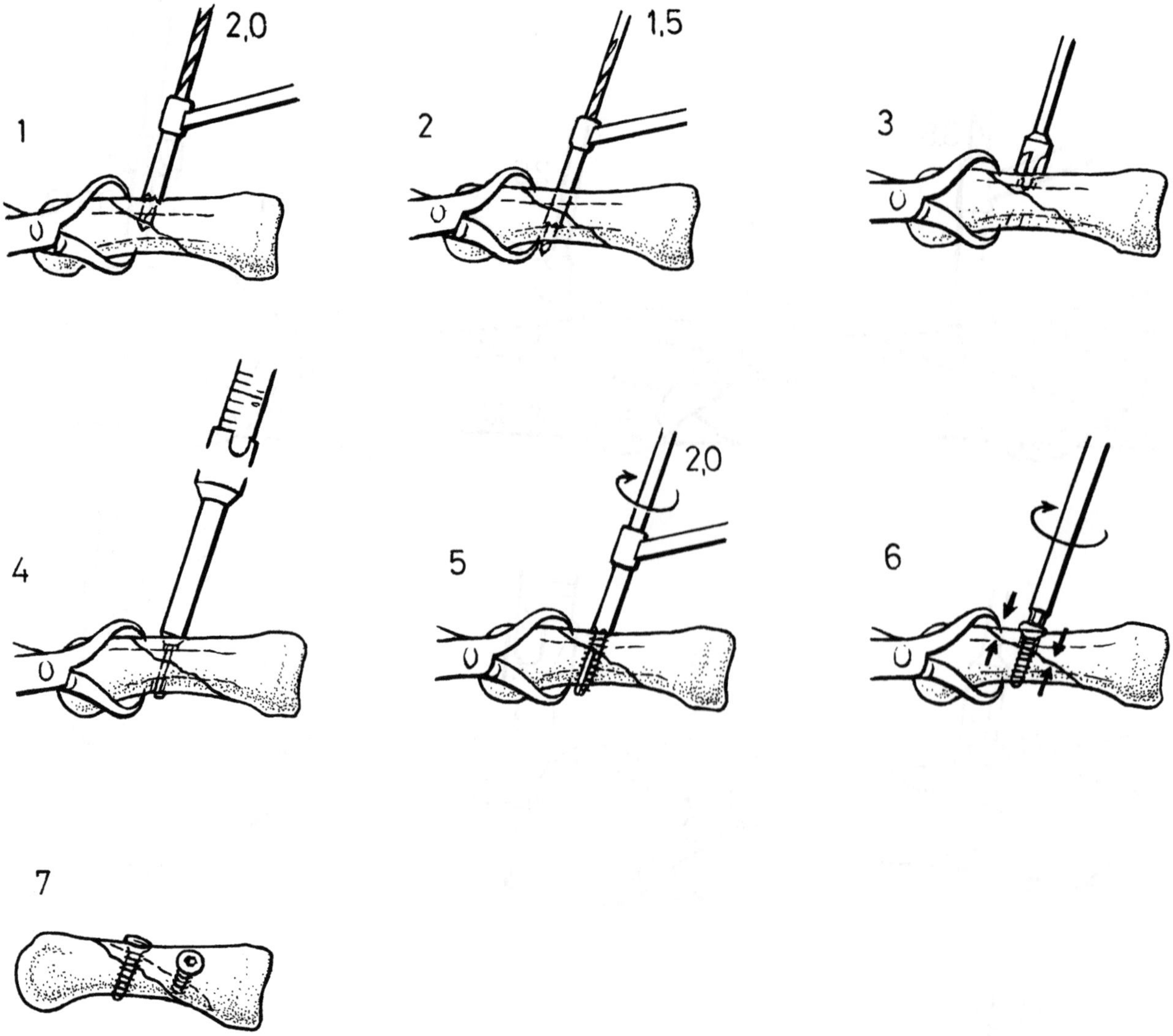

Fig. 24. Fixation with 2.0-mm mini screws

The technique is like that for 3.5-mm cortex screws. The gliding hole is drilled through the 2.0-mm sleeve of the double drill guide (1), and the narrow end of the guide is used as an insert sleeve for drilling the 1.5-mm thread hole (2). The mini countersink is used (3), screw length is determined with the mini depth gauge (4), the thread hole is tapped through the large end of the double drill guide (5), and the screws are inserted (6, 7).
When the 1.5-mm mini screw is used, the gliding hole is 1.5 mm, and the thread hole is 1.1 mm

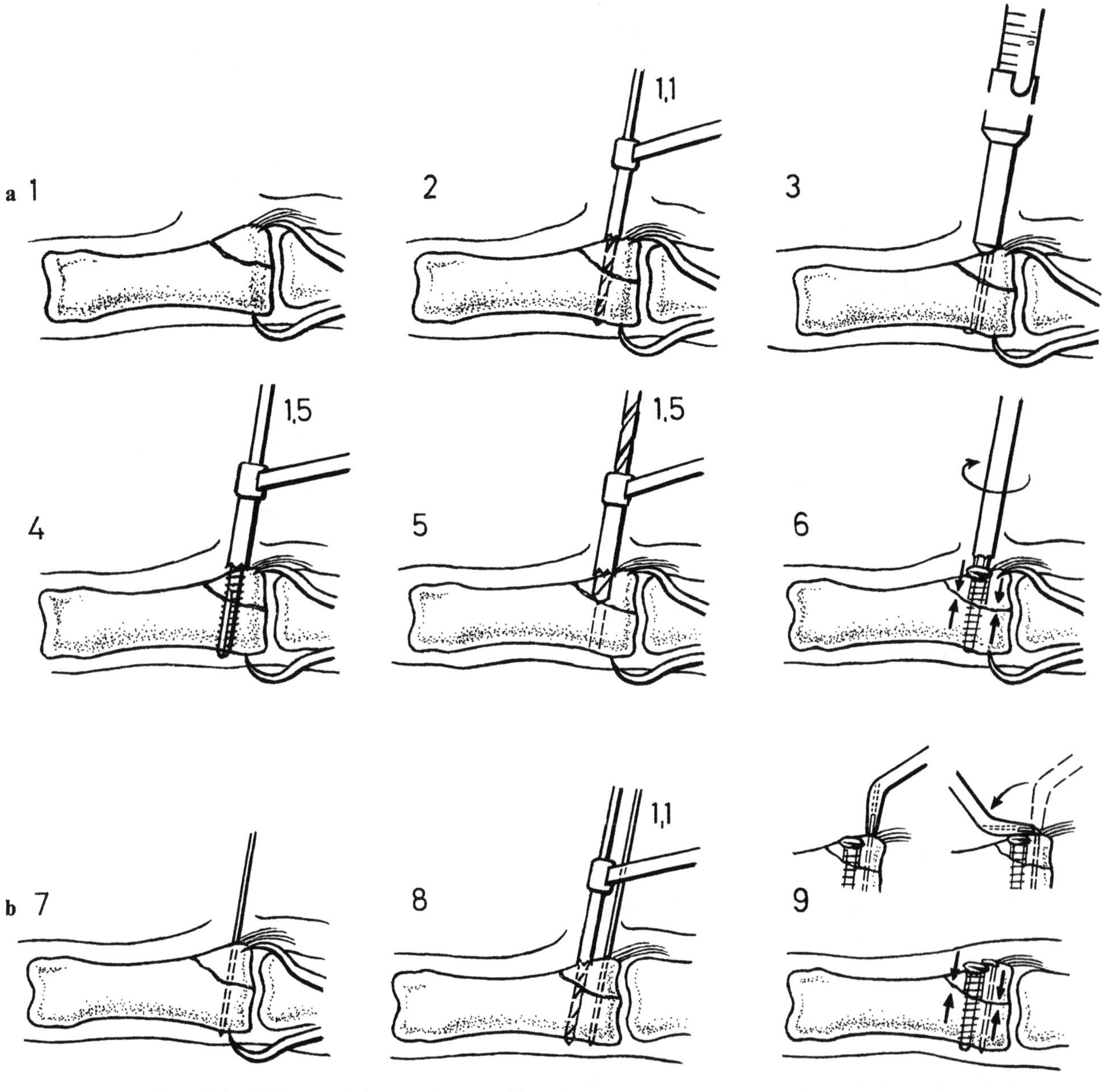

Fig. 25a, b. Use of the 1.5 mm mini screw in cancellous bone

a The fracture is reduced and temporarily fixed through a unilateral incision with the fine reduction forceps, which is applied percutaneously on one side (1). The entire metaphysis is perforated with the 1.1-mm bit through the corresponding drill guide (2). The screw length is determined (3), and the hole is threaded with the 1.5-mm tap through the double drill guide (4). The same sleeve is used to make the gliding hole in the near fragment (5). The screw is inserted (6)

b Alternative technique: After reducing and temporarily fixing the fracture with the fine forceps, the latter is replaced with a thin Kirschner guide wire (7). The appropriate end of the double drill guide handle is threaded over the wire, and a parallel 1.1-mm hole is drilled through the entire metaphysis (8). The rest of the procedure is as described in **a**. The screw is definitively tightened after removal of the Kirschner wire. If desired, the wire may be left in place to check rotation; in this case it is shortened and bent close to the bone with the bending iron (9)

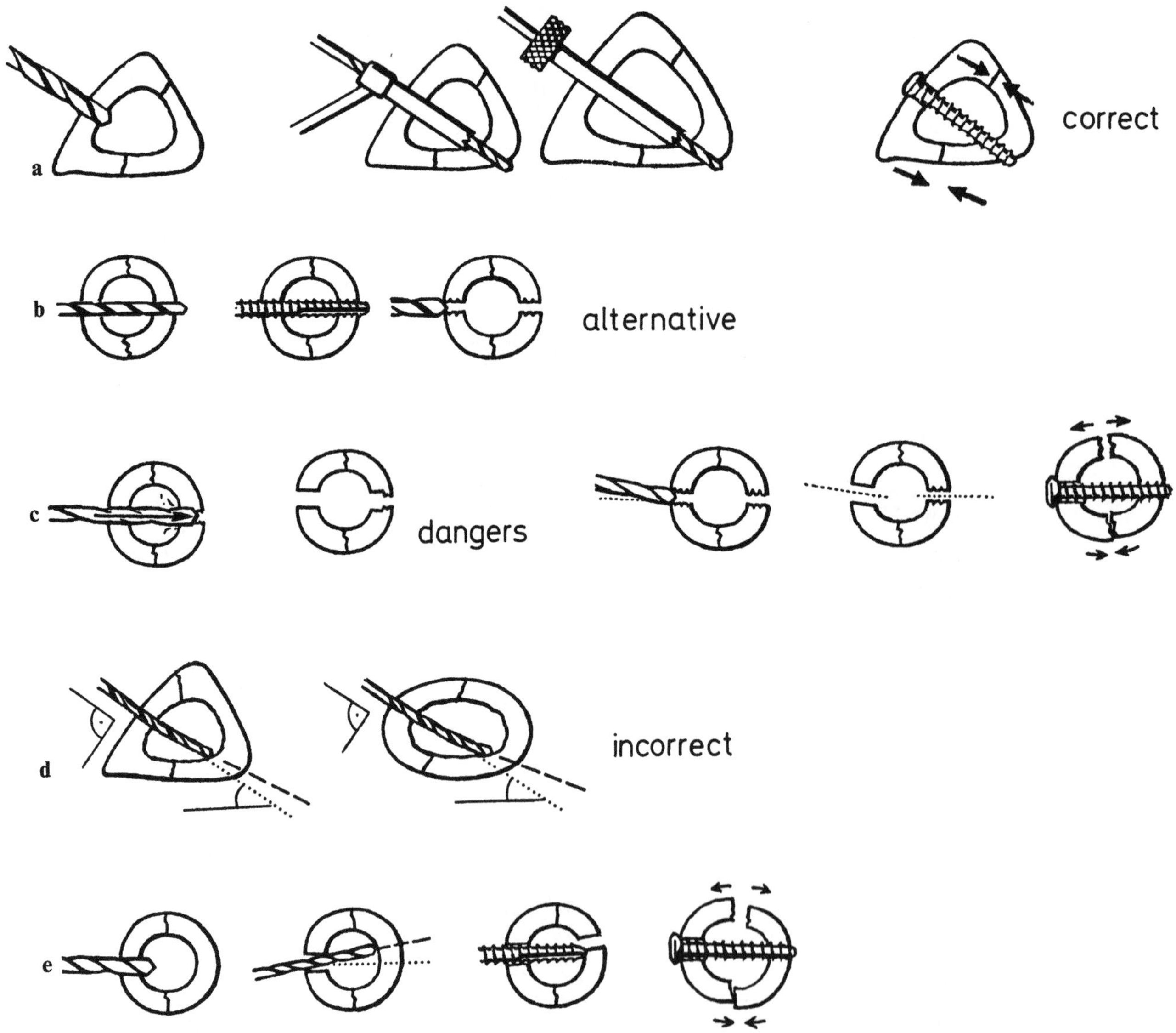

Fig. 26 a–e. Problems of lag screw fixation in cortical bone (cross-sections)

a Correct technique: The gliding hole is drilled first, and the thread hole is drilled through an insert sleeve

b Alternate technique (the "small fragment technique"): The thread hole is made through both cortices, both the cortices are tapped, and the hole in the near cortex is enlarged to form the gliding hole

c Dangers of this technique: Inserting the larger bit too deeply will damage the threads in the far cortex. Drilling the gliding hole at an angle will lead to displacement of the fragments and uneven compression

d, e Two examples of faulty technique: Drilling a small thread hole through both cortices in bone with a wide medullary cavity: The oblique far cortex deflects the bit off the correct axis (**d**). A thread hole drilled without an insert sleeve may not be coaxial with the gliding hole. In both cases it is difficult to locate the thread hole with the tap or screw, and the fragments are liable to displace (**e**)

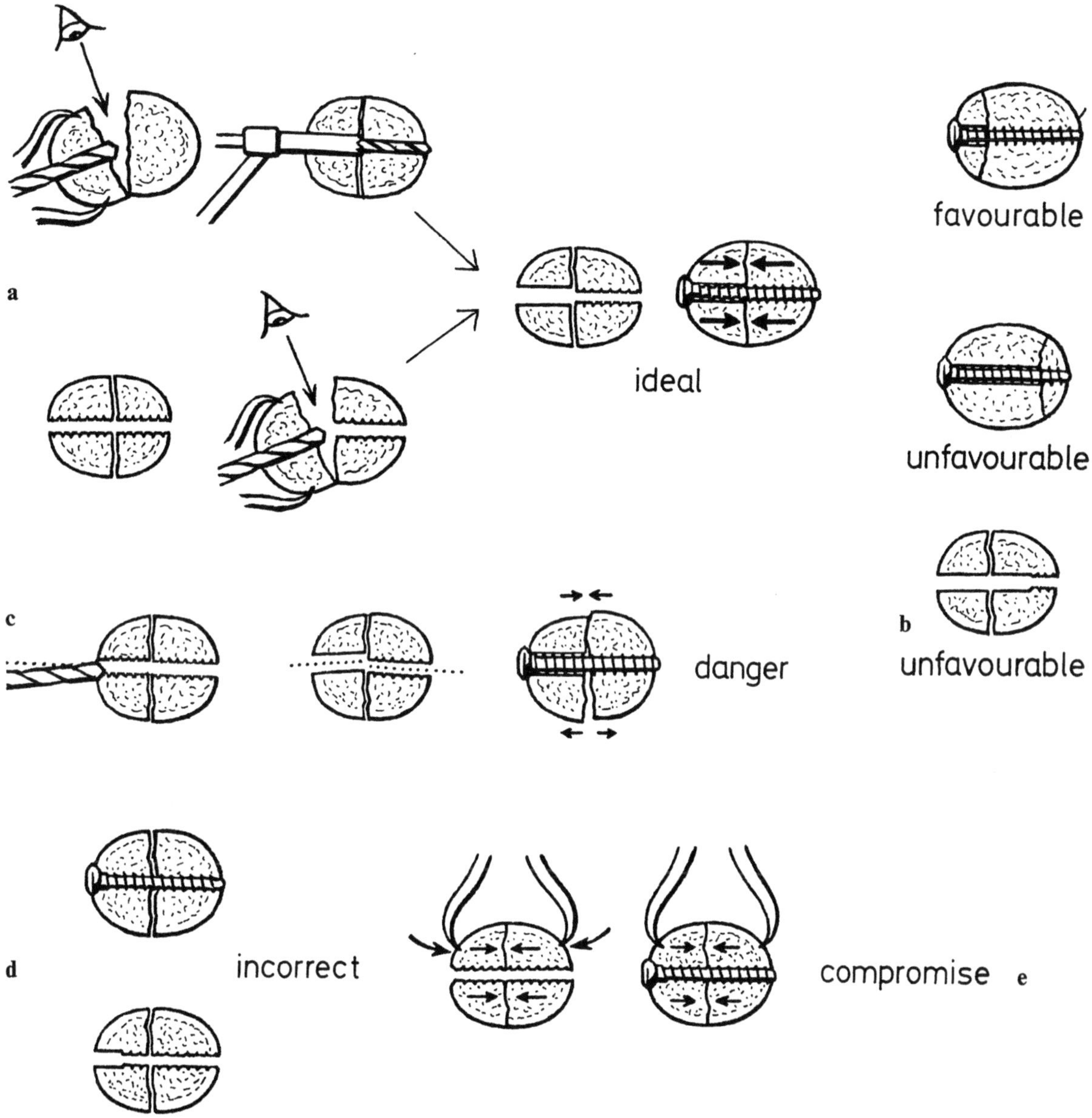

Fig. 27 a–e. Problems of lag screw fixation in cancellous bone for the 2.7- to 1.5-mm screw sizes

The main problem in producing good interfragmental compression is estimating the correct depth of the gliding hole

a Ideal situation: Make the gliding hole with vision of the fracture surface either before performing the reduction, or by reopening the fracture after tapping the full length of the pilot hole.These conditions are rarely met. The screw hold is better with a small near fragment than with a small far fragment, which can accommodate only a short thread

b A gliding hole drilled too deeply damages the thread and weakens interfragmental compression. The screw may strip the hole

c When the gliding hole is made secondarily, there is a danger of axial discrepancy, leading to asymmetric compression and displacement

d No interfragmental compression is produced without a gliding hole or when the gliding hole is drilled too superficially

e A compromise technique in small fractures is to compress the fracture with the reduction forceps before tapping. This yields a reduced interfragmental compression corresponding to the magnitude of the forceps pressure

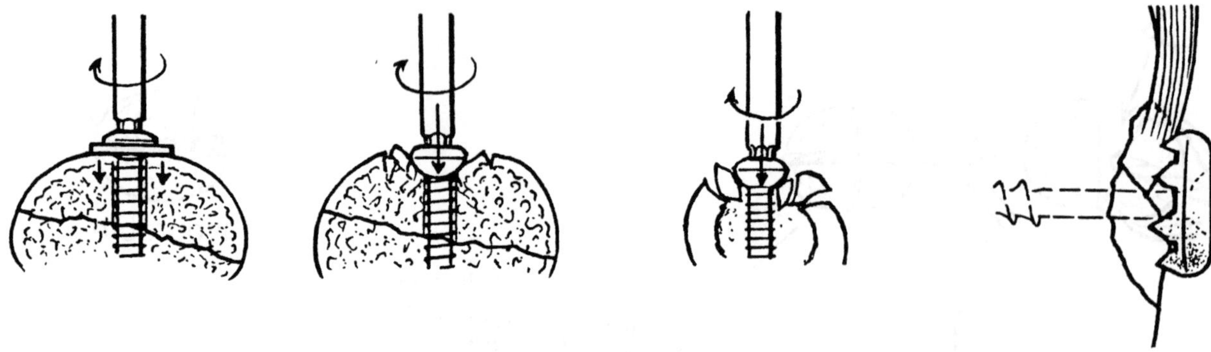

Fig. 28. The function of washers

The washer keeps the screw head from sinking into cancellous bone or cracking thin cortex. The spiked plastic washer can grip and apply pressure to small comminuted areas and ligament attachments

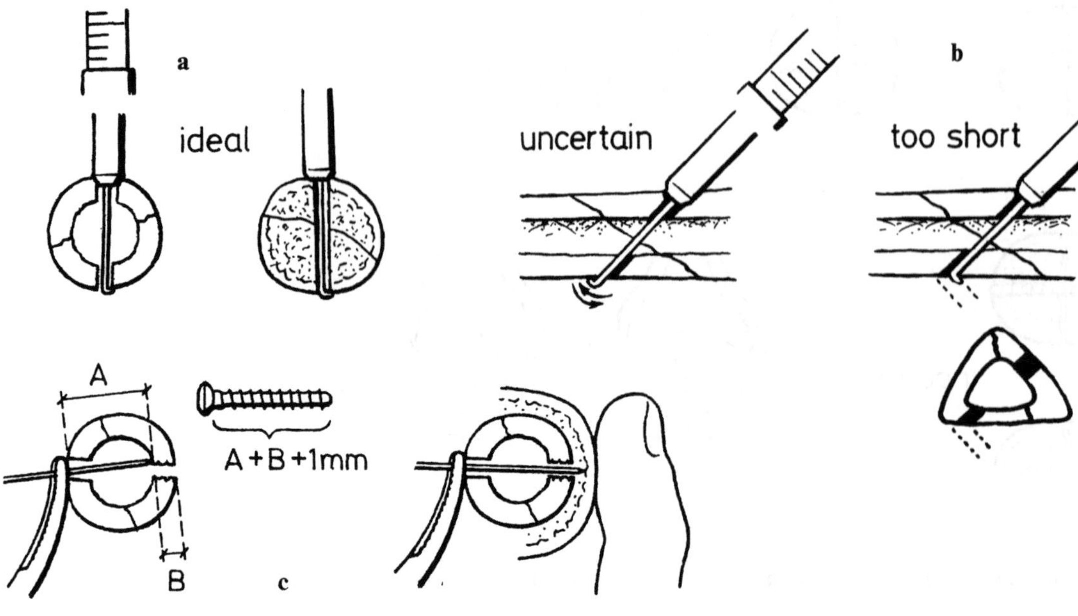

Fig. 29a–c. Problems of screw length measurement

a Correct measurement of screw length: The depth gauge is used in cortical bone after countersinking and *before* tapping. In cancellous bone the depth gauge is inserted without use of the countersink

b Problems with an oblique hole: The small hook of the depth gauge will tend to slip off the obtuse-angled lip of the thread hole, even though this is the correct site for making an accurate measurement. The acute-angled lip of the thread hole is more easily engaged with the hook, but it does not provide an accurate measurement

c One way to measure the depth of a very narrow screw hole is with a Kirschner wire gripped in a hemostat. The tip of the wire abuts against the far cortex. To that distance is added the thickness of the far cortex, plus 1 mm (safety margin). The distance can be measured directly if the wire tip is palpable through the tissues on the opposite side of the bone

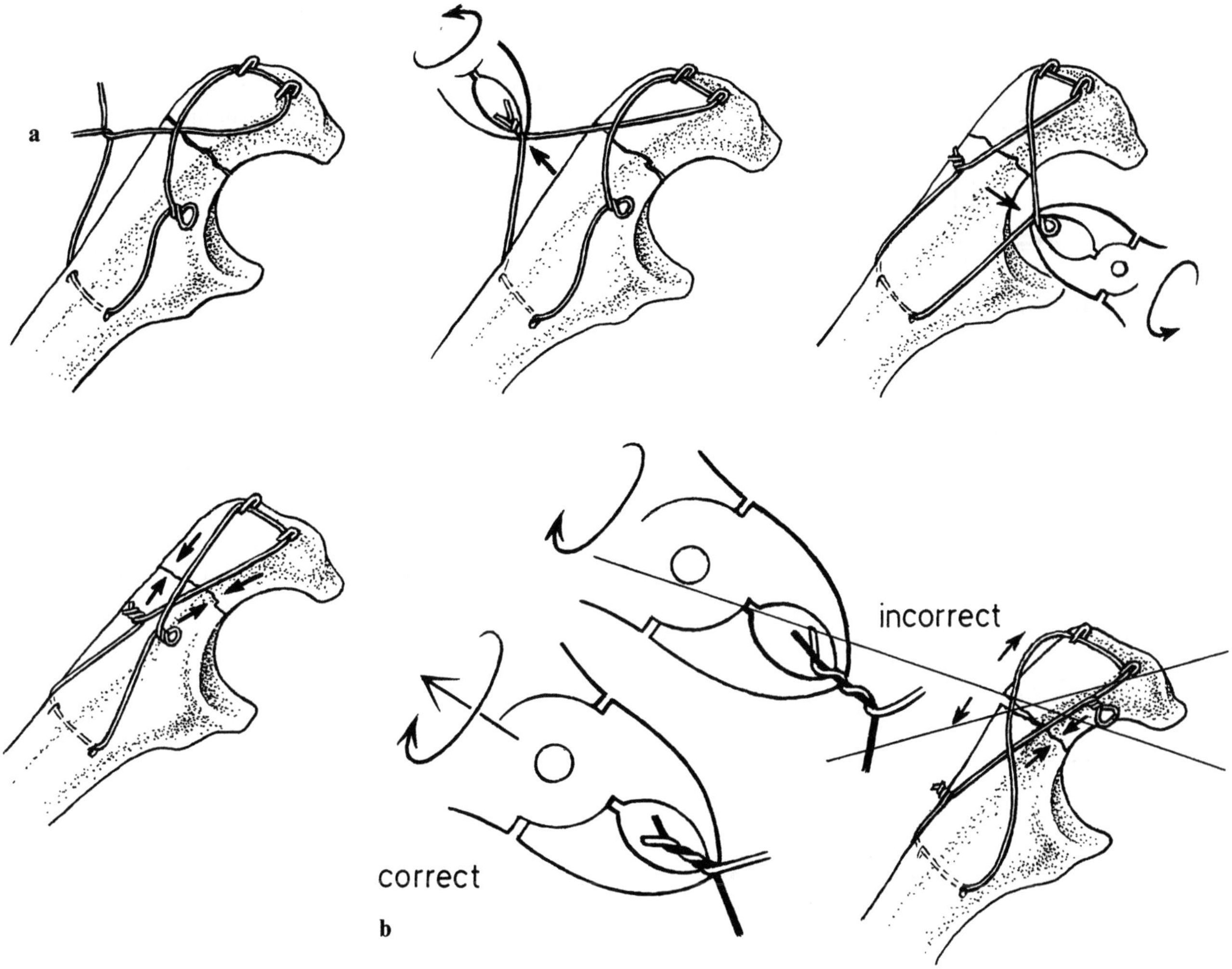

Fig. 30 a, b. Technique for tightening tension-band wires (shown here for the olecranon)

Reduction has been accomplished, axial parallel Kirschner wires have been inserted, and a transverse hole has been drilled through the cortex of the distal fragment. A long wire with a prepared loop has been applied and its free ends provisionally twisted by hand

a The lower limb of the wire is pulled up from the bone with the wire twisting pliers and is twisted as vertical tension is released. The tension has kinked the wire loop at the drill hole and Kirschner wires. The same is done on the opposite side. The maneuver is repeated until both limbs of the wire are tight against the bone, and corresponding interfragmental compression is produced

b Detail of technique: The wire is twisted systematically by grasping the twist at its base and pulling upward before rotating the pliers.Failure to do this can lead to irregular twisting or breaking of the wire. Both limbs must be tightened to obtain symmetrical pressure; two twists in the same limb are of no value

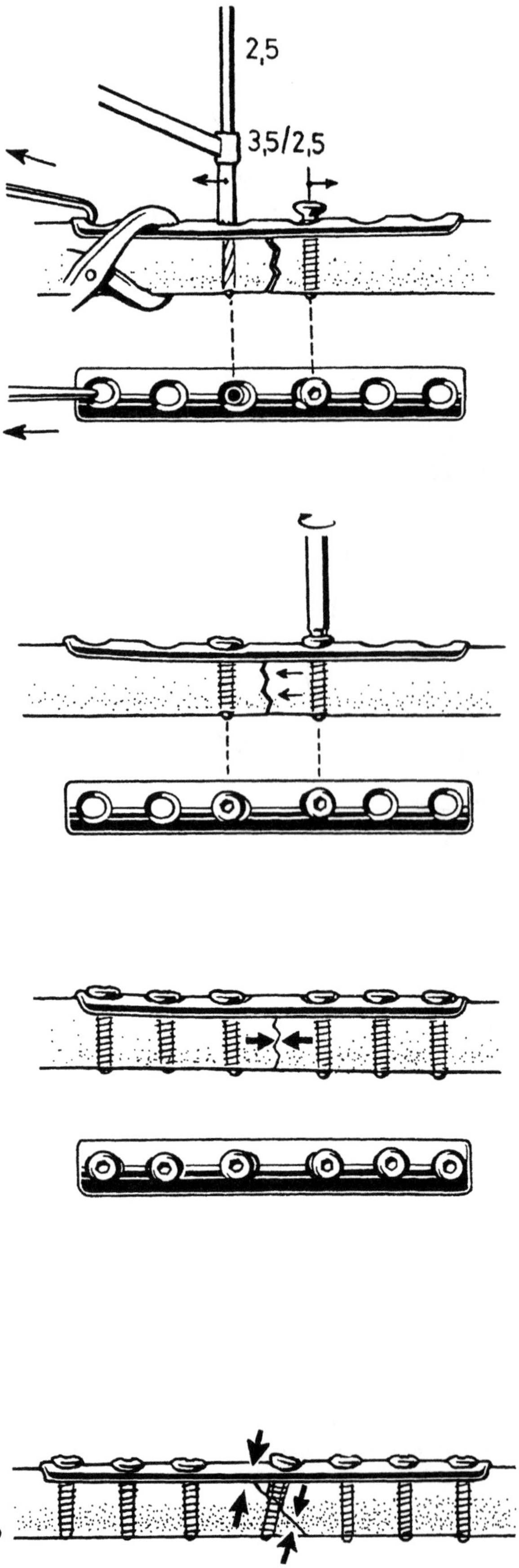

a

b

Fig. 31 a, b. Axial compression with the one-third tubular plate

For fixation of the 3.5-mm plate size, both cortices are perforated with the 2.5-mm drill bit and threaded with the 3.5-mm *cortex* tap

a The plate is loosely fixed to one fragment with a screw placed close to the fracture. The plate is then pulled toward the other fragment with a hook. An eccentric hole (away from the fracture line) is drilled in the other fragment, and a second screw is inserted. Tightening the screws exerts tensile stress on the plate and presses the fragments together. The remaining screws are inserted after axial compression has been obtained. This technique corresponds to the DCP principle, although the thinness of the plate lessens the compressive effect somewhat

b In an oblique fracture, the additional placement of an interfragmental lag screw through the plate greatly increases the stability of the fixation

Fig. 32a–d. Axial compression with the 3.5-mm dynamic compression plate

a The fracture is reduced and the plate held in place with a forceps. The first, 2.5-mm hole is drilled through an adjacent plate hole using the green (neutral) end of the DCP drill guide. The hole is tapped with the 3.5-mm *cortex* tap, and the first screw is inserted

An eccentric drill hole is made in the opposite fragment using the yellow end of the DCP drill guide, making sure the arrow points to the fracture. Correct placement of the bit can be checked by looking at the lower part of the drill guide. The hole is tapped and the screw inserted. Tightening the screw moves it 1 mm toward the fracture and compresses the fragments

b Twice as much compressive displacement can be obtained by inserting a second screw by the same technique.The screw adjacent to the fracture should be loosened before tightening the second screw to reduce friction between the plate and bone

c Stability in an oblique fracture is markedly increased by inserting an interfragmental lag screw through the plate. This is preceded by compression of the plate with only one eccentric screw

d Ranges of angulation of plate screws on the longitudinal and transverse planes: Screws can be angled through 30° on the plate axis, and through 15° transversely. This may be done, for example, to avoid collision with a separate lag screw placed on a different plane

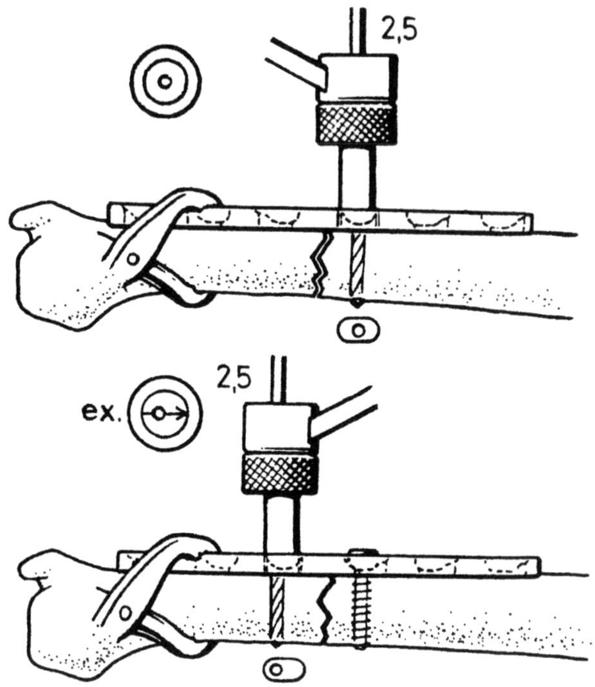

a

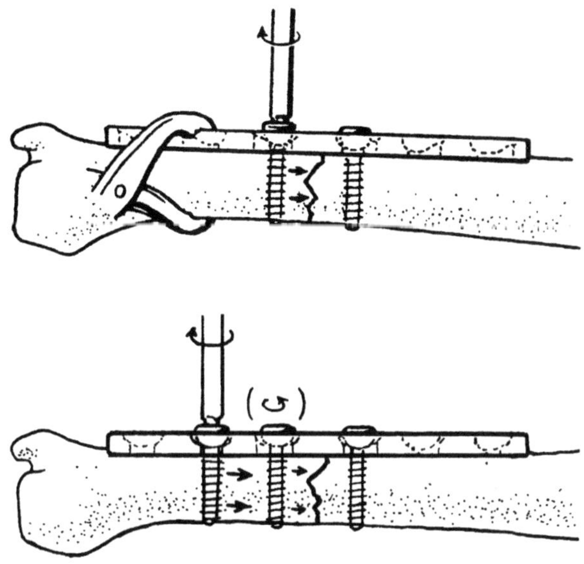

b

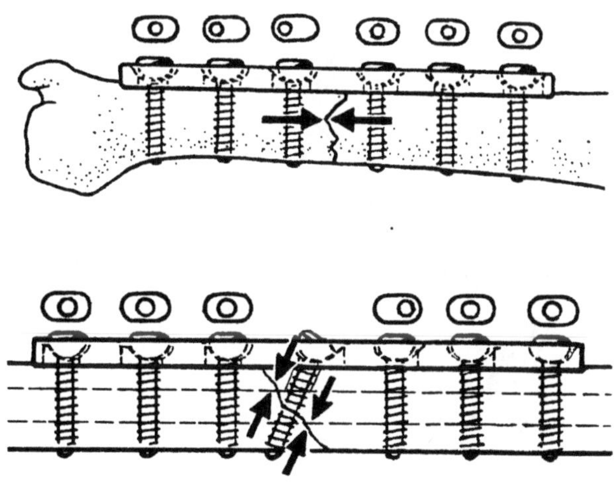

c

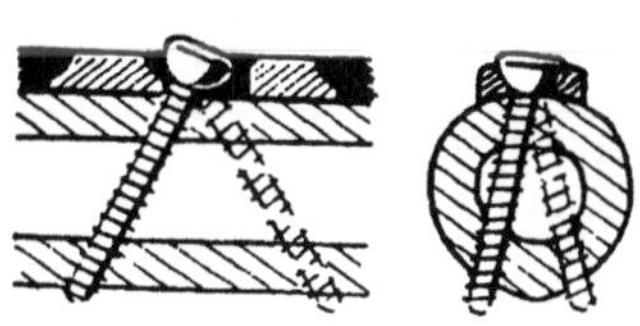

d

Fig. 33a–e. Functions of the tension device and small compression forceps

The tension device can perform functions in addition to classic interfragmental compression (Fig. 18b)

a The tension device is a useful reduction aid in cases where there is marked separation of the bone ends

b The tension device permits better fine reduction of interdigitating fragments as well as fine rotational adjustments. The reduction forceps is loosened during this maneuver

c The articulated tension device can be tilted aside during compression to facilitate maneuvers such as the insertion of an oblique lag screw

d The hook of the tension device can be reversed to apply distraction, as in a lengthening osteotomy

e The small compression forceps for plates of the 2.7/1.5-mm system. Compression is applied by fitting the angled tips of the forceps into a cortical drill hole and into an adjacent plate hole

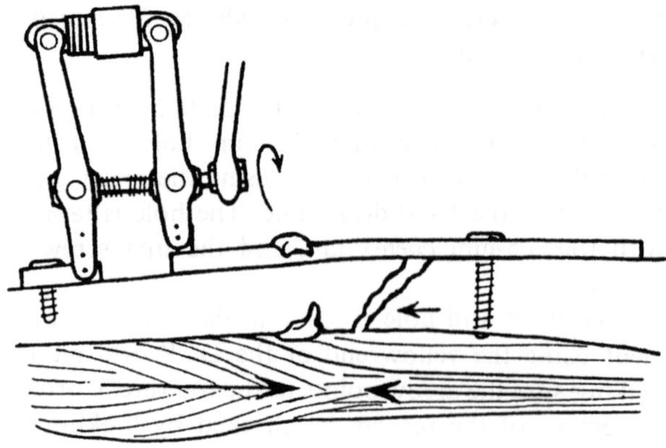

a

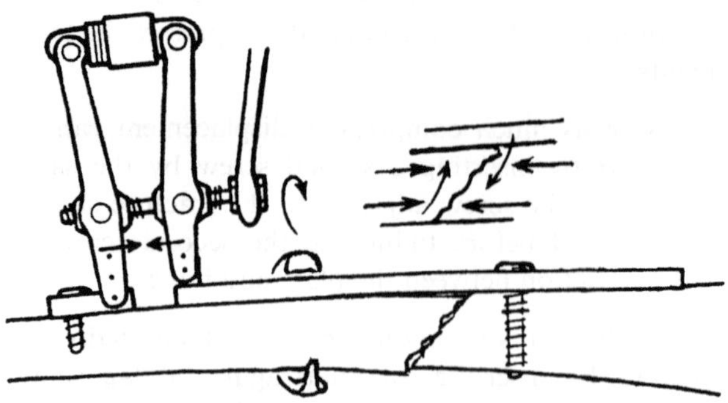

b

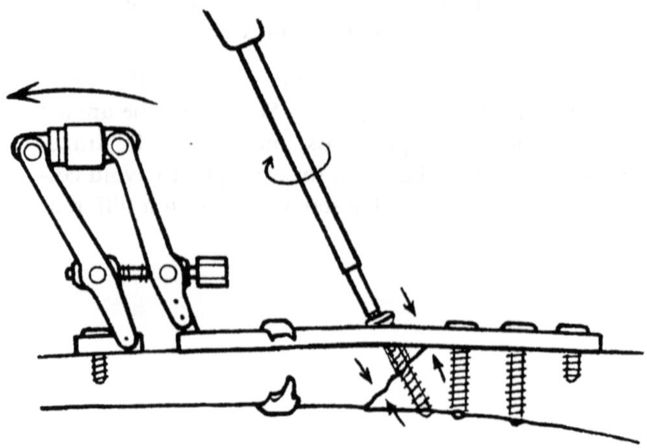

c

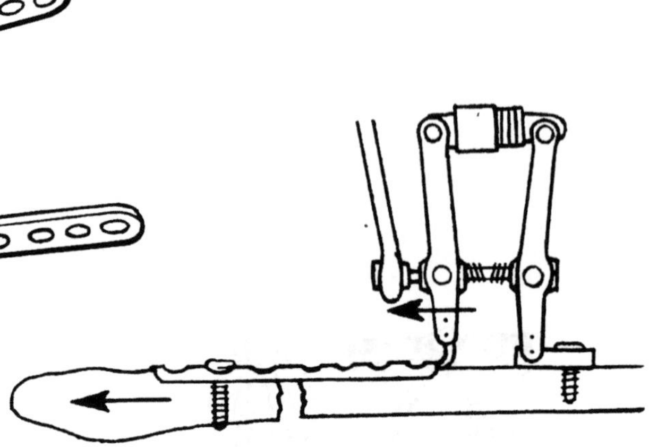

d

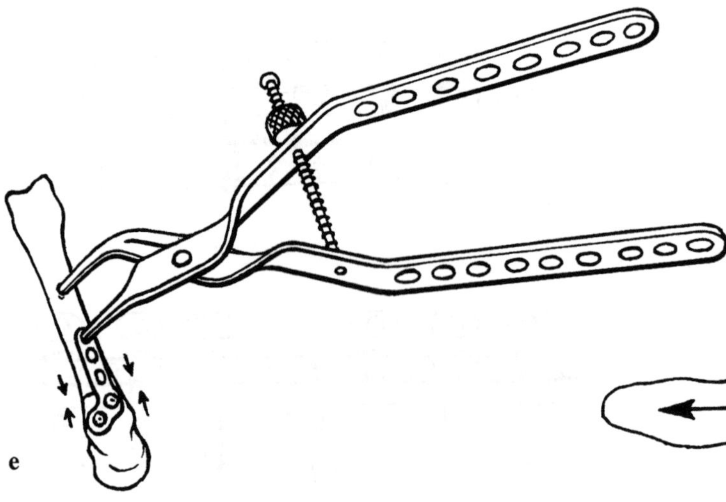

e

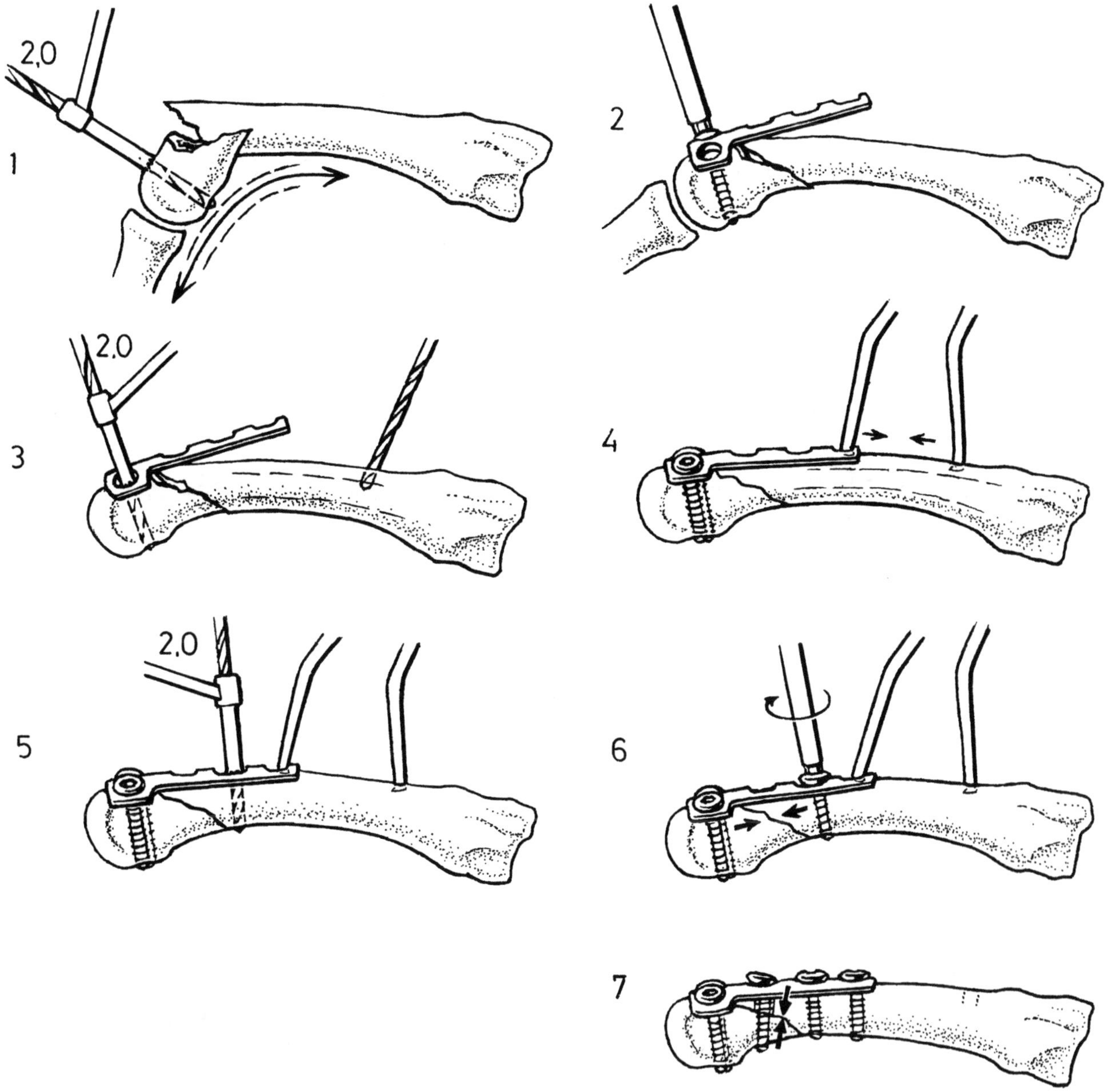

Fig. 34. The small T plate as a tension band and reduction aid

Oblique metaphyseal fracture with volar angulation. After axial alignment is checked, the plate is attached to the peripheral fragment with one screw (1, 2). The plate is used as a lever to tentatively reduce the fracture. For fine reduction, a hole is drilled in the proximal cortex (3), the tips of the mini compression forceps are inserted into the drill hole and adjacent plate hole, and pressure is applied (4). Axis and rotation are rechecked after insertion of the second screw in the plate head and before inserting a third screw in the proximal fragment (5). Axial compression is initiated by tightening the proximal screw (6) and is increased by inserting an interfragmental lag screw through the plate (7)

a

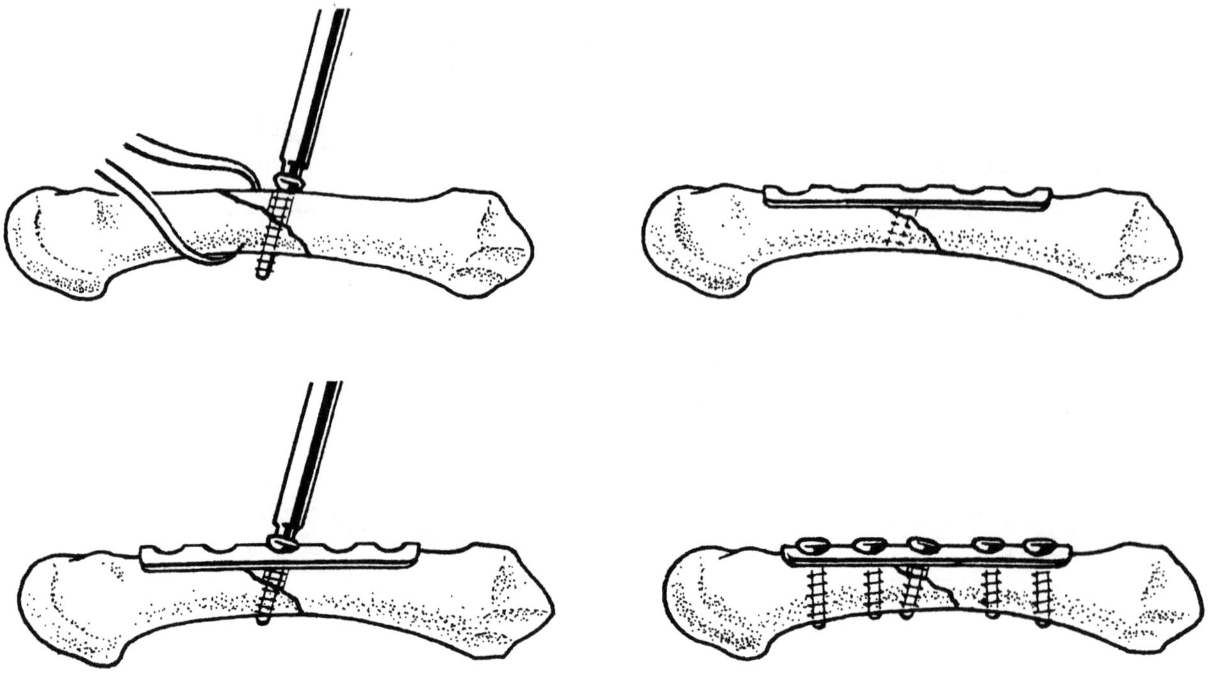

b

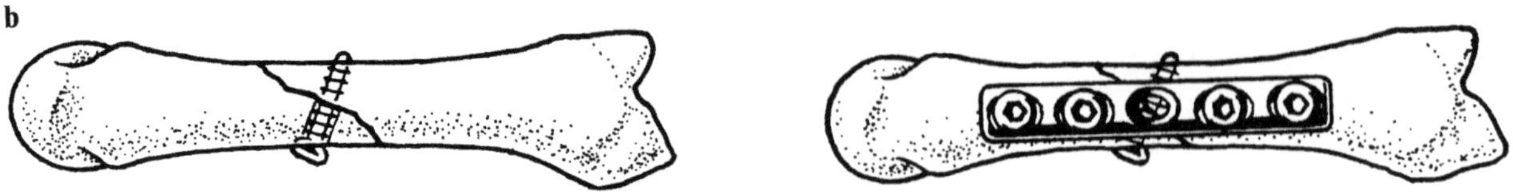

Fig. 35a, b. Combination of a lag screw and neutralization plate on a small bone

In an oblique fracture, a plate attached on the incision plane can hide the fracture line, and displacement is apt to occur when the plate screws are inserted. There are two ways of avoiding this:

a If the fragment tip is on the plane of the plate, the fracture is tentatively fixed with a lag screw that is slightly too long. The reduction is checked, and the plate is contoured to the bone. Then the screw is removed and reintroduced through the center of the plate. The remaining plate screws are inserted

b If the fragment tips are not on the plane of the plate, reduction and interfragmental compression are achieved with a preliminary lag screw. The neutralization plate is then applied separately on the incision plane

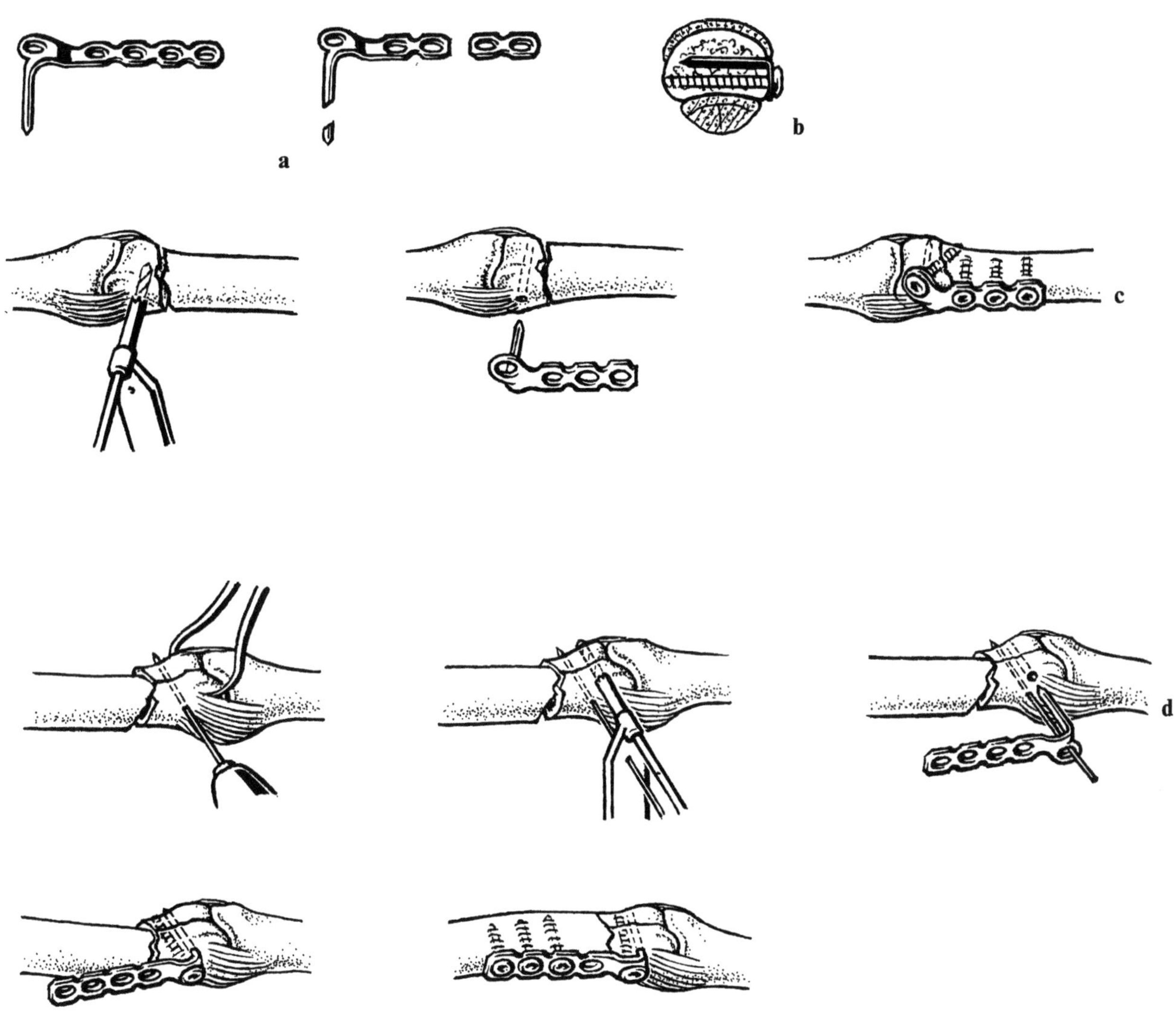

Fig. 36a–d. Technique for applying the mini condylar plate (2.0- and 1.5-mm sizes)

a The length of the intraosseous pin and the diaphyseal part of the plate must be adapted to local anatomy.They may have to be shortened with the plate cutting forceps

b Topography of the plate (cross-section through the metaphysis): Applying the plate laterally avoids interference with the extensor apparatus and flexor tendon

c Transverse metaphyseal fracture: A transverse hole for the pin is predrilled in the distal fragment parallel to the joint line, sparing the collateral ligament.The pin is tentatively inserted to check and if necessary correct the pin angle, and the plate is contoured with bending pliers. The pin is inserted. The reduction is checked for axial and rotational alignment and secured with a small forceps. Then the distal plate screw is inserted and tightened; this screw may be lagged across the fracture if desired.Finally the diaphyseal screws are inserted to produce interfragmental compression

d The bicondylar fracture is reduced under vision and tentatively fixed with a Kirschner wire, which serves as a guide for pin insertion.The guide hole at the end of the drill guide is threaded over the Kirschner wire, and the pin channel is drilled at right angles to the shaft with a 2.0- or 1.5-mm bit. The rest of the procedure is as described in **a**

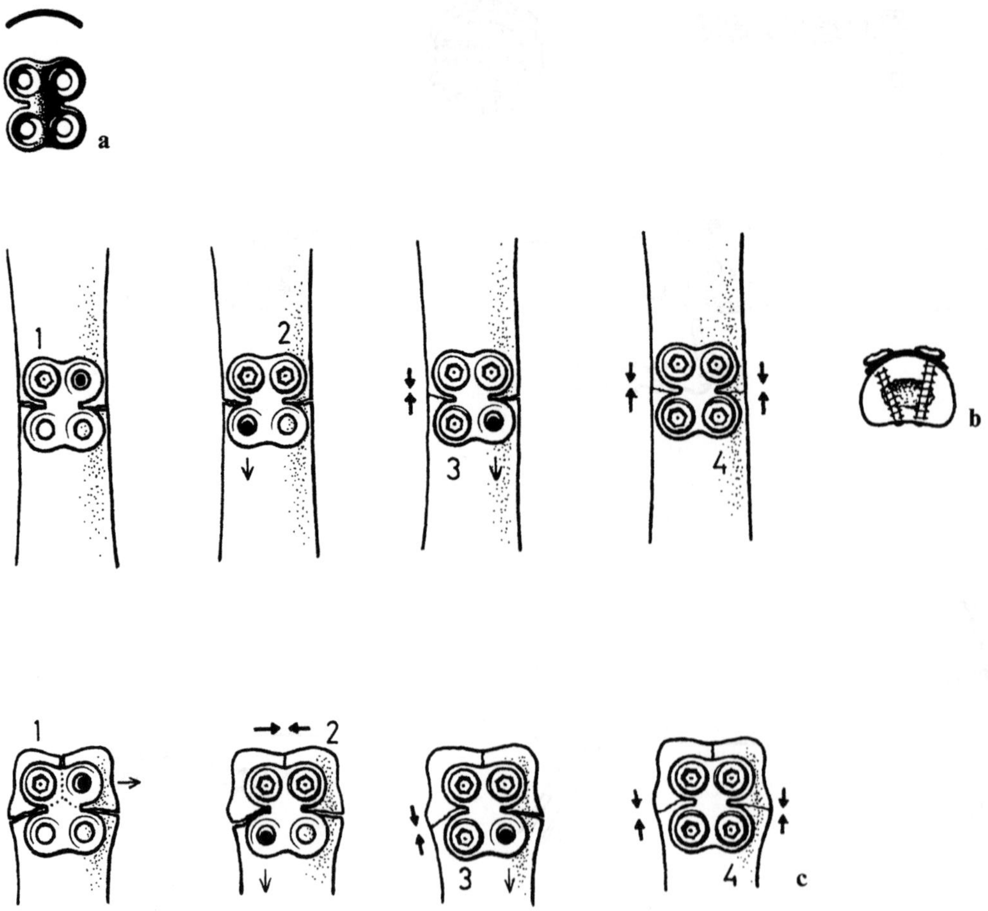

Fig. 37 a–c. Technique for applying the mini H plate (2.0- and 1.5-mm sizes)

a Top view and cross-section

b Technique (sequence of screw insertion) for a transverse fracture: Screws 1 and 2 are inserted in one fragment. Eccentric holes for screws 3 and 4 are alternately drilled to provide symmetric interfragmental compression. Caution: When drilling the holes, make sure the tips of the screws do not touch owing to the convexity of the bone

c Technique for a Y fracture: Screw 1 is inserted in one fragment through a centered drill hole, and screw 2 is placed eccentrically to compress the condylar fragments. Then eccentric holes are alternately drilled for screws 3 and 4 to provide symmetric, axial interfragmental compression between the condyle assembly and the proximal part of the fracture

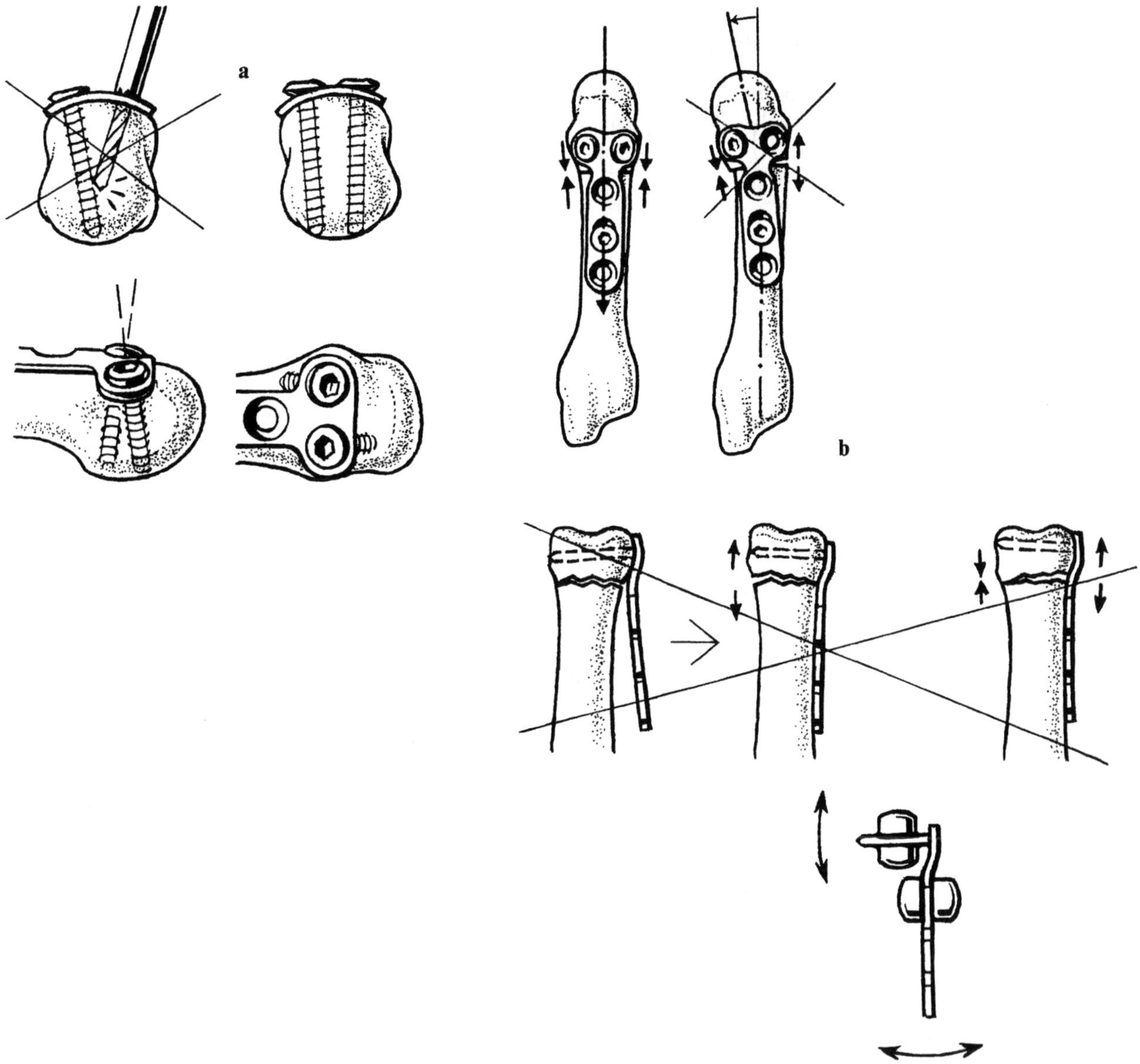

Fig. 38 a–d. Dangers and problems of internal fixation with small shaped plates

a Screw collision at the head of the plate–first noticed during insertion of the tap–is avoided:
- by parallel placement of the screws. In this case the screw heads will not be completely flush with the plate holes
- by drilling the holes obliquely but on different planes. Directional orientation is provided by the screwdriver or by the lighter screwdriver attachment

b Axial malalignment:
- In the T plate this occurs when only one screw is placed initially through the head of the plate. The asymmetric compression causes the fracture to gape on the side opposite the screw. The correct technique is to insert both screws through the plate head before compressing the fracture
- In the mini condylar plate this occurs when the pin is not inserted parallel to the joint line. Avoid this by partially inserting the pin, estimating the correct angle, and then contouring the plate with bending pliers before definitive insertion of the pin

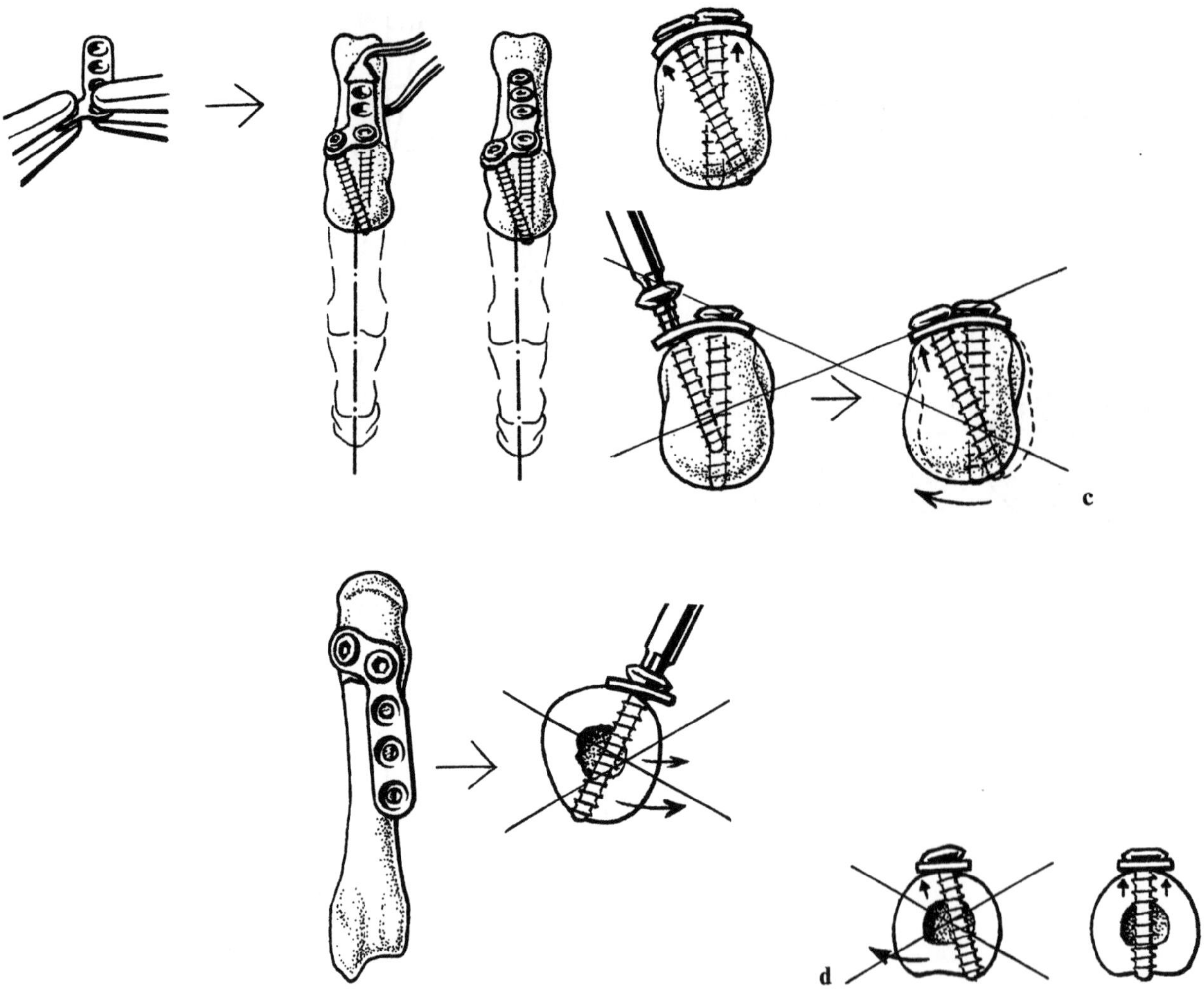

Fig. 38 cont.

c Rotational malalignment at the head of the plate:

- This occurs when the head of the L plate is not perfectly contoured to the bone. Insertion of the lateral screw pulls the bone in that direction and rotates the fragment. The remedy is to contour the head of the plate accurately with bending pliers before inserting the screws

d Rotational malalignment at the shaft of the plate:

- This is *always* a danger when a plate is placed eccentrically. Tightening the screw rotates the fragment toward the side on which the plate stands away from the bone. Avoid this by confirming plate-bone alignment *before* drilling the hole for the second screw in the plate head. Existing malrotation is corrected by loosening or removing the plate and twisting it. The screws are then replaced in the existing holes
- It can result from angled screw insertion in plates with a flat shaft (especially oblique radial T plates and mini plates). The unilateral pressure from the screw head tends to pull the bone toward that side. Avoid this by drilling the screw hole perpendicularly. Existing malrotation is corrected by loosening or removing the plate and twisting it

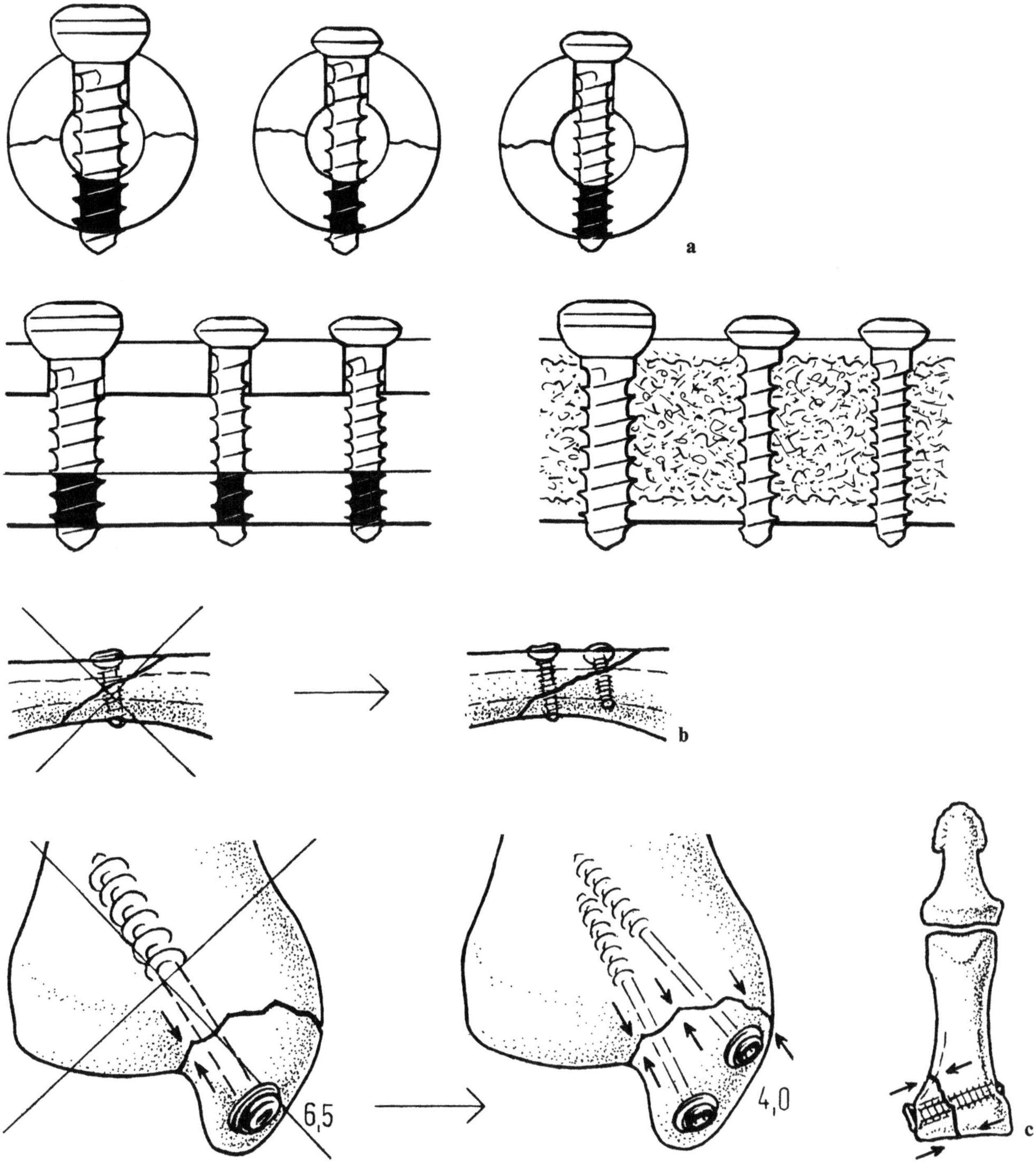

Fig. 39 a–c. Stabilization rule 1: Screw fixation

a Comparison of the bony contact areas of different screws:
- Reduction of the pitch from 1.75 mm to 1.25 mm in the new 3.5-mm cortical screw increases the number of active threads from 2 to $3^1/_2$
- This effect is not as significant in cancellous bone

b Uniform compression of oblique fracture surfaces by two small screws vs. a single, larger screw

c A single screw is acceptable *only* for an interdigitating fracture or avulsion

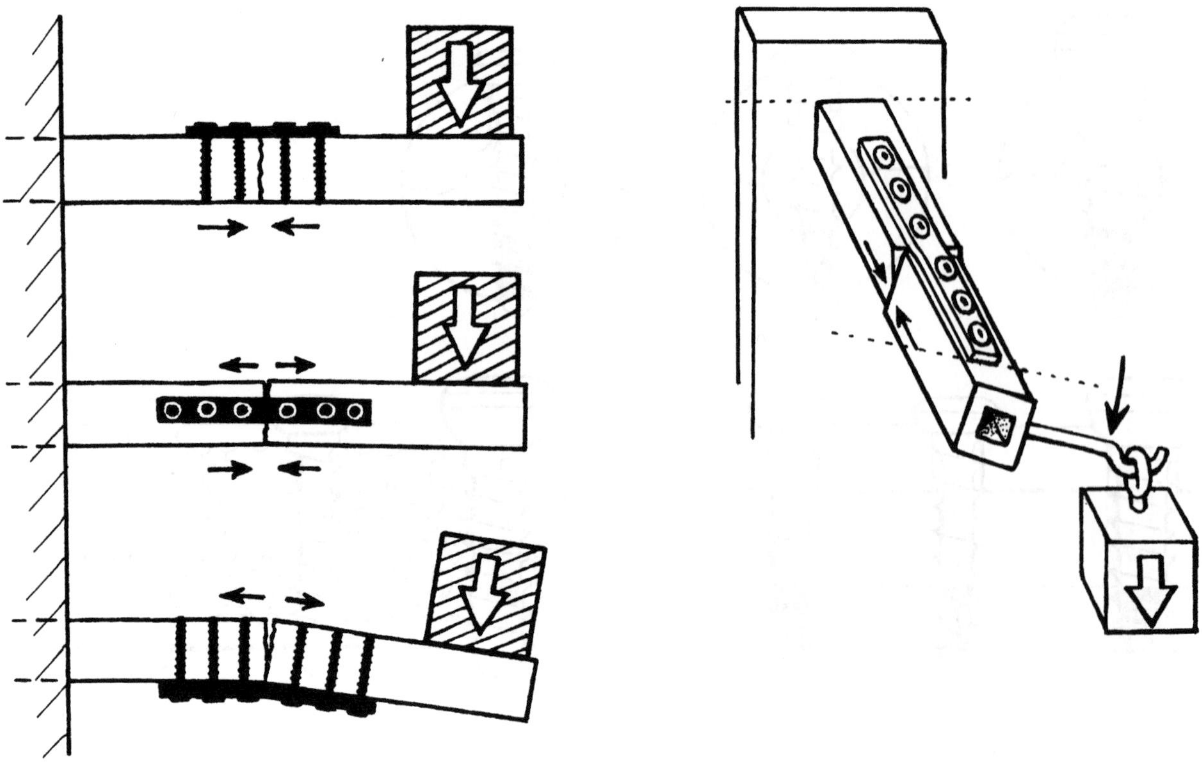

a

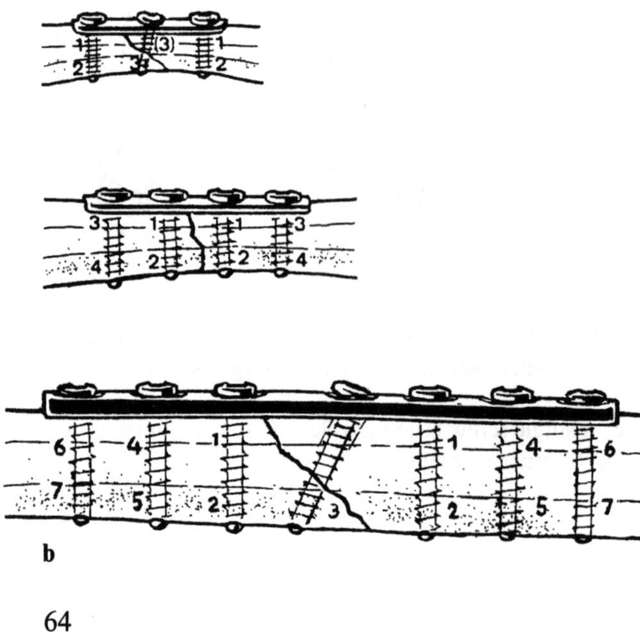

b

Fig. 40 a, b. Stabilization rule 2: Plate stability

a Relationship of plate size and plate length to the force imposed:A short plate is sufficient on the tension side of the bone (tension-band effect). A plate applied laterally is loaded in tension and compression and needs to be longer. On the pressure side of the bone, even an oversized plate is unable to provide sufficient strength. The plate length also affects rotational stability. The plate itself must have adequate torsional strength to withstand rotational forces

b The number of threaded cortices recommended for plate fixation increases in the distal-to-proximal direction

Fig. 41 a, b. Stabilization rule 3: Vassal rule

a Mechanical dependence between multiple fractures: In the example, the dominant fracture of the 5th metatarsal is fixed with a lag screw and neutralization plate. When this is done, the subordinate (vassal) fracture of the 4th metatarsal reduces spontaneously. It may be left alone, or it may be secured with an axial Kirschner wire or single screw

b A vassal fracture in a larger bone is illustrated by a fibular fracture accompanying a spiral fracture of the tibia. The fibular fracture reduces spontaneously when the tibia is fixed and does not require treatment

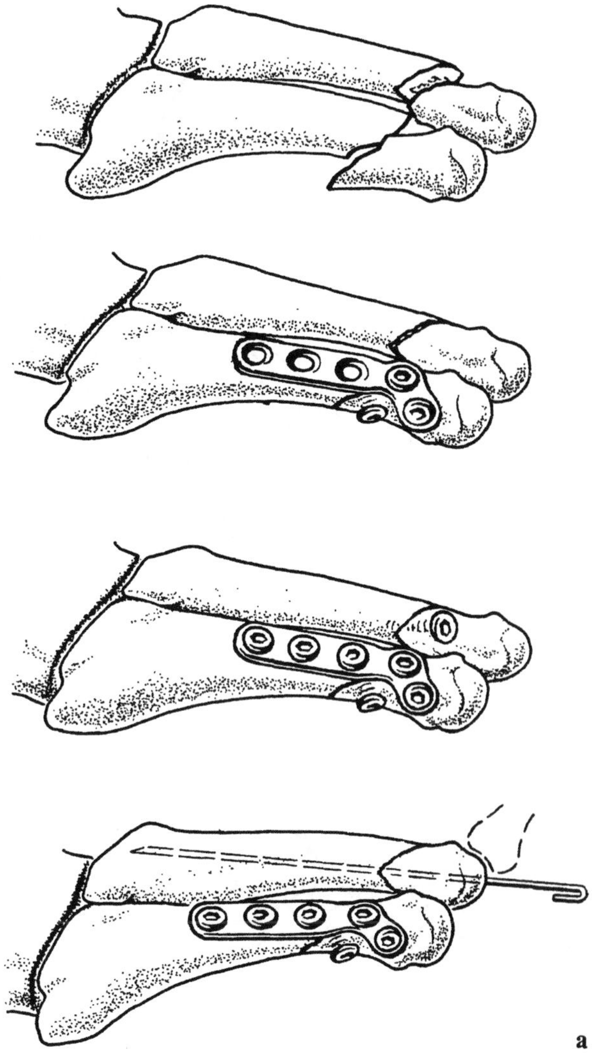

a

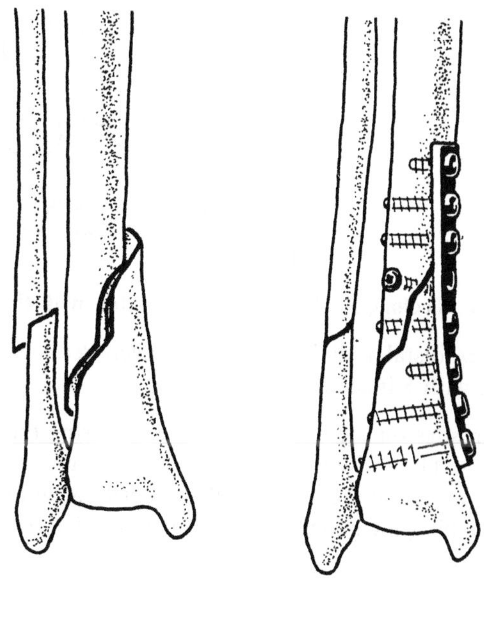

b

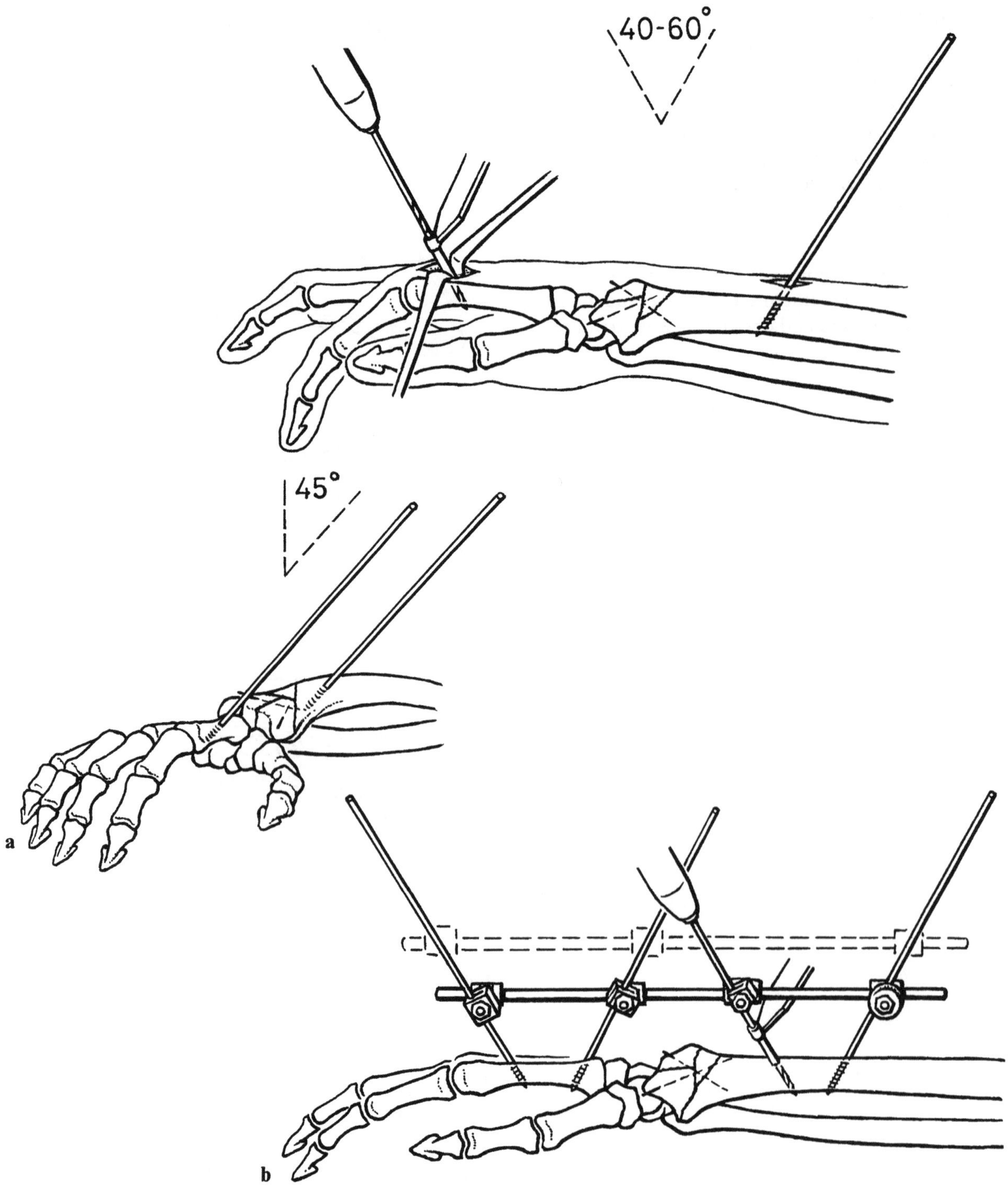

Fig. 42a, b. Technique of wrist immobilization with the small external fixator applied as a half-frame

A complex distal radial fracture has been reduced and fixed with Kirschner wires

a The pin sites on the bone are exposed, sparing the soft tissues. The end wires (2.5 mm, with thread) are drilled in at the appropriate angle. Predrilling with a 2.0-mm bit (not shown) is recommended. Lateral and anterior view

b A 4.0-mm connecting rod carrying four 4.0/2.5-mm clamps is mounted over the end wires and hand tightened. The central pin sites are exposed, and two more Kirschner wires are inserted through the central clamps, which serve as guides. The assembly is reinforced by mounting a second connecting rod on the wires

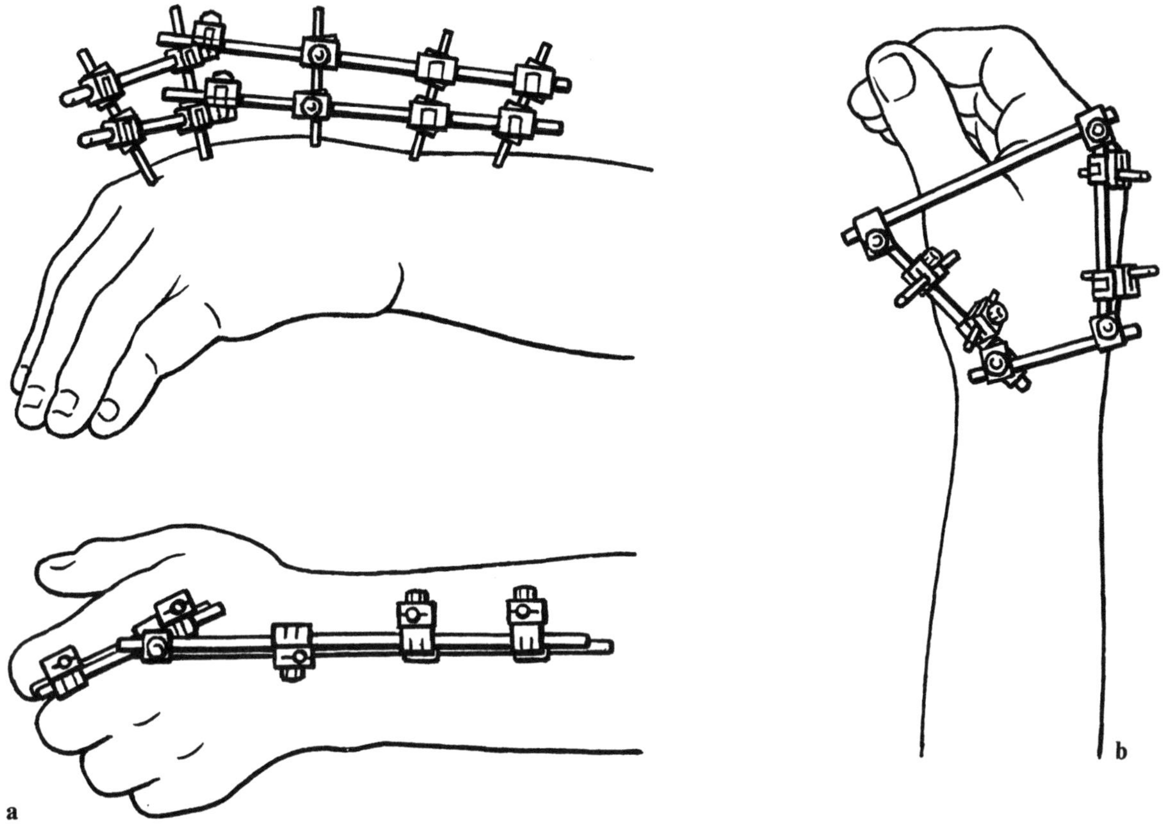

a

b

Fig. 43 a, b. Other methods of assembling the small external fixator about the wrist

a Transarticular half-frame with the wrist in ulnar or palmar flexion: Shorter connecting rods are used between the distal and proximal threaded wires and are interconnected with 4x4-mm clamps. This permits the desired angles and positions to be maintained

b Quadrilateral frame assembly with four connecting rods, anchored in the 1st and 2nd metacarpals

IV. Preoperative, Operative, and Postoperative Guidelines

The peripheral areas of the extremities are very susceptible to *post-traumatic swelling*, and this must be taken into account when timing operative treatment. The procedure either should be performed right away, before swelling appears, or it should be delayed for several days until swelling has subsided. This should be hastened by appropriate elevation of the injured limb. When surgery is postponed, it is our practice to clean the operative site thoroughly on the eve of the operation and cover it with a sterile antiseptic dressing. There is no scientific proof that this improves asepsis, but it at least directs the attention of the staff toward optimum preparation of the operative site.

The standard "shave prep" has fallen into disfavor in recent years. Shaving should be limited to the proposed area of the incision and should be done immediately before the operation. Shaving produces multiple tiny breaks in the epidermis which, if made on the day before surgery, could become infected and spoil asepsis. Constraints of time and personnel may necessitate some compromise of these requirements. A cream depilatory may be used in place of shaving.

We no longer use plastic incise drapes, and we have never used them on the hand, where it is important to be able to observe the relative movements of the individual joints during the operation. Thorough mechanical cleansing of the hand is done on the day before surgery, and the fingernails are carefully trimmed. The areas around the nails are always contaminated on both the dorsal and volar sides, and it is a good precaution to cover the fingertips with sterile drapes (e.g., a sterile surgical glove or glove fingers).

A *pneumatic tourniquet* is applied to obtain a bloodless field. The tourniquet should not be kept inflated more than 2 h in younger patients. In older patients and patients with circulatory problems, this period should be shortened, or else a tourniquet should not be used.

The peripheral skeleton is invested by a thin, delicate, and poorly distensible soft-tissue envelope. Preservation of these tissues is of critical importance, and special care is taken to protect the skin from pressure or tension injury. Overeager assistants should be specifically cautioned about this, since surgical access is usually quite restricted, and opportunities for extension are limited.

Problems of scar formation are another major concern. For one thing, scars on the dorsal aspect of the upper limb (the "social side" that is seen and displayed) are so conspicuous that cosmetic considerations are a factor in patient selection. For another, poorly placed skin incisions can result in hypertrophic scars or desmogenic contractures. In the foot, incisions must be placed to allow comfortable ambulation and the wearing of shoes.

Hemostasis: Careful attention is given to hemostasis throughout the approach phase of the operation. Small blood vessels are not divided unless absolutely necessary.Standard electrocoagulation is not without hazards, as it produces necrotic zones of indeterminate extent which serve as media for bacterial growth. Larger veins that cannot be spared should be divided between ligatures. Bleeding from arterioles is best controlled with bipolar microcoagulation. The simple pneumatic tourniquet is superior in this regard to an Esmarch bandage, for it allows some amount of blood retention in the small vessels, making them easier to identify.

At the conclusion of the osseous phase of the operation, the tourniquet should be released so that definitive hemostatis can be achieved.

The *reduction* should be performed openly under direct vision, especially with intra-articular fractures. The resolving power of the image intensifier is limited and often is insufficient for procedures on the peripheral skeleton. As far as radiation exposure is concerned, the main hazard is the cumulative exposure to the surgeon's hand. But the use of apparatus for manipulations prolongs the operation and might compromise asepsis.

Provisional fixation of the fragments can be quite difficult. We use special forceps for this purpose or very fine Kirschner wires, especially in cancellous areas. Larger Kirschner wires damage the delicate articular cartilage and can cause thermal necrosis of bone, predisposing it to infection. Cerclage wires should be avoided due to the danger of tendon and nerve trauma.

Sometimes none of these devices are suitable, and we have to perform a "freehand" reduction with the help of a reliable assistant. In these cases the fracture is stabilized using the techniques described above.

During *wound closure* the joint capsule and fibrous layers are reapproximated separately with absorbable sutures. The fascia and subcutaneous tissue are not sutured.

Generally the skin is closed with vertical mattress sutures. An especially atraumatic closure is obtained with the unilateral intracutaneous modification of this technique. This is helpful in maintaining blood supply to a precarious skin flap. A different type of suture is preferred for the thick skin on the flexor surface of the hand or foot. Here it is better to coapt the skin margins accurately with fine interrupted sutures of a nonabsorbable, synthetic monofilament material.These sutures are not removed until the 12th postoperative day.

Drainage: The Jost-Redon type of suction drainage has proved generally effective in preventing postoperative hematoma.The suction drainage is maintained under supervision for 24-36 h and then removed. It may be used only in the presence of a watertight wound closure. Otherwise air will be sucked into the wound through the dressing, ruining asepsis. For this reason a classic, well-padded pressure dressing with conventional short-term drainage (24-36 h) is commonly preferred in the hand and foot. We have had good results with ribbed plastic films and microdrains, although some surgeons prefer to leave the skin open at selected sites

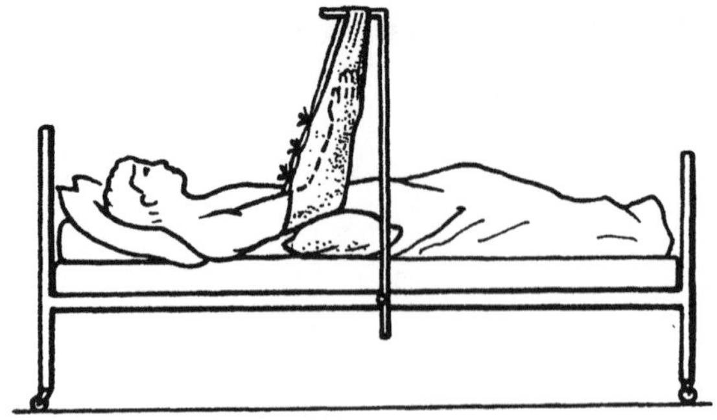

a

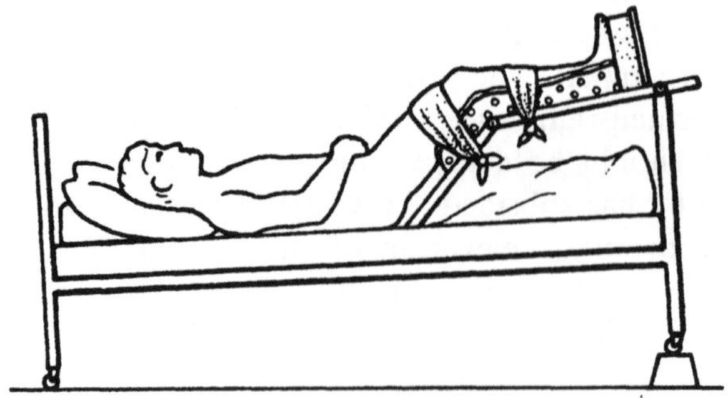

b

Fig. 44a, b. Postoperative elevation

a The upper limb (hand and forearm) is suspended from a pole in a reversed pillowcase. The elbow rests on a cushion. This provides elevation without pressure and allows free inspection of the fingertips, which are free of the compression dressing

b Classic elevation of the lower limb on a splint padded with sponge rubber. The ankle is flexed 90°, and the knee is slightly flexed. The leg is tied loosely to the splint with wide bandages

or to make separate incisions for the drainage of deeper secretions.

Postoperative elevation is of major importance and should be continued until swelling subsides.The classic sponge-rubber padded splint is satisfactory for the lower limb, and the arm is conveniently and comfortably suspended in a pillowcase (Fig. 44). A tricot stocking also can be used provided it does not restrict finger movements. Elevation should be supplemented by active postoperative mobilization according to the following routine: After recovering from anesthesia, the patient is instructed to raise his arm at least once per hour and actively flex and extend his fingers for 1 to 2 min. The dressing will prevent undesired or potentially damaging excursions. This routine should be memorized and reinforced by the entire therapy team (nurses, ward physician, etc.) so that it will become second nature to the patient and he will continue to practice it at home.

When the patient is mobilized from bed, the forearm should never be allowed to dangle, and the pressure dressing should remain intact. To be safe, we still often prescribe a sling, making sure that adequate shoulder and elbow exercises are performed to avoid loss of motion.

Active mobilization relies on the stability of the fixation, which must exceed the forces that accompany active mobilization and must be sufficient to cope with the subsequent partial loading of the fracture site after removal of the dressing.

In the lower limb, a tight elastic bandage should be applied before the patient gets out of bed. After the first attempt at ambulation, the wounds should be checked for secondary swelling or hematoma formation.

Particular attention is given to the mobilization of distant joints that are subject to reflex stiffening (shoulder!). Passive movement of these joints should be maintained from the start of postoperative therapy.

An attempt is made during the postoperative course to adjust the level of weight bearing to the degree of stability achieved. The leg should bear 10-15 kg of weight and never more than 20 kg under any circumstances. Excessive loading is fairly easy to avoid in the leg, where the applied weight can be measured with a step-on scale. In the upper limb, however, actions such as sitting up in bed can impose considerable stresses on the operative site and on the fixation, increasing the danger of secondary displacement. Personality factors (carelessness, obstinacy, indolence, etc.) can also lead to surprises, and individualized management is essential. Many patients will have to be held back rather than encouraged, but the reverse is generally true in the hand, where psychogenic inhibition is a factor.

The surgeon estimates the time for commencing weight bearing, which progresses incrementally to full weight bearing over a period of 3-4 weeks. Definitive approval for initiating weight bearing is contingent on monthly X-ray examinations. The consolidation of shaft fractures is generally complete between 6 and 12 weeks. Full weight bearing on the lower limb means ambulating without crutches, whereas full loading of the upper limb generally coincides with the resumption of work.

V. Removal of Implants

It is widely agreed that metallic implants should be removed when their function, considered to be temporary and auxiliary, has been satisfactorily assumed by the healed and reconstructed bone. However, a number of controversies persist that cannot be definitively resolved by scientific means. It is recommended, therefore, that the removal of implants be considered on an individualized basis.

Three problems are posed by the implantation of metallic foreign objects in the human body:

The Volume Factor. Especially in the periphery, skeletal implants tend to be bulky and may disturb or displace surrounding soft tissues. Foreign bodies that must be placed directly beneath gliding tissues, such as tendons, or close to joints and associated capsuloligamentous tissues may cause relative shortening of these structures. They promote the formation of adhesions between the gliding planes and can produce a bursa-like irritation. Consequently, these devices can interfere with rehabilitation, and they should be removed when they are no longer of benefit. This will provide increased space and length and will also afford an opportunity to perform a tenolysis or capsulotomy if such a procedure is indicated.

Implant Compatibility: Incompatibility may relate to corrosion or allergy.

Corrosion is possible whenever an implanted, metallic foreign body comes in contact with tissue fluids. The corrosion of individual screws is minimal owing to the metallurgic quality of modern implant materials. But corrosion increases markedly when different metallic components are placed in contact with each other, especially if their physicochemical properties are dissimilar.

Another factor that promotes corrosion is friction between different implants, as in the

Table. Average interval (in months) from operation to implant removal for various implants and localizations. S – screws, P – plates, K – Kirschner wires, TB – tension-band wires. These figures apply to typical fractures with uncomplicated healing

Fracture of clavicle	P	12-14
Nonunion of clavicle	P	20-24
Scapula	S	4-6
	P	8-12
Tuberosity of humerus	TB	4-6
	S	4-6
Head of humerus	P	12-14
Distal humerus	S	8-12
	P	12-16
Shaft of forearm	P	24-28
Distal radius	K	1-2
	S	6-8
	P	8-12
Scaphoid	S	12-14
Metacarpals and phalanges	K	1-2
	S	4-6
	P	4-6
Tibial tuberosity	S	6-8
	P	6-8
Intercondylar eminence	S	6-8
Reattached ligamentous insertions	S	3-5
Type C malleolar fracture (cortical)	P	12
Type A and B malleolar fracture (metaphyseal)	S	6-8
	P	6-8
Talus and calcaneus, including avulsions	S	6-8
	P	6-12
Metatarsals and great toe	K	1-2
	S	4-6
	P	8-12

contact zone between a plate and a screw. The areas of contact between small plates and screws are very small, and clinical experience shows that frank corrosion is extremely rare. Some amount of corrosion must be expected, however, when the thicker DCP is used.

Until recently, the question of *allergy* was thought to be clinically irrelevant. But recent observations suggest that some patients develop subclinical and even clinical allergic manifestations to alloy components. Studies also are being done on the link between allergy and resistance to infection.Subclinical manifestations are a particularly important motivation for the timely removal of metallic implants.

Alterations of Bony Structure: These vary with the type of implant used. The medullary nail and medullary wire (used chiefly in the peripheral skeleton) are not very stable and tend to produce callus. Simple screw fixation causes minimal changes. The most pronounced bony changes occur in connection with plating. For some time it was thought that the plate acted as an external, load-bearing splint, and that rarefaction of the underlying bone was a response to this protective effect. More recent studies indicate that the active remodeling of the bone under the plate is partly a result of vascular disturbances. These processes are inconsequential in the peripheral skeleton.

Implants that are not causing irritation or complaints do not need to be removed, nor do very deeply situated implants whose removal would entail unacceptable risk or difficulty. Implants also may be left in older patients or persons with a limited life expectancy if the devices are not causing irritation. In younger patients, plates should be removed whenever possible, giving particular consideration to cosmesis.

Finally, implant removal may be the only opportunity for the surgeon to reexamine a patient living far away and document the functional outcome. In this way it can provide the surgeon with valuable feedback that can help him in assessing the efficacy of his procedures.

When removing an implant, it may be unnecessary to reopen all of the original incision. Subcutaneous screws are easily removed through small stab incisions. Subcutaneous plate ends are exposed through a somewhat larger incision. However, in cases where delicate soft tissues such as tendons and nerve branches are vulnerable to injury between the skin and implant – especially in the hand – this method is not acceptable.

The identification and removal of screws having an hexagonal socket is considerably easier than with the older cross-slotted head screws. Cancellous screws with unthreaded shafts should be removed slowly and carefully, since fracture can occur at the junction between the 1.9-mm core of the threaded part of the screw and the 2.3-mm shank. Recently the back surface of the threads has been sloped in an effort to prevent this complication.

The *optimum time* for implant removal is somewhat earlier in the peripheral skeleton than in the larger bones, and it is earlier in cancellous bone than in pure cortex. The *table* shows the average interval from surgery to implant removal for different implants and anatomic sites.

VI. Autogenous Bone Grafts

The transplantation of cancellous bone or mixed corticocancellous grafts is often necessary when treating injuries of the peripheral skeleton. As experience has grown, indications for use of these grafts have expanded. Besides the classic indications of bone loss and comminution (tibial pilon, distal radius, etc.), attention has been directed to small defects of biomechanical importance in the radial head, the base of the first metacarpal, the tarsus, metatarsus, and other areas. Cancellous bone grafts speed fracture union and help to prevent secondary displacement and implant loosening.

In larger bone defects where the soft tissues are partially intact and retain significant functional value – as in dorsal defects of the thumb and fingers – the primary insertion of bridging corticocancellous grafts has proved successful. The graft is anchored to the surrounding bone with screws, a small plate, or a tension band.

When secondary internal fixation is performed for a delayed union, nonunion, osteotomy, or arthrodesis, the biologic status of the fragments must be considered. If a strong callus is present in association with a hypertrophic (reactive) nonunion, bone grafting usually is not required, and it is necessary only to stabilize the site in order for bony consolidation to occur.

However, if osteoporosis exists and the bone fragments are nonreactive, fixation with metallic implants is insufficient. The site will require an autogenous cancellous graft, possibly combined with decortication of the bone.With extreme osteoporosis, a corticocancellous graft may be necessary to provide sufficient anchorage for plate screws.

Preparations for harvesting of the grafts are made prior to the operation. The proposed donor site is designated. Access to this area is taken into account when positioning the patient, and the area is aseptically prepared and draped (Fig. 45). It is worthwhile to carry out these preparations even if there is doubt as to the need for a bone graft. Because this means extra work for the operating team, it is important that personnel appreciate the importance of this phase so that proper motivation can be engendered and maintained.

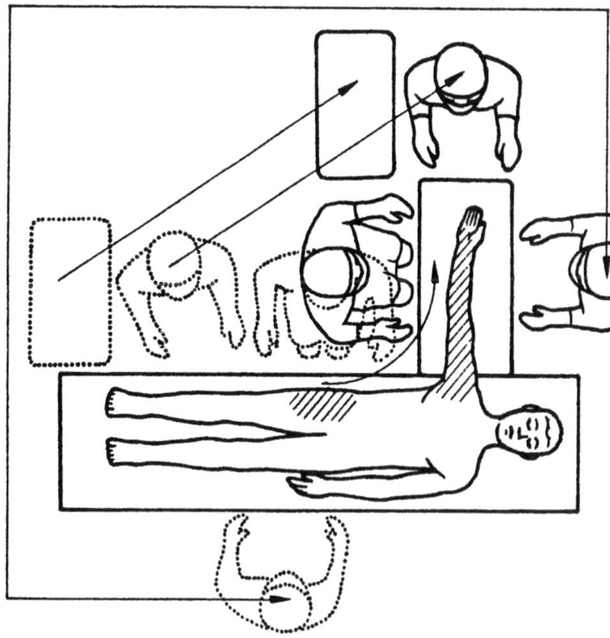

Fig. 45. Disposition and movements of the surgical team for taking a cancellous bone graft (iliac crest) in an internal fixation of the upper limb

For removal of the bone graft (*dotted lines*), the assistant stands opposite the surgeon (*seated*), and the scrub nurse stands at the surgeon's right
Changing positions for the main procedure (*solid lines*): The surgeon turns 90°, the assistant moves opposite the surgeon, and the scrub nurse stands between the assistant and surgeon. The instrument table is on the nurse's right and surgeon's left
For operating on the lateral side of the arm or dorsum of the hand, the positions of the surgeon and assistant are reversed

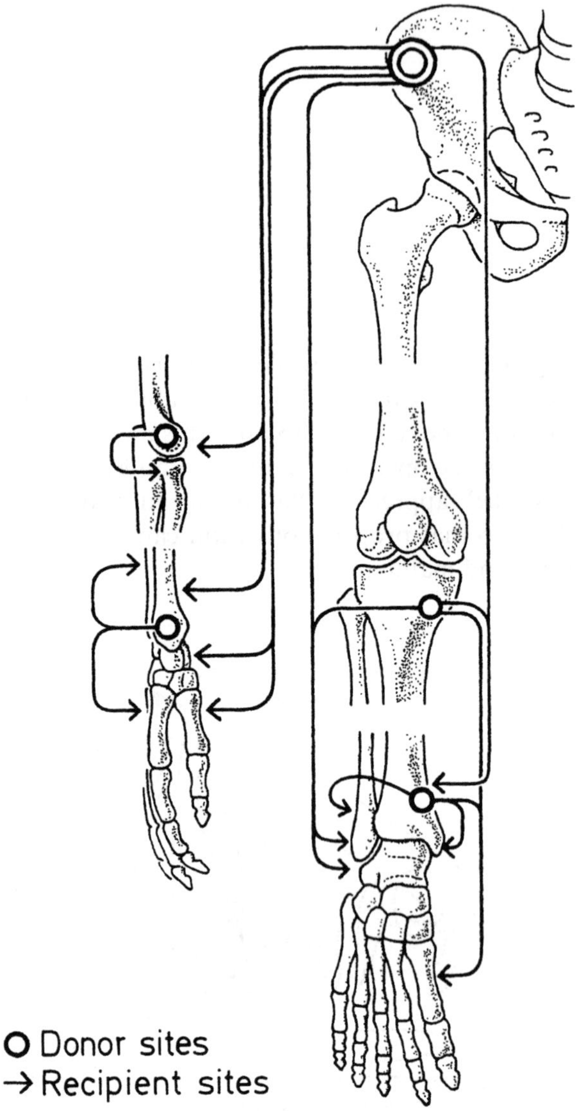

Fig. 46. Autogenous bone grafting: donor and recipient sites for internal fixations of the extremities

The ilium (iliac crest, iliac fossa, posterior outer table) is the biologically optimum source for autogenous cancellous bone
Less common donor sites are the radial metaphysis of the humerus, the olecranon, the distal radial metaphysis, the upper, and the distal tibial metaphysis

It is best from a biologic standpoint to use pure cancellous bone taken from the iliac crest and corticocancellous bone taken from the inner table of the anterior iliac wing or outer table of the posterior iliac wing. Even in elderly patients these areas contain hematopoietic bone marrow and have a very fine trabecular structure.

There are other factors that must be considered when selecting a donor site: The volume of harvested cancellous bone should be commensurate with the demand, and it should be readily accessible. Also, given the need to maintain asepsis and keep tourniquet time to a minimum, it is best to select a nearby donor site if possible. This is especially important in view of the increasing use of regional anesthesia. Small grafts may be taken from areas close to the defect that have a separate blood supply.

Occasionally these considerations lead to the selection of donor sites that would not be suitable for operations on larger bones. These include the capitulum of the humerus for depressed fractures of the radial head, the distal radial epiphysis for the hand and forearm, the tibial head for tibial pilon fractures, and the medial distal tibial metaphysis for the fibula and foot. The various combinations of donor and recipient sites are illustrated in Fig. 46. The selection is more limited in juveniles due to the presence of unfused growth plates and apophyses.

VII. Reconstructive Surgery

Many peripheral fractures are far from spectacular, and their presence may be overlooked initially or their functional significance unappreciated. Moreover, effective methods of conservative treatment, especially in the hand, are not widely known or have actually been forgotten. We find that deformities of rotation, angulation, or shortening are a more frequent indication for secondary operative intervention than nonunions. The pain of traumatic arthritis and rheumatoid disease can be relieved by arthrodesis of the affected joint. Fixation with small implants has proved very useful for these procedures and gives far better stability than Kirschner wires alone, which often produce a distractive effect. In most cases it is unnecessary to apply external fixation after surgery. Intensive, active mobilization of neighboring joints and immediate partial weight bearing lead to surprisingly good functional results–especially in patients who have mobile, pain-free joints prior to undergoing an osteotomy. This is far less likely if there has been previous surgery or prolonged immobilization, or if significant osteoporosis or dystrophy exists. This particularly applies to nonunions after failed attempts at internal fixation, and to chronic infections.

In our experience, autogenous bone grafting combined with metallic fixation is definitely the most reliable procedure. There are many other cases that do not require bone grafting owing to the presence of a good blood supply, broad contact between the bone ends, and excellent stability through interfragmental compression. Various surgical options are available, and we may select the one that is most appropriate for a given situation.

All operations to correct deformity must be preceded by meticulous planning that includes not only the study and measurement of radiographs in relation to the healthy side, but also an assessment of the stability that will be needed for postoperative mobilization.

In performing these procedures, certain standard techniques have proved effective and will be briefly described below. Details may be found in corresponding chapters of the Special Section.

Dowel Graft Combined with a Plate (Fig. 47a): Because of limited access, the corticocancellous dowel graft usually can be inserted into the reamed medullary cavity of one fragment only. The graft is then inlaid into a slot cut in the cortex of the other fragment. Rotational alignment can still be adjusted after the dowel graft has been placed. The graft is secured with a plate.

This technique is suitable for the fixation of osteotomies and nonunions.

Interposed Graft (Fig. 47b): The interposition of solid corticocancellous grafts is mainly used for bone lengthening when less than 1 cm of length gain is required (fibula, foot, hand). Forcible distraction is potentially harmful to the soft tissues, especially the nerves and blood vessels. When distracting the fragments after an osteotomy, care is taken to avoid axial and rotational displacement. The lever arm situation is unfavorable, and the internal fixation device must have a secure hold in both main fragments (see Stabilization Rule 2, p. 37).

If more than 1 cm of lengthening is required, it generally cannot be achieved in one sitting. A small distractor is applied and left in place for a prolonged period as the fragments are gradually separated by the desired amount over a period of several weeks.

Compressed Bridge Graft (Fig. 47c, 48d): This is similar to the dowel graft, except that the graft is inlaid into slots cut in the cortices of both fragments. The graft should project slightly above the bone surface, and it is compressed by the implant, which may be a plate or wire tension band. Rotational alignment cannot be adjusted after the graft has been placed, but minor angular corrections are possible.

This technique is appropriate for arthrodeses of the wrist and the carpometacarpal joint of the thumb, for partial arthrodeses of the carpus, and for nonunions.

Arthrodeses and Internal Fixations of Nonunions in Well Vascularized Areas (Fig. 48): These are usually done without bone grafting, but we like to use resected callus or periarticular cancellous material to obliterate small defects or to make slight positional corrections in situ.

Arthrodesis with a tension-band plate or wire is particularly appropriate for the metacarpophalangeal joint of the thumb.Screw fixation and tension-band wiring are both possible for the proximal interphalangeal joints of the fingers. The screws may be inserted from the proximal or distal direction, or small tension-band wires may be applied from the proximal side.

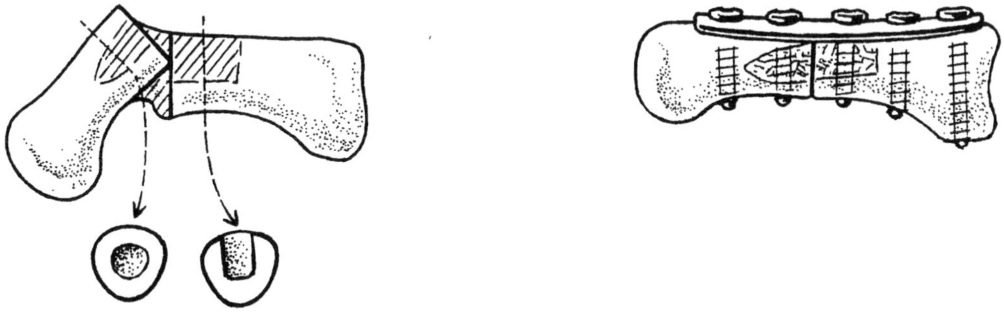

a

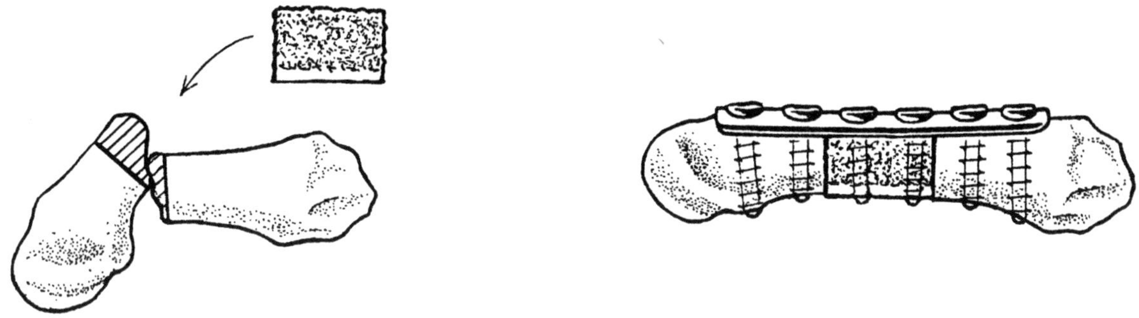

b

c

Fig. 47 a–c. Osteotomy and nonunion

a Osteotomy of the diaphysis fixed with a dowel graft and plate:
The osteotomy is performed with a fine osteotome or oscillating saw, and the bone is realigned. The distal medullary cavity is drilled open, and a wide slot is made in the proximal dorsal cortex. A cortico-cancellous graft is inserted and secured with a plate

b Interposed graft for a nonunion with bone loss:
The fragments are mobilized and freshened, the desired length is established, and a full-thickness corticocancellous graft is interposed with its cortical side opposite the plate. The plate should solidly engage the main fragments with two screws in each, and additional screws should secure the cancellous block

c Compressed bridge graft for an atrophic nonunion:
The bony margins are sparingly decorticated and freshened, and the bone is realigned. The corticocancellous graft is slotted dorsally into both cortices; it projects slightly above the bone surface and is compressed by the plate

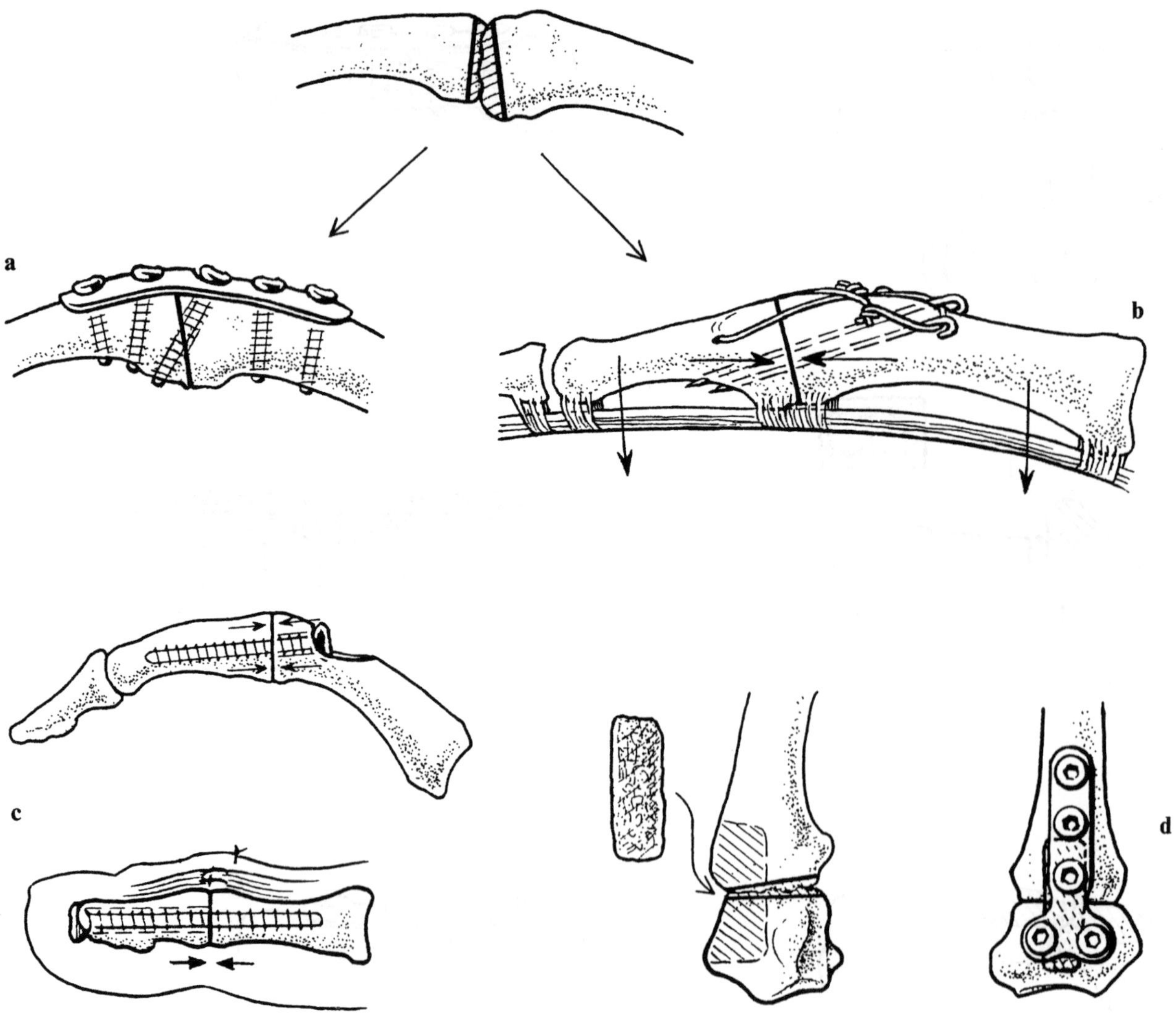

Fig. 48 a–d. Arthrodeses

a Joint resection and plating:
The joint surfaces are sparingly resected with the oscillating saw or osteotome in the desired position of arthrodesis. A plate is applied in the tension-band position and incorporates a central interfragmental lag screw

b Joint resection and tension-band wiring:
The joint is resected as in **a**. An initial, splinting Kirschner wire is inserted, rotation is checked, and a second, parallel wire is inserted (to block rotation). A wire-loop tension band is then applied for interfragmental compression, which is distributed evenly across the arthrodesis under the pull of the flexor tendon. Danger: impalement of the volar soft tissues

c Screw arthrodesis of the interphalangeal joints:
Arthrodesis of the PIP with a lag screw inserted from the proximal side (gliding hole), and arthrodesis of the DIP with a lag screw inserted from the distal side (gliding hole)

d Arthrodesis with a compressed bridge graft:
This is recommended in joints that have a relatively poor vascularity or are subject to large mechanical loads (e.g., the first carpometacarpal joint). The joint is sparingly resected as in **a**. The bridge graft is slotted across the arthrodesis dorsally and is secured with a plate that engages each fragment with two screws and compresses the graft in its bed

Special Section

VIII. Introduction and Overview

Fractures of the peripheral bones and joints are regular indications for use of the SFS, and so we shall take a systematic look at the types of injury that can occur in those areas. Because it is possible to apply small implants to larger bones, examples from the more proximal regions will also be described.

It should be understood that small plates and screws are not appropriate for all internal fixations of peripheral bones. Thus, the semitubular plate is frequently placed in areas where small implants would ordinarily be used. Also, tension-band wiring is commonly used on the olecranon, malleoli, and other peripheral areas, where it gives excellent results.

It is inevitable, therefore, that some of our material will overlap with that presented in the *Manual of Internal Fixation*, and, indeed, we have adapted a number of illustrations from that text. Positioning, surgical approaches, and aftertreatment are dealt with only to the extent that they differ from those described for standard-size implants in the *Manual of Internal Fixation*.

Experience has demonstrated the need for depicting surgical approaches and techniques as accurately as possible. Thus we have devoted considerable space to semischematic drawings, which make it easier to portray the essential elements of a given technique.

We also felt it necessary to draw on cases from our own files, and so each chapter concludes with a series of illustrative X-rays. These demonstrate the variability of individual cases and how they may differ from the ideal solutions depicted in drawings.

- Most of the examples were taken from the 2nd edition of the *Small Fragment Set Manual* and retain their technical validity. We were particularly interested in reviewing the late results of patients operated 8–11 years earlier. The internal fixations were performed with the older implants.
- New indications and technical refinements caused us to add a number of new clinical examples. Even so, we have been able to document only a few of the newest types of implant.

IX. The Shoulder Girdle

Fractures about the shoulder have become more prevalent as a result of traffic accidents and sports-related injuries. Scapular fractures and fracture-dislocations of the humeral head have become particularly common. Conservative treatment is still preferred for most of these injuries, and the preservation of shoulder function continues to be the major goal.The period of immobilization should be as brief as possible; abduction splints and shoulder spicas become less acceptable the longer they need to be worn. Operative treatment is indicated for the rare open fractures of the shoulder girdle and also for avulsion fractures, unstable fracturedislocations, and severely displaced fractures.

1. Clavicle

a) Fractures of the Middle Third

Ninety to ninety-five percent of these fractures are still treated conservatively with a figure-of-eight bandage.This method requires frequent position checks and continual monitoring of shoulder function. The few indications for primary operative fixation include the rare open fractures, impending perforation of the skin by a sharp irreducible fragment, fractures with concomitant injury to the subclavian artery and brachial plexus, and a coexisting fracture of the scapular neck (instability). Internal fixation may also be appropriate in multiply injured patients to facilitate nursing care and position changes, in patients with concomitant chest wall injury to improve active respiration, and in patients with coexisting peripheral fractures in the same arm (summation of immobilization injury).

Approach and Internal Fixation. We approach the clavicle through a vertical incision ("saber-cut" or "suspender" incision) made over the fracture site. This incision may be extended as desired, and it gives the best cosmetic result in an area that is prone to hypertrophic scarring. The lateral and medial fragments are alternately exposed (Fig. 49a). Great care is taken to avoid vascular trauma when dissecting medially on the inferior surface. Reduction can be difficult if comminution is present and can be aided by the preliminary screw fixation of butterfly fragments to the main fragments. But the great majority of fractures are simple oblique types that are easily reduced. Temporary maintenance of the reduction with forceps can be considerably more difficult. We usually plate the fracture (or nonunion) with a 7- or 8-hole DCP for 3.5-mm screws. There may be problems in contouring the plate to the clavicle, and flexible aluminum templates cannot always be used. In this case we proceed as follows: The plate is first contoured to one main fragment, is tentatively attached to it with screws, and is used as a lever arm. The necessary shape is easily determined when the plate is attached to the second fragment. At this time the first screw usually has to be removed once or even twice along with the plate until adaptation to the second fragment is satisfactory (Fig. 49b). The soft tissues deep to the clavicle are protected with a Hohmann retractor while the bone is drilled and tapped. If a bone defect or devitalization is noted, autogenous cancellous bone grafting is performed.

A variation of the technique is to attach the plate to the anterior aspect of the clavicle, rather than superiorly. This eliminates the danger of vascular injury, but it poses some threat to the brachial plexus and makes it more difficult to contour the plate to the anatomic curve of the bone.

b) Fractures of the Lateral Clavicle

An undisplaced or minimally displaced lateral clavicular fracture may be treated with a figure-of-eight bandage, the same as mid-third fractures.Internal fixation is indicated if significant displacement exists (especially if there is upward displacement due to a tear of the coracoclavicular ligament), in comminuted fractures predisposed to nonunion, or if there is anatomic involvement of the acromioclavicular joint.

Approach and Internal Fixation. The approach is the same as for mid-third fractures, and reduction is usually straightforward.Provisional fixation is obtainable with transacromial Kirschner wires.Depending on the size of the fragments, definitive fixation can be accomplished with a small T plate or one-third tubular plate (Fig. 51). With upward displacement of the clavicle, we recommend driving an extra-long plate screw through the clavicle and into the coracoid process. The hole for this screw is overdrilled to 4.5 mm (larger than a normal gliding hole) to ensure that the screw will not break under bending loads during postoperative mobilization of the shoulder. The coracoclavicular ligament, usually clearly visible, should be repaired before the screw is inserted.

Alternative technique: Instead of placing a screw in the coracoid process, pass a loop of wire, absorbable suture material, or tendon graft around the coracoid process and fix it to the clavicle. Note, however, that the coracoid projects farther anteriorly than the clavicle, and that this can cause oblique tension to be exerted on the clavicle.

Screws placed in the thin acromion are unstable and loosen very quickly.

Fractures of the lateral end of the clavicle can also be stabilized with a wire tension band. To avoid articular disc injury, this fixation should not encroach upon the acromioclavicular joint (Fig. 51 a).

Recently, various special implants have been introduced for fixation of the acromioclavicular joint. An example is shown in Fig. 58. This development shows that these injuries are being seen with increasing frequency, and that they can present problems of treatment as well as diagnosis.

c) Secondary Operations

The main indications for secondary operations on the clavicle are nonunions of the middle third and post-traumatic shortening with deformity. The major goals of surgery are pain relief and improvment of shoulder function.

Osteotomy of the clavicle is recommended to improve access for reconstructive surgery in cases of brachial plexus injury. The osteotomy is fixed with a previously contoured plate. Osteotomy to correct shortening requires the interposition of a corticocancellous graft.

With a clavicular nonunion, which is nearly always hypertrophic, the technique corresponds to that for a fresh fracture. However, the potentially small area of contact between the bone ends can make contouring of the plate more difficult. The fragments must be apposed without force and without malrotation to prevent traumatic arthritis in the acromioclavicular joint. The anatomic length of the clavicle should be accurately restored. Reference to preoperative radiographs of the healthy side is helpful in avoiding deformity.

With a hypertrophic nonunion, the soft callus tissue that is excised to mobilize the bone ends can be utilized as an autogenous graft material. With an atrophic nonunion, autogenous cancellous bone chips must be applied.

Our favorite implant for fixation is the 3.5-mm DCP. We can also recommend the 3.5-mm reconstruction plate, which is easier to contour than the DCP, but is not as strong.

2. Scapula

a) Fractures of the Glenoid Rim

Isolated fractures of the anterior and inferior glenoid rim may occur in association with shoulder dislocations. Larger rim fragments should be temporarily stabilized with Kirschner wires and fixed with one or two 4.0-mm cancellous screws, which may be used with metal washers (Fig. 60).

b) Fractures of the Glenoid Fossa

Undisplaced fractures are usually managed nonoperatively. Markedly displaced glenoid fractures are anatomically reduced and fixed in a functionally stable manner.

c) Fractures of the Neck of the Scapula

Minimally displaced fractures that are unaccompanied by other injuries of the ipsilateral shoulder or thoracic skeleton usually can be satisfactorily treated with early functional exercises.

– Isolated Fractures of the Scapular Neck

Traction of the triceps muscle on the infraglenoid tubercle can pull the glenoid distally and tilt it laterally. The fracture can be fixed with individual lag screws driven into the tubercle from the posterior side. Larger fragments should be fixed with a one-third tubular plate, also applied posteriorly, which buttresses or presses the articular fragment against the proximal lateral border of the scapula. This may be combined with 3.5-mm cortex lag screws introduced separately or through the plate (Fig 62).

– Coexisting Scapular Neck Fractures

Rarely, fractures of the clavicle or ribs will be accompanied by a fracture of the ipsilateral scapular neck. This type of fracture is very unstable and allows the entire shoulder girdle to glide medially. The degree of displacement and instability depends upon the integrity of the coracoclavicular and acromioclavicular ligaments. In most cases simple internal fixation of the clavicle with a 3.5-mm DCP will correct the displacement and instability and will enable functional exercises to be performed. Separate fixation of the scapular neck fracture is usually unnecessary (Fig. 61).

d) Fractures of the Acromion and Spine

Operative treatment is indicated only for markedly displaced fractures and painful nonunions.

A lateral fracture of the acromion is fixed with Kirschner wires and a tension-band loop (Fig. 53a). More medial fractures are stabilized with a one-third tubular plate (possibly with a small hook) applied as a tension band. Small fragments may be excised and the detached deltoid muscle reattached in transosseous fashion.

e) Fractures of the Coracoid

Fractures of the coracoid process are very rare. Surgery is indicated if the fracture is associated with marked coracoclavicular displacement or if there is compression of the neurovascular bundle.

A more common indication for internal fixation is osteotomy of the coracoid to gain access to the anterior part of the shoulder joint. Fixation may be accomplished with a 6.5-mm cancellous screw, a malleolar screw, or a small 4.0-mm cancellous screw combined with a tension-band wire (Fig. 60).

f) Approaches

– **Anterior Approach** (Fig. 52a)

We use the anterior approach through the delto-pectoral groove for anterior and inferior glenoid rim fractures. The coracobrachial muscle and short head of the biceps are retracted medially, and the joint is opened after medial retraction of the subscapularis. Adequate exposure may require osteotomizing the coracoid and notching the deltoid at its clavicular insertion. Both structures are repaired at the end of the operation.

– **Posterior Approach** (Fig. 52b)

The posterior approach is generally used for fractures of the scapular neck. The skin incision extends from the palpable posterior border of the acromion medially along the scapular spine and then curves toward the inferior angle of the scapula.

The deltoid is released from the scapular spine leaving a narrow rim of tissue. The shoulder joint and lateral margin of the scapula are approached between the infraspinatus and teres minor muscles. All released muscles are reattached at the time of wound closure.

3. Proximal Humerus

a) Avulsion of the Greater Tuberosity

Relatively undisplaced tuberosity avulsions are not an indication for operative treatment. These fractures heal well with a few weeks' conservative therapy and are solid in about 4–6 weeks. Open reduction is necessary only for significant displacement of the tuberosity fragment, and especially for subacromial impingement. The openly reduced fragment is fixed with small cancellous screws and washers supplemented by a tension band (Fig. 54).

Approach is generally made through an incision in the deltopectoral groove, stripping deltoid fibers from the lateral clavicle as required.

b) Subcapital Comminuted Fractures

Internal fixation is definitely indicated for irreducible fracture-dislocations in this area. A relative indication exists in cases of extreme displacement and instability, especially in younger individuals. The cloverleaf plate has occasionally proved useful in comminuted fractures of the humeral head, permitting the atraumatic fixation of multiple fragments to the upper humerus and their secure attachment to the shaft.

These fractures are approached through a long incision in the deltopectoral groove. Usually the coracoid process is osteotomized. A difficult reduction may also require division of the subscapularis tendon and long biceps tendon (which later is reapproximated to the short biceps tendon). Osseous defects must be obliterated with cancellous grafts.

4. Illustrative Clinical X-Rays (Figs. 55-63)

Pages 98–106

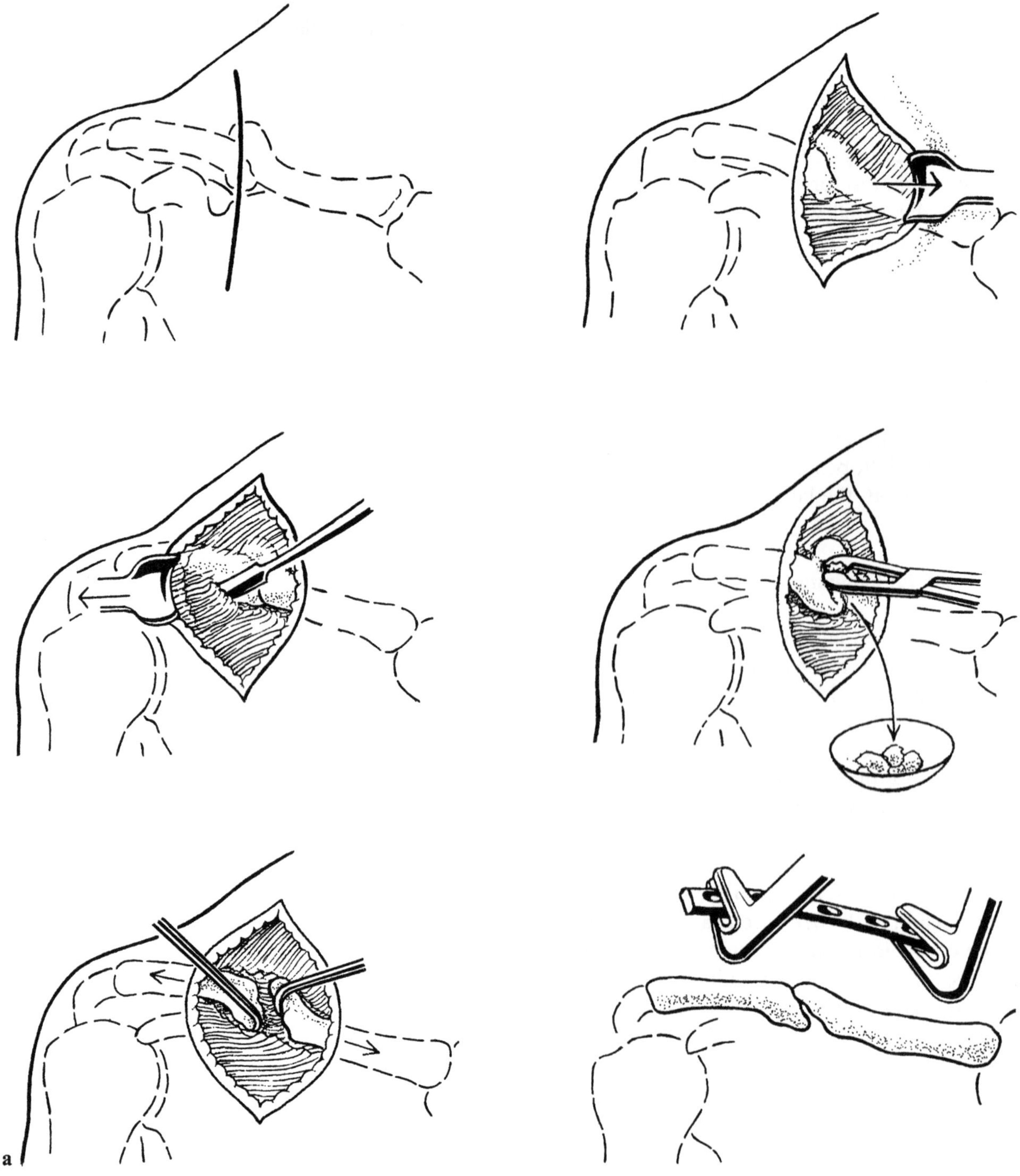

a

Fig. 49 a–c. Internal fixation of a hypertrophic nonunion in the middle third of the clavicle

a A vertical incision is made over the nonunion, and the fragments are alternately exposed by retraction of the wound edges. Attached muscle is stripped with a periosteal elevator. The hypertrophic callus mass is removed with a ronguer, saving the pieces. The bone ends are elevated and their posterior surfaces are carefully dissected.Then the reduction is carried out, restoring a normal length and alignment. A 3.5-mm DCP is contoured and temporarily fixed to one fragment with a screw, using a Hohmann retractor to protect the underlying soft tissues. At this time the surgeon estimates the contour of the second fragment, removes the first screw, and finishes contouring the plate, which is then definitively attached with screws. The callus pieces removed earlier are packed around the bone ends. A suction drain is inserted, the muscles are reattached with approximating sutures, and the skin is closed

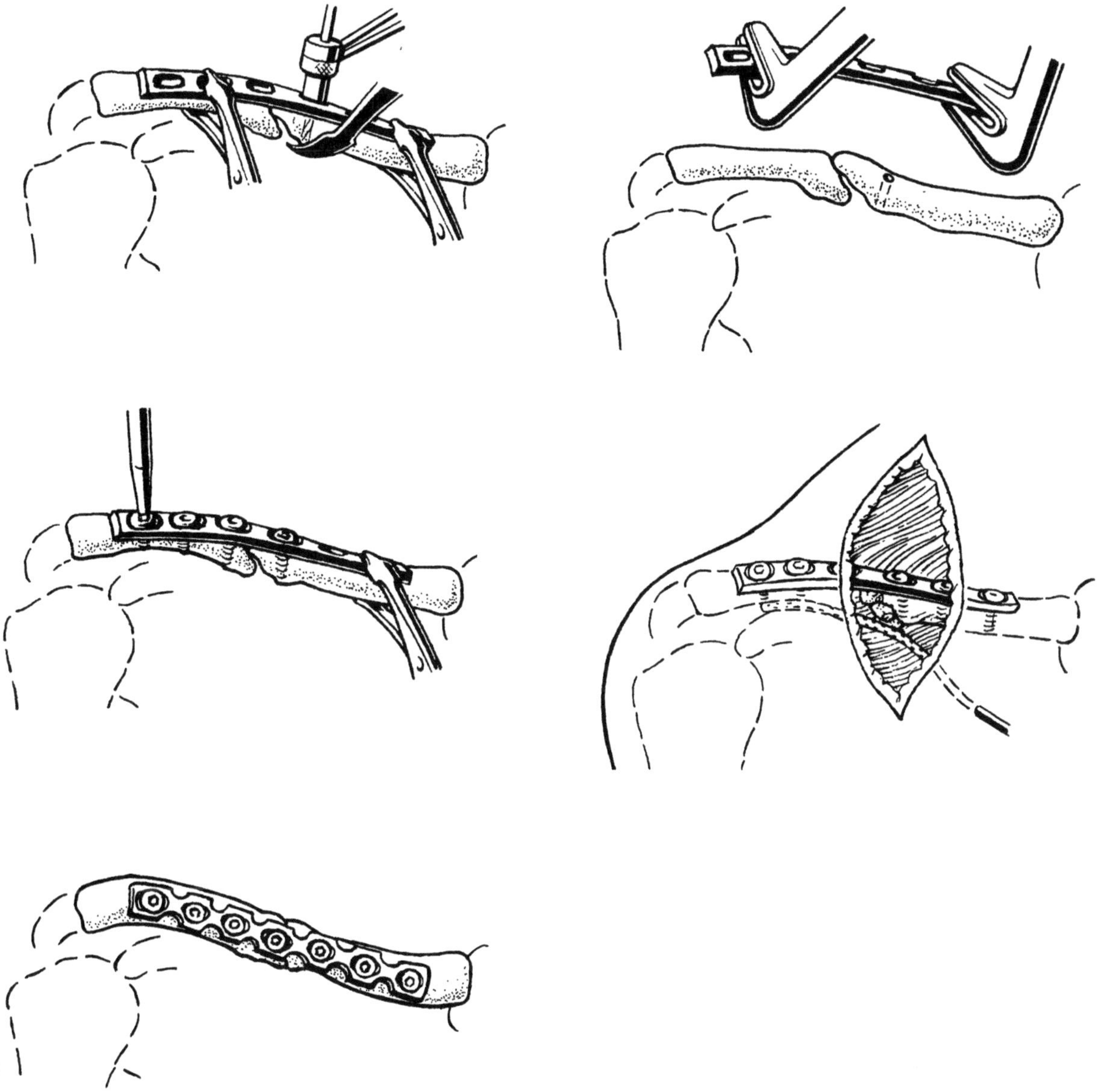

b

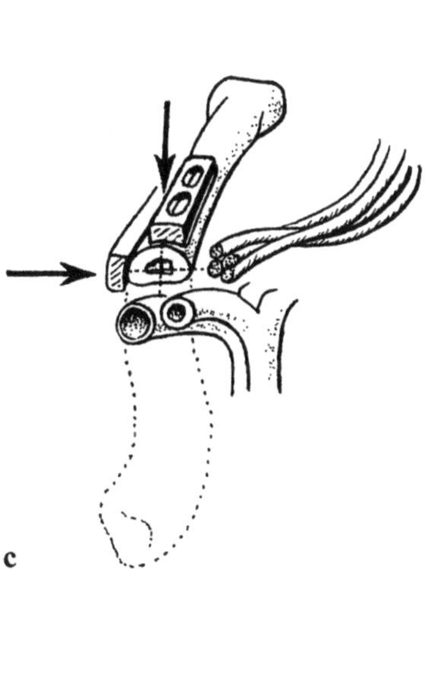

c

b Anterior application of the 3.5-mm reconstruction plate

c Cross-section through the clavicle mid-third: Blood vessels are threatened by a plate applied superiorly, and the brachial plexus by a plate applied anteriorly

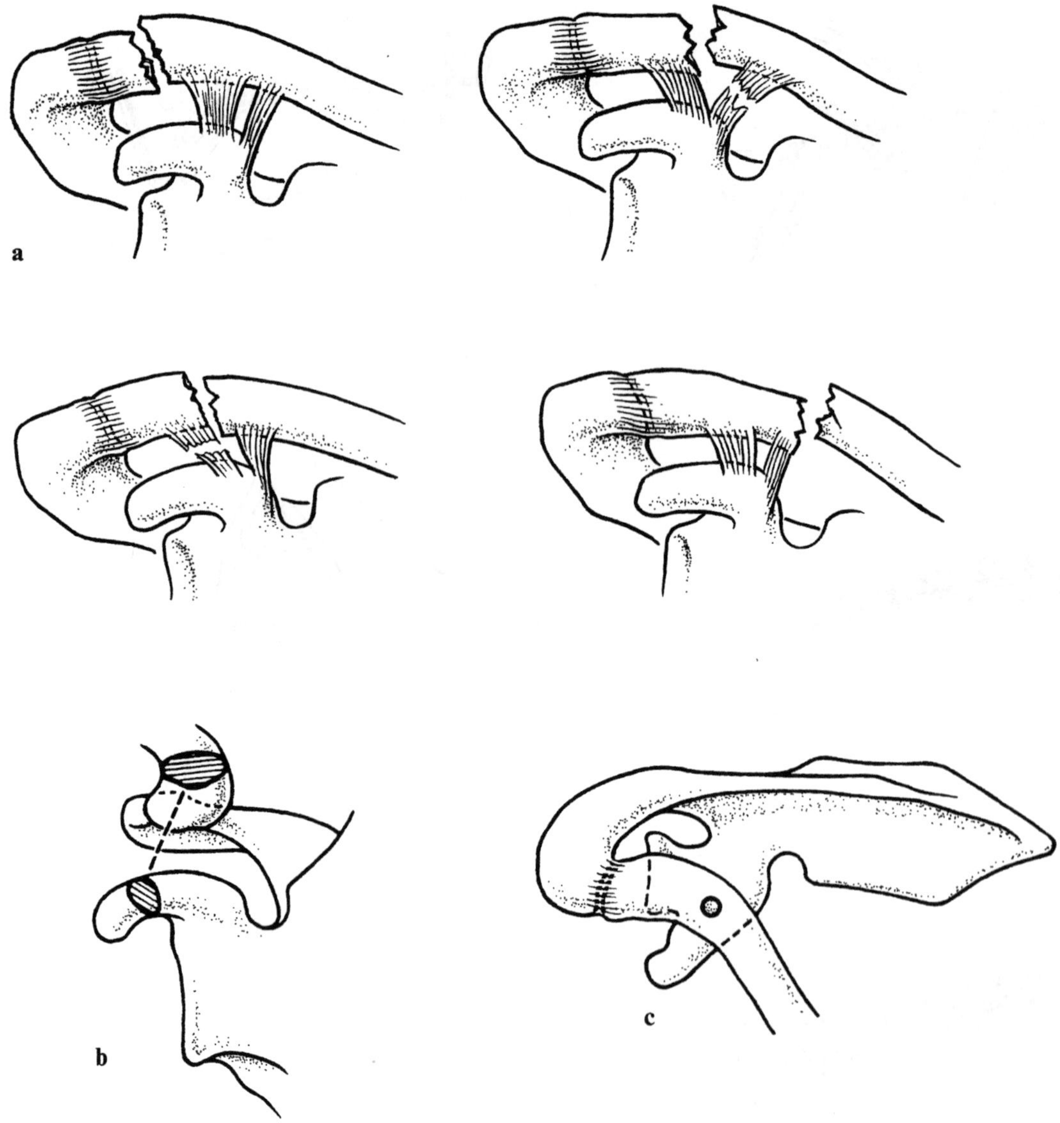

Fig. 50 a–c. Classification of lateral clavicular fractures and topography of the clavicle and coracoid

a Contrast between semistable and unstable lateral clavicular fractures associated with different tears of the coracoclavicular ligaments, after Jäger

b Topography of the clavicle and coracoid: The tip of the process is anterior to the lateral clavicle. Mobile connections between the two bones tend to displace the clavicle forward, causing subluxation at the acromioclavicular joint

c Top view: A connecting screw centered in the lateral clavicle pierces the coracoid behind its tip

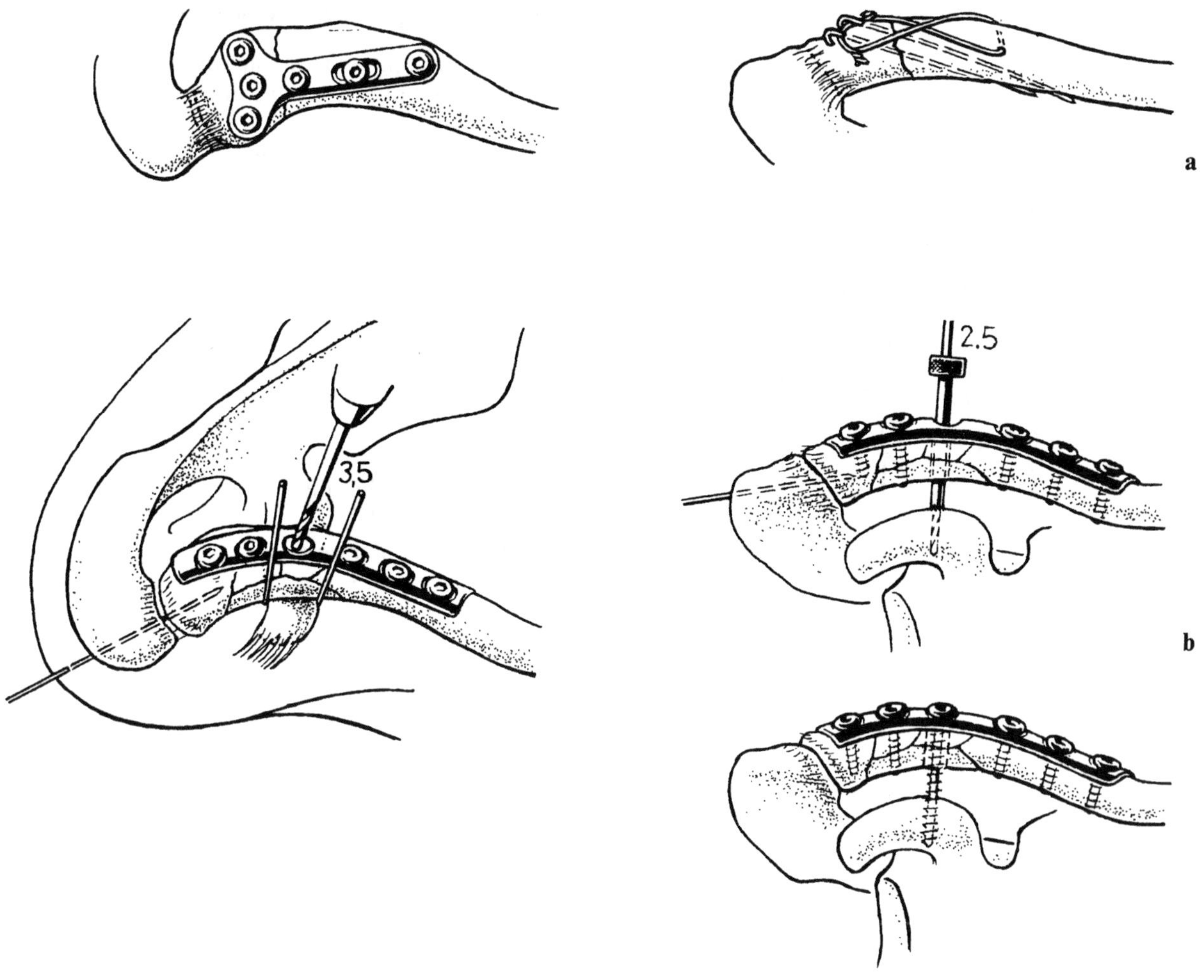

Fig. 51 a, b. Internal fixation of a lateral clavicular fracture

a The fracture may be stabilized with an extra-articular transverse or oblique T plate or with a wire-loop tension band

b A comminuted lateral fracture is stabilized with a one-third tubular plate incorporating a screw anchored in the coracoid process. The fracture is reduced, and if acromioclavicular instability exists, the fracture is temporarily transfixed with an axial Kirschner wire. A long one-third tubular plate is contoured to the clavicle and temporarily attached with screws. The coracoid process is identified and its borders marked with two Kirschner wires. A 3.5-mm gliding hole is drilled through the plate toward the coracoid, the straight drill sleeve is inserted, and the coracoid is perforated with the 2.5-mm bit. A 3.5-mm cortex screw or 4.0-mm cancellous screw is driven in, drawing the plate toward the coracoid. The gliding hole in the clavicle must be sufficiently width to prevent screw breakage during movements of the shoulder. If a larger-gauge screw has to be used in the coracoid for better stability, the diameter of the gliding hole must be increased accordingly

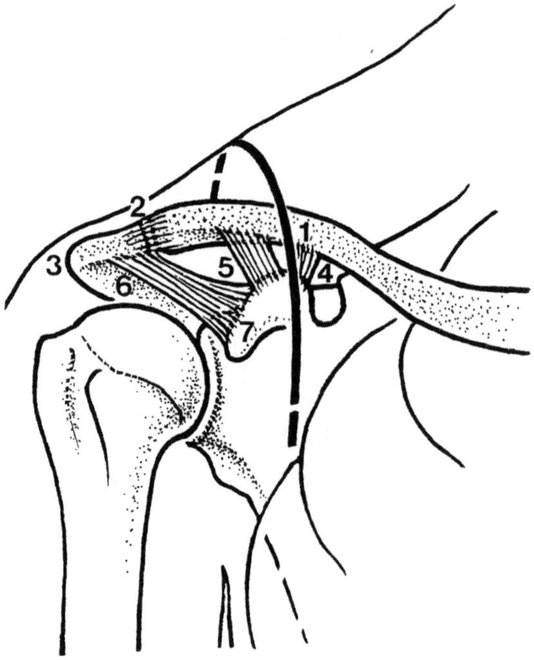

a

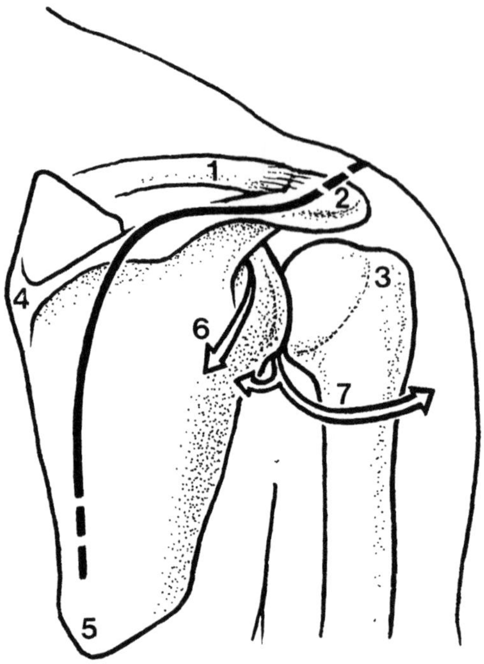

b

Fig. 52 a, b. Approaches to the scapula

a Anterior approach for fractures of the anterior and inferior glenoid rim (details in text)
1 – Clavicle
2 – Acromioclavicular joint
3 – Acromion
4 – Conoid ligament
5 – Trapezoid ligament
6 – Coracoacromial ligament
7 – Coracoid process

b Posterior approach (details in text)
1 – Clavicle
2 – Acromion
3 – Greater tuberosity
4 – Trigone of the spine
5 – Inferior angle
6 – Suprascapular nerve
7 – Axillary nerve

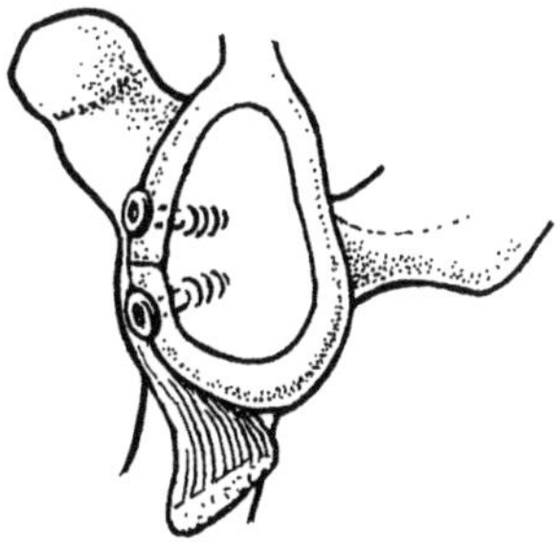

a

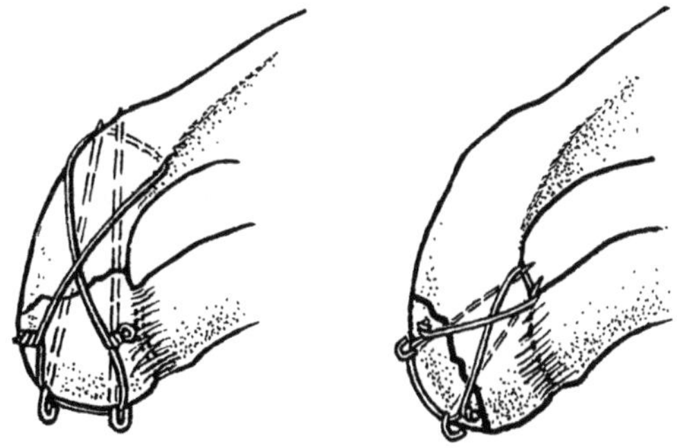

b

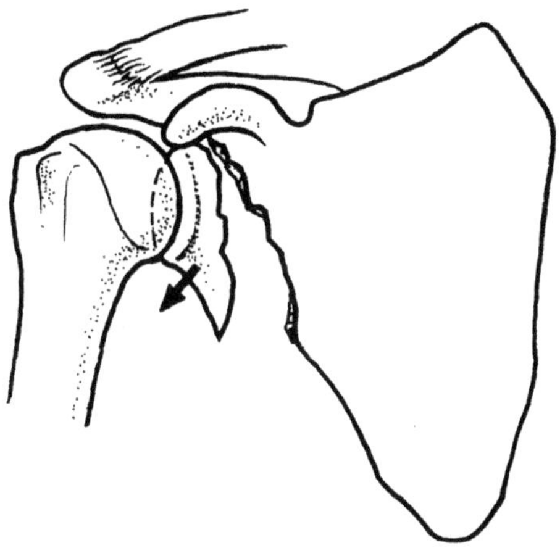

c

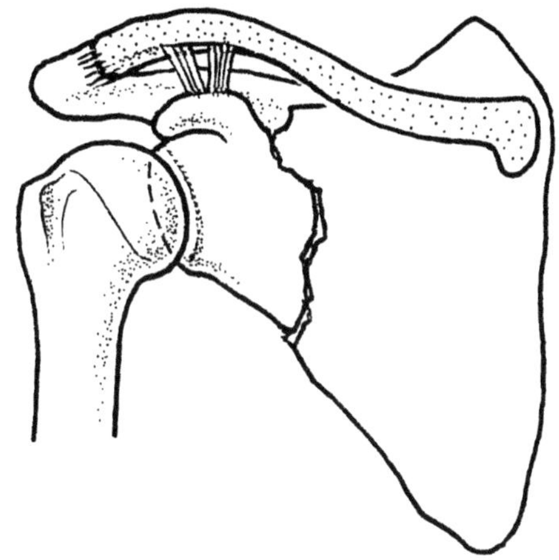

d

Fig. 53 a–d. Internal fixations of the scapula

a Screw fixation of the glenoid rim. Osteochondral shear fragments are fixed with small cancellous screws

b Tension-band wiring of an acromion fracture

c The displaced, mobile scapular neck fracture is an indication for screw or plate fixation through a posterior approach

d Coexisting fractures of the scapular neck and clavicle. Internal fixation of the fractured clavicle is sufficient to stabilize the shoulder girdle (Fig. 61)

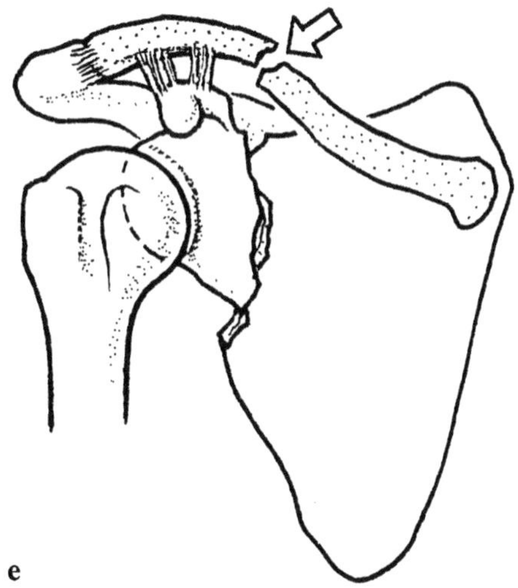

e

Fig. 54a, b. Internal fixations of the proximal humerus

a Combined screw and tension-band fixation of a markedly displaced tuberosity avulsion

b An irreducible, unstable subcapital fracture or fracturedislocation of the humerus is stabilized with a cloverleaf plate whose upper tab has been removed

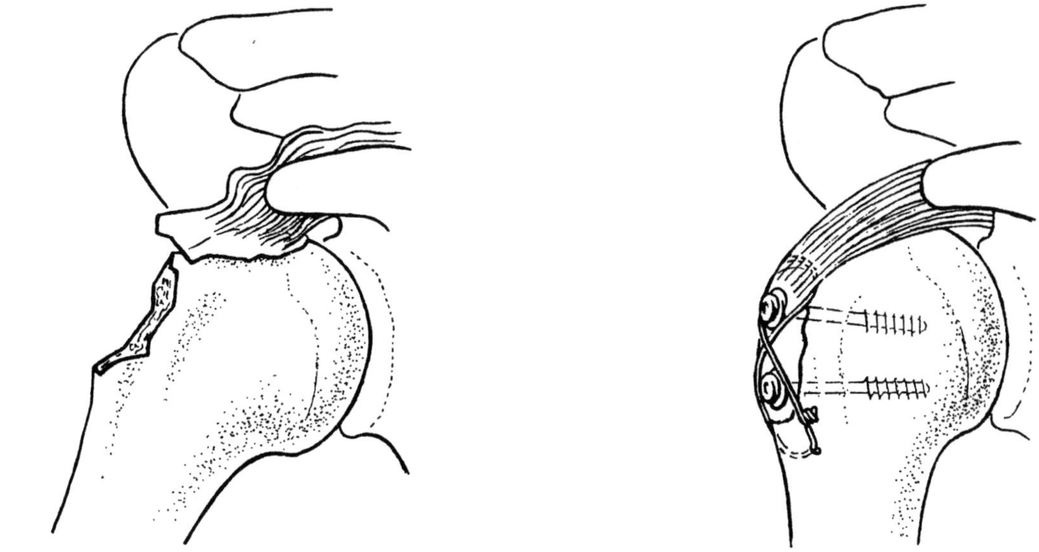

a

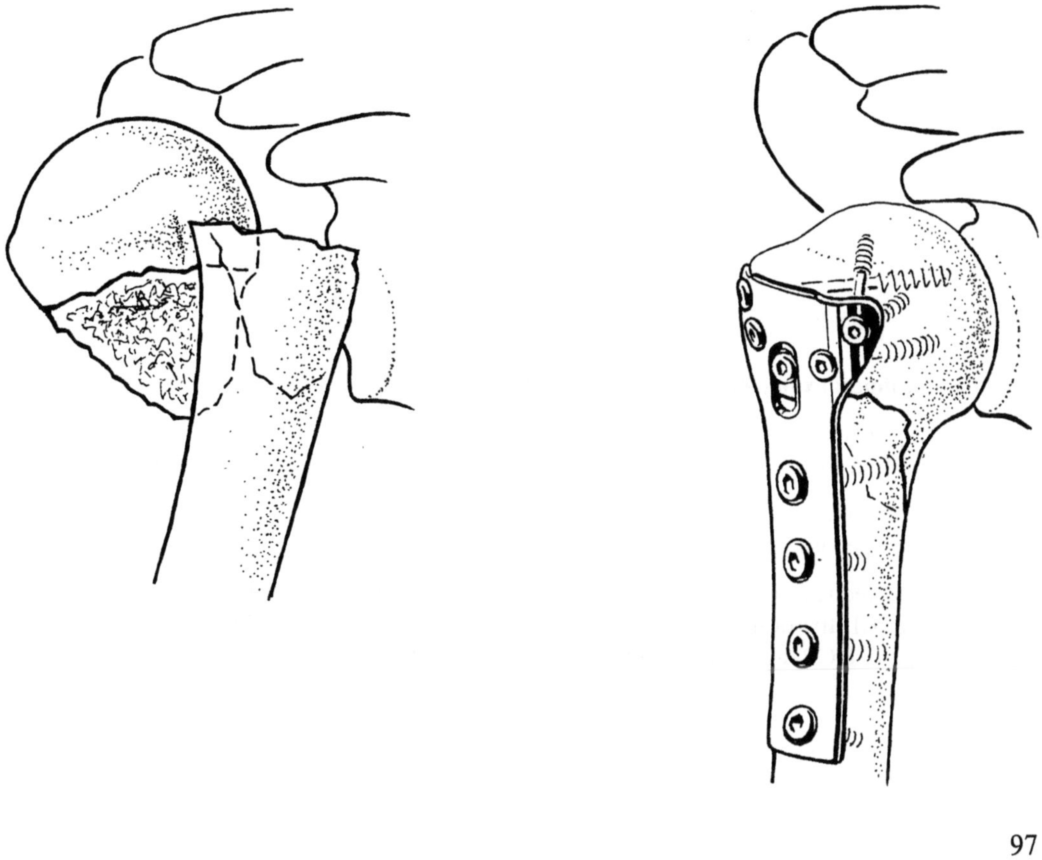

b

a
b
c
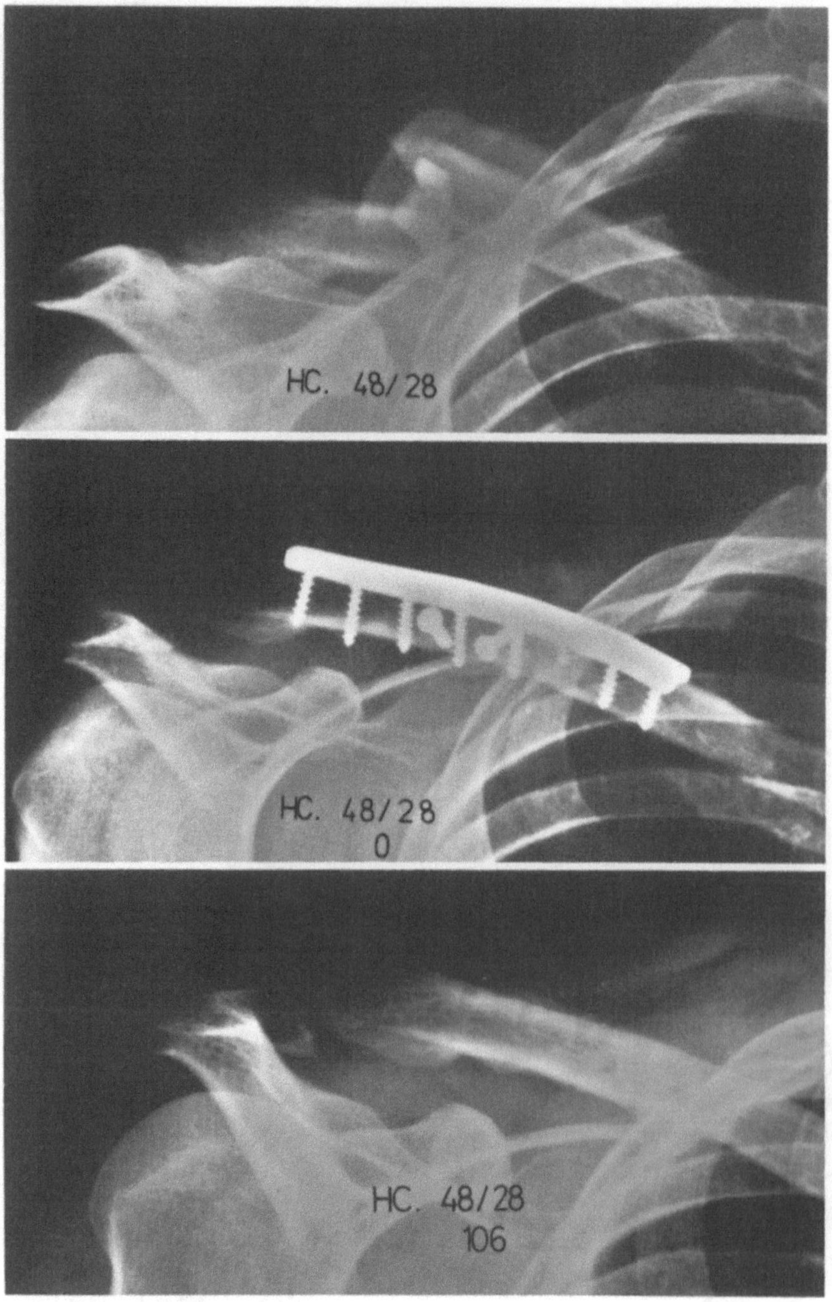

Fig. 55a–c. Clinical example: fracture of the middle third of the clavicle

Karl B., 42-year-old civil servant, fell on the right shoulder during a soccar game on 6/23/79

a Comminuted fracture of the middle third of the clavicle with impending perforation of the skin

b After closed reduction was tried unsuccessfully on 6/24/79, internal fixation was performed with a 3.5-mm, 8-hole DCP and two 3.5-mm cortex lag screws. The postoperative course was uneventful, and functional exercises were initiated. Patient returned to work at 2 weeks and had unrestricted shoulder motion at 8 weeks

c Implants were removed at 2 years.Patient had no pain, full shoulder motion, and a minimal scar.The cortex appears solid on X-rays

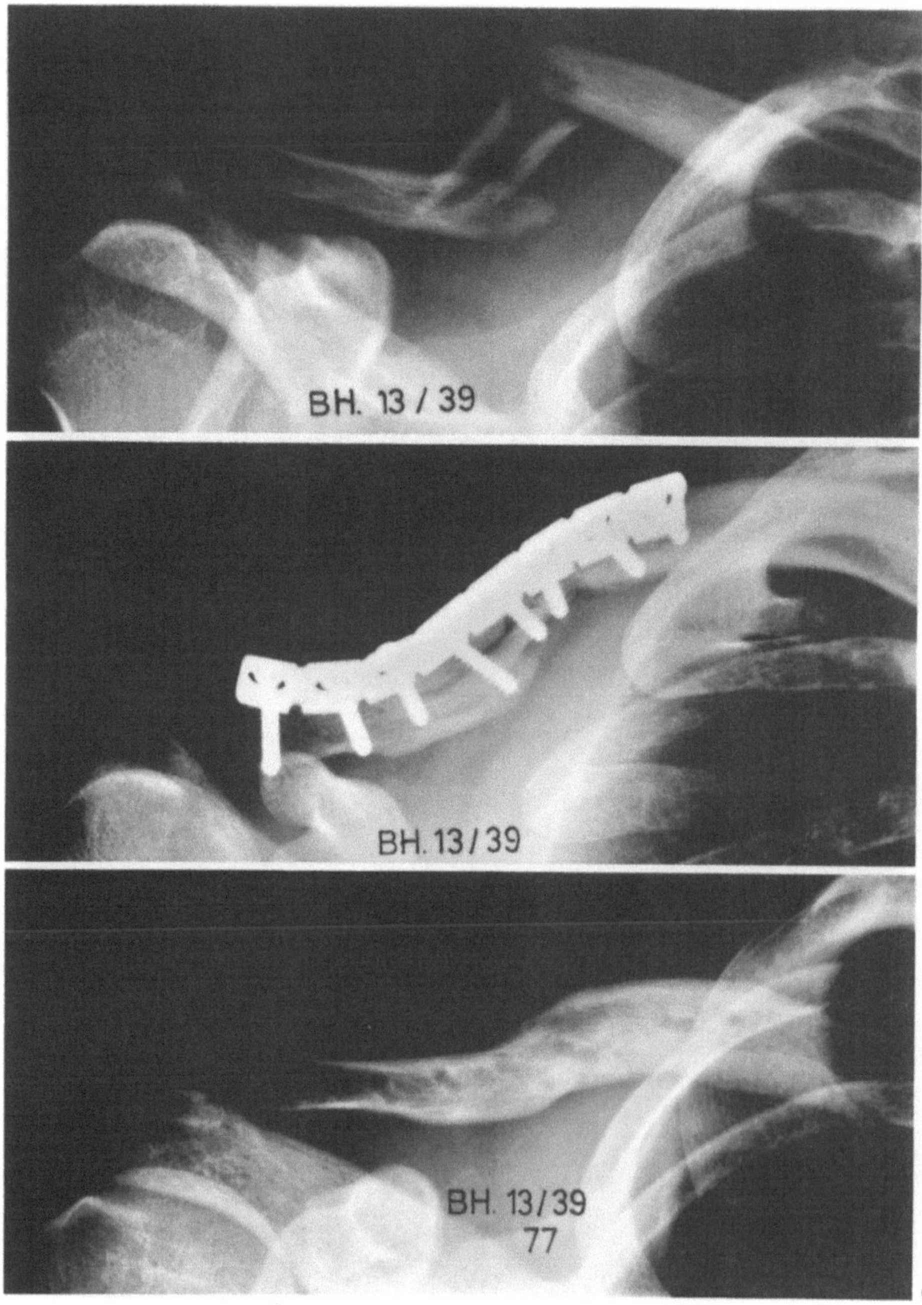

Fig. 56 a–c. Clinical example: primary internal fixation of the clavicle with a reconstruction plate

Giovanni S., 18-year-old auto mechanic, injured in a collision with another motorcycle on 6/17/84

a Segmental fracture of the right clavicle with impending skin perforation, cerebral concussion

b Internal fixation was performed 2 days later with a 3.5-mm reconstruction plate applied anteriorly. A seroma was drained at 2 weeks. The 3rd screw from the medial side loosened and was subsequently removed. Patient returned to work at 7 weeks with full shoulder motion. Fracture was solid at 4 months

c Implants were removed at 18 months on 1/31/86 at the request of the patient (who was bothered by the plate when wearing a knapsack). The fracture had healed; shoulder function was painless and equaled that on the unaffected side

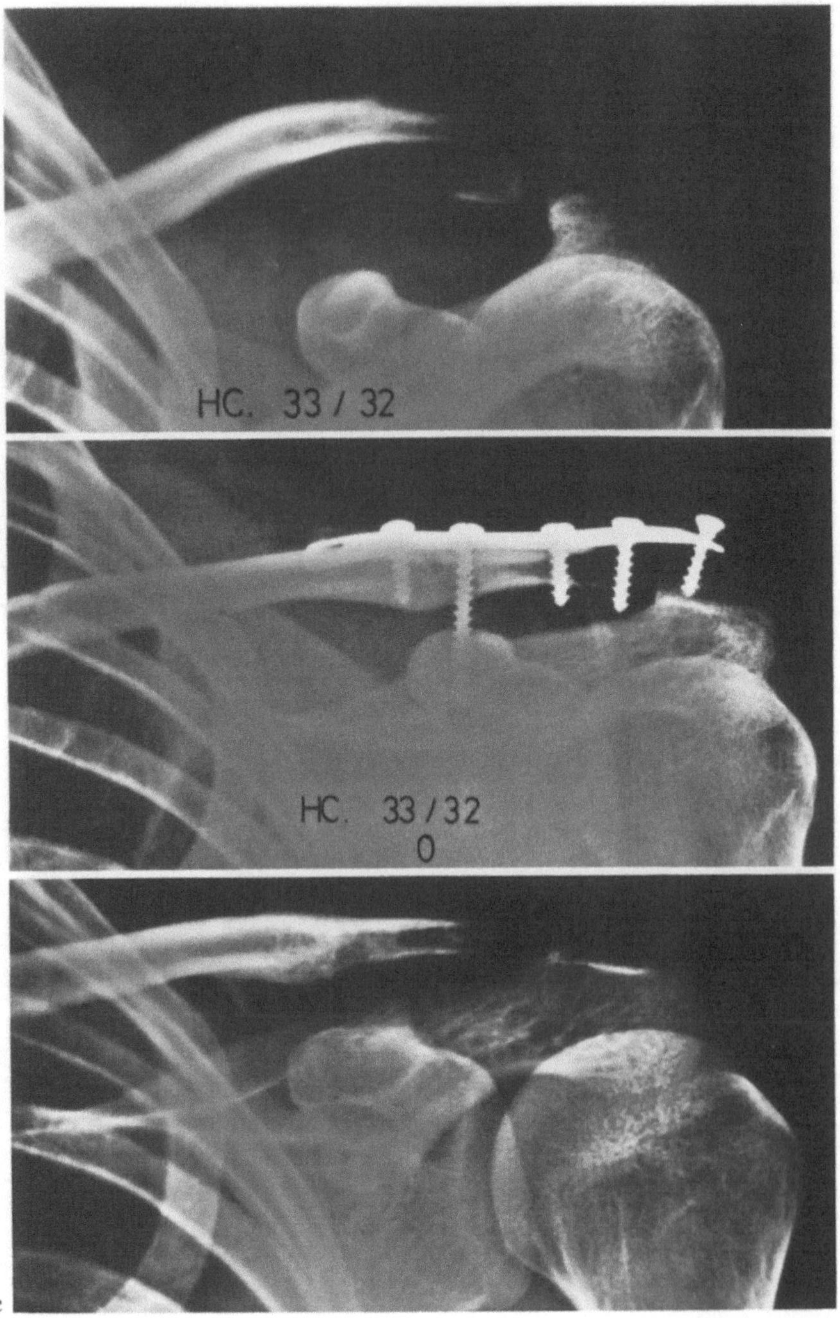

a
b
c

Fig. 57 a–c. Clinical example: lateral clavicular fracture with acromioclavicular joint injury

Anita M. P., 26-year-old needlework teacher, fell on the left shoulder during gymnastic exercises on 12/0/76; concussion

a Lateral fracture of the left clavicle with upward displacement due to rupture of the coracoclavicular ligament

b Internal fixation was performed 2 days later with a contoured one-third tubular plate. One plate screw was anchored in the coracoid process. With active mobilization the acromial screw loosened and was removed through a stab incision at 3 weeks. Patient had full shoulder motion at 6 weeks and returned to work. Implants were removed at 4 months

c Follow-up at 3 1/2 years on 3/19/80 showed unrestricted motion and a minimal scar. Patient was fully active in gymnastics

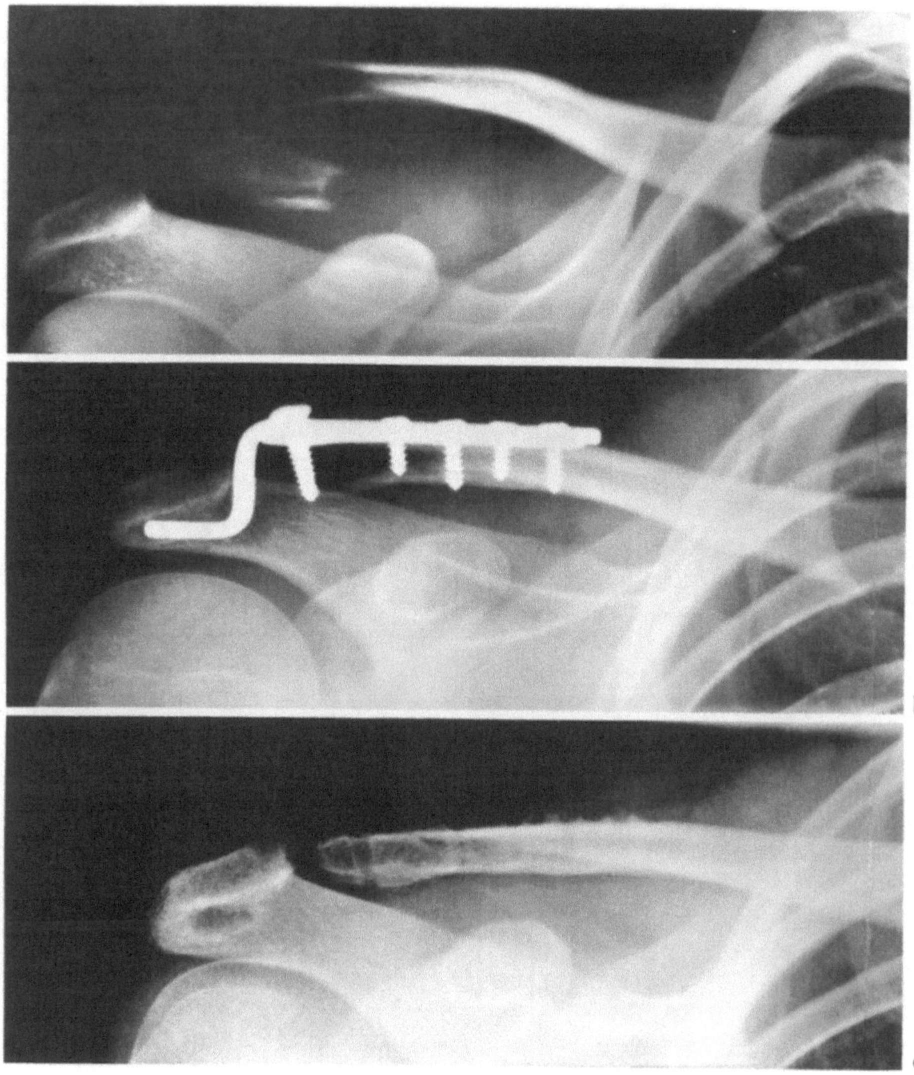

a

b

c

Fig. 58 a–c. Clinical example: unstable lateral clavicular fracture fixed with a special plate

Jose-Manuel S., 19-year-old bartender, injured in a fall from a bicycle

a Markedly displaced lateral fracture of the right clavicle, not amenable to closed reduction

b Internal fixation was performed with a Balser plate with an S-shaped subacromial extension. The shoulder was mobilized shortly after surgery. Patient resumed partial work load at 6 weeks and full load at 9 weeks

c Implants were removed at 14 months. Patient had full shoulder function with no pain or degenerative arthritis

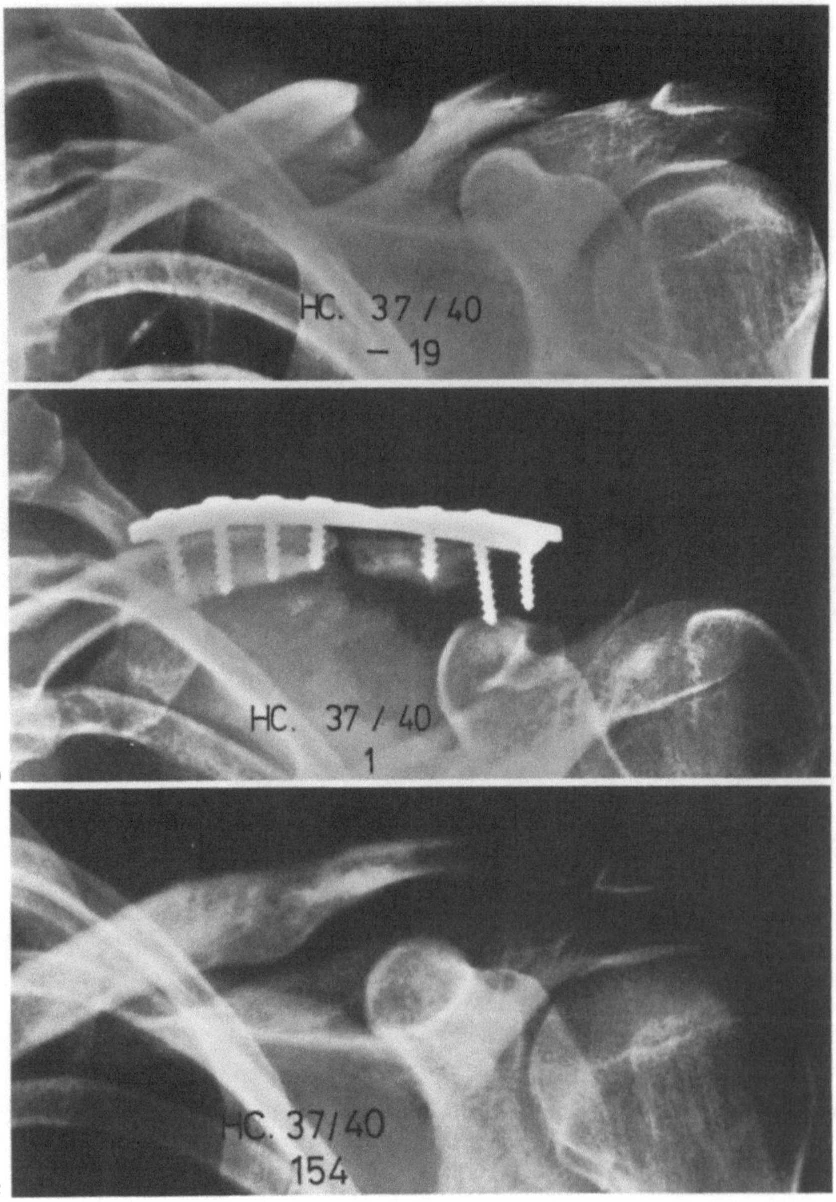

a

b

c

Fig. 59 a–c. Clinical example: nonunion of the clavicle with bone loss

Pius B., 28-year-old policeman, injured in a motorcycle accident on 7/12/75, sustaining a cerebral concussion and a fracture of the left clavicle that was not treated. Patient presented in spring of 1977 with pain and weakness of the left arm; nonunion was diagnosed

a Nonunion of the left clavicle with bone loss

b Internal fixation with a 3.5-mm 8-hole DCP was performed on 6/14/77. The screws grip six cortices in each main fragment, and the defect is bridged with iliac cancellous bone, visible on X-ray as a cloudy density.
Postoperative course was uneventful, and patient returned to work with full shoulder function at 8 weeks. Implants were removed at 1 year; patient had no pain, complete function, and a linear scar

c Follow-up at 3 years on 6/30/80 demonstrated normal structure of the clavicle. Patient has participated in two marathon races

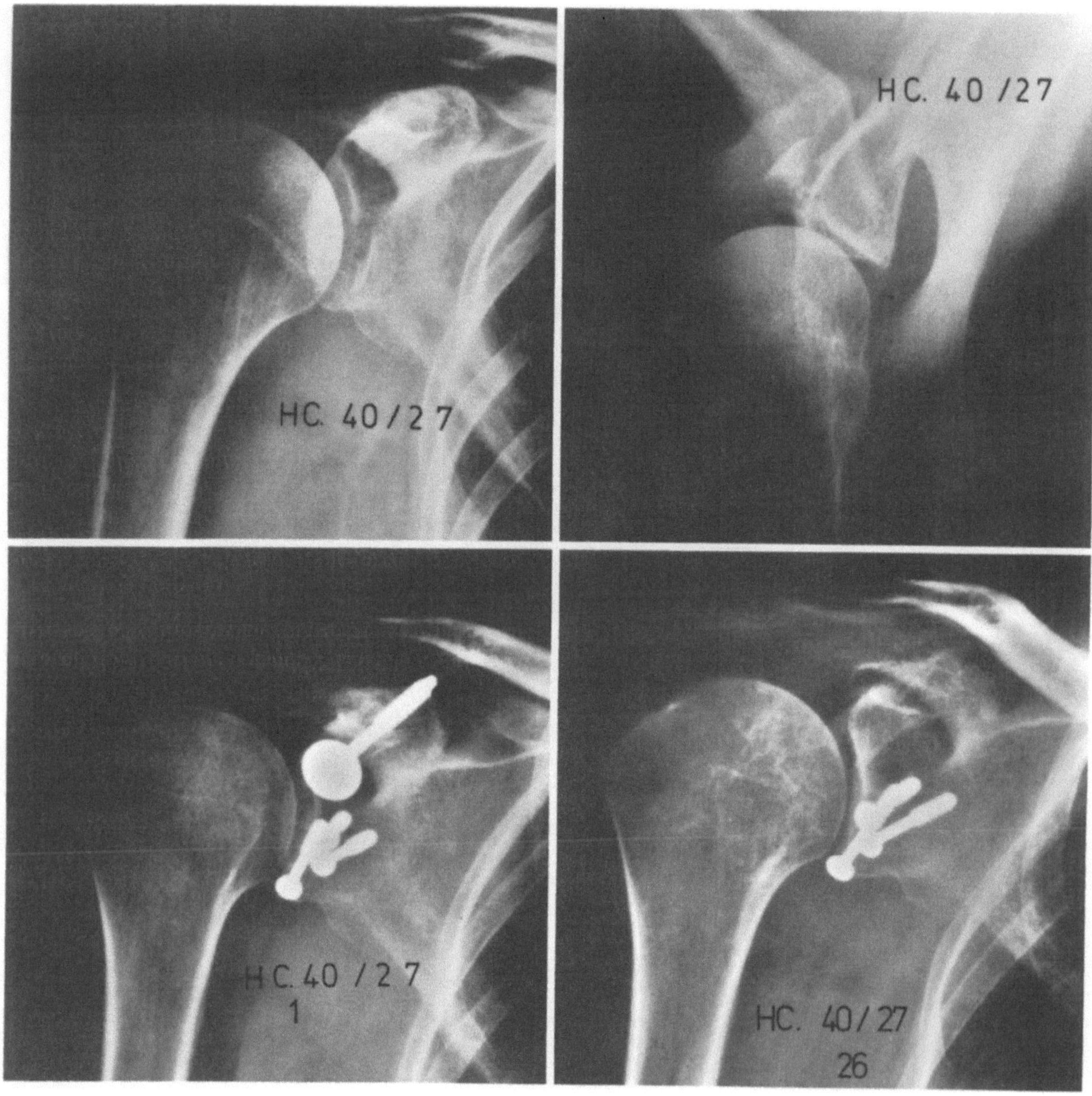

Fig. 60 a–c. Clinical example: fracture of the anterior glenoid rim

Liselotte N., 43-year-old secretary, fell on right shoulder while ice skating on 1/18/78. She saw her physician 2 days later and was referred for emergency treatment

a Fracture of the anterior rim of the right glenoid fossa

b Internal fixation was performed on 1/21/78. The mobile, markedly displaced rim fragment was reattached with three small cancellous screws. The coracoid process was osteotomized and reattached with a malleolar screw and washer.
The postoperative course was uncomplicated. Pendulum exercises were started at 2 weeks, active mobilization at 3 weeks

c Six months' follow-up on 7/17/78 showed slight residual limitation of shoulder elevation and rotation and a small linear scar. The osteotomy screw was removed from the coracoid; removal of the deep screws is not proposed

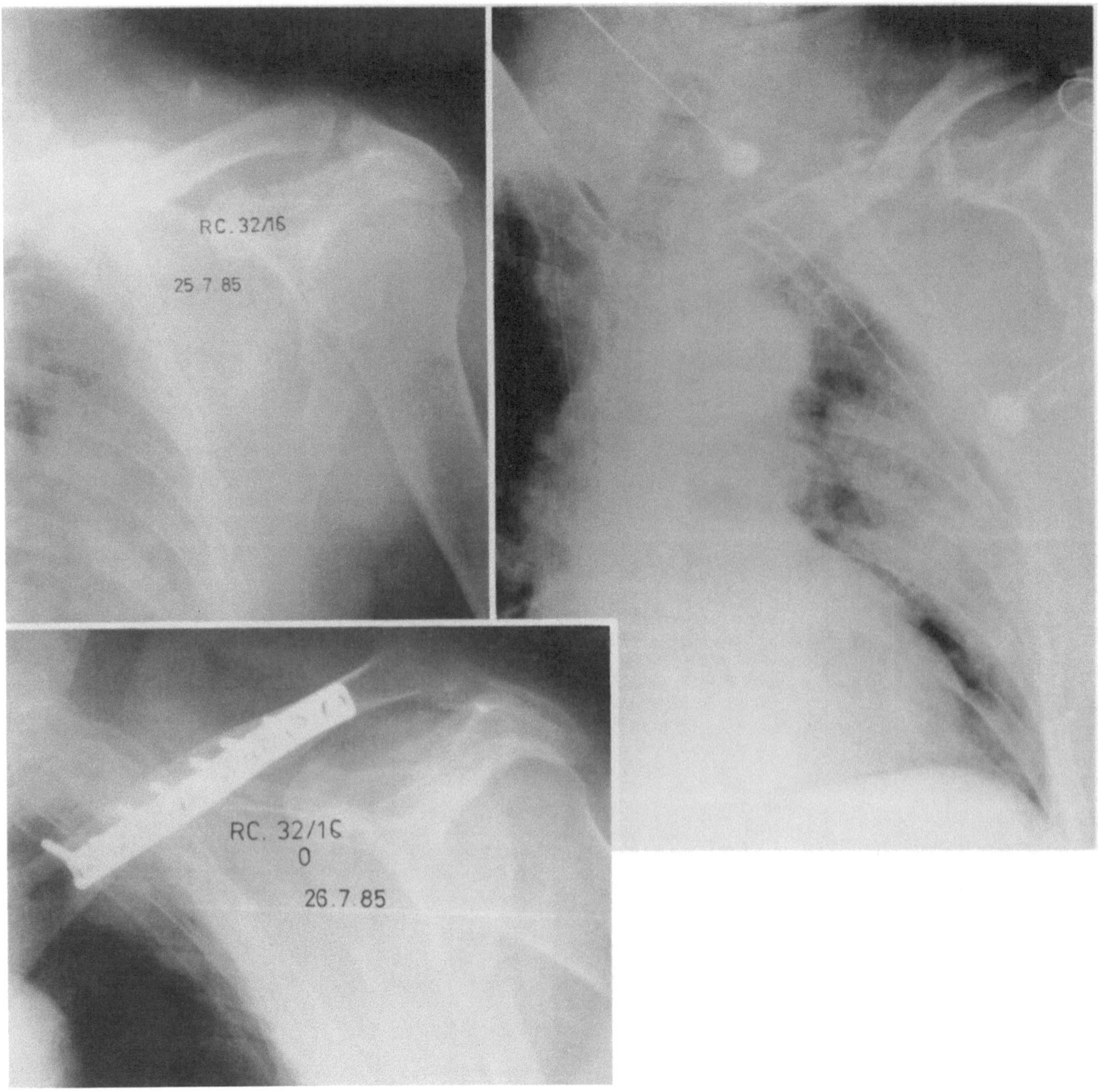

a

b

c

Fig. 61 a–c. Clinical example: medial scapular neck fracture, open fracture of the clavicle, serial rib fractures with left hemopneumothorax

Christian G., 61-year-old railway worker, struck curb with motorcycle on 7/25/85

a The fractures resulted in an unstable left shoulder girdle with skin penetration by the medial clavicular fragment

b Hemopneumothorax was evacuated with a Bülau drain

c Emergency stabilization of the shoulder girdle was accomplished by internal fixation of the clavicle with a 3.5-mm 8-hole DCP applied anteriorly. A Gilchrist bandage was worn for 1 week, with pendulum exercises started on day 4. Patient was discharged at 3 weeks with an irritation-free wound.The shoulder was rehabilitated with functional exercises. There were no pulmonary sequelae

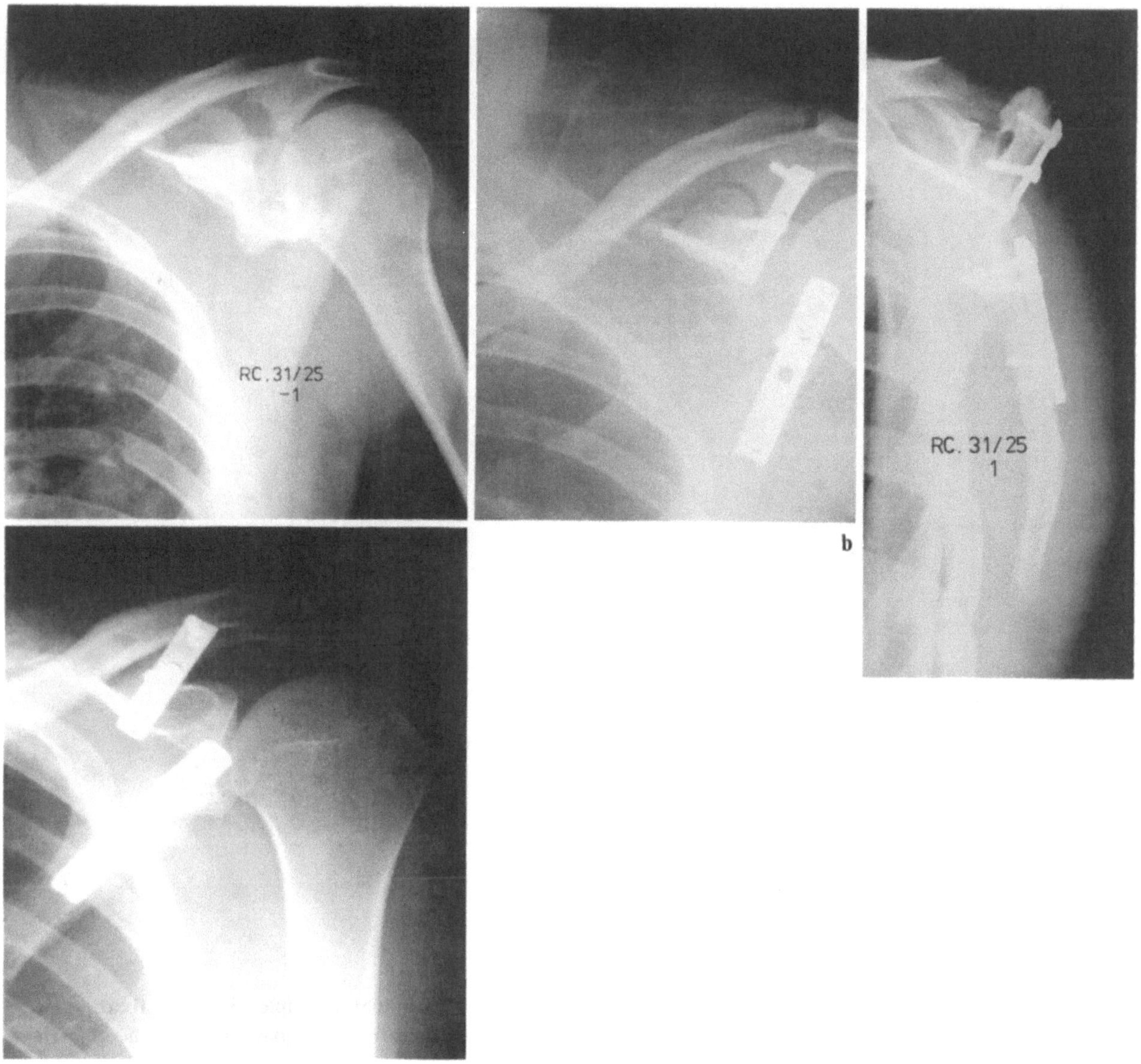

a b b′ c

Fig. 62a–c. Clinical example: displaced medial scapular neck fracture with a fracture of the scapular spine and ipsilateral serial rib fractures

Robert J., 24-year-old dairy employee, injured in auto accident on 9/27/85

a Postinjury radiograph of scapular and rib fractures

b Internal fixation was delayed until 10/4/85 due to multiple excoriations about the left shoulder girdle. The lateral border of the scapula was fixed with a 3.5-mm DCP, and the scapular spine with a 3-hole one-third tubular plate. Functional exercises were started after surgery

c Follow-up at 1 year showed complete fracture union and functional recovery. Removal of the implants is not proposed

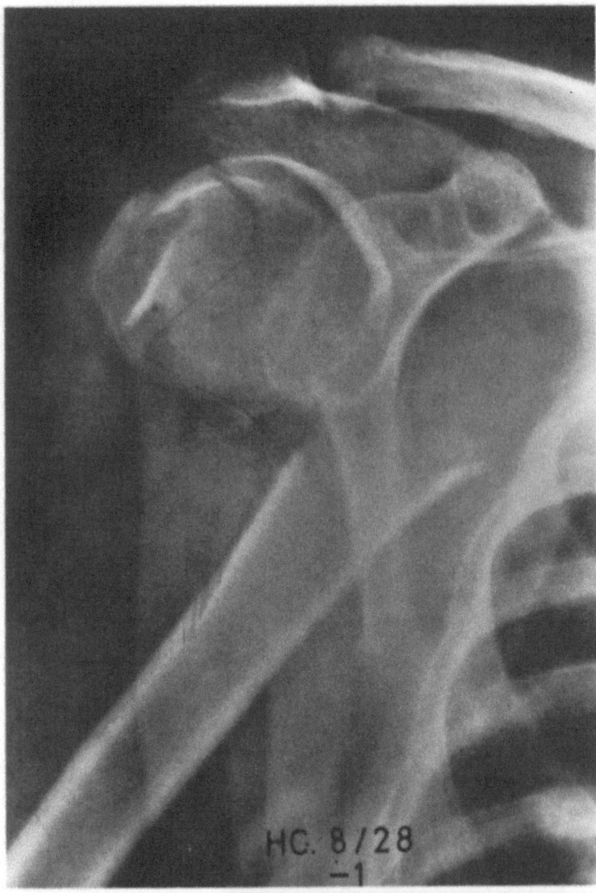

a

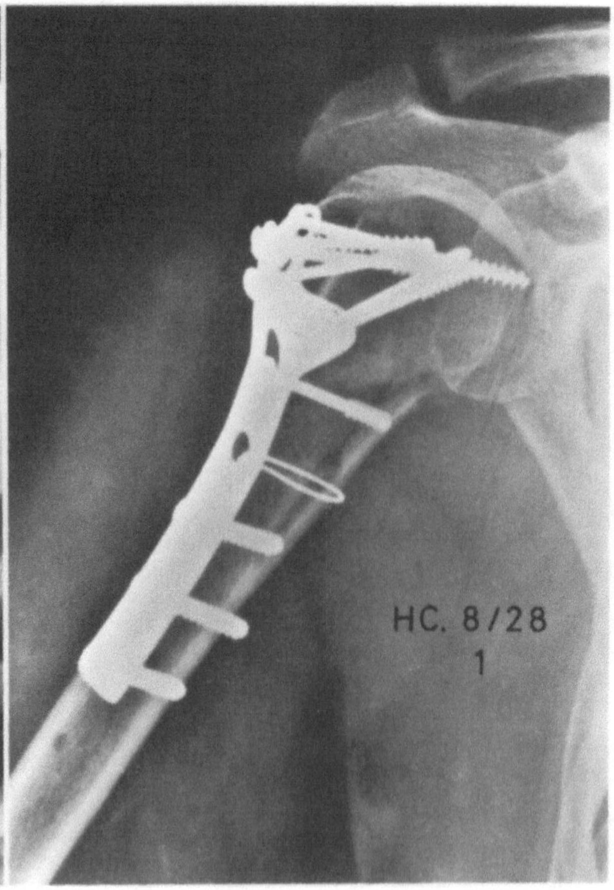

b

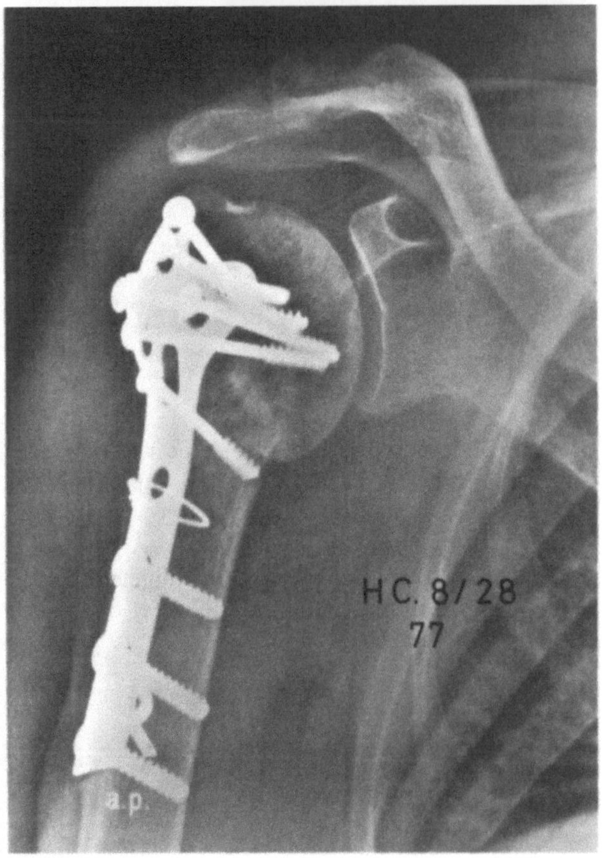

c

Fig. 63a–c. Clinical example: internal fixation of a subcapital fracture of the humerus with the cloverleaf plate

Rosa W., 58-year-old housewife, fell on icy steps on 2/25/72

a Grossly displaced and very mobile subcapital fracture of the humerus; also an ununited Colles fracture of the ipsilateral radius, with restricted motion and moderate circulatory impairment

b Internal fixation with a cloverleaf plate was performed on 2/29/72. The postoperative course was uneventful, and functional exercises were initiated

c X-ray at 18 months showed union of the fracture in slight varus. Patient declined to have the implants removed.
When contacted by telephone in July of 1980, the patient stated that her shoulder was painless and functioned very well. She will not present for clinical or X-ray examination, which she considers unnecessary in view of her condition

X. The Elbow

The elbow joint comprises three articulations: the hinge joint between the trochlea and proximal end of the ulna (olecranon, trochlear notch, coronoid process), which allows flexion and extension; the humeroradial joint between the capitellum and the concave articular surface of the radial head, which follows this movement; and the proximal radioulnar joint, consisting of the radial notch of the ulna, the circumference of the radial head, and the annular ligament, which binds the proximal end of the radius dynamically to the ulna and enables it to rotate about the ulna in any position of flexion or extension. The disc-like surface of the radial head transmits forces to the capitellum under axial loads and contributes much to the stability of the elbow joint on the radial side.

Whereas losses of terminal extension and flexion at the elbow can generally be well compensated for by the patient, limitations of pronation and supination can cause significant disability. Slight incongruities of the articular surfaces and the sequelae of fracture-dislocations with persistant instability can lead to traumatic arthritis. This explains the current tendency to favor anatomic reduction for displaced intra-articular fractures.

The various proven operative techniques are described below in some detail.

1. Distal Humerus

a) Fractures and Avulsions of the Condyles and Epicondyles

These fractures, which are most common in children and adolescents, must be accurately reduced to avoid later deformity. With dislocation, bony fragments may become incarcerated between the joint surfaces (e.g., entrapment of the common flexor origin after an avulsion fracture of the medial epicondyle in adolescents) (Fig. 65). Generally these fractures are stabilized with Kirschner wires in children, and with screws in adolescents and adults–usually two small cancellous or cortex lag screws (Fig. 76).

b) Intra-articular Fractures of the Distal Humerus

Open reduction and internal fixation are definitely indicated for these fractures, which are of two different types:

Simple Y Fracture

Bilateral exposure with lag screw fixation is often sufficient for this type of injury. A small cancellous screw is used for the trochlea, and long 3.5-mm cortex screws fix the reassembled articular fragment to the shaft (Fig. 65b).

Complex Comminuted Fracture Involving the Trochlea

Reduction of these fractures can be extremely difficult but generally is possible if done systematically:

Preparations. Preparations are made for harvesting iliac cancellous bone, and a pneumatic tourniquet is applied to the proximal upper arm.

Positioning. Positioning is done carefully to avoid neurapraxia of the brachial plexus. Either of two positions may be used: prone or lateral decubitus. In the prone position the elbow is flexed over a carefully placed, well-padded roll.

In this way the elbow will remain mobile and can be flexed past 90° during the operation (Fig. 64d). When the patient is on his side, the upper arm is supported on a roll at the level of the pneumatic tourniquet so that the elbow can be flexed to about 120° (Fig. 64c).

In older patients and in patients with multiple injuries, anesthetic constraints may require that the operation be performed in the lateral or supine position under regional anesthesia.

Incision. The skin incision is 25-30 cm long and curves around the radial side of the olecranon. It must afford complete exposure of the dorsal aspect of the joint (Fig. 66). The ulnar nerve is identified in the sulcus, snared with a tape, and gently retracted. In some circumstances subcutaneous or volar transposition of the nerve may be necessary at the end of the procedure.

Approach with Osteotomy of the Olecranon (Fig. 67). This is necessary to gain optimum exposure of the trochlea. Our experience is that this metaphyseal osteotomy heals rapidly and without sequelae.Today we recommend a V-shaped osteotomy in preference to a straight cut, and we generally reconstruct with parallel Kirschner wires and a tension-band wire. The ends of the Kirschner wires are bent 180°, and absorbable sutures are placed to check dorsal migration of the wires.

Technique of the V Osteotomy. Under the protection of two Hohmann retractors, a deep, V-shaped notch is made in the olecranon at the level of the trochlea with an oscillating saw. The cut is continued into the joint with a fine osteotome. The olecranon is reflected proximally to expose the distal humerus and fractured trochlea.

Alternative. A straight, oblique osteotomy is made toward the joint center. The olecranon is reattached with a 3.5-mm cortex lag screw and wire-loop tension band (Fig. 67f).

Reconstruction of the Trochlea (Fig. 68). This is the most important step of the internal fixation. Often the fragments are markedly displaced, but even isolated or devitalized fragments should be accurately replaced rather than removed.True osseous defects are rare in these cases and should be grafted with autogenous cancellous bone.

Kirschner wires are used for reduction and provisional fixation. The first wire serves as a guide, so its accurate placement is critical. The blunt end of the wire is sharpened for retrograde insertion. First the wire is drilled through the center of the radial fragment from the ulnar side (i.e., through the fracture surface). It is then used as a lever to assist the reduction and is drilled back through the central trochlear fragment(s) in retrograde fashion. A 2.5-mm hole is drilled parallel to this wire, and a small cancellous screw is inserted to produce interfragmental compression (Fig. 68b). The usual screw length is 45–50 mm. The original Kirschner wire may be left in place to enhance rotational stability, or it may be replaced with a second screw. If part of the articular surface is missing, a 3.5-mm cortex screw is used in place of a cancellous screw to maintain the anatomic width of the trochlea (Fig. 69c).

Joining the Trochlea to the Humeral Metaphysis (Fig. 69). The trochlea having been stabilized, it is necessary to unite the articular assembly with the distal humeral metaphysis. This may be accomplished with long one-third tubular plates (5- to 7-hole) or with the 3.5-mm reconstruction plate, depending on the extent of the fracture, its location, and the number of fragments. It is essential that the plate be accurately contoured and fitted to the bone. Today the reconstruction plate is used with increasing frequency owing to its excellent stability and ease of contouring.Internal fixation material should be kept out of the olecranon fossa and coronoid fossa so that it will not restrict terminal flexion and extension. Medially the plate should be kept away from the ulnar nerve; it is advantageous to place the ulnar plate on the medial ridge and the radial plate dorsolaterally. Most surgeons no longer recommend interconnecting the plates proximally with a central screw or the use of a Y plate, as this increases the technical difficulty of the procedure and of implant removal.

In simpler fractures, the second plate may be replaced with a single long screw uniting the trochlea and distal shaft.

After the internal fixation is completed, the olecranon is reattached as described above.

Wound Closure. A suction drain is inserted, and the wound is closed in one layer with cutaneous sutures. Scarification may be advisable if contusion is severe. Initially the limb is placed in about 80° flexion in a removable, padded plaster splint and is elevated to avoid pressure injury about the wound.

Aftertreatment. This depends on the stability achieved. It is recommended that a removable plaster splint be worn for several weeks. We use a "slip-on" splint that is open dorsoradially and permits active assisted exercises. Comminuted fractures take 12 weeks or more to become solid enough to withstand loading. Flexion generally is recovered more rapidly than extension, and some limitation of terminal extension may persist. If implant removal is necessary, it usually is done in two stages. First the ulnar nerve is examined clinically and perhaps tested by electromyography. If there is evidence of irritation or residual paresis, anterior transposition of the nerve and neurolysis generally can be performed at the time the ulnar implants are removed. In any case, the ulnar nerve must be reidentified and protected whenever it is necessary to remove an implant from the ulnar side.

Secondary Operations. Nonunions of the distal humerus are uncommon. Persistent pain should raise suspicion of instability and justifies reintervention. Post-traumatic deformities are often complex since both the radial and ulnar pillars are involved. Corrective surgery must be planned with utmost care. Autogenous corticocancellous bone grafts are mandatory following decortication and freshening of the bone ends. Nonunions are fixed either with the 3.5-mm DCP, which is relatively difficult to contour, or with the 3.5-mm reconstruction plate (Fig. 86). Both are preferred over the one-third tubular plate.

2. Radial Head

Today it is widely recognized that the radial head plays a key role in the transmission of forces from the wrist to the upper arm and shoulder ("radial pillar") and is an important stabilizer of the elbow. Further experimental studies are needed, however, to determine the magnitude of these forces.

"Isolated" fractures of the radial head are almost invariably caused by a fall onto the extended and pronated hand. In this injury triceps innervation brings the elbow reflexly to a defensive position of subtotal extension (30° flexion) and slight valgus. On impact the joint is subjected to a peak load of very brief duration (10–20 ms) occurring before innervation of the muscular stabilizers that protect the joint.

The recent literature uses the classification of radial head fractures proposed by Mason in 1954:

Type 1 = undisplaced fracture
Type 2 = wedge fracture with displacement
Type 3 = comminuted fracture
Type 4 = posterior fracture-dislocation with associated ulnar fracture

Many years of experience suggest a need to supplement types 2 and 3, particularly with regard to patient selection and operative technique (Fig. 71):

- The displacement in a wedge fracture may consist of a step or a gaping fissure with cartilage interposed (Fig. 71a).
- Comminuted fractures in the true sense are rare and are far less common than depressed fractures of the articular surface in which one wall of the head is still intact and the fragments are viable (Fig. 71b).
- We also must differentiate fractures of the radial neck, in which there is marginal compression of the cancellous bone and the disc-like articular face is angulated and requires realignment (Fig. 71c).

Undisplaced radial head fractures should be treated conservatively with functional exercises (early mobilization from a removable splint).

Displaced radial head fractures are generally considered to be an indication for surgery. The following problems should be noted:

- Biplane spot films are necessary to evaluate the displacement. Following the injury the elbow is painful and cannot be extended. AP projections should be taken perpendicular to the radial head, not the humerus (Fig. 70).
- One must be alert for coexisting injuries. An "isolated" fracture can occur only if there has been stretching or rupture of capsuloliga-

mentous structures. The possibility of a spontaneously reduced dislocation should not be overlooked. The valgus force can produce ligamentous tears or small avulsion fractures on the ulnar side which affect the stability of the entire elbow. These injuries are easily overlooked on primary evaluation. Untreated ligamentous tears can later lead to restricted motion and calcification (Fig. 71).

- Tears of the interosseous membrane, which is essential to forearm stability, are visible only on arthrograms; they are not apparent clinically.Interosseous tears should be suspected if the radial head is found to be unusually mobile and easily exposed when internal fixation is carried out. These tears probably account for the secondary changes in the distal radioulnar joint that have been reported by various authors, and which often are clinically significant.

Clinical experience suggests that the tears will heal without sequelae under a program of nonstrenuous postoperative exercise. In any case, we have seen no limitations of pronation and supination following internal fixations in our patients.

Radial head fractures also may be one component of a fracturedislocation of both forearm bones.In a Monteggia fracture with anterior dislocation of the radial head, the head remains intact and generally will reduce spontaneously with internal fixation of the ulna. Suturing of the capsule and ligaments, especially the annular ligament, is necessary only if dislocation persists.

With a posterior fracture-dislocation (Mason type 4), the ulna is usually fractured in its proximal third, and a shear fracture or comminuted fracture of the radial head is frequently present. It is very important to get an anatomic reconstruction in these cases to prevent instability and arthritic change in the elbow.

Partial excision of the radial head has been shown to promote degenerative arthritis and has been abandoned by most surgeons. Total excision of the radial head should be reserved for the exceptional situations in which an anatomic reconstruction is not possible, or significant devascularization has occurred.

We classify the fractures into four types from the standpoint of operative reconstruction:

a) Wedge Fractures (Fig. 71 a)

These are by far the most common type and account for approximately two-thirds of cases.

In these fractures a marginal segment of the radial head has been sheared off by an asymmetric load, leaving a portion of the head intact. Displaced fractures are fixed operatively with screws.

Pieces of cartilage are frequently sheared off from the humeral articular surface by the trauma and become entrapped between the radial head fragments, posing an obstacle to reduction. Sometimes they are manifested on X-rays by a gaping fracture line.

b) Depressed Fractures (Fig. 71 b)

Marginal, cap-like depressions of the radial head as well as central depressions of the articular surface, combined with a wedge fracture, are common and are difficult to appreciate on X-ray films. Defects should be filled with cancellous bone to improve stability and encourage revascularization. Only a small amount of bone graft is needed and may be obtained from the adjacent lateral epicondyle of the humerus. This site is readily accessible in the extended approach (Fig. 72b).

c) Comminuted Fractures

Generally an anatomic reconstruction is possible even in complex fractures. Usually one wall of the radial head is intact and periosteal connections are preserved, making it possible to stabilize the fracture with screws. Defects are grafted with cancellous bone.In exceptional cases we have used mini plates to stabilize comminuted fractures. Because these devices interfere with pronation and supination, they should be removed at the earliest opportunity. This reconstructive procedure is definitely superior to resection, although resection remains an option if late complications arise.

If resection is unavoidable, we generally recommend replacing the radial head with a prosthesis to preserve stability and avoid secondary valgus, even though the complex anatomy and function of the radial head do not make it particularly amenable to prosthetic replacement. In our experience and that of other authors, the silastic prosthesis of Swanson appears to give good results. A new model is being produced that has an extra long head. The flexible implant is able to adapt well to the surrounding skeleton, but it yields to impact and pressure and does not transmit forces well. Various metallic and plastic prostheses are also available which are either cemented into place or have locking mechanisms for their attachment. Presumably these devices would be better able to transmit forces.

d) Radial Neck Fractures (Fig. 71 c)

These are common in children, and many are amenable to closed reduction.

In adults, it is necessary to realign the angulated head. The resulting marginal defect is filled with cancellous bone. The head is stabilized with oblique screws that are placed in the fashion of supporting or retention screws (Fig. 84).

e) Approach and Internal Fixation

Standard Approach (Figs 64 a, 72 a). The radial head is approached through a longitudinal incision starting at the lateral epicondyle. The extensor muscles are split in line with their fibers, respecting the proximity of the deep branch of the radial nerve. This nerve courses more anteriorly, passing over the joint capsule of the radial head. The annular ligament presents as a thickening of the joint capsule and is rarely identifiable as a separate structure. The fracture is exposed by rotating the forearm. Hohmann retractors should not be placed on the ulnar side of the head, as this might cause pressure injury to the radial nerve (Fig. 72a); the assistant should be instructed accordingly. The radial head may, however, be gently elevated with a blunt retractor braced against the lateral epicondyle. Material interposed between the fragments is removed with a small hook. Depressed areas are elevated, and detached fragments are replaced while preserving periosteal attachments. Temporary fixation is obtained with the fine, pointed forceps that are ordinarily used for hand surgery (termite forceps, stag-beetle forceps) or with fine Kirschner wires. Definitive fixation is obtained with at least two screws or as many as three to five screws inserted parallel to the joint on different planes. In recent years we have used 1.5-mm mini screws almost exclusively, which come in lengths up to 20 mm and can be driven into the articular surface of the proximal radioulnar joint without concern. The screw heads are countersunk in the cartilage slightly so that they will not hinder rotation (Fig. 73).

The joint is closed in one layer with absorbable through-andthrough sutures that encompass the joint capsule and the fibrous layers (Fig. 73 d). It is unnecessary to place a separate suture in the annular ligament, which usually presents as a thickening of the capsule. Postoperative exercises will not stretch the ligament if an anatomic reconstruction has been achieved. A suction drain is inserted.

Extended Approach (Fig. 72b). In complex fractures or when exposure is inadequate, the original incision may be extended dorsoproximally with an angled cut. The epicondyle is exposed, drilled and tapped, and a small cancellous screw 24–28 mm long is inserted over a spiked metal or plastic washer. After solid seating of the screw is confirmed, the screw is twisted back out of the bone, and the epicondyle is osteotomized with a small chisel. The fragment is then reflected to the side along with the adherent radial capsule and muscular origins. This affords excellent exposure of the entire radial head. Very good-quality cancellous bone can be harvested from the osteotomized humeral surface with a small curet and packed into radial head defects; this should not interfere with the reconstruction. Following internal fixation of the radial head, the osteotomized fragment is reattached with the original cancellous screw. The joint is closed as in the standard approach.

Posterior Approach (Fig. 74d). We favor the prone position for operations on posterior fracture-dislocation of the elbow. Preparations are the same as for comminuted fractures of the distal humerus. An incision is made for exposing the olecranon and ulnar fracture. The first structure to appear in the field is the prominent, dislocated radial head. The radial head fracture is reduced and reconstructed using the technique described above. Next the ulnar fracture is reduced, at which time the dislocated radial head will return spontaneously to its anatomic position. As a rule, we do not advise later implant removal from the radial head because of the deep exposure that would be required.

f) Aftertreatment

The arm is elevated and immobilized in a removable posterior plaster splint with the elbow placed in 90° flexion and intermediate rotation.

Active exercises are started after the wound has healed, beginning with pronation/supination and later progressing to flexion and extension (which involve greater muscular traction). The removable splint is discarded after 4–8 weeks, depending on the type of fracture and the stability. Full loading is not allowed before 10–12 weeks in patients with depressed and comminuted fractures. Implant removal is necessary only if the patient finds the palpable screw heads to be troublesome. Fairly early implant removal (i.e., at 4–5 months) is recommended for purely cancellous fractures.

g) Secondary Operations

Indications for secondary operations include traumatic arthritis after conservative treatment of displaced radial head fractures and painful deformity secondary to rheumatoid disease. Reconstructive measures are no longer feasible in these cases, and the radial head has to be excised. Prosthetic replacement is recommended to preserve the length of the radius and the stability of the elbow. We prefer the Swanson silastic prosthesis.

3. Olecranon

The great majority of olecranon fractures are fixed primarily with tension-band wires, followed by functional aftertreatment. A detailed discussion of these fractures is presented in the *Manual of Internal Fixation*. Use of the SFS is limited to the following special indications:

a) Oblique Fracture

A classic tension-band system will produce an asymmetric compressive force in this type of fracture, so an additional lag screw should be used to obtain uniform interfragmental compression (Fig. 74b).

Simple screw fixation may be acceptable for long oblique fractures and simple undisplaced fissures, especially in children (Fig. 254).

b) Fracture of the Coronoid Process

Small chip fractures of the coronoid process may occur during a dislocation of the elbow or during its reduction.These do not require internal fixation, but temporary immobilization in a plaster splint is advised.

More extensive avulsions of the coronoid process disrupt the congruity of the hinge joint. Usually the fragment is displaced by muscular traction, and anatomic reduction and internal fixation are indicated. Generally this can be accomplished with a small cancellous screw inserted through an ulnar approach (Fig. 74c).Exposure is optimized by combining this with an epicondyle osteotomy that spares the muscular origins.The procedure then resembles that described in the extended approach to the radial head. Care is taken at operation to identify and protect the ulnar nerve.

c) Comminuted Fractures

Simple tension-band wiring may be insufficient for many of these fractures. Good results have been obtained with the one-third tubular plate. The plate should be of sufficient length (6–8 holes) and anatomically contoured. The first screw is driven into the tip of the olecranon. Then tension is applied to the plate either by means of an eccentric drill hole or with the articulated tension device (Fig. 74a). Usually it is necessary to place additional screws on different planes. Bony defects are grafted with autogenous cancellous bone.

d) Approach and Operative Technique

General inhalation anesthesia or a plexus block is used. The patient is positioned supine with a pneumatic tourniquet applied to the upper arm and the forearm placed across the chest. The wrist is secured with a towel that may be held by an assistant, clamped to the drapes, or held taut by a weight on the opposite side of the table (Fig. 64a).

An alternative is to place the hand and forearm on a padded rest (infusion board) mounted transversely above the chest so that the elbow is raised above the level of the upper arm (Fig. 64b).

The approach is made through a skin incision that curves gently around the olecranon on the radial side. In complex fractures it is crucial to identify and protect the ulnar nerve. The fracture is reduced and fixed temporarily with forceps, hooks, or fine Kirschner wires.

e) Fracture-Dislocations

In a posterior fracture-dislocation involving both forearm bones, a fracture of the radial head is generally present. Generally the patient is positioned prone with the arm flexed over a side rest (Fig. 64d). If the patient's general condition prohibits this, the supine position is an acceptable alternative (Fig. 64b). The incision is the same as that used for distal humeral fractures. First the radial head is stabilized using the technique described above. With reduction of the ulna, the radial head will reduce spontaneously in most cases. Fixation of the ulnar or olecranon fracture follows the technique described for comminuted fractures.

If the ulnar fracture is located farther distally on the diaphysis, where greater bending and shear forces are imposed, a long DCP for 3.5-mm screws should be used in preference to the one-third tubular plate.

f) Secondary Operations

Nonunions of the olecranon are rare and are managed by the same techniques described above, using either the one-third tubular plate or 3.5-mm DCP applied under appropriate tension. An atrophic nonunion additionally requires autogenous bone grafting, possibly combined with decortication.

4. Illustrative Clinical X-Rays (Figs. 75-86)

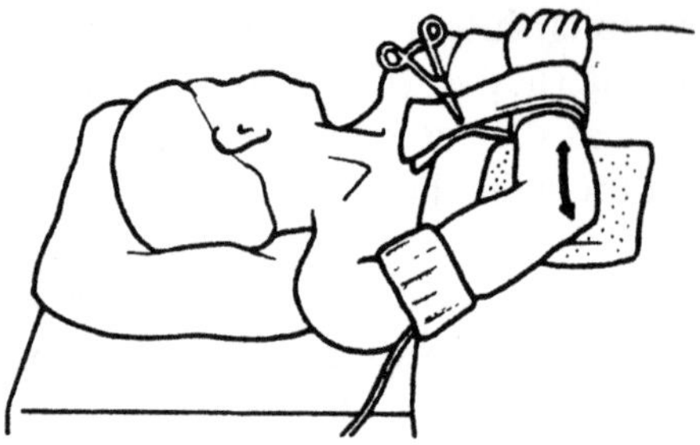

a

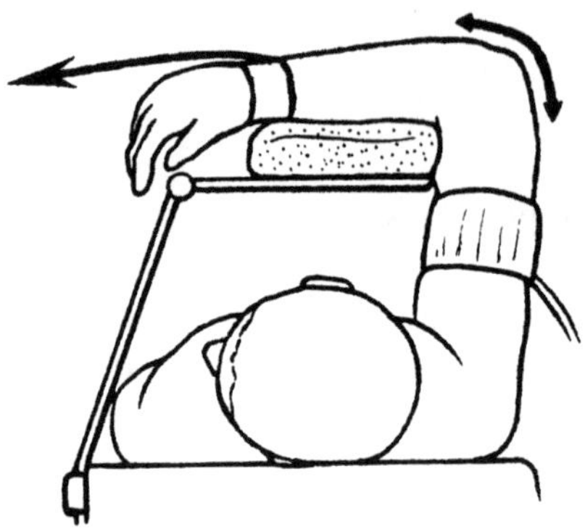

b

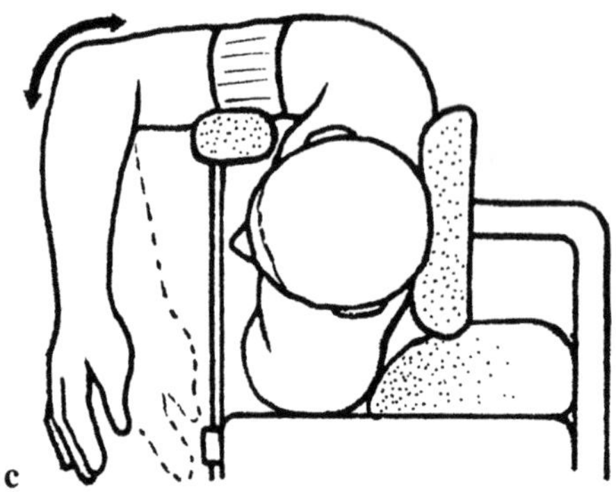

c

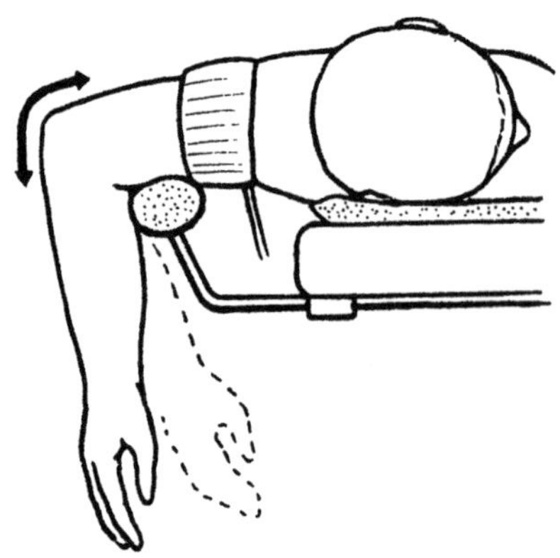

d

Fig. 64 a–d. Standard positions for internal fixations about the elbow

Positions **a** and **b** are suitable for exposures of the radial head and olecranon, **c** and **d** for complex fractures of the distal humerus and fracture-dislocations of the radius and ulna

a Supine position with a pneumatic tourniquet and the flexed elbow supported by a pad on the chest. The wrist may be fastened to the sheet with a sling and towel clip, or it may be pulled toward the opposite side by a traction weight

b Supine position with the elbow elevated on a padded arm board. The wrist sling is held to one side by a traction weight

c Lateral decubitus with the elbow flexed and supported by a padded rest under the tourniquet. The elbow may be flexed past 90°

d Prone position with the elbow flexed over a padded rest. Flexion is unrestricted

Fig. 66. Comminuted intra-articular fracture of the distal humerus: incision

The incision and approach bypass the olecranon with the elbow flexed. The ulnar nerve is retracted with a tape. The line of the olecranon osteotomy is shown

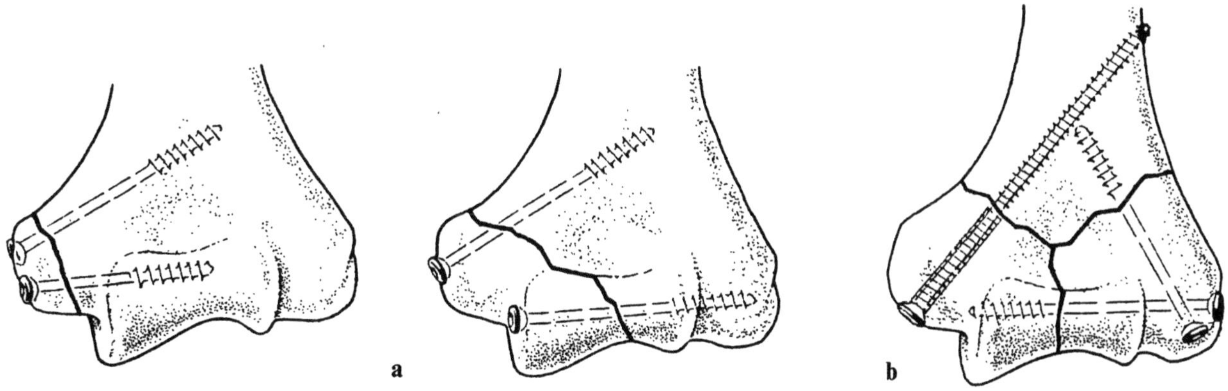

Fig. 65 a, b. Internal fixation of simple fractures of the distal humerus

a Fixation of condylar and epicondylar fractures in adults through a unilateral approach. The ulnar nerve must be identified and protected on the ulnar side

b A minimally displaced intra-articular Y fracture is approached bilaterally, and the trochlea is fixed with a small cancellous screw. The pillars are repaired with a cancellous or long 3.5-mm cortex screw

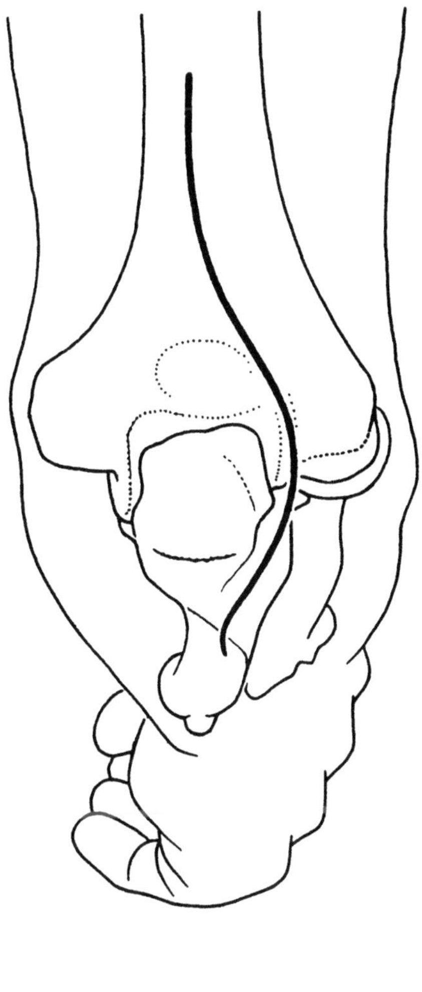

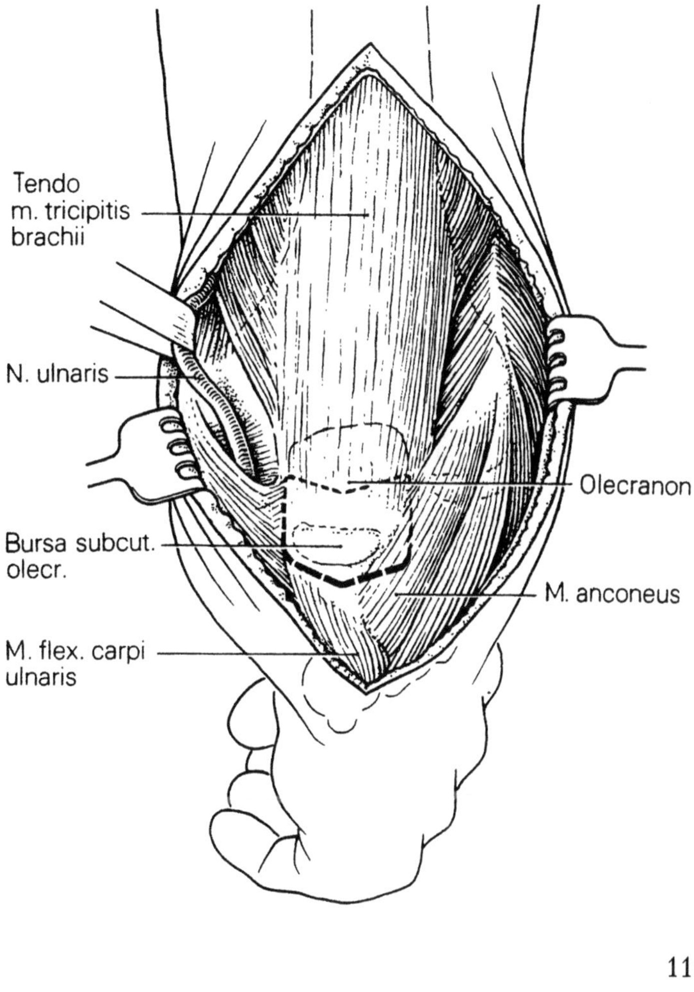

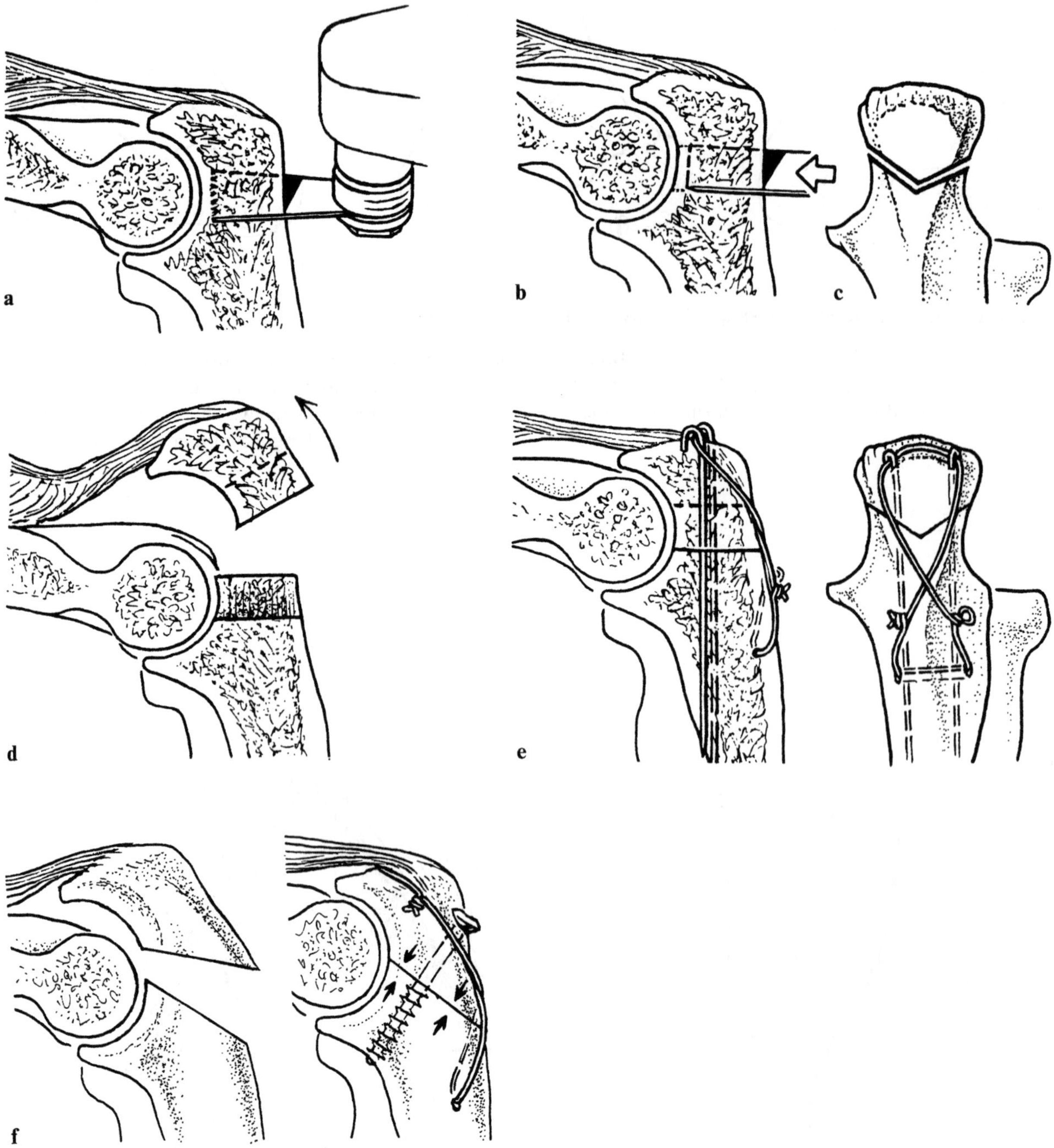

Fig. 67 a–f. Osteotomy of the olecranon for access to the trochlea

a A deep, V-shaped notch is cut with the oscillating saw

b The cut is continued into the joint space with a fine osteotome

c Dorsal view of the saw cut

d The osteotomized olecranon is reflected upward

e The olecranon is reattached with a wire tension band

f Alternative: straight oblique osteotomy toward the center of the hinge joint. The fragment is later reattached with a lag screw and tension band

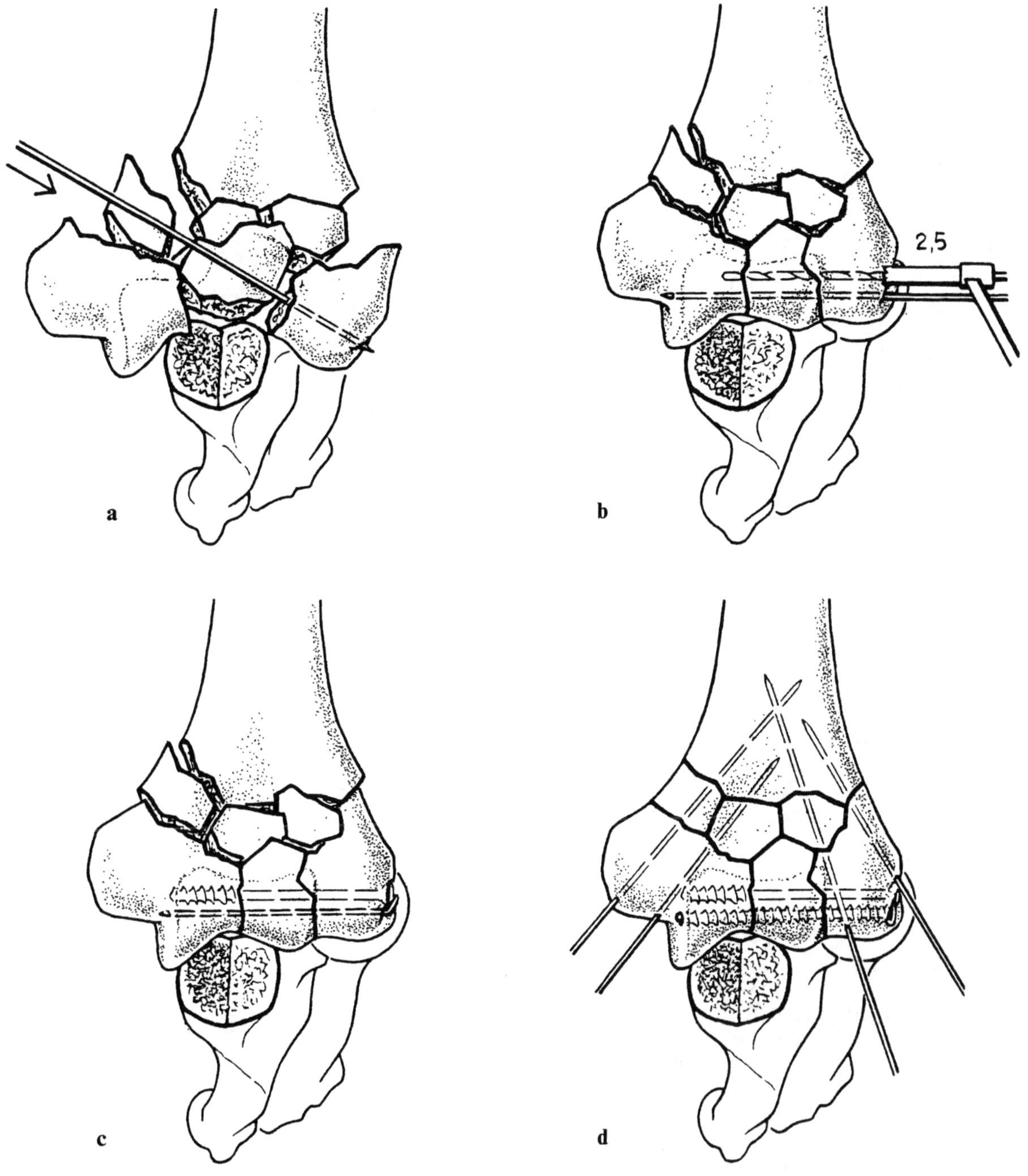

Fig. 68 a–d. Reconstruction of the trochlea in a comminuted intra-articular fracture

a A Kirschner guide wire (1.6-mm diam.), sharpened at both ends, is twisted into the radial fragment from the ulnar side

b The guide wire, serving as a lever, is drilled back into the reduced trochlear fragments.The guide hole in the handle of the drill guide is threaded over the wire, and a parallel 2.5-mm hole is drilled through the fracture

c The hole is tapped, and a compressive cancellous screw is inserted

d The Kirschner wire may be left in place for rotational stability, or it may be replaced with a second screw (3.5-mm cortex)
The reassembled trochlea is reduced to the humeral metaphysis and tentatively fixed with Kirschner wires

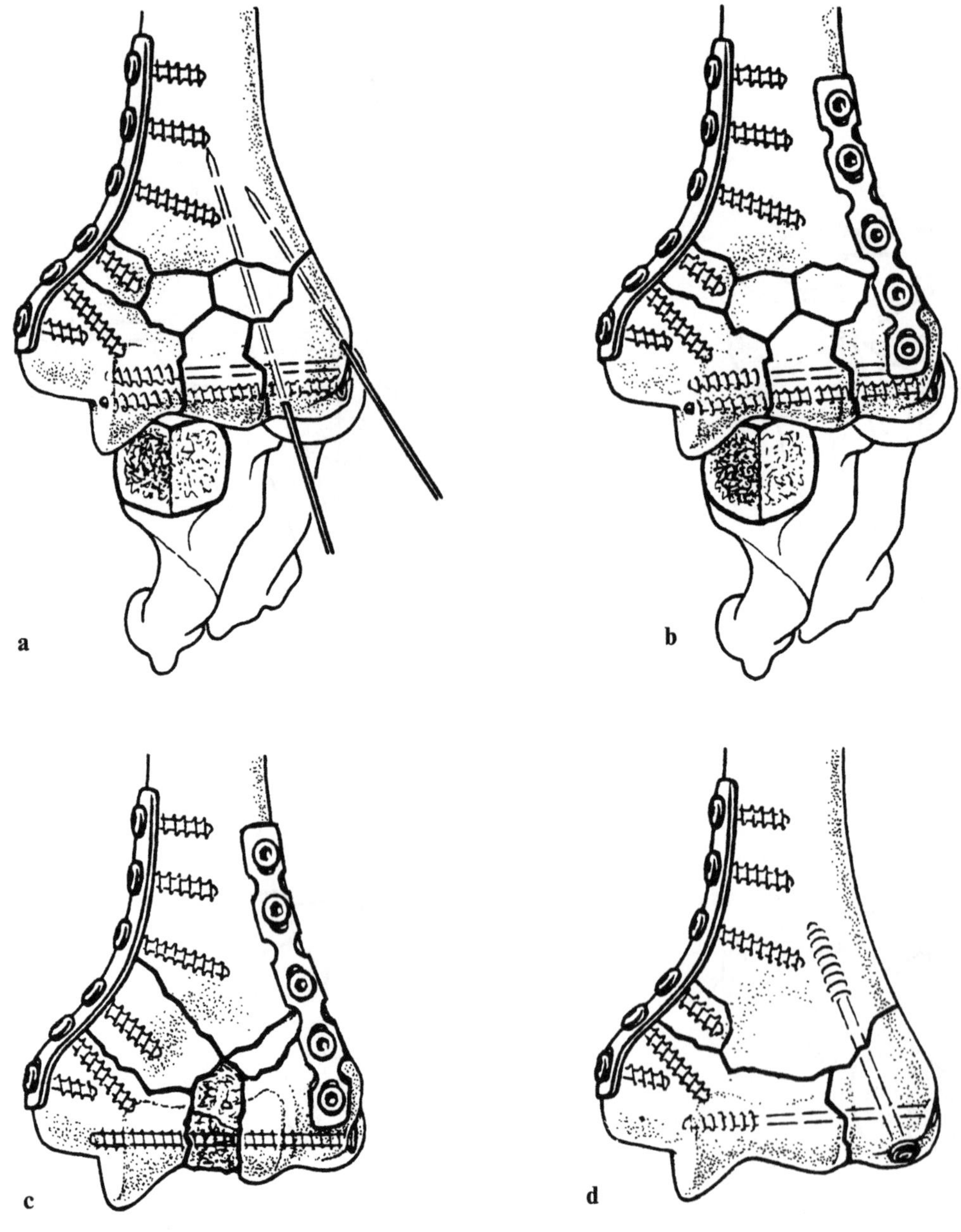

Fig. 69 a–d. Joining the trochlea to the humeral metaphysis

a A contoured one-third tubular plate is attached to the ulnar border

b A contoured reconstruction plate is attached on the radiodorsal side

c A defect in the articular surface is bridged with a corticocancellous graft, and the trochlea is stabilized with a 3.5-mm cortex screw inserted without a gliding hole (retention screw)

d Alternative: In a simple fracture the radial side may be stabilized with screws alone

Fig. 70. AP spot films of the radial head

The X-ray beam must strike the radial head vertically, not the distal humerus. Usually the elbow cannot be fully extended in the postinjury period

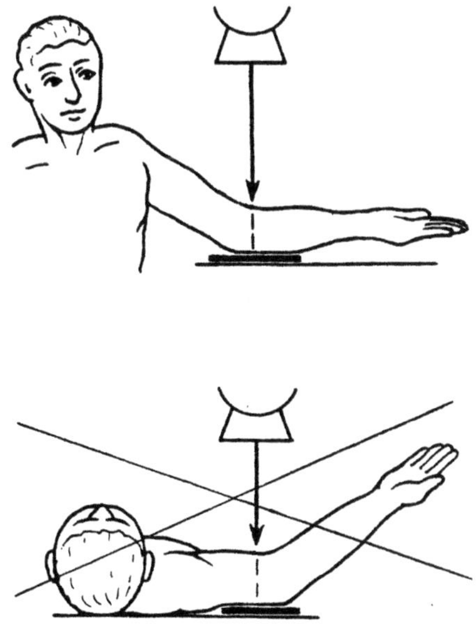

Fig. 71 a–c. Typical fractures of the radial head

a Displaced wedge fracture. It is common for cartilage sheared from the humeral articular surface to become interposed between the fragments

b Comminuted fracture with central depression that spares one wall of the head

c Impaction of the neck with angulation of the intact articular surface. This is accompanied by avulsion of the ulnar collateral ligament

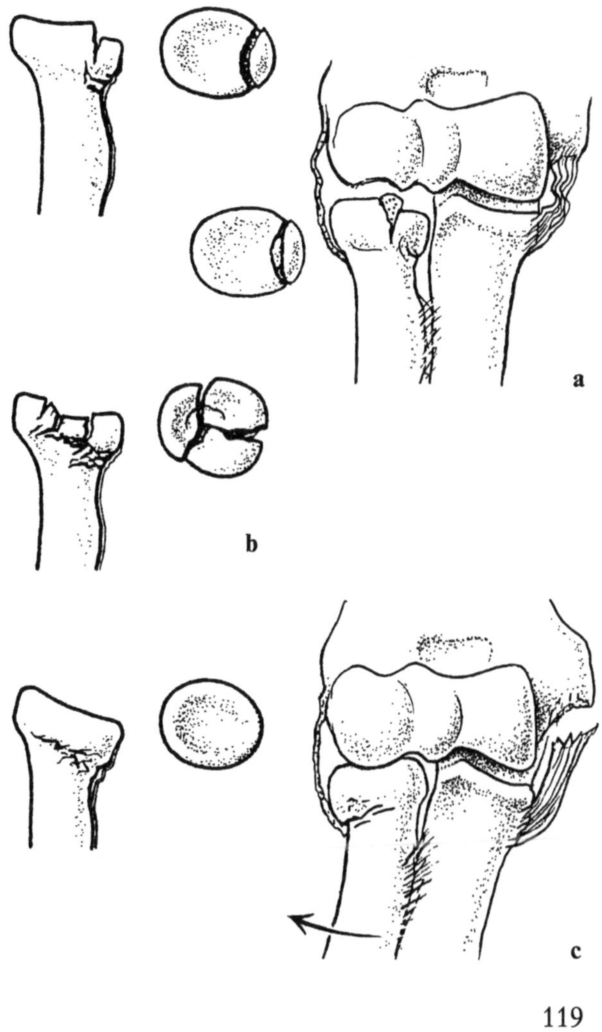

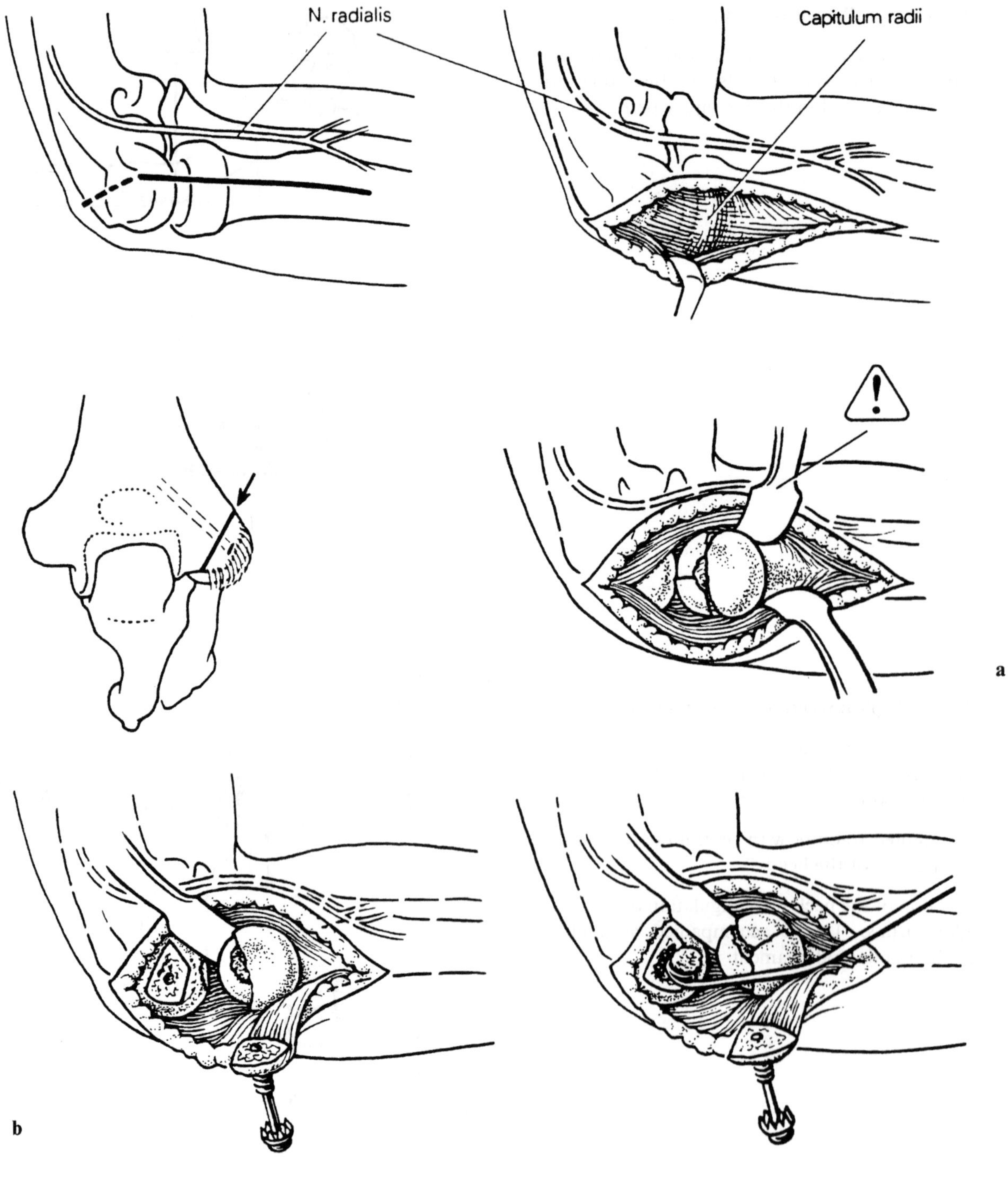

Fig. 72 a, b. Approach to the radial head

a The longitudinal radiodorsal incision may be extended proximally as shown. The muscle fibers and joint capsule are divided along with the annular ligament, avoiding undue pressure on the deep radial nerve branch from the Hohmann retractor

b Extended approach with osteotomy of the epicondyle, which is reflected on the collateral ligament after first inserting a small cancellous screw with a spiked plastic washer. Almost the entire circumference of the radial head is exposed by this maneuver. The Hohmann retractor is braced against the condyle. Cancellous bone is harvested from the osteotomy site

Fig. 73a–d. Screw fixation of radial head fractures

a After removal of entrapped cartilage, the central area is reduced with a fine hook and lateral pressure and is retained with a small forceps or thin Kirschner wire. The screws are introduced from the lateral joint surface (1.5-mm screws, slightly countersunk)

b Fixation of a depressed fracture with multiple screws. The central defect is grafted beforehand with cancellous bone

c Treatment of a neck impaction: If one wall is still intact, the fragment is elevated (on the intact periosteum) and fixed with a screw. With a torn periosteum or larger defect, this is supplemented by cancellous grafting of the metaphysis.If the wall opposite the impaction is not intact, grafting is performed and the site reinforced with an oblique retention screw

d The joint capsule, annular ligament, and overlying muscles are closed in one layer, and the skin is sutured

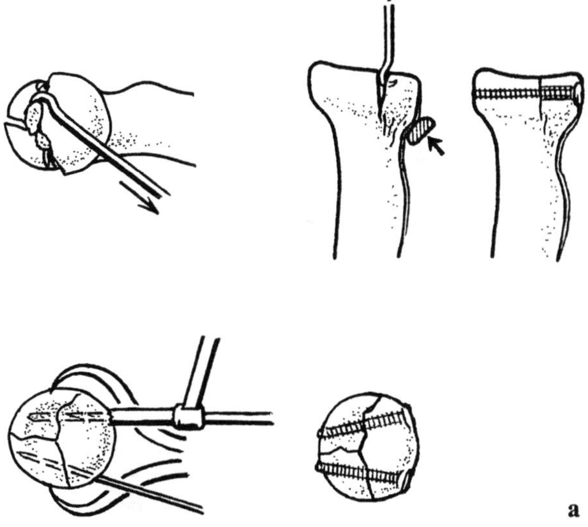

a

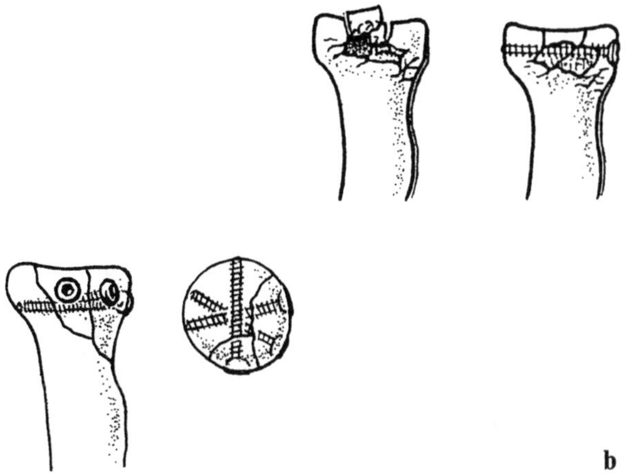

b

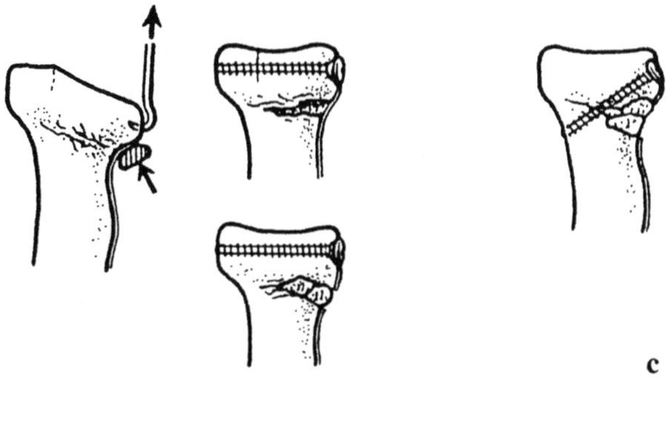

c

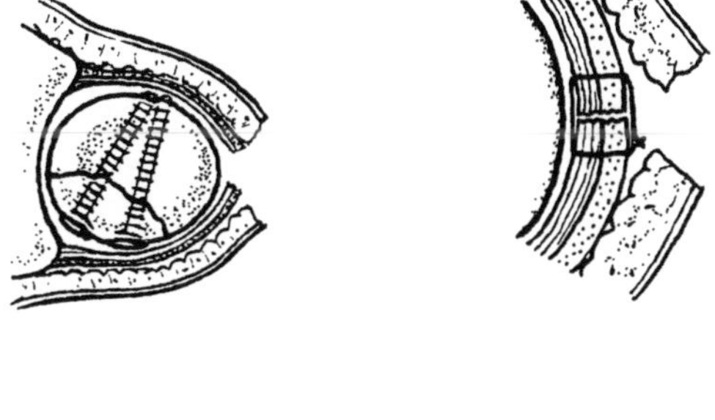

d

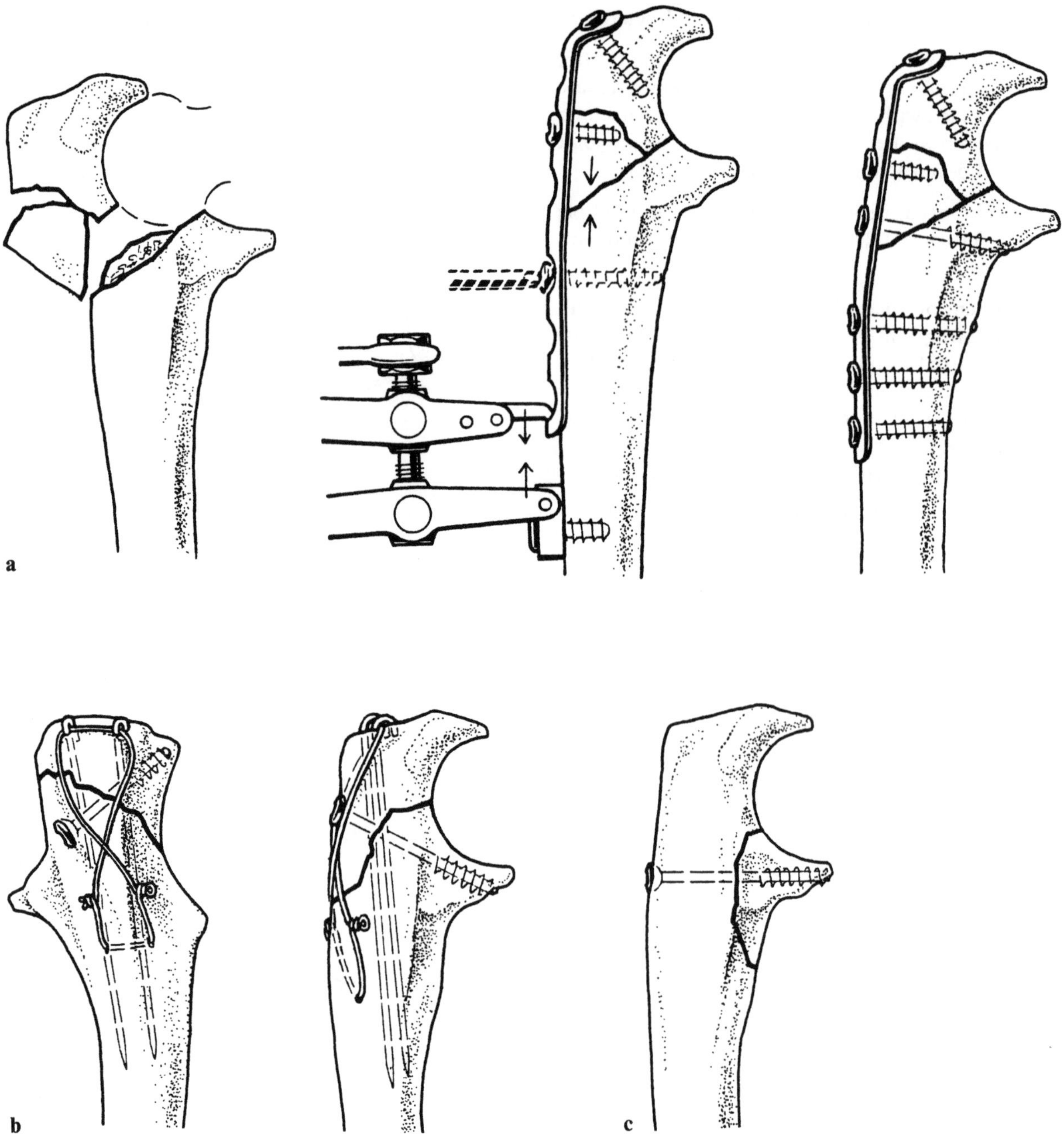

Fig. 74 a–c. Fixation of olecranon fractures with lag screws and the one-third tubular plate

a A three-part fracture of the olecranon is fixed with a long one-third tubular plate applied as a tension band. The tension device is used to obtain fine reduction and optimum compression

b For an oblique fracture, a lag screw is combined with a wire tension band

c Fixation of the coronoid process with a cancellous screw

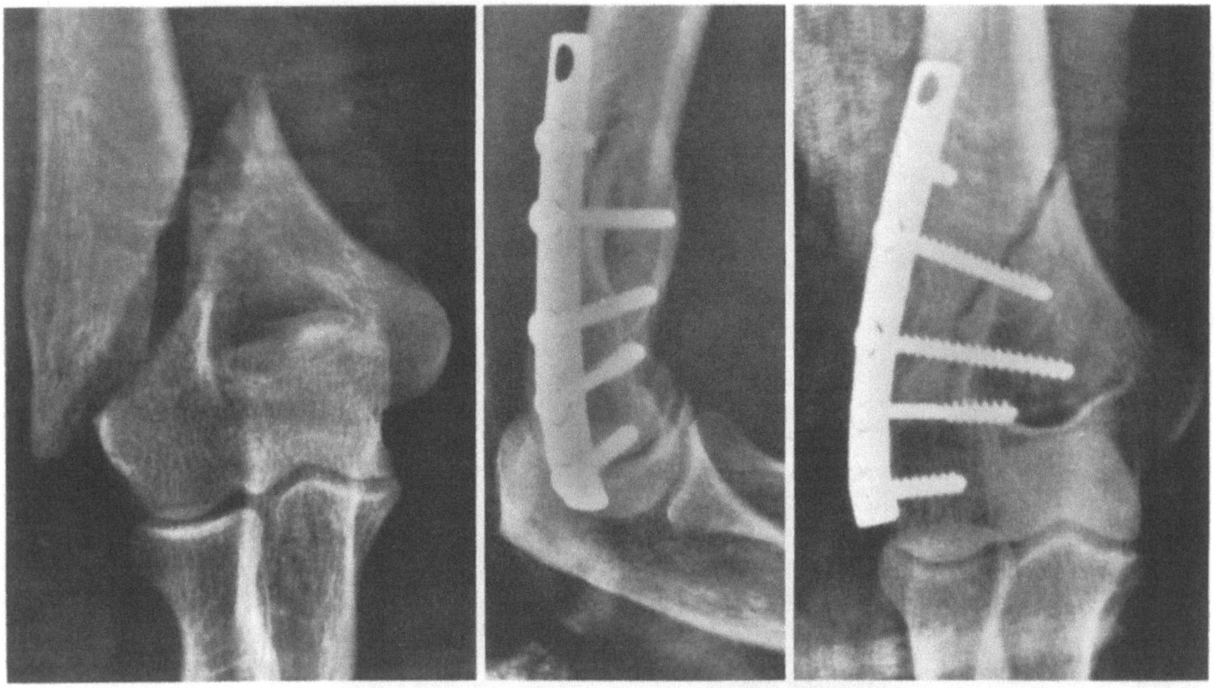

a b b′

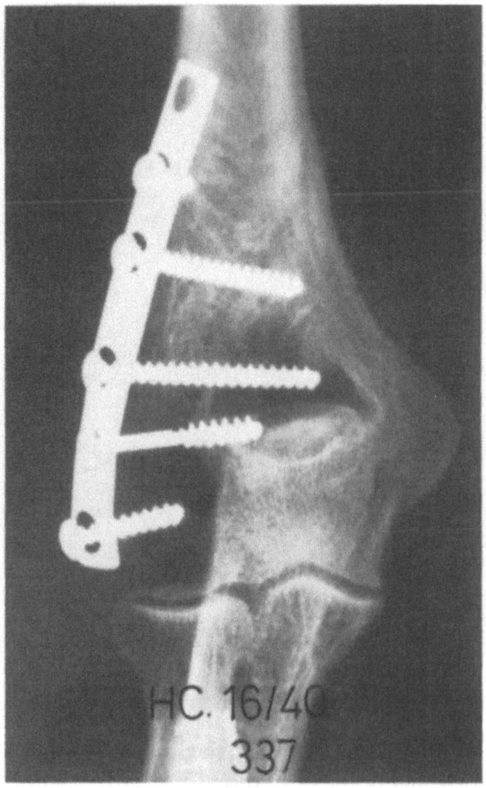

c

Fig. 75a–c. Clinical example: internal fixation of a supracondylar fracture of the humerus with a one-third tubular plate

Lilly W., 50-year-old housewife, injured in household accident on 9/7/73

a Displaced, oblique supracondylar fracture of the humerus

b Emergency internal fixation was performed through the radial approach, using the one-third tubular plate.The screws were placed outside the olecranon and coronoid fossae.
The postoperative course was uneventful, and a dorsal plaster splint was worn for 4 weeks. Patient was lost to initial follow-up and did not have the implants removed

c When seen 7 years later on 3/24/80, the patient had no complaints, a 10° flexion deficit, and unrestricted extension, pronation, and supination. The implant was palpable through the skin, and X-rays showed loosening of several screws. The patient declined removal

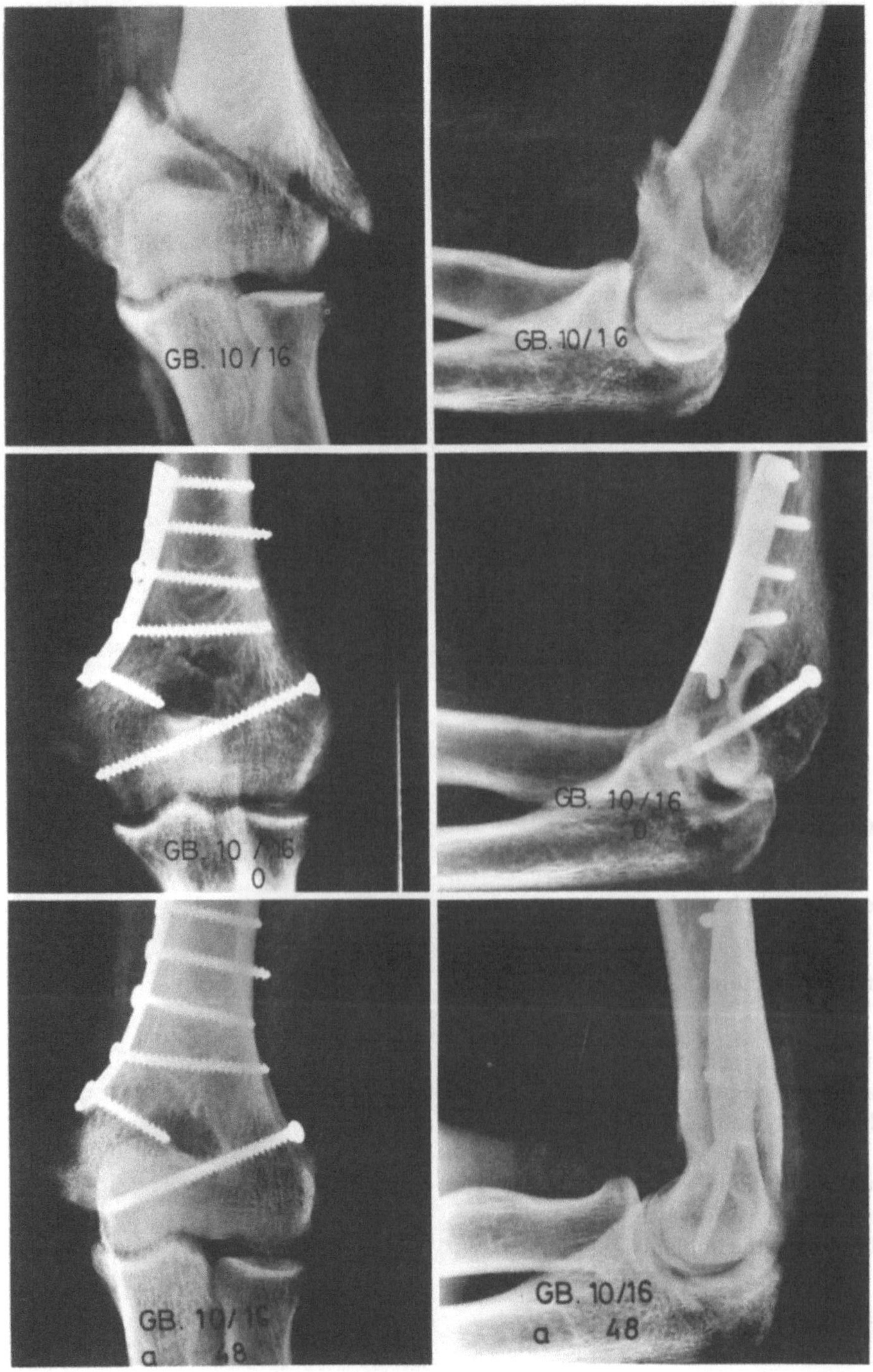

Fig. 76a–c. Clinical example: supra- and transcondylar fracture of the distal humerus

a Oblique fracture of the distal humerus directly proximal to the olecranon fossa, with radial extension into the condyle

b Internal fixation was performed through a bilateral approach. Ulnar component was fixed with a one-third tubular plate incorporating a short distal screw. A separate, long lag screw was inserted obliquely through the trochlea from the radial side

c Result at 11 months: primary fracture union. Removal of the implants is not proposed

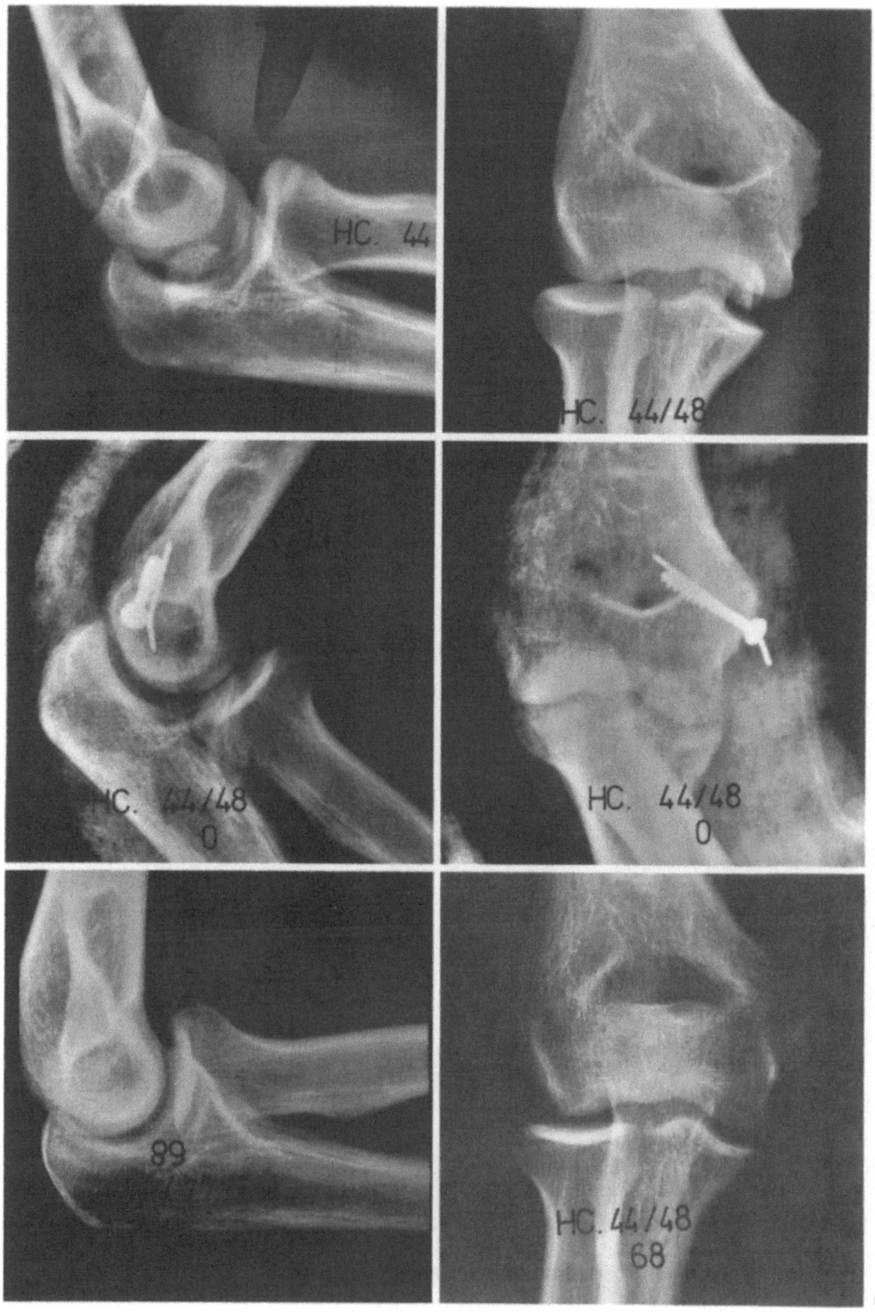

a

b

c

Fig. 77a–c. Clinical example: avulsion fracture of the ulnar epicondyle with intra-articular entrapment of the fragment

Rene B., 15-year-old school boy, injured in skiing accident on 12/27/78

a Avulsion fracture of the ulnar epicondyle. The fragment is displaced into the medial compartment of the joint. Patient reported paresthesia in the area of the ulnar nerve

b Emergency internal fixation was performed on the day of the injury. The ulnar nerve was exposed, and the epicondyle fragment was reduced and fixed with a cancellous screw and Kirschner wire for rotational stability
The postoperative course was uncomplicated. A dorsal plaster splint was worn for 3 weeks, followed by functional exercises. The implants were removed elsewhere

c At follow-up on 4/18/80 the patient had no complaints, full function, and normal X-ray findings

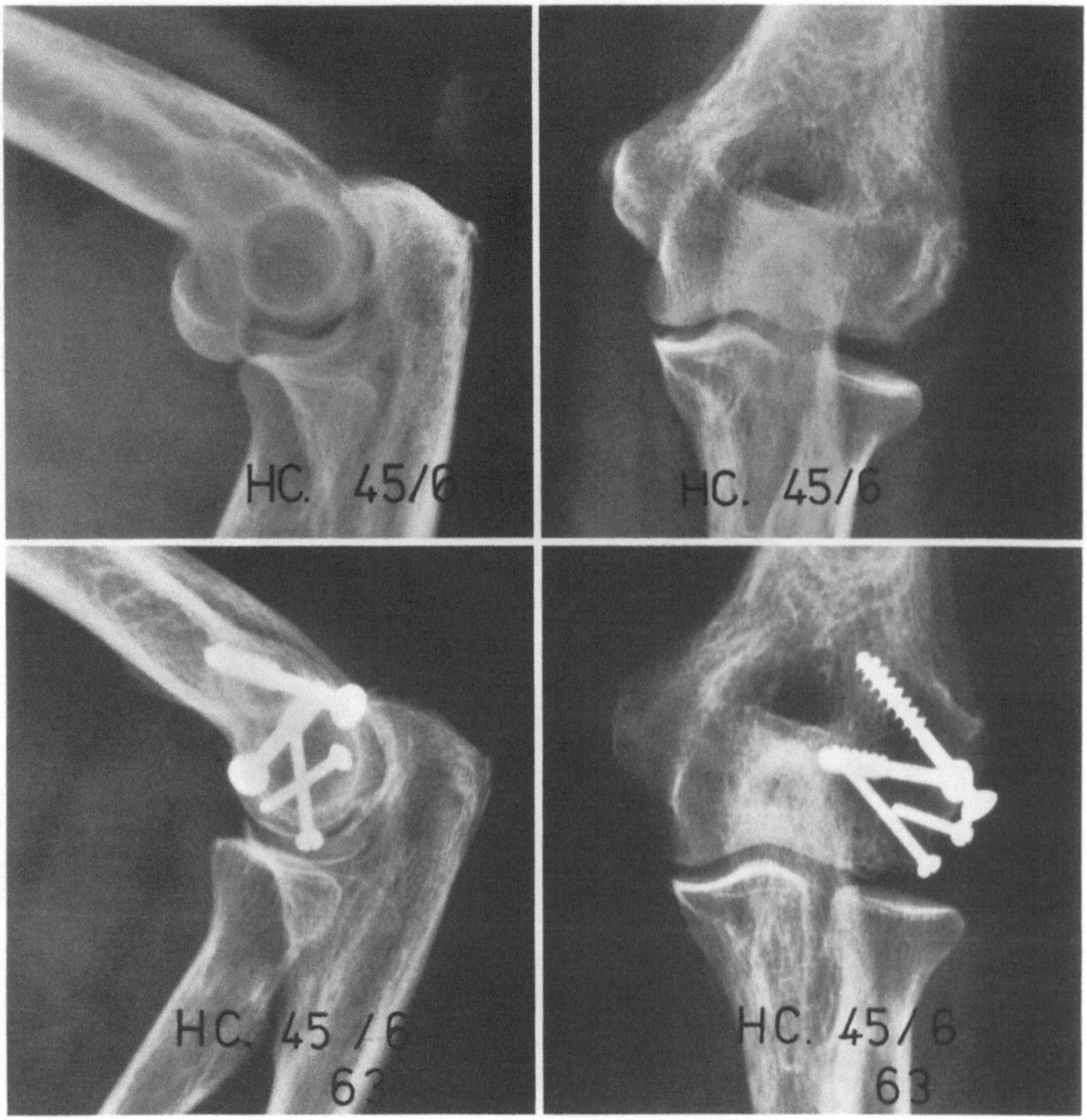

a

b

Fig. 78 a, b. Clinical example: condylar shear fracture

Ursula S., 69-year-old farmer's wife, injured in a household accident. High pain tolerance in this patient delayed diagnosis by 2 weeks

a Shear fracture of the lateral condyle with anterior displacement. Internal fixation with screws was performed at 2 weeks through a radial approach. A dorsal plaster splint was worn for 6 weeks. By 4 months, patient was able to do unlimited lifting and farming work

b Follow-up at 14 months showed no complaints, full work fitness, and unrestricted motion with no evidence of degenerative arthritis. Patient has declined implant removal

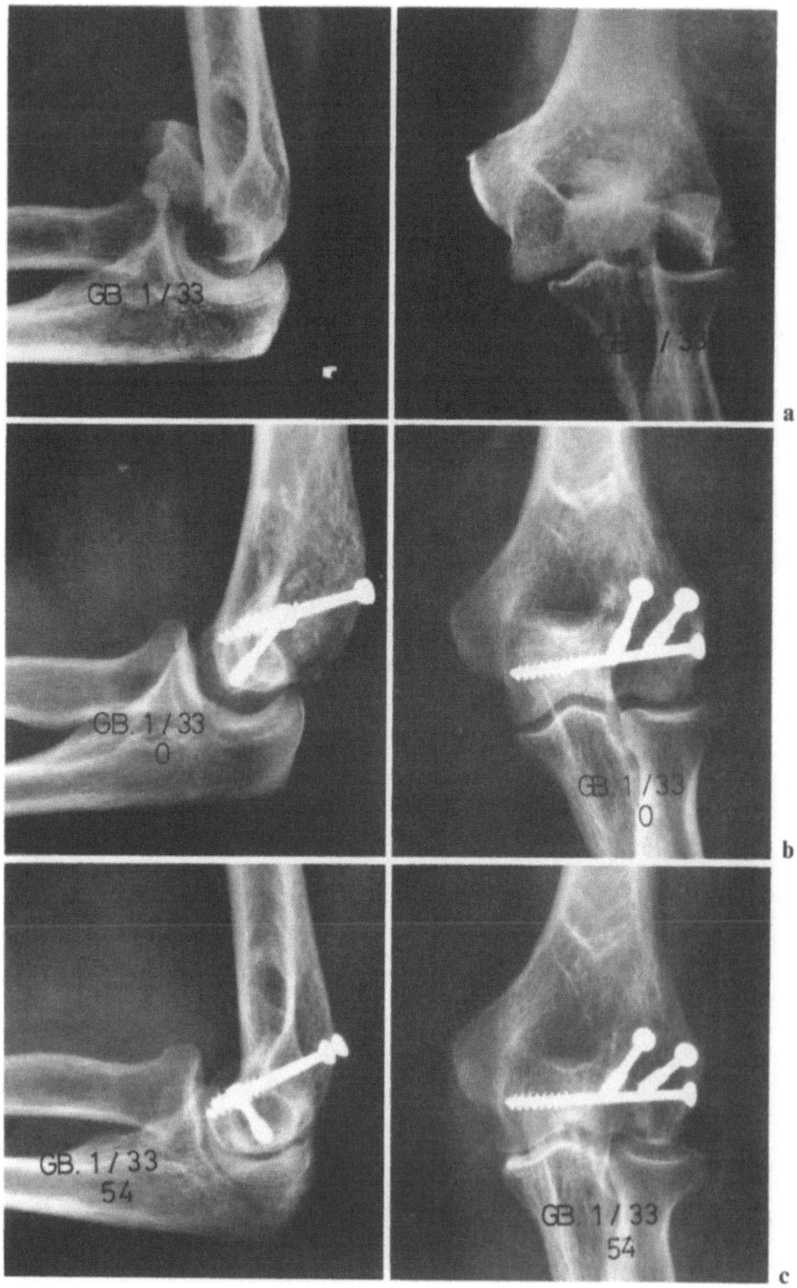

Fig. 79 a–c. Clinical example: screw fixation of a trochlear fracture

a Displaced fracture of the trochlea and capitellum with radial subluxation

b Fracture was exposed through the dorsoradial approach, reduced, and fixed with small cancellous screws inserted parallel to the joint

c Follow-up at 1 year showed fracture union with slight dorsal angulation of the trochlea. Implant removal is not contemplated

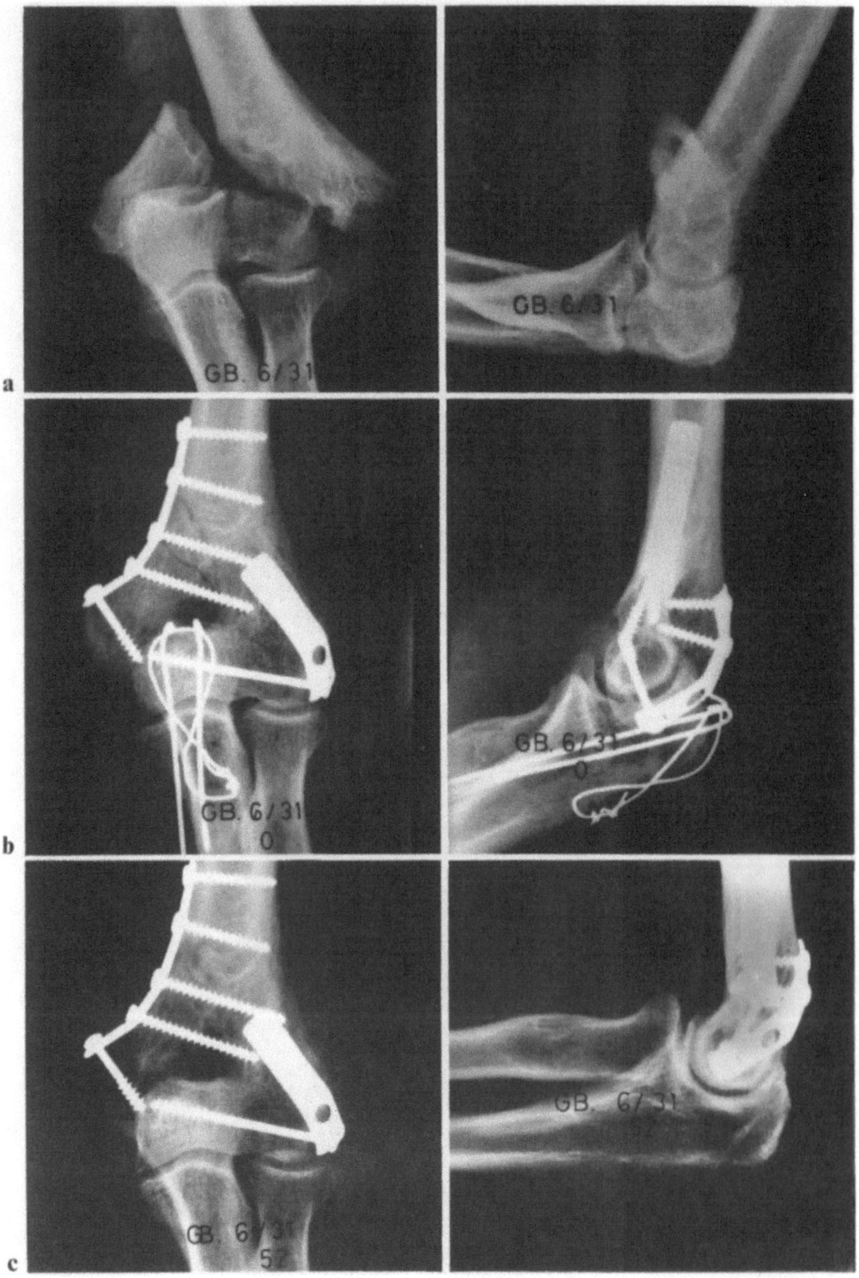

Fig. 80 a–c. Clinical example: intra-articular T fracture

a Supracondylar fracture of both pillars extending through the olecranon fossa, with splitting of the trochlea

b Internal fixation was performed through a dorsal approach that included osteotomy of the olecranon (reattached with a tension band).

A one-third tubular plate was attached to the ulnar border, and a shorter radial plate to the dorsal side of the condyle. The distal cancellous screw in the plate compresses the articular part of the fracture

c Follow-up at 1 year confirmed fracture union. Implant removal is not proposed

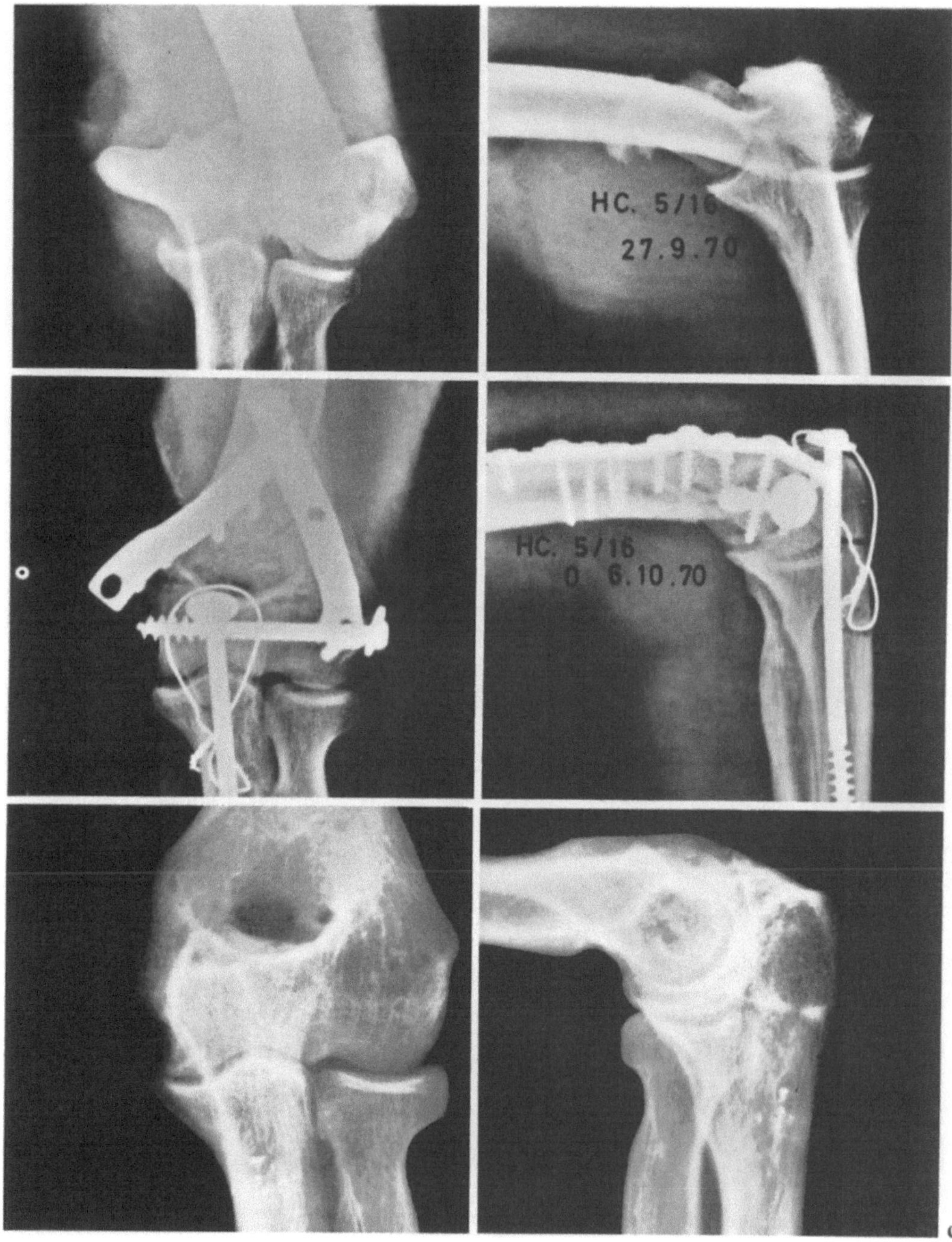

a
b
c

Fig. 81 a–c. Clinical example: comminuted intra-articular fracture of the humerus

Rene H., 30-year-old resort manager, fell while playing soccer on 9/29/70

a Comminuted intra-articular fracture of the distal humerus

b Emergency internal fixation was performed with osteotomy of the olecranon. The trochlea was fixed with a cancellous screw, and one-third tubular plates were applied on the sides. A dorsal plaster splint was worn for 6 weeks, and at 9 months the implants were removed and the ulnar nerve transposed anteriorly

c Ten years later (3/29/80) the patient had no complaints other than slight weakness of the left arm; slight muscular atrophy was noted. There was a 20° extension loss, 5° flexion loss, and unrestricted pronation and supination. X-rays showed mild degenerative arthritis

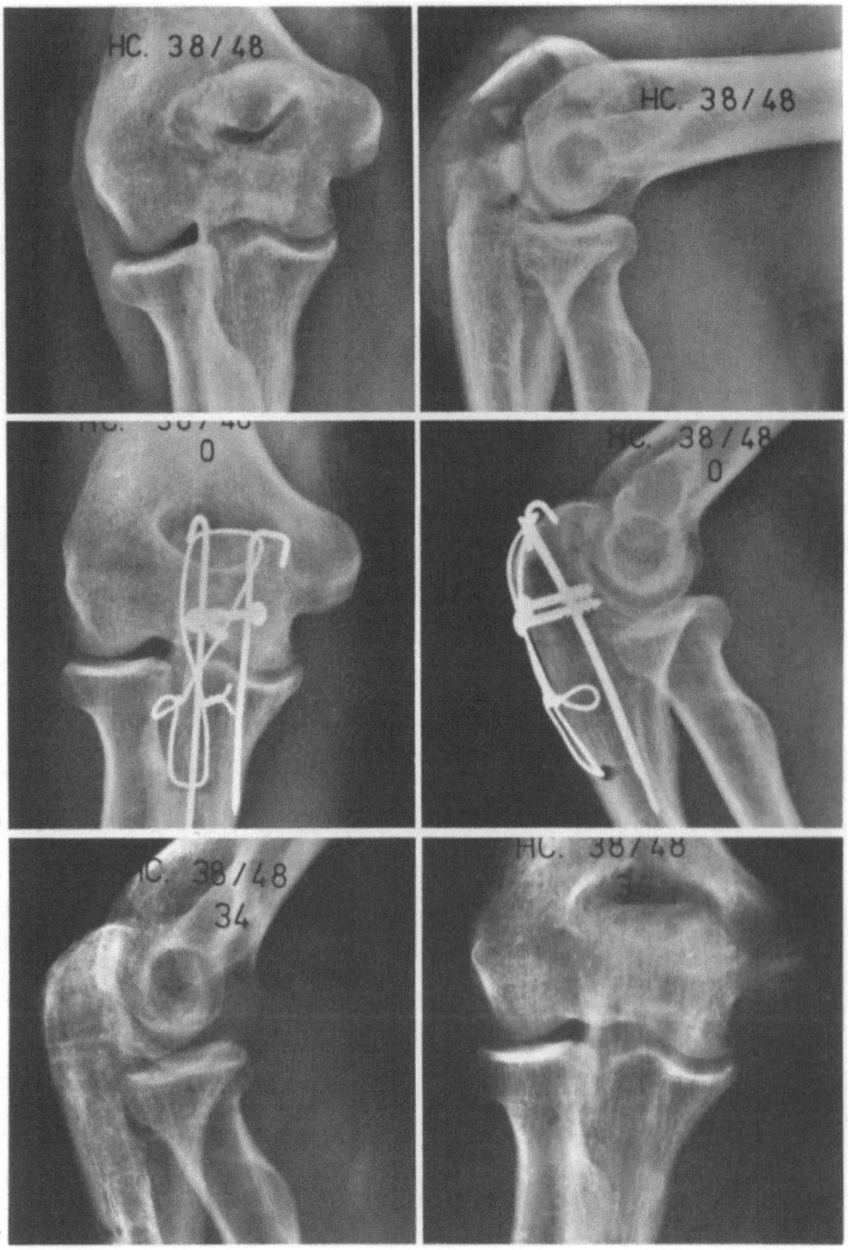

a

b

c

Fig. 82a–c. Clinical example: multiple fracture of the olecranon

Anton L., 46-year-old retail employee, fell from motorcycle when struck by a car

a Multiple fracture of the right olecranon

b Emergency internal fixation was performed with two parallel Kirschner wires and a figure-of-eight wire tension band with two twists. The oblique fracture lines and additional fragment were fixed with small cancellous screws.

Postoperative course was uneventful, and patient was discharged with a removable plaster splint to be worn for 4 weeks. Full loading of the arm was commenced at 8 weeks. Patient returned to work at 9 weeks

c Follow-up and implant removal at 8 months on 6/20/78: no complaints, full function, primary fracture union without degenerative arthritis

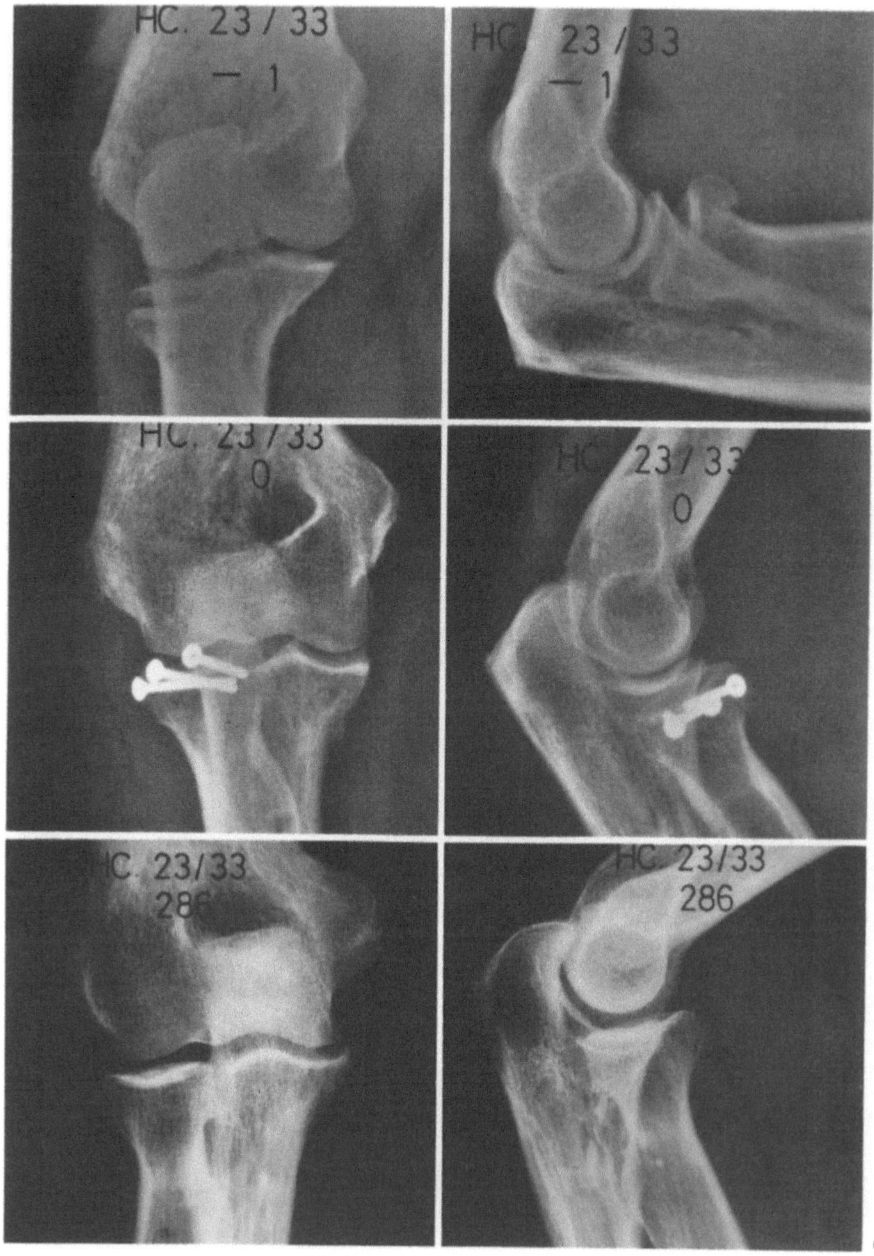

a

b

c

Fig. 83a–c. Clinical example: wedge fracture of the radial head

Maria C., 61-year-old florist, fell on a flagstone on 12/23/74

a Markedly displaced wedge fracture of the right radial head. Fracture was initially fixed in plaster; patient was hospitalized 1 week later

b Internal fixation was performed on 1/3/75. Interposed articular cartilage from the humerus was removed, and the fracture was reduced and fixed with three 1.5-mm screws.

A removable plaster splint was worn for 4 weeks, and full loading was permitted at 10 weeks. Patient resumed work at 12 weeks. Implants were removed at 5 months

c Follow-up at $5^1/_2$ years (6/30/80) showed no subjective or objective changes. The arm was painless and fully mobile. There was no evidence of atrophy or degenerative change

Fig. 84a, b. Clinical example: depressed fracture of the radial head

Pia S., 23-year-old retail employee, fell on an icy street on 1/22/78

a Depressed fracture of the radial metaphysis with an articular wedge fracture and marked displacement.
Emergency internal fixation was performed through an extended approach (osteotomy of the epicondyle). The radial head was realigned, reduced, grafted with cancellous bone (from the epicondyle), and fixed with two oblique 1.5-mm retention screws.Plaster splint was worn 8 weeks. Full loading was permitted at 10 weeks

b When seen at 10 months, prior to implant removal, the patient had no complaints and a stable elbow with full function. Primary union was confirmed. Calcification of the medial epicondyle was noted as evidence of the primary ligament avulsion. Patient left the country and was lost to further follow-up

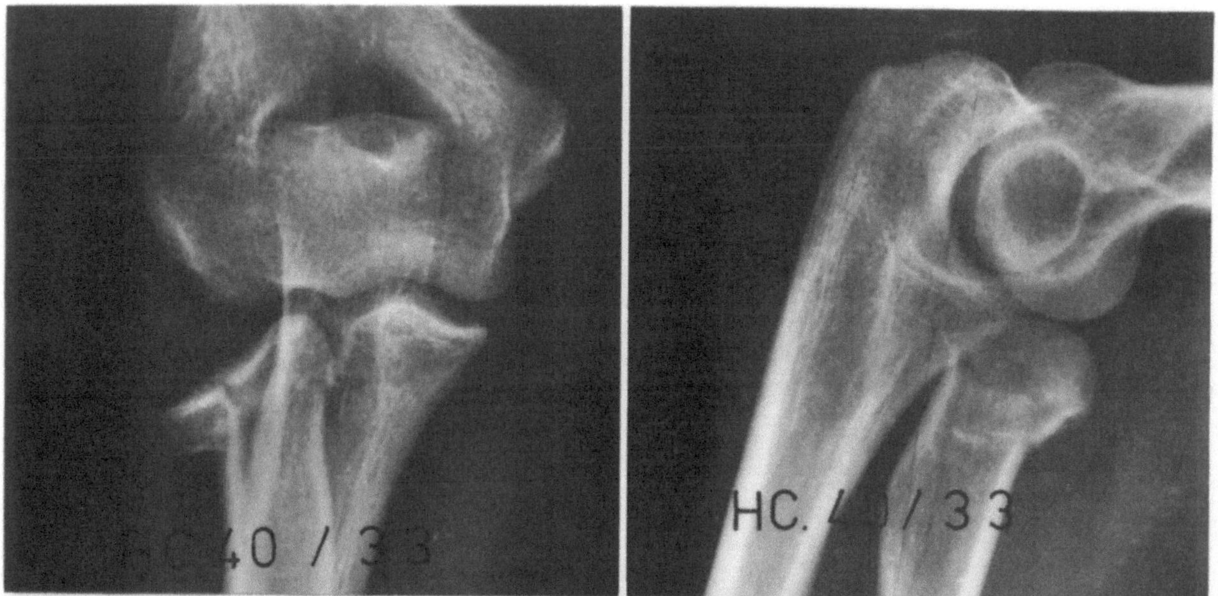

a

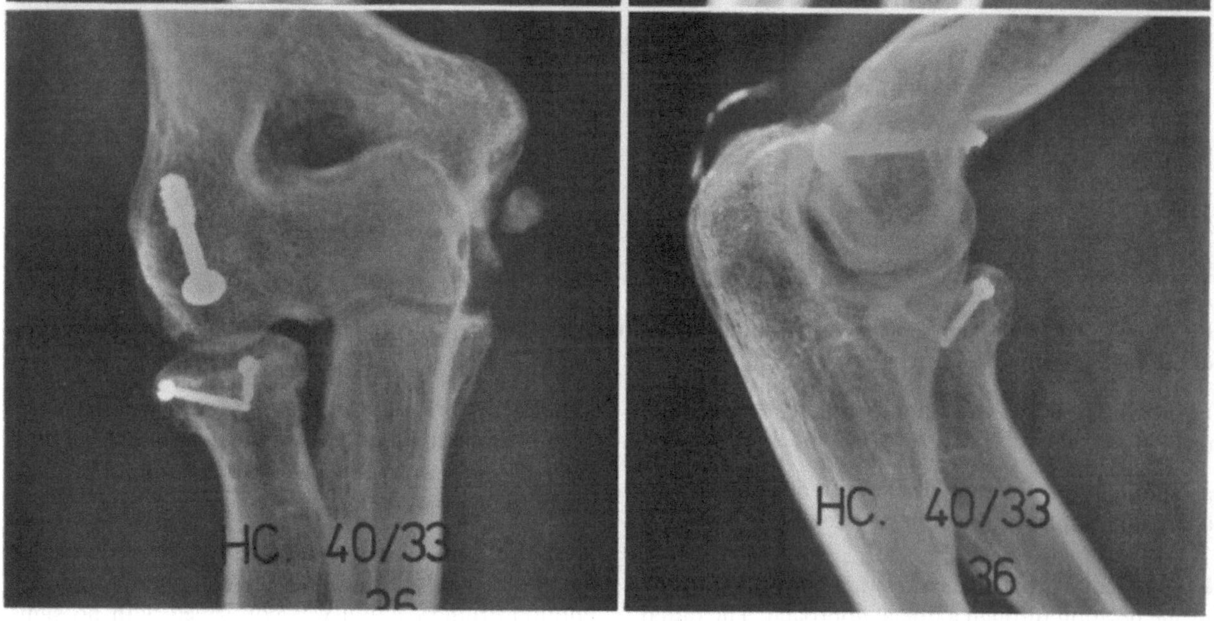

b

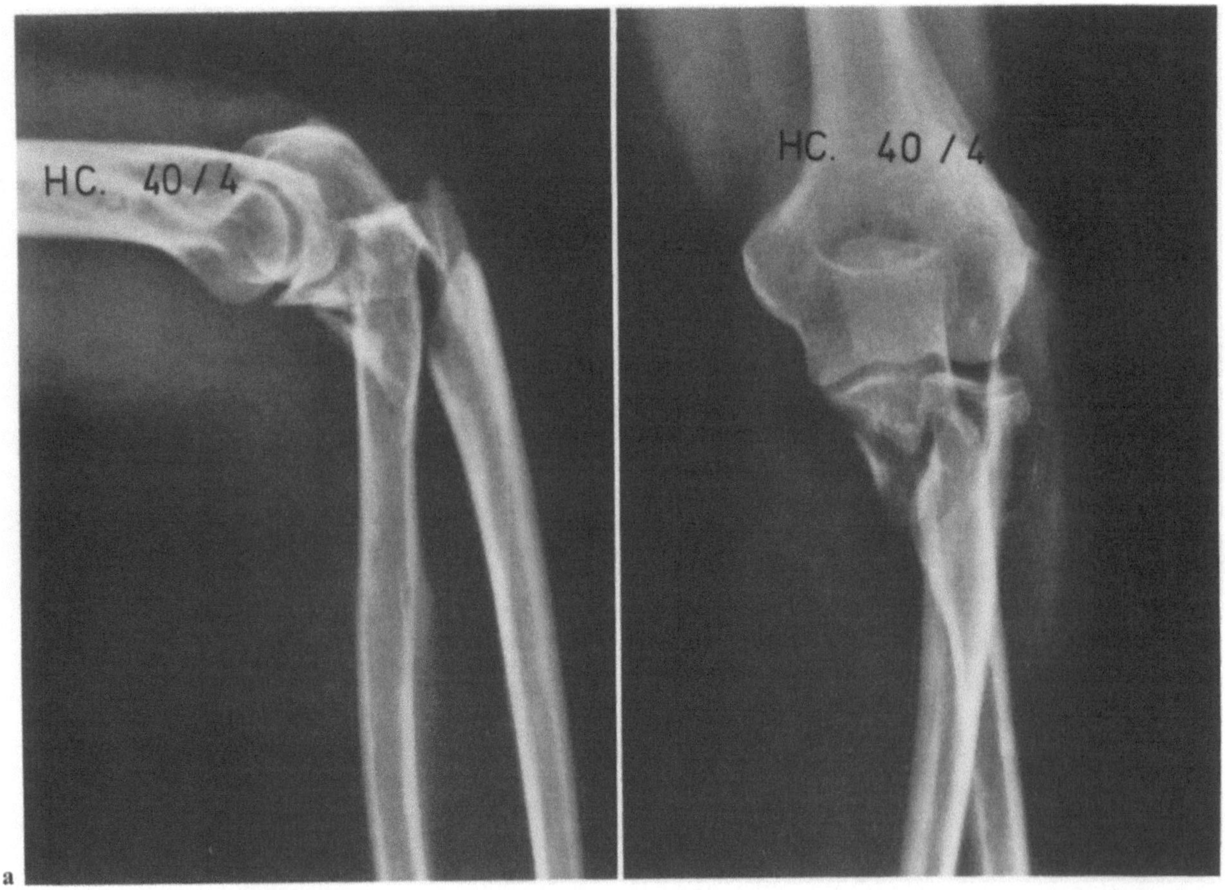

a

Fig. 85a–c. Clinical example: reverse Monteggia fracture, comminuted olecranon fracture, fracture-dislocation of the radial head

Elisabeth C., 60-year-old housekeeper, fell on stairs on 1/11/78

a Comminuted fracture of the left olecranon with a dorsally displaced radial head fracture

b Emergency internal fixation was performed in the prone position through a dorsal approach. The radial head was fixed with three 1.5-mm screws. The dislocation was reduced and the ulna stabilized with a 6-hole one-third tubular plate and 2 lag screws
The postoperative course was uncomplicated. A full arm cast was worn for 6 weeks after wound healing, then exercises were begun

c At 15 months the patient was reexamined and the implants removed.She had no complaints and full motion.Primary union was confirmed with no signs of degenerative arthritis. One screw resisted removal and was left behind

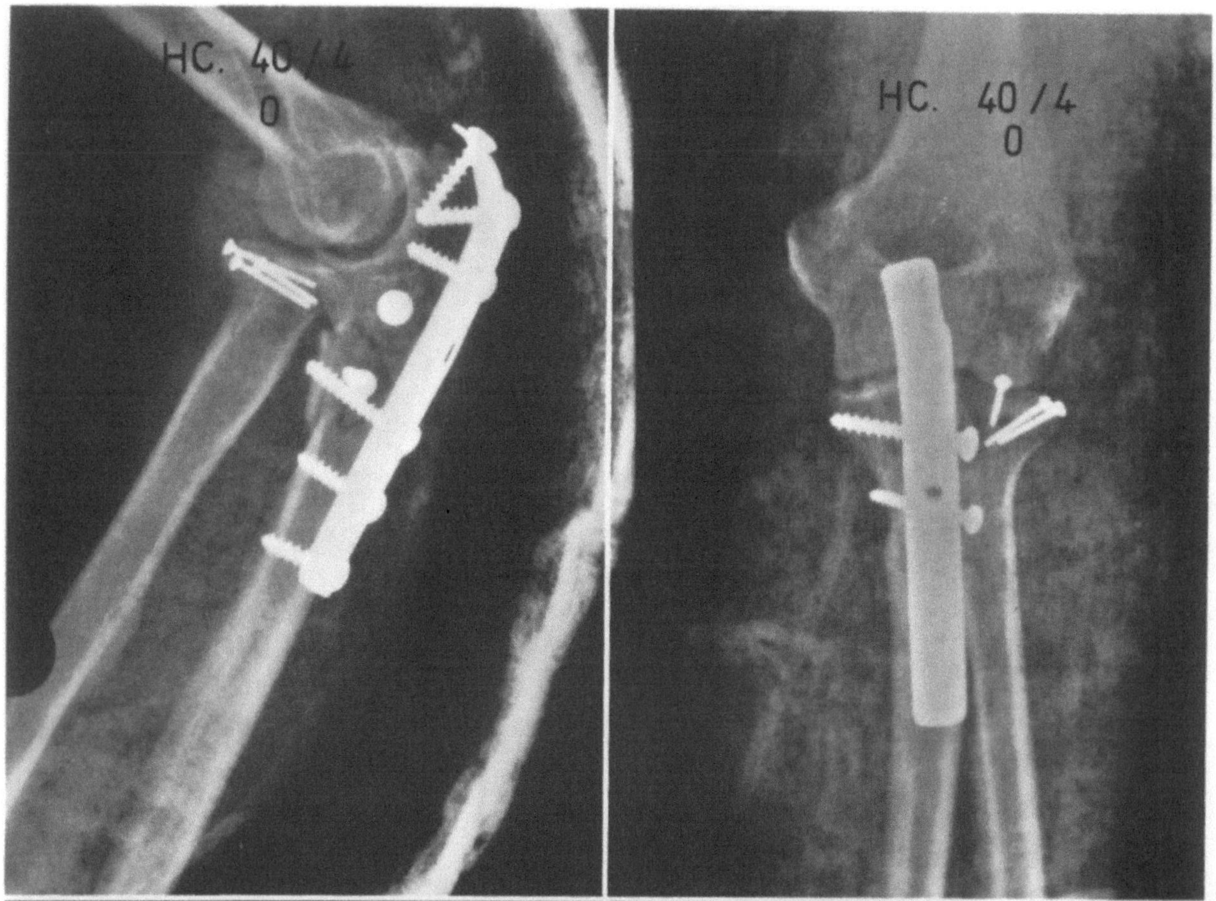

b

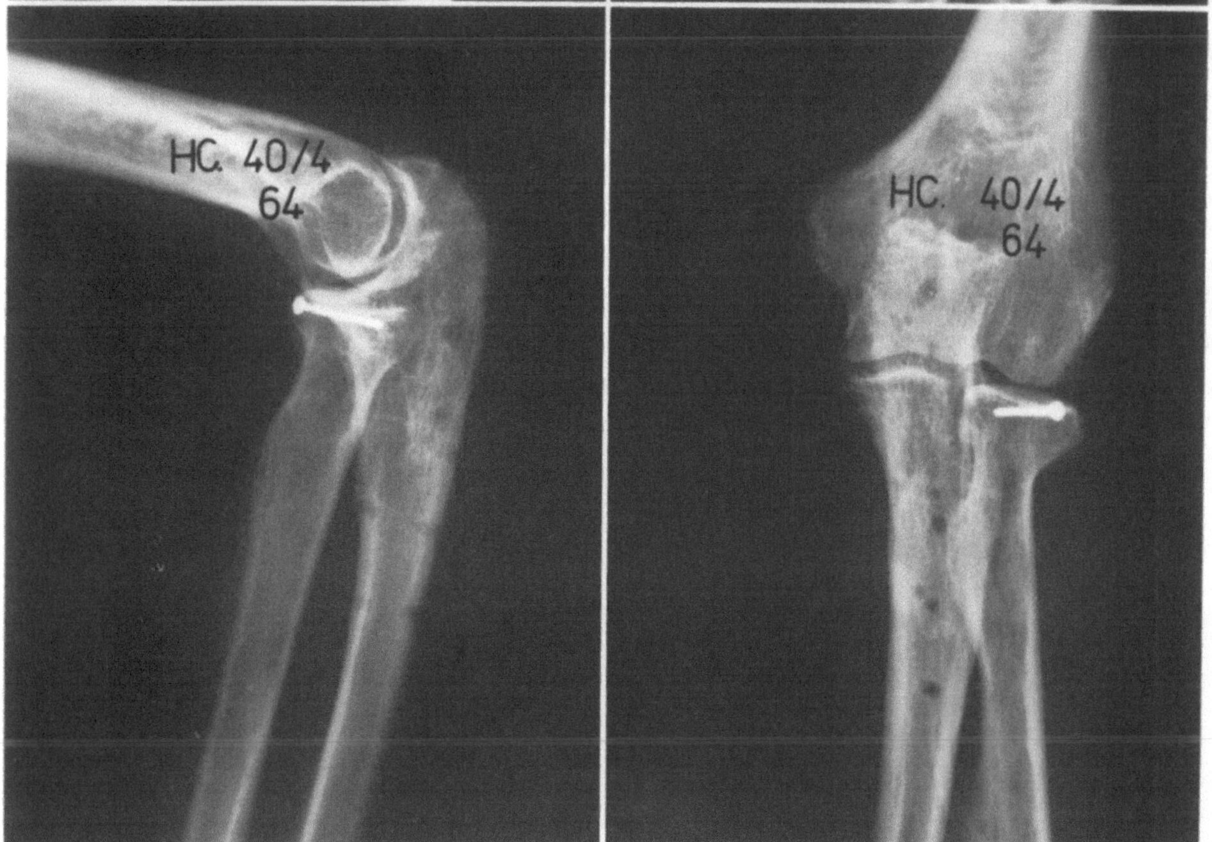

c

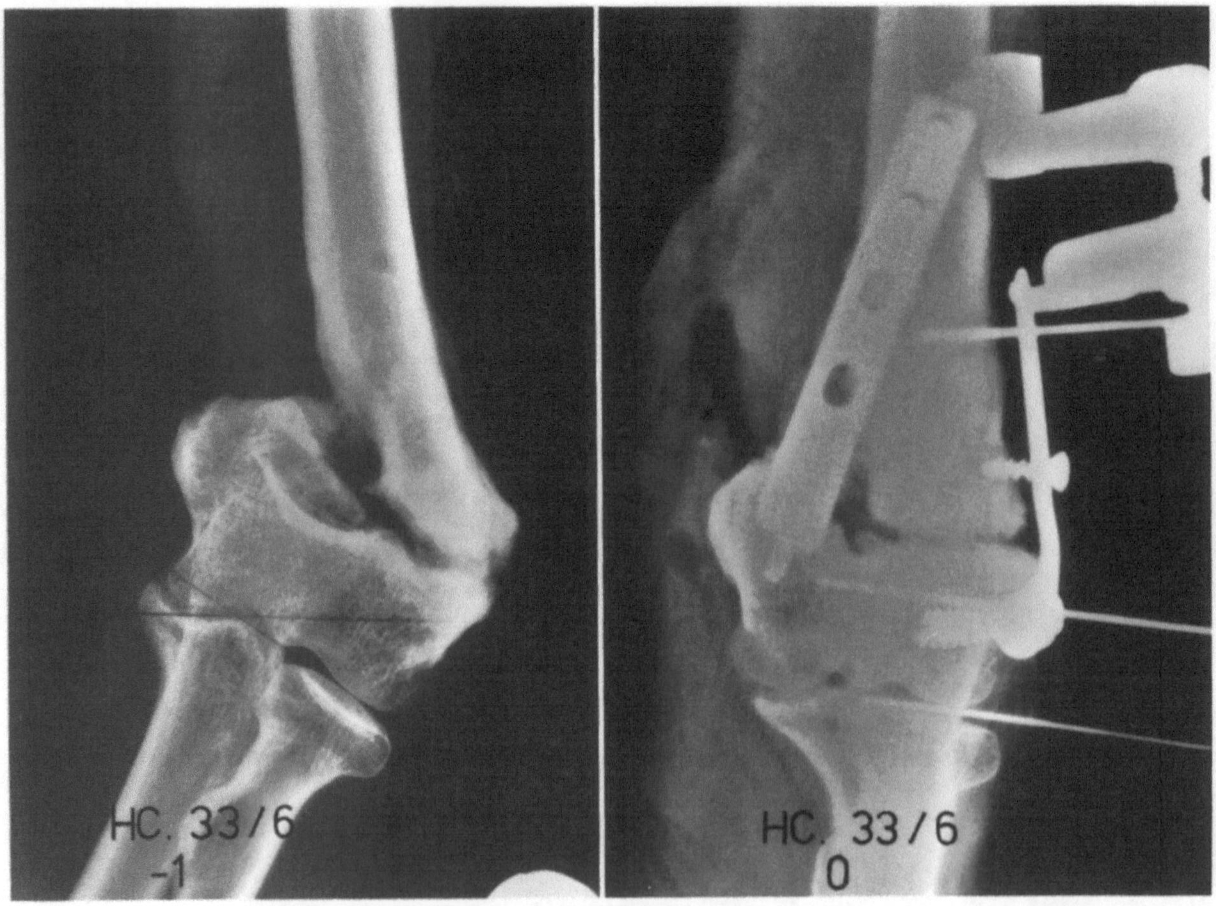

a b

Fig. 86a–c. Clinical example: nonunion of the distal humerus

Ilse G., 36-year-old physician, sustained an open supracondylar fracture of the left humerus in a fall from a horse in 1973. (Patient is left-handed.) Primary, nonrigid internal fixation was followed by chronic infection and prolonged cast immobilization, culminating in a mobile, painful nonunion

a Supracondylar nonunion with varus and internal rotation deformity (September, 1976)

b Internal fixation was performed on 10/1/76. Ulnar pillar was buttressed with a 3.5-mm DCP placed over an interposed corticocancellous graft. Fracture was compressed radially with a small T plate (intra-operative film shows tension device applied to the radial side)

c Postoperative film shows perfect restoration of alignment

Postoperative course was uneventful. Removable plastic splint was worn for 3 months, followed by incremental loading.Full work fitness was achieved at 5 months. Implants were removed elsewhere after 1 year

d When seen again at 2 years, the patient had no complaints or disability. There was a 10° extension deficit, 35° flexion deficit, and full pronation and supination. The nonunion was solid, and there were no signs of degenerative arthritis

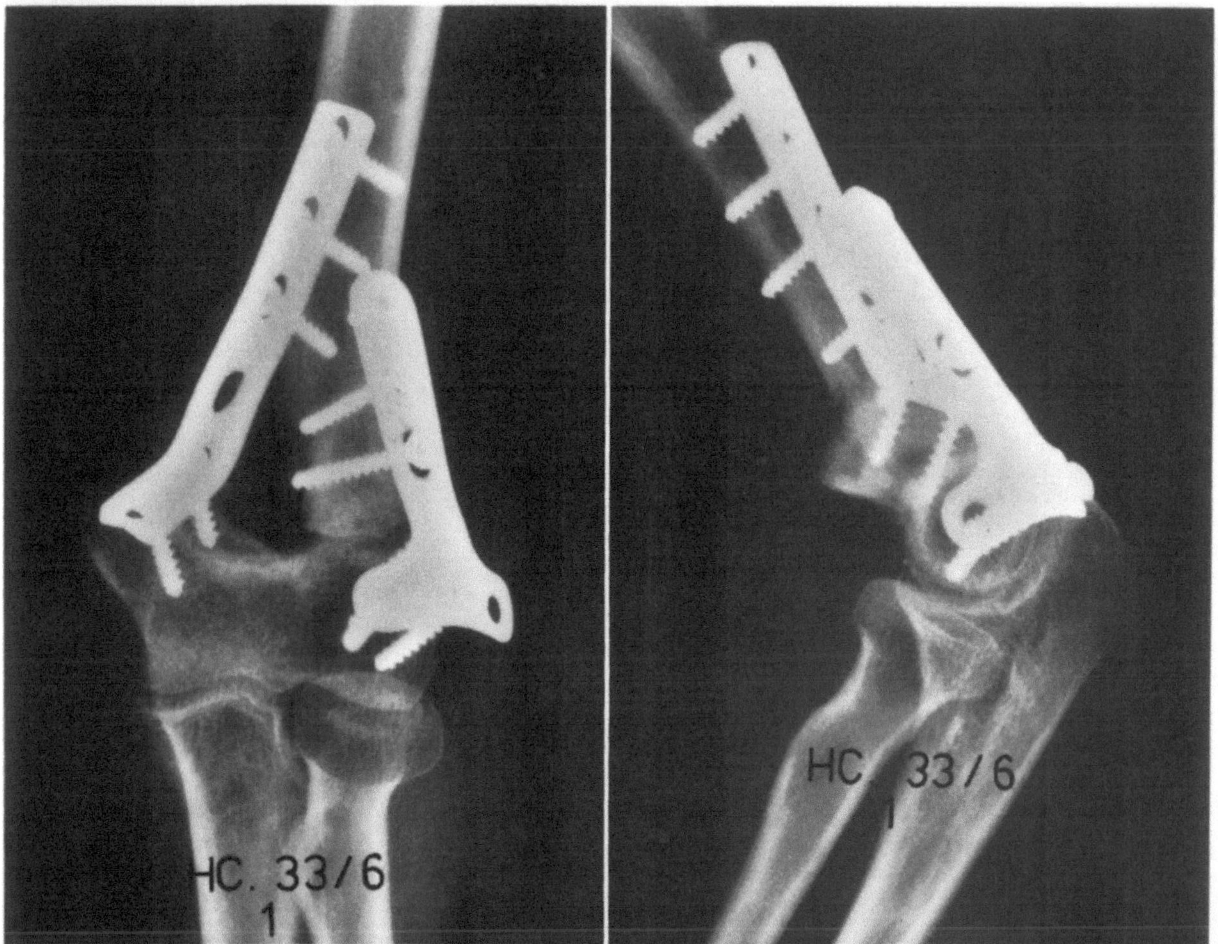

c

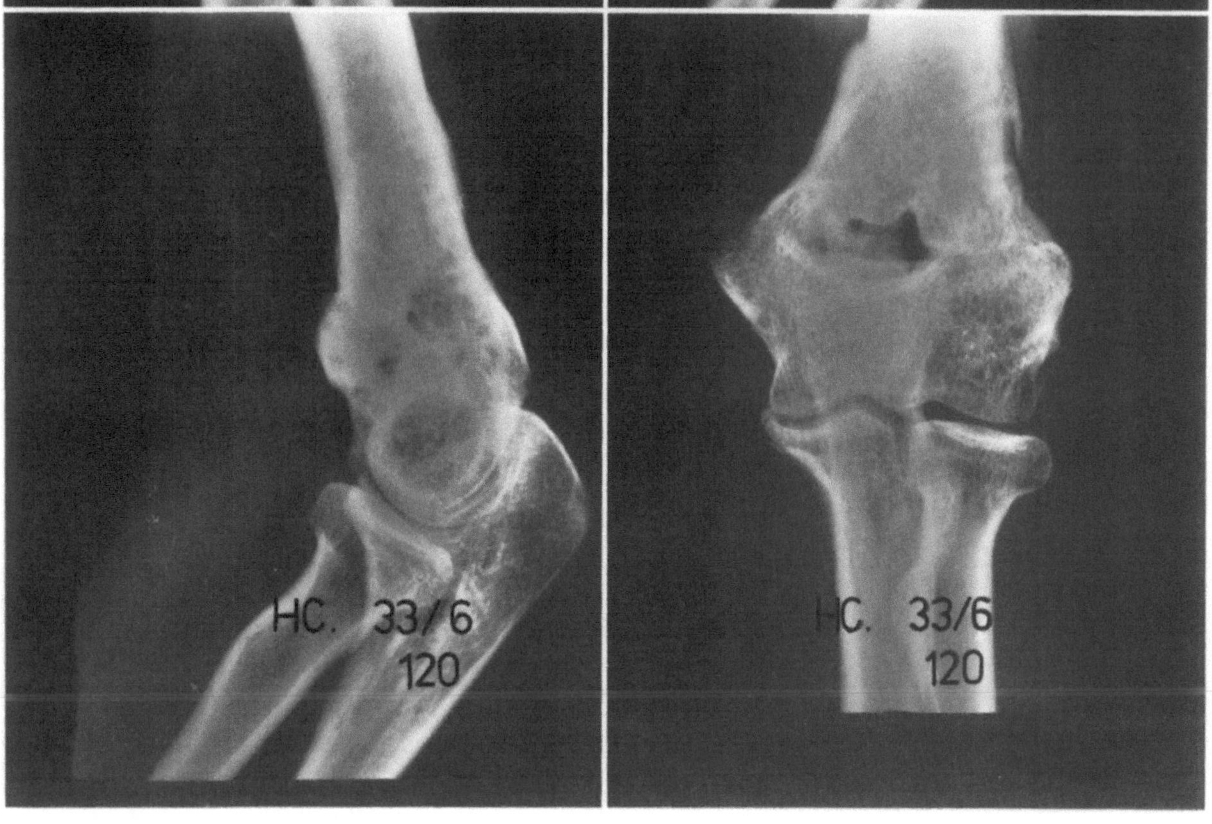

d

XI. The Shafts of the Radius and Ulna

Today, internal plating is generally acknowledged as the treatment of choice for diaphyseal fractures of one or both forearm bones and for fracture-dislocations of the Monteggia or Galeazzi type. It is the only way of achieving early mobilization, which is necessary to ensure recovery of pronation and supination.

For general technical information on the approach, internal fixation, and aftertreatment, we refer the reader to the *Manual of Internal Fixation*.

The shafts of the radius and ulna are very slender bones, even in males. The older, straight plates with round, widely spaced holes and the 4.5-mm cortex screws often proved to be too bulky. Sometimes the screws produced additional fissure fractures when tightened, and the wide plates blocked vision of the fracture site and made it difficult to assess the reduction. In some cases the sheer volume of the plates interfered with rotation or hampered skin closure.

These problems are avoided by use of the 3.5-mm DCP. Its 3-mm thickness gives good stability and occupies little space. The holes are closer together, so an 8-hole plate of the 3.5-mm system has the same length as a 6-hole plate of the 4.5-mm system. The 3.5-mm DCP is also easier to adapt to bone anatomy and especially to the curvature of the radius. The new 3.5-mm cortex screws are an ideal size and do not traumatize the bone.

At least a 7-hole plate is recommended for simple oblique fractures, and an 8- to 10-hole plate for fractures that are multiple or segmental. In the pure transverse fracture, use of the articulated tension device aids fine reduction and permits finer control of axial compression–although space limitations often preclude its use. In oblique fractures, stability is optimized either by inserting a separate lag screw on a different plane, or by inserting a central plate screw across the fracture site in the fashion of an interfragmental lag screw (Figs. 32, 33). If there is bone loss or devascularization, autogenous cancellous bone grafting is mandatory.

The 3.5-mm DCP also has proved stable enough for use in secondary operations (refractures and nonunions).

Use of the small external fixator, mounted across the wrist, has given good results in cases where a fracture of the ulnar shaft coexists with comminution of the distal radius (Fig. 42). This is also true in cases where soft-tissue injuries contraindicate the primary internal plating of a diaphyseal fracture. This applies more frequently to the exposed ulna than to the radius, which occupies a more protected position. The external fixator effectively prevents secondary displacements, especially shortening. Compression plating is deferred until the soft-tissue lesions have healed or have been definitively repaired by a graft or flap technique.

Illustrative Clinical X-rays (Figs. 87–90)

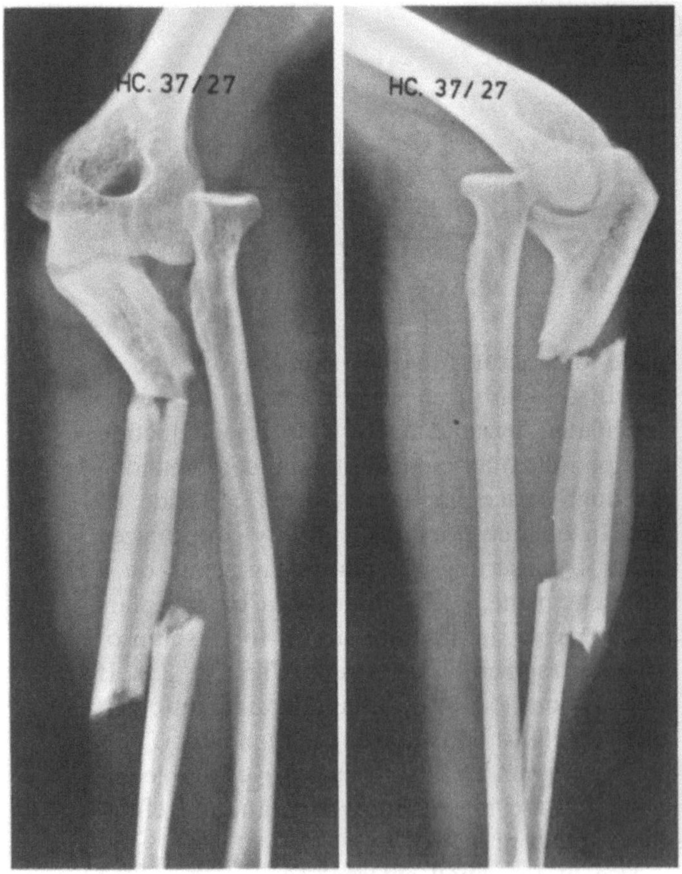

a

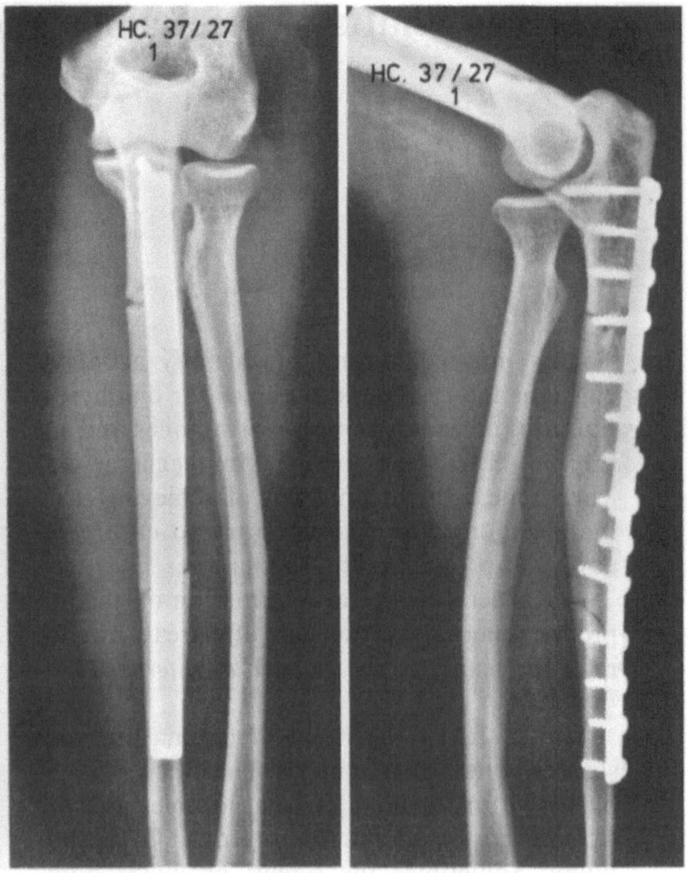

b

Fig. 87 a–e. Clinical example: Monteggia fracture, nonunion of the ulna

Luigi M., 50-year-old factory worker, caught left arm in machinery on 4/29/77

a Monteggia injuries with dislocation of the radial head and segmental fracture of the ulna

b Immediate internal fixation of the ulna was performed with two superimposed 8-hole one-third tubular plates; the radial head reduced spontaneously. The annular ligament was not repaired. A dorsal plaster splint was applied
Postoperative course was uneventful, and functional exercises were started at 3 weeks

c The proximal fracture remained painful and caused disability. Five months after primary internal fixation, a rigid nonunion of the proximal fracture was diagnosed due to faulty screw placement in the proximal one-third tubular plate

d Revision was performed at 5 months. The proximal plate was removed and replaced with a 3.5-mm DCP. Bone grafting was not performed. The nonunion consolidated within 3 months.The implants were removed 16 months after the second operation

e When seen 3 years postinjury on 3/24/80, the patient has no complaints and full function.The proximal scars were slightly adherent to underlying tissues. Patient was able to work with no disability

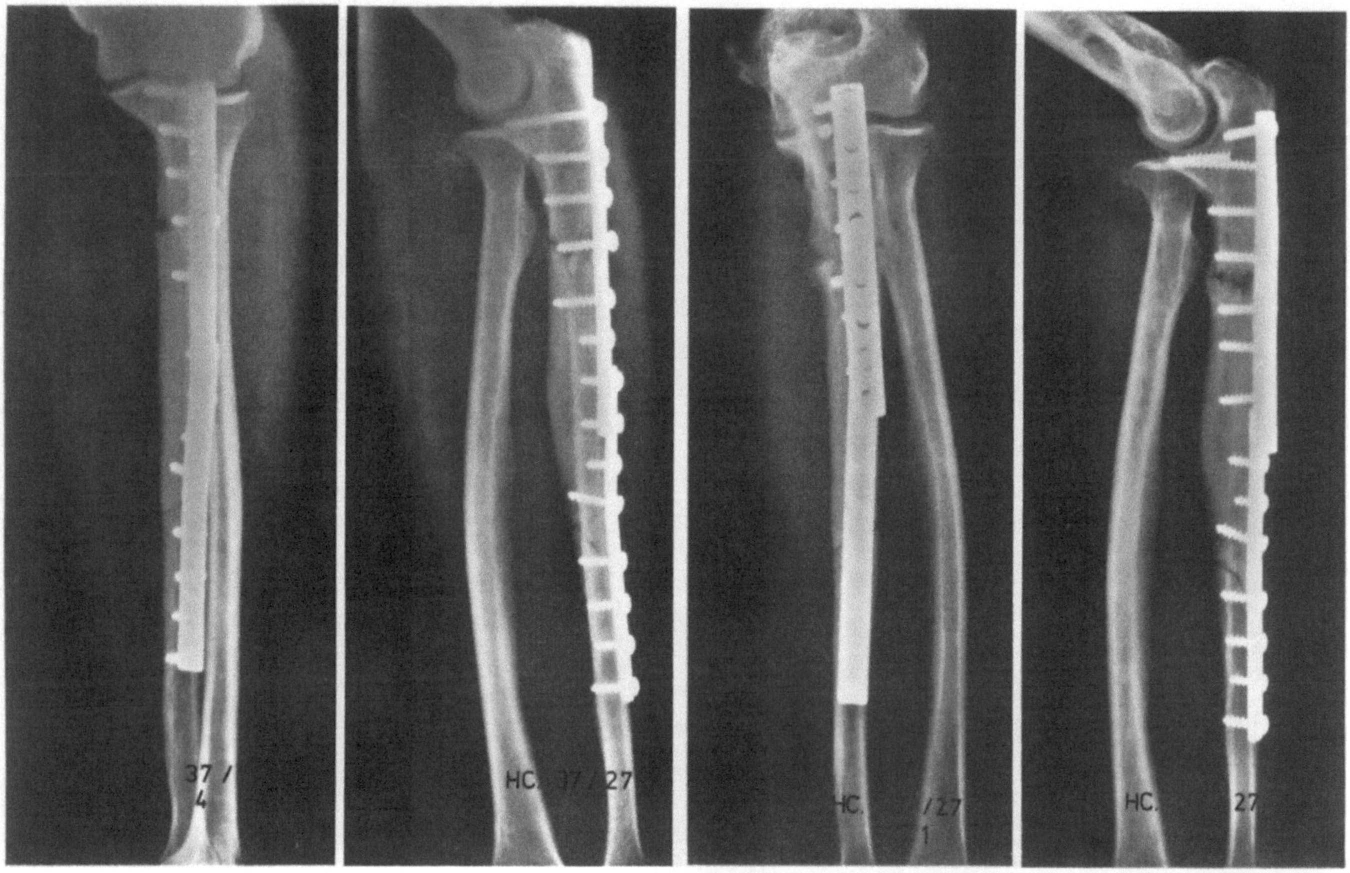

c, d

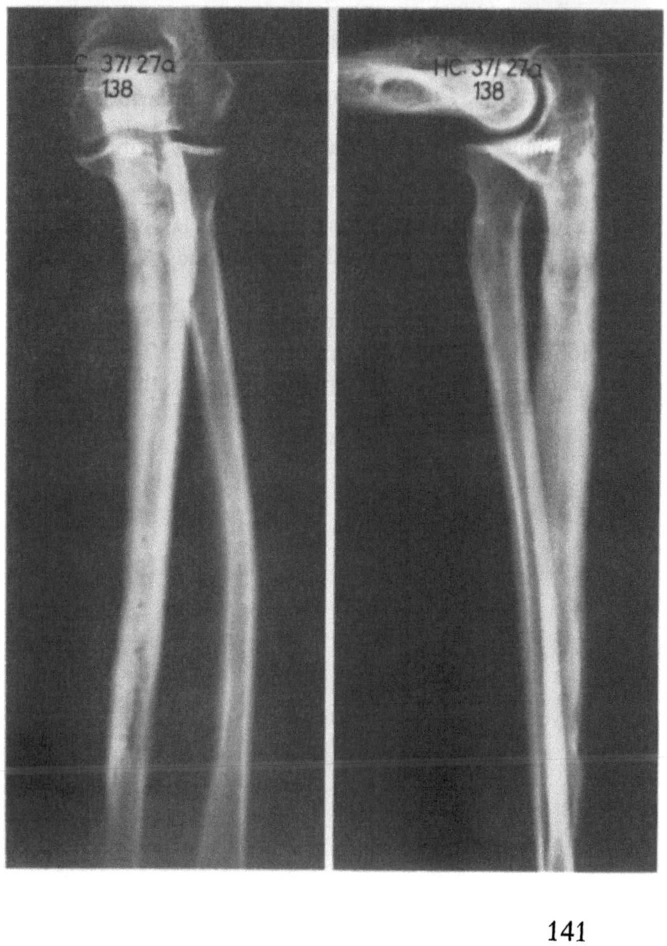

e

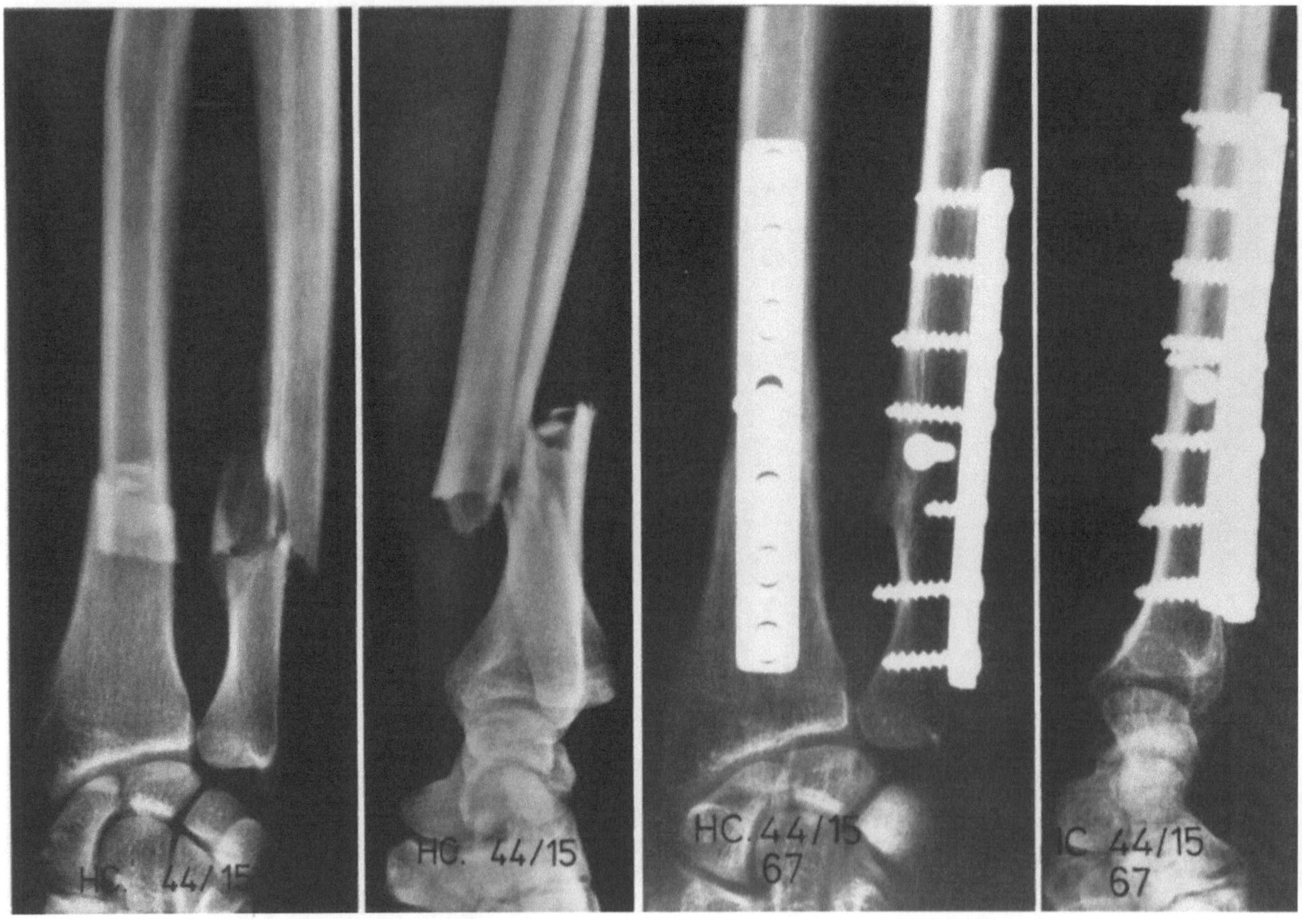

a b

Fig. 88a, b. Clinical example: distal forearm fracture

Tibor D., 42-year-old lathe operator, caught left forearm in machinery on 11/29/78

a Oblique fracture of both forearm bones with butterfly fragments and dislocation of the distal radioulnar joint.
The fractures were immediately exposed through two longitudinal incisions, and two 3.5-mm 7-hole DCPs were applied. The butterfly was fixed to the ulna with a separate screw. Swelling necessitated a fasciotomy. Postoperative course was uneventful, and a removable plaster splint was worn for 6 weeks. Full work fitness was achieved at 26 weeks

b On follow-up at 14 months, the patient had no complaints and full function. Primary union was confirmed.Implants were removed on 8/14/80

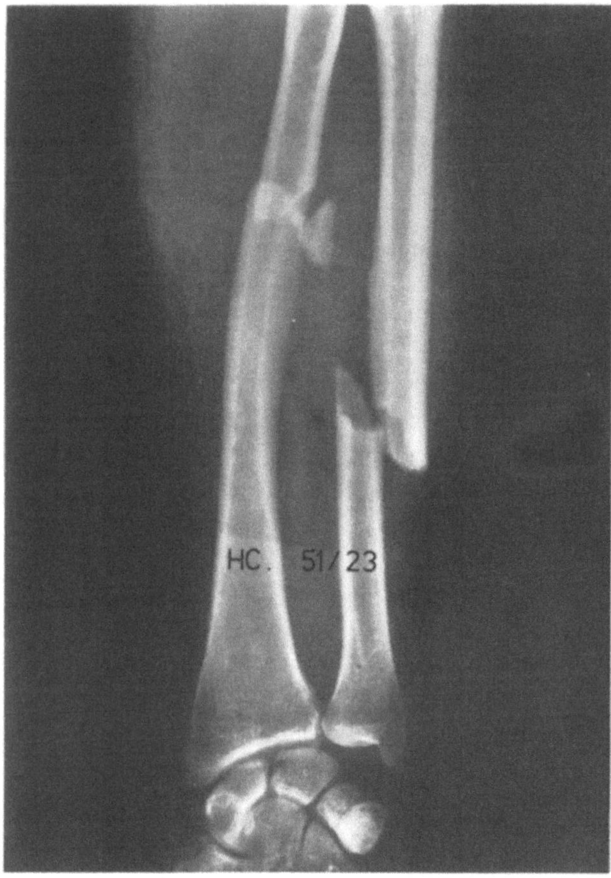

a

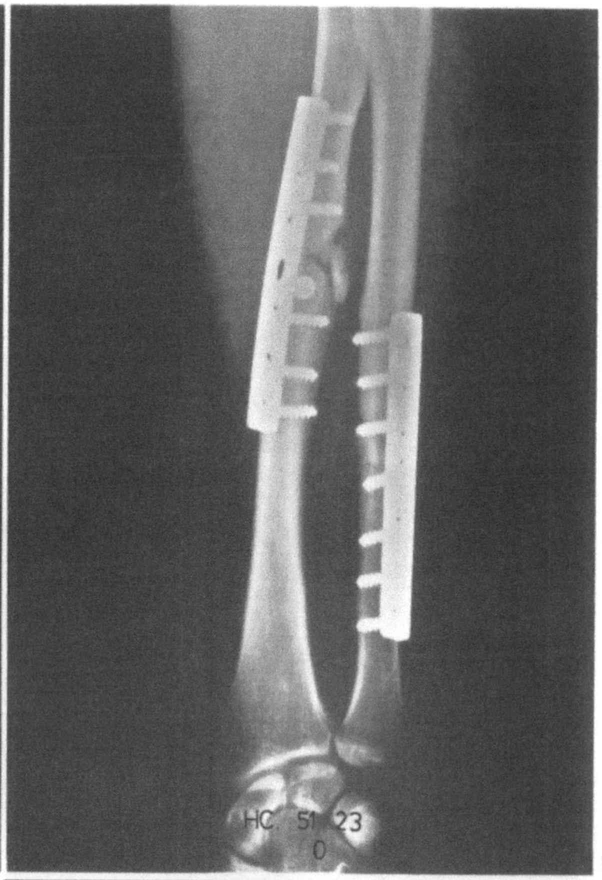

b

Fig. 89a–c. Clinical example: open forearm fracture

Rosa E., 46-year-old farmer's wife, fell while skiing on 2/20/80

a Grade-one open fracture of the left forearm with a radial butterfly and a fissure fracture of the ulna

b The radius and ulna were exposed through separate incisions, and each was fixed with a 3.5-mm 7-hole DCP; a separate lag screw was used in the radius
Postoperative course was uncomplicated. A removable plaster splint was worn for 3 weeks, followed by functional exercises
Patient resumed her farming work at 4 months. The implants were removed at 2 years

c When seen $6^1/_2$ years later, the patient had no complaints, full function, and good cortical structure on X-rays

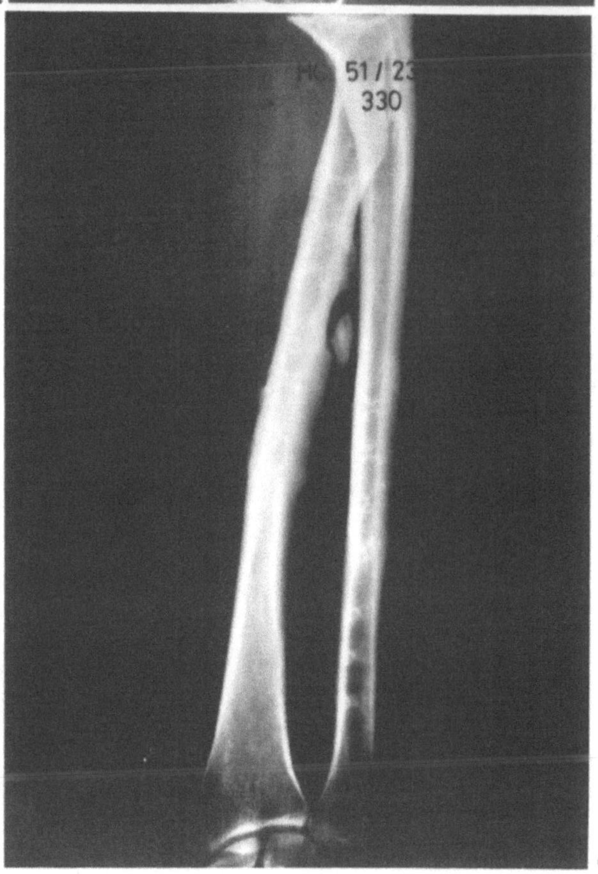

c

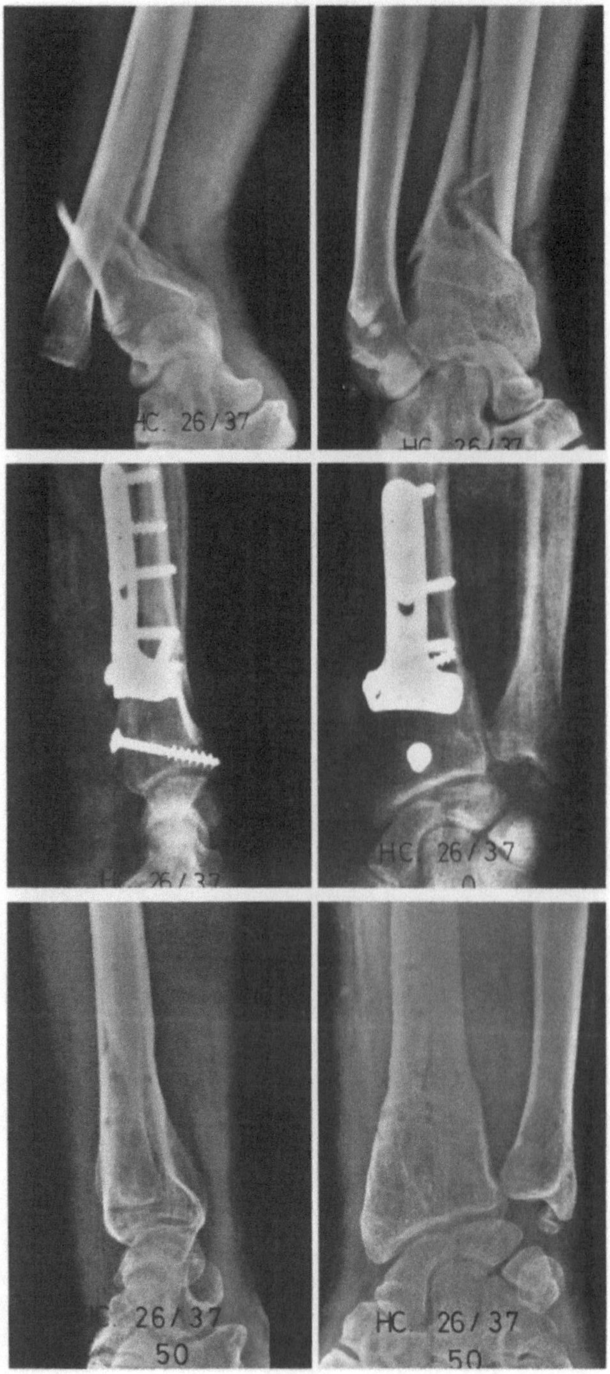

a
b
c

Fig. 90 a–c. Clinical example: Galeazzi fracture

Hans V., 52-year-old civil servant, injured while skiing on 3/19/75

a Complex distal fracture of the radius with dislocation of the ulna and avulsion of the ulnar styloid process

b Emergency internal fixation was performed, stabilizing the radius with a dorsal T plate and separate screw. The ulna reduced spontaneously
Removable plaster splint was worn for 9 weeks. Full loading and work fitness were achieved at 12 weeks

c At 1-year follow-up the implants were removed. Patient had no complaints, full function, no muscular atrophy, and a linear scar

XII. The Wrist and Carpus

1. Distal Radius

The most common fracture in this region, and probably the most common fracture of the human skeleton in general, is the Colles fracture. This is a compression fracture of the distal radius in which the distal radial articular surface is tilted dorsally (extension fracture) and also radially, with corresponding shortening. The great majority of these fractures are treated conservatively, but serious disability can result if the reduction is inexact or if secondary displacement occurs, which some authors describe in approximately half of cases. This injury should not be considered trivial just because it predominantly affects elderly women whose disability may have little impact on their work or earnings.

In 1981 the ASIF adopted the ABC system for the classification of these fractures. This system has proved very useful in the selection of patients for operative treatment (Fig. 91). Type A fractures are extra-articular fractures of the metaphysis. Type B fractures involve the articular rim and only partially disrupt the continuity of the joint, metaphysis, and diaphysis. Type C fractures are epiphyseal-metaphyseal fractures that destroy this continuity.

When assessing the need for operative treatment, one needs to distinguish among the options that are available: percutaneous Kirschner wire fixation, open reduction and internal fixation, and transarticular fixation with external pins and rods.

Percutaneous pinning with Kirschner wires has proved effective for simpler, unstable fractures (Fig. 92a), but it cannot prevent secondary displacement in all cases.

In younger patients with steplike incongruities in the joint suface, closed reduction by manipulation often is impossible, and there is no acceptable alternative to rigid internal fixation.

Operative treatment is also indicated for Smith type 2 or reverse Barton fractures ("Goyrand fracture" in French). These are flexion fractures in which all or part of the articular surface is displaced proximally and volarly, and the proximal carpal row is subluxated. These fractures are extremely unstable (Fig. 93).

Fractures that have both an extension and a flexion component and appear Y-shaped on lateral radiographs, as well as comminuted fractures, represent borderline situations. Each case must be evaluated and treated individually. Internal fixation, while limited in its indications, can give excellent results in experienced hands.

Follow-ups of numerous internal fixations in our patients have shown that functional outcomes are significantly better after volar plating for flexion fractures than after dorsal plating for extension or mixed-type fractures.

The internal fixation can be stable only if the screws solidly engage the distal fragment – especially a large fragment of the radial styloid or the radial volar rim. For complex fractures, good results have been obtained in recent years with the small external fixator applied in a transarticular configuration (Fig. 42, 103).

Open reduction and internal fixation has demonstrated its efficacy in the following types of fracture:

a) Fractures of the Radial Styloid

Many of these fractures are minimally displaced, but almost all are unstable. Sometimes they are the visible manifestation of a transnavicular-perilunar fracture-dislocation that has reduced spontaneously. Thus, one should always consider the possibility of a coexisting scaphoid fracture. Internal fixation has a better success rate than cast immobilization and is most effectively accomplished with two 4.0-mm cancellous or 3.5-mm cortex screws (Fig. 92c). With a very small fragment, a preliminary Kirschner wire may be left in place to stabilize against rotation.

b) Comminuted Articular Fractures

These fractures most commonly occur in younger individuals as a result of motor vehicle accidents and sports-related injuries. Often the fragments are impacted and are not amenable to closed reduction. It is imperative that steps in the articular surface be eliminated and congruity reestablished. Most of these fractures are of the extension type and are stabilized with an oblique T plate applied dorsally (Fig. 92d).

c) Flexion Fractures (Goyrand, Smith, Reversed Barton)

The volar fragments are difficult to reduce by closed manipulation and are not maintained well in a cast. They exert pressure on the flexor tendons and median nerve. These fractures are a classic indication for the buttress plate. The radial T plate is designed specifically for this site and conforms perfectly to the bone.Bony defects are uncommon and require autogenous cancellous grafting. The radial styloid cannot be solidly engaged in these cases, so in comminuted fractures it may be necessary to insert separate oblique or transverse screws or Kirschner wires to obtain sufficient stability (Fig. 93).

d) Y Fractures

These are mixed fractures having both a flexion and an extension component. It can be difficult to select a single approach for internal fixation. A plate applied to one side cannot adequately support the opposing fragment, which may redisplace.

Experience has shown that the plate should be applied to the least stable side, which is the side of greatest comminution. In this way a screw can be driven more securely into a larger, shell-like opposing fragment, while smaller fragments are easier to visualize and are compressed by the plate itself. We recommend using an image intensifier while carrying out the fixation. With the fracture site exposed, reduction is effected by continuous traction on the thumb. The unseen, opposing fragment is kept from displacing by pressing the wrist down against a hard surface or, preferably, by passing the index finger or a Hohmann retractor beneath it on the volar side. The first extensor tendon sheath is opened for this maneuver so that the finger or instrument can be passed around the radius without trauma. Pressure against the opposing fragment is maintained while the plate is applied and the screws inserted.The screws in the crosspiece of the T plate must be long enough to engage the thin opposite cortex (cancellous or cortex screws 22-28 mm long). Screws hold best in the volar articular margin of the radius.

The first screw is placed through the oval hole of the T plate if possible, as this will temporarily buttress the fracture while still allowing plate adjustments. Defects in the metaphysis are grafted with cancellous bone. With a simple oblique fracture, one plate screw is lagged across the main fragments to effect compression.

e) Approaches and Technique of Internal Fixation

Experience shows that surgeons are reluctant to operate on the wrist joint because of its complex anatomy. Especially on the dorsal side of the radius, the bone is overlaid by many tendons and nerves coursing at diverse angles, and it would appear difficult to gain access without causing unacceptable soft-tissue injury. Below we shall describe in some detail approaches that have been tested specifically for internal fixations about the wrist and have proven successful.

Approach to the Radial Styloid

The landmark for the incision is the tip of the styloid process on the radial border of the anatomic snuffbox.

A slightly curved incision is made on the dorsoradial aspect of the wrist. The superficial branch of the radial nerve is identified and retracted to the dorsoulnar side. The styloid process is approached between the tendons of extensor pollicis brevis and extensor carpi radialis longus. The extensor retinaculum is incised, and the first three extensor tendon sheaths are opened. The tendons of extensor pollicis brevis and abductor pollicis longus are retracted to the radiovolar side, and the fracture is exposed by splitting the periosteum and opening the joint dorsally (Fig. 94a1).

Dorsal Approach to the Distal Radius

A lazy S- or Z-shaped skin incision is made from the base of the second metacarpal over the wrist to the distal forearm (Fig. 94 a2). After epifascial mobilization of the radial skin flap, the superficial branches of the radial nerve are retracted radially. The extensor retinaculum is split longitudinally over the first tendon sheath of abductor pollicis longus and is dissected around toward the ulnar side, sharply dividing its attachments to the dorsal ridges of the radius. This is done more easily with a scalpel than with a periosteal elevator. Next the tendons of abductor pollicis longus, extensor pollicis brevis, extensor carpi radialis longus and brevis, and extensor pollicis longus are retracted radially, while the tendons of extensor indicis and extensor digitorum communis are retracted to the ulnar side.

Extension of the approach for exposing the volar side of the radius is described under **d** above.

The oblique T plate for 3.5-mm screws is excellent for this region. The screw holes are designed so that the plate can be inverted for use on either the right or left extremity. The plate was modified so that the crosspiece would extend farther toward the styloid process of the radius (Fig. 92).

Following attachment of the plate, the divided extensor retinaculum usually can be reapproximated over the tendons without tension (Fig. 94). The danger of tendon abrasion by the round screw heads is minimal. Alternatively, half or all of the extensor retinaculum may be interposed between the plate and the extensor tendons, as is done in rheumatoid surgery. In younger patients with strong dorsal extensors, we have sometimes seen troublesome bulging of the tendons beneath the skin in the absence of retinacular coverage. With appropriate functional aftertreatment, there is virtually no danger of extensor function impairment by tendon adhesions.

Approach to the Distal Radius from the Volar Side

The landmark for this approach is the flexor carpi radialis tendon. A wide exposure is needed so that the median nerve can be decompressed in the carpal tunnel at the time internal fixation is carried out. For this reason the flexor retinaculum should be completely divided in all internal fixations of this area. The large incision also helps protect the deep soft structures (tendons, nerve, vessels) from intraoperative pressure injury and postoperative edema.

A slightly angled incision is made over the distal forearm and is extended onto the thenar crease of the palm (Fig. 95). The median nerve is identified on the ulnar side of the prominent flexor carpi radialis tendon and is carefully dissected to the flexor retinaculum. Particular care is taken to spare its sensory palmar branch coursing to the thenar. This branch may arise some distance proximal to the wrist and run parallel to the main trunk for several centimeters, crossing the flexor carpi radialis tendon dorsally or perhaps volarly on its way to the skin of the thenar.

The flexor retinaculum is divided at its ulnar margin (Fig. 95c). Usually the median nerve is gently retracted to the radial side along with the flexor carpi radialis tendon, or possibly to the ulnar side together with the long flexor tendons (taking care to protect the palmar branch of the nerve). The flexor tendons within their sheath are retracted to the ulnar side. At this point the distal volar border of the radius and the wide band of the pronator quadratus muscle just proximal to it should be visible in the field. The muscle is incised as far radially as possible under the retracted flexor carpi radialis tendon and is stripped to the ulnar side with a periosteal elevator to expose the fracture site (Fig. 96). The radiocarpal joint can be marked with a hypodermic needle or thin Kirschner wire, or if necessary the joint may be opened transversely under vision to perform the reduction. Access to the radial styloid, however, is relatively difficult from this approach.

Variation: When exposure of the distal radioulnar joint is needed, the flexor tendons are retracted radially along with the median nerve, while the flexor carpi ulnaris is retracted to the ulnar side together with the ulnar artery and nerve (Fig. 96c).

Closure

On both the volar and dorsal sides, the skin is closed over a suction drain placed at the fracture site. A well-padded plaster splint is applied with the wrist slightly extended to protect wound healing and hold the wrist in a physiologic position.This permits elevation of the limb and mobilization of the fingers. If stability is questionable, the splint may be worn for a longer period. Active mobilization of the fingers is started right away.

Implant Removal

The original incisions are largely reopened for removal of the plates. Subcutaneous scar formation can make it difficult to spare the superficial radial nerve branch dorsally. In most cases it is surprisingly easy to remove volar plates, although care must be taken to spare the sensory palmar branch of the median nerve.

f) Secondary Operations

Secondary Internal Fixation

The most frequent indication for dorsal plating is deformity secondary to a malunited extension fracture. The procedure is easier to perform if consolidation is not yet complete (prior to the 12th week). Satisfactory peripheral circulation and trophism are essential to a good functional outcome. Corrective surgery is performed through the dorsal approach described above, the object being to restore the physiologic angle of the radial joint surface and eliminate radial deviation and shortening. Defects in the metaphysis are grafted with autogenous cancellous bone. A corticocancellous graft may be needed if significant osteoporosis exists. We stabilize the bone with a suitably contoured T plate or with the special oblique T plate.

Nonunions of the distal radius are uncommon and are fixed with a dorsal T plate or DCP.Defects are filled with autogenous cancellous bone.

Osteotomy

Osteotomy is mainly indicated for the correction of deformity secondary to the nonoperative treatment of extension fractures with associated dorsal and radial impaction of the articular surface and shortening. The correction must be secured by the insertion of iliac corticocancellous wedge grafts that are stable under compression. The decision for corrective surgery is based not on the degree of deformity, but on the deficits of hand and wrist function and associated complaints. Chronic compression of the median nerve in the carpal tunnel may be one component of the syndrome, and this should be evaluated before surgery is performed. Electromyography is recommended in doubtful cases. If median nerve compression exists, one must combine the skeletal operation with nerve decompression by incision of the flexor retinaculum. The procedure follows the technique described for secondary internal fixations, and the same implants are used.

As a rule, steplike incongruities in articular surfaces cannot be corrected secondarily. If complaints are referrable to incipient traumatic arthritis, no benefit will be derived from corrective osteotomy.

In an elderly patient presenting with a marked limitation of pronation and supination due to relative lengthening of the ulna, a shortening osteotomy of the ulna or simple resection of the ulnar head is preferable to a corrective operation on the radius.

Shortening osteotomies of the distal radius are indicated mainly for the early stage of lunate malacia. Either a dorsal or volar approach may be used. The osteotomy is made obliquely so that an interfragmental lag screw can be inserted through the plate. The osteotomy is fixed with one of the shaped plates described earlier, or less frequently with a straight DCP.

2. Distal Ulna

The narrow, distal part of the ulnar shaft is occasionally a site of transverse or short oblique fractures, which may occur in isolation or in conjunction with fractures of the radial shaft or metaphysis. These fractures are subject to heavy bending and shear loads during pronation and supination and consequently are unstable. They are an absolute indication for operative treatment.

Because the ulna is subcutaneous, exposure should pose no difficulties. The sensory branch of the ulnar nerve, which passes to the dorsal side close to the styloid, must be protected.

The one-third tubular plate may occasionally be too flimsy for distal ulnar fractures, and the stronger 3.5-mm DCP too bulky. An alternative would be to use the 2.7-mm DCP or perhaps two one-third tubular plates of different lengths placed one atop the other.

Secondary Operations

Indications for secondary operations on the distal ulna are relatively frequent. Most relate to deformities of the distal radius. Troublesome subluxations of the distal radioulnar joint in older patients and ulnar head syndrome in the rheumatoid hand are indications for resection of the distal ulna. Generally this will not significantly compromise wrist stability.It is necessary to reconstruct a sheath for the extensor carpi ulnaris tendon, possibly by using a tendon graft or a pedicle flap from the extensor retinaculum.

In some cases shortening osteotomies are recommended in younger patients as adjuncts to corrective procedures on the radius. The goal is to improve pronation and supination while preserving the distal ulna. Successful lengthenings in cases of lunate malacia have been described.

3. Scaphoid (Navicular)

a) Indications

Undisplaced fractures of the scaphoid or navicular bone of the carpus are treated conservatively, and most will heal in 8–12 weeks with proper cast immobilization. Solitary tubercle fractures will unite in 3–4 weeks.

Years of clinical experience have limited the role of primary internal fixation in the management of these cases. It is justified for displaced and unstable fractures of the middle third. Survey radiographs and even spot films do not always give enough information on these injuries, and we supplement X-rays with a functional examination of the carpus using nerve block anesthesia and an image intensifier, comparing it with the uninvolved side. Many seemingly acceptable reductions are associated with a partial collapse of the carpus or deformity of the scaphoid, leading to poor functional results.

The classic indication for primary internal fixation is the perilunar, transnavicular fracture-dislocation described by de Quervain, which proceeds to nonunion in about half of cases. Internal fixation is also indicated for the rare vertical oblique fracture which, like the Pauwels type 3 fracture of the neck of the femur, is subject to very large shear forces and accordingly shows a six times higher incidence of nonunion than other types of fracture.

We fix these fractures with a screw inserted under vision from the dorsoradial side, using a screw size that is matched to the size of the fragments. The 4.0-mm cancellous screw (formerly called the "navicular screw") is usually too bulky, and increasingly we prefer the 2.7- and 2.0-mm sizes. A second implant is useful for checking rotation; the provisional Kirschner wire may be sufficient for this purpose.

b) Approach and Internal Fixation from the Dorsoradial Side (Fig. 97)

The standard approach is made through a curved incision in the anatomic snuffbox. The superficial branches of the radial nerve are retracted dorsally with the extensor pollicis longus tendon. The tendons of extensor pollicis brevis and abductor pollicis longus are retracted distally and volarly together with the radial artery. As an alternative, one may use a right-angled incision starting at the dorsal base of the second metacarpal, extending radially through the anatomic snuffbox, and turning dorsally and proximally at the level of the abductor pollicis tendon. This incision may be extended in Z fashion as required. Its scar is less prone to hypertrophy than that of the standard incision. The wrist is opened at the dorsal edge of the radial styloid while the hand is positioned in strong volar and ulnar flexion. The fracture is exposed and reduced using an atraumatic elevator, fine forceps or small hook, taking great care to preserve the articular cartilage (Fig. 98). A thin Kirschner wire of known length is drilled through the fracture site from the tubercle, and its position is checked radiographically. This enables the correct screw length to be determined. Next a hole for the screw is drilled parallel to the Kirschner wire through the appropriate guide. The hole is tapped, a gliding hole is made in the distal fragment, and the screw is introduced. The guide wire may be left in place for rotational stability, or it may be replaced with a second screw (Fig. 98e).

The primary partial excision of the radial styloid to improve exposure of the fracture site is controversial due to the danger of circulatory compromise.

Postoperatively we recommend that even a stable internal fixation be supplemented by external cast immobilization for 4–6 weeks.

Recently Herbert has recommended performing internal fixation on the scaphoid axis through a wide volar approach using a special screw with two terminal threads of different pitch. The indications for this technique are broad. Subsequent implant removal is seldom possible.

c) Secondary Operations

The delayed union of a conservatively treated scaphoid fracture is a good indication for screw fixation. The decision for operation may be based on a tomogram taken at eight weeks. Success depends on a viable proximal fragment, and the screw fixation should always be supplemented by external immobilization.

True nonunions are characterized by sclerosis of the bone ends, possibly accompanied by cyst formation, deformity, and shortening. Screw compression by itself is definitely unsuitable in adults. We manage most cases with bone grafting by the technique of Matti and Russe, followed by plaster immobilization.

Angular deformity and shortening of the scaphoid generally are associated with a painful collapse of the entire carpus and diminished wrist motion. These circumstances must be considered when selecting an internal fixation technique. The length and axes of the scaphoid can be reestablished only by realigning the bone and interposing a wide corticocancellous graft. In favorable cases this will realign the carpus and significantly improve wrist function. Generally the bone is stabilized with transfixing Kirschner wires, although screws, H plates, or small condylar plates may also be suitable. Attention should be given to the scapholunar ligamentous connection, as concomitant damage to this structure is not unusual. Rupture-related instabilities must be corrected to ensure painless wrist function.

4. Other Carpal Bones

Fractures of other carpal bones are rare.Larger fragments that are easily accessible are an indication for rigid internal fixation when displacement or diastasis exists. Longitudinal fractures of the trapezium combined with Bennett's fracturedislocation are most commonly seen and are amenable to screw fixation. Fractures of the remaining carpal bones may be accessible to screw fixation, depending on the location of the fracture plane. Otherwise they may be stabilized with a Kirschner wire, a wire suture, or perhaps an H plate.

5. Arthrodesis of the Wrist (Fig. 99)

Fusion of the wrist has proved beneficial for severely comminuted carpal fractures, for severe traumatic arthritis, and for chronic inflammatory diseases (rheumatic fever, tuberculosis, etc.) that are associated with painful instability and dislocation. The arthrodesis may be secured with a plate attached to the distal radius and to the third (or second) metacarpal. The DCP for 3.5-mm screws (8- to 9-hole) is best for this purpose. After the removal of small bone fragments and tissues showing inflammatory change, or following cartilage removal in patients with degenerative arthritis, the defects are grafted with an appropriate volume of cancellous bone. In addition, the carpus is bridged from the radius to the base of the metacarpal with a rectangular corticocancellous iliac graft. The cancellous surface of the graft should face the carpus. Before the plate is attached, the carpus is drawn against the radial styloid with a lag screw to keep the distal radioulnar joint out of the fusion area. The screw holds best in the capitate bone. With this technique, good pronation and supination can be preserved without excision of the ulnar head.

6. Illustrative Clinical X-Rays
(Figs. 100–112)

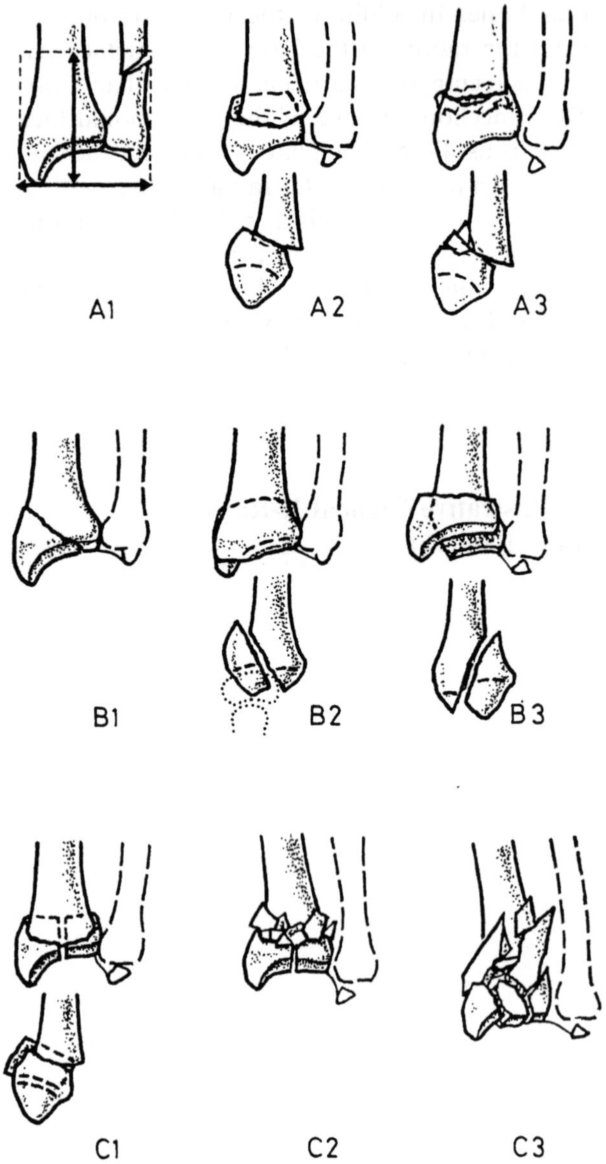

Fig. 91. ASIF classification of distal forearm fractures, based on the ABC system (subgroups are not shown)

A = Extra-articular metaphyseal fracture
Junction of the metaphysis and diaphysis is identified by the "square" or "T" method (greatest width on frontal plane of distal forearm; illustrated on A1)
A1 = Isolated fracture of distal ulna
A2 = Simple radial fracture
A3 = Radial fracture with metaphyseal impaction

B = Intra-articular rim fracture (preserving the continuity of the epiphysis and metaphysis)
B1 = Fracture of radial styloid
B2 = Dorsal rim fracture (dorsal Barton)
B3 = Volar rim fracture (reverse Barton = Goyrand-Smith type 2, Letenneur)

C = Complex intra-articular fracture (disrupting the continuity of the epiphysis and metaphysis)
C1 = Radiocarpal joint congruity preserved, metaphysis fractured
C2 = Articular displacement
C3 = Diaphyseal-metaphyseal involvement

It should be considered that injury of the distal radioulnar joint is possible in any of these fractures

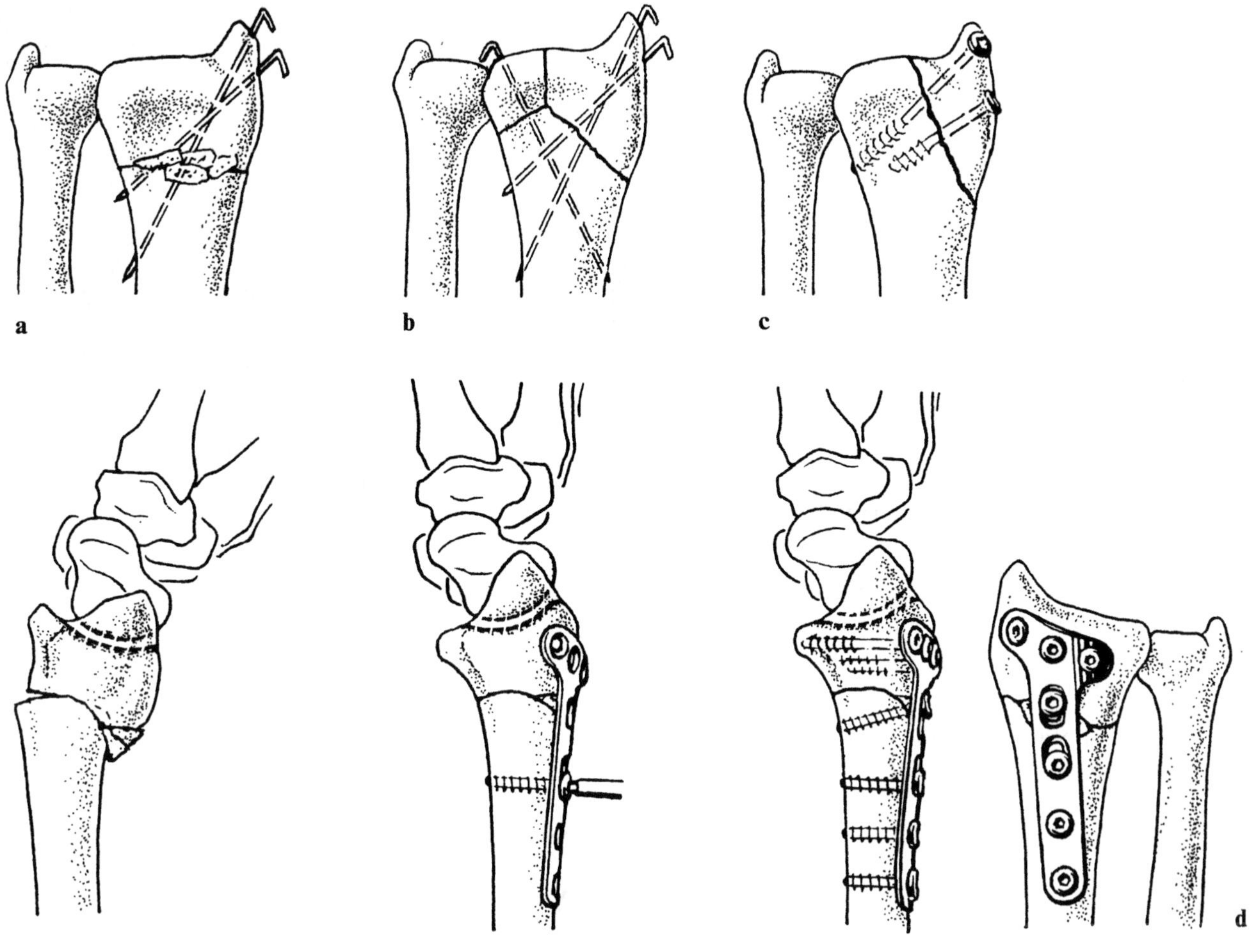

Fig. 92 a–d. Typical internal fixations of distal radial fractures

a Unstable extra-articular fracture fixed with percutaneous Kirschner wires introduced from the radial side

b Arrangement of Kirschner wires for an intra-articular fracture with a dorsoulnar fragment

c Screw fixation of a radial styloid fracture

d Internal fixation of a dorsally angulated type A fracture with an oblique T plate applied to the dorsal radius (rare indication for primary surgery see p. 145.) After preliminary reduction, the plate is temporarily attached with a screw in the oval plate hole. Fine reduction is carried out, and the remaining plate screws are inserted

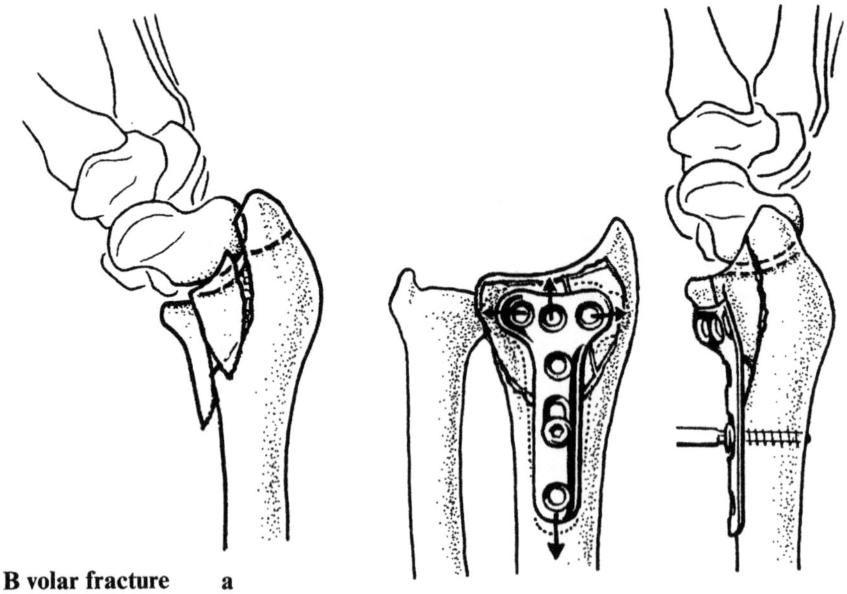

a

Fig. 93 a, b. Internal fixation of a type B volar fracture

a A T plate buttresses the fracture on the volar side. The first screw is placed through the oval plate hole and provisionally tightened. Fine reduction is carried out, and the plate is contoured. Then the remaining screws are inserted

b Finished appearance of the internal fixation with a right-angled or oblique T plate

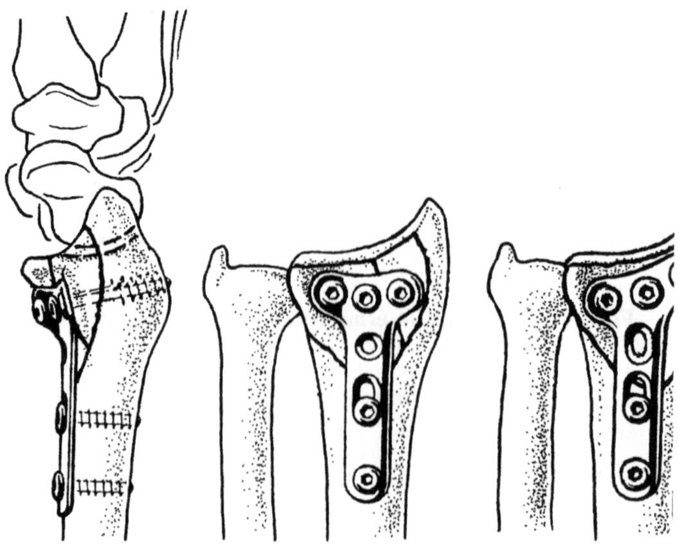

b

Fig. 94. Radiodorsal approaches to the distal radius

a S-shaped skin incisions:

1 The radial styloid is approached through a short skin incision between the tendons of extensor pollicis brevis (EPB) and extensor carpi radialis longus (ECRL)

2 The distal radial metaphysis is approached by dividing the extensor retinaculum and reflecting it upward

3 Combined approach for dorsal plating and volar control of reduction: The extensor retinaculum is divided at the volar margin of the abductor pollicis longus (APL) tendon sheath and reflected to the dorsoulnar side. The surgeon passes his left index finger beneath the pronator quadratus muscle to assist the reduction and stabilization from the volar side

b The approaches in cross-section:

1 Between the tendons of extensor pollicis brevis (EPB) and extensor carpi radialis longus (ECRL)

2 Between the tendons of extensor carpi radialis brevis (ECRB) and extensor pollicis longus (EPL), elevating the tendon sheaths from the periosteum

3 At the volar edge of the abductor pollicis longus tendons (APL), reflecting the extensor retinaculum to the dorsoulnar side

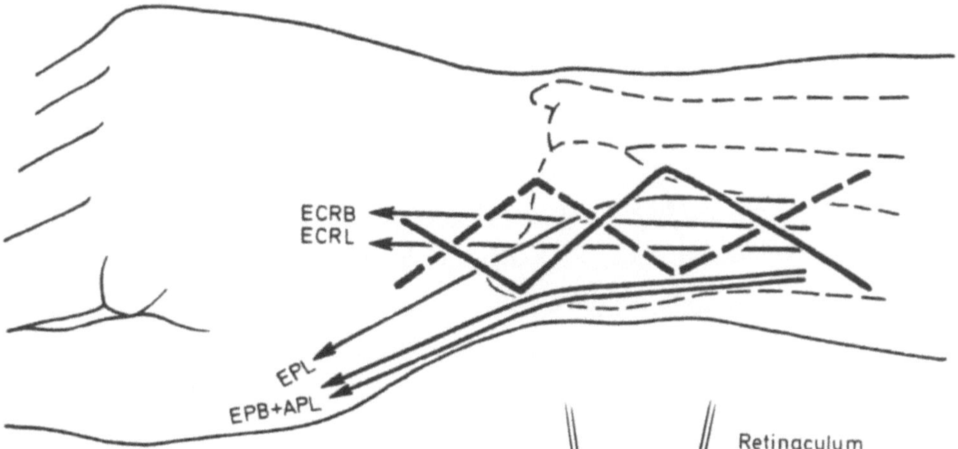

a

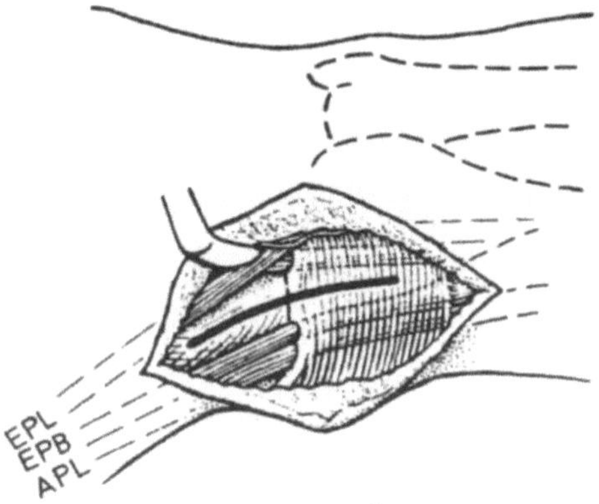

1

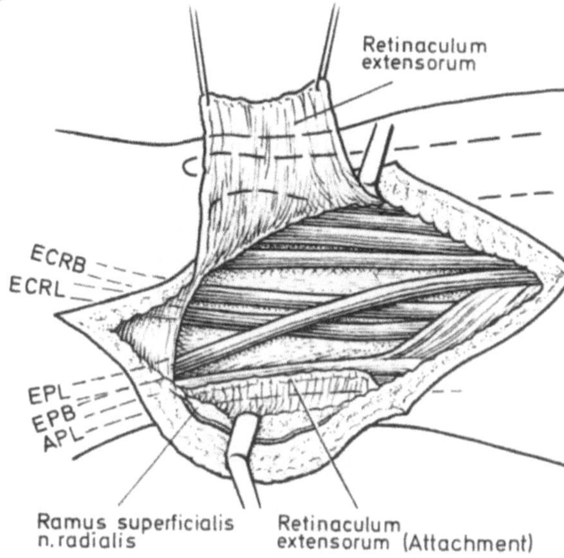

2

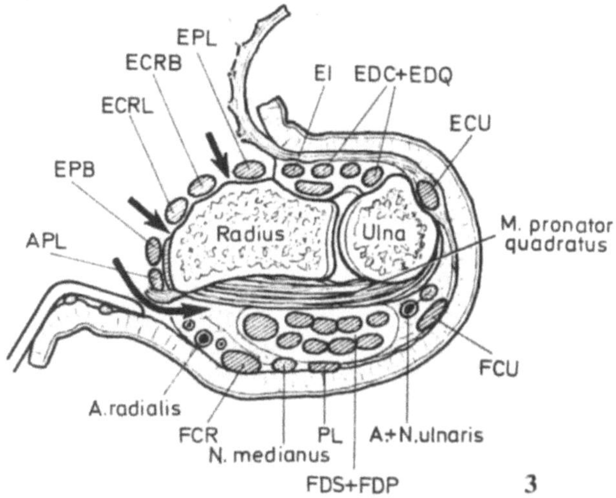

3

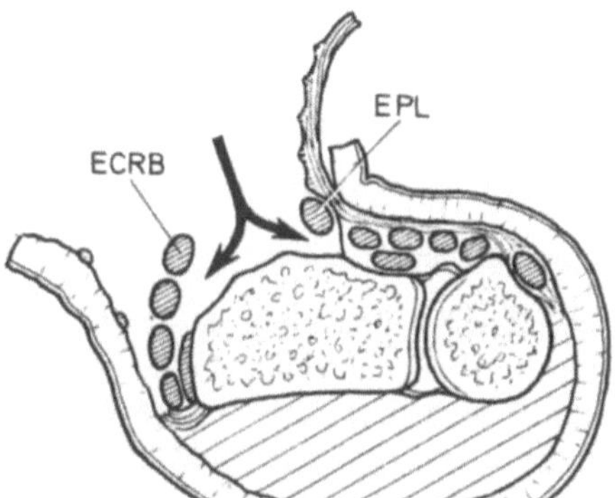

b

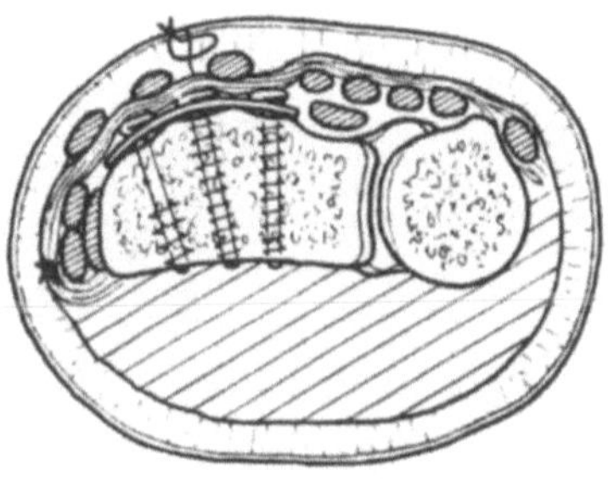

c

c Following the internal fixation, the extensor retinaculum can be split and a portion passed beneath the tendons to protect them from abrasion by the implants

EI Extensor indicis proprius tendon
EDC Extensor digitorum communis tendon
EDQ Extensor digiti quinti tendon
ECU Extensor carpi ulnaris tendon
FCR Flexor carpi radialis tendon
PL Palmaris longus tendon
FDS Flexor digitorum superficialis tendon
FDP Flexor digitorum profundus tendon
FCU Flexor carpi ulnaris tendon

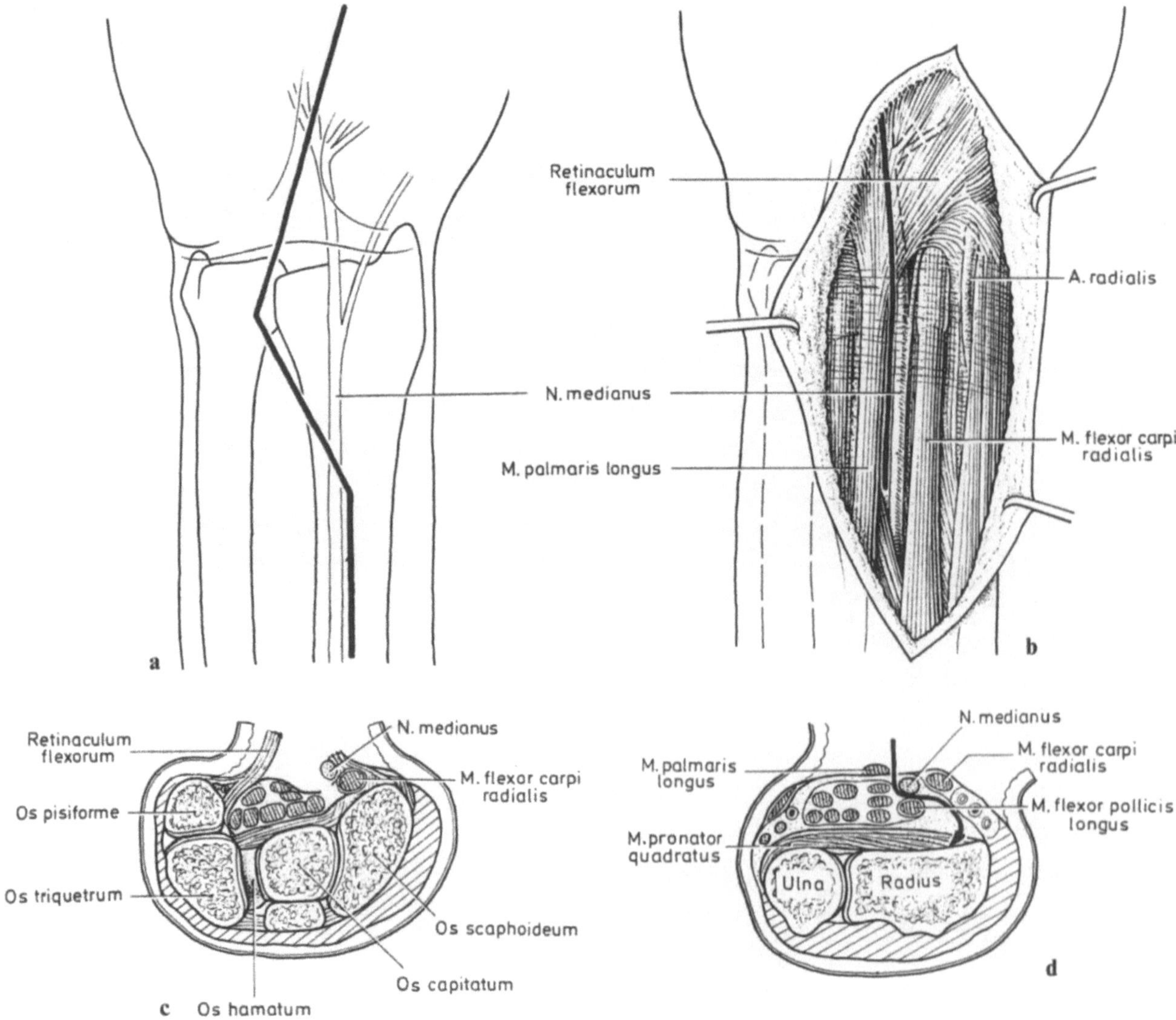

Fig. 95a–d. Volar approaches to the distal radius

a Long, angled skin incision

b The flexor retinaculum is divided, and the distal radius is approached ulnar to the flexor carpi radialis tendon. The median nerve is retracted radially to protect the sensory palmar branch arising proximal to the wrist

c Distal cross-section at the level of the flexor retinaculum. The median nerve is retracted to the radial side

d Proximal cross-section at the level of the distal radius, showing approach to the radial attachment of pronator quadratus

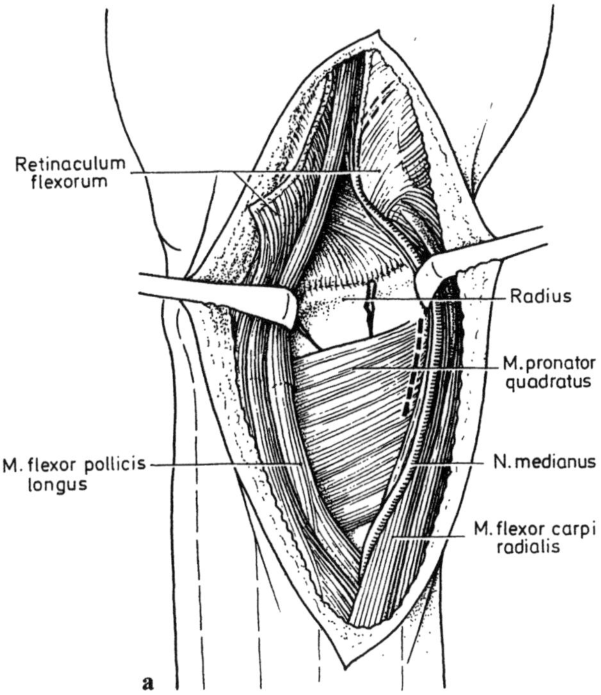

a

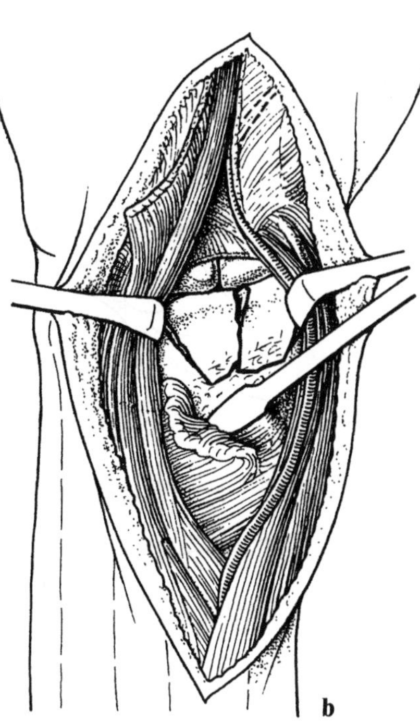

b

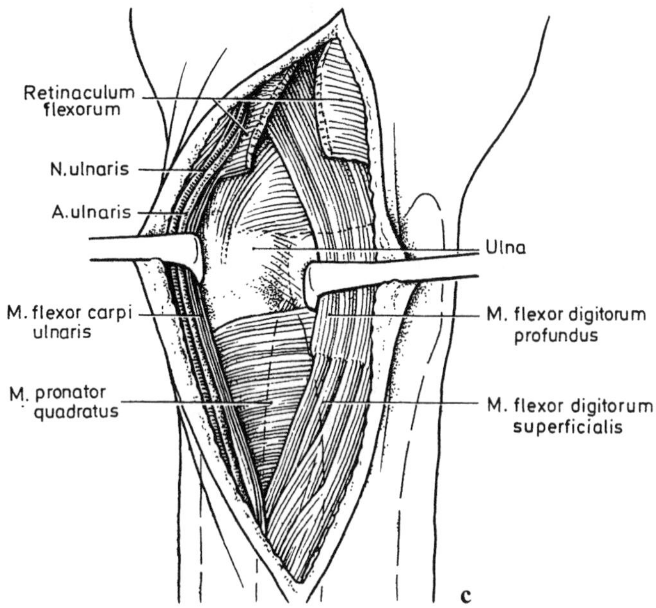

c

Fig. 96 a–c. Volar approach to the distal radius (deep layer)

a The median nerve and flexor carpi radialis are retracted radially to expose the fracture and pronator quadratus muscle

b The pronator quadratus is incised at its radial attachment. The radiocarpal joint is opened if this is necessary for reduction under vision

c Variation: The flexor tendons are retracted radially for exposure of the distal radioulnar joint

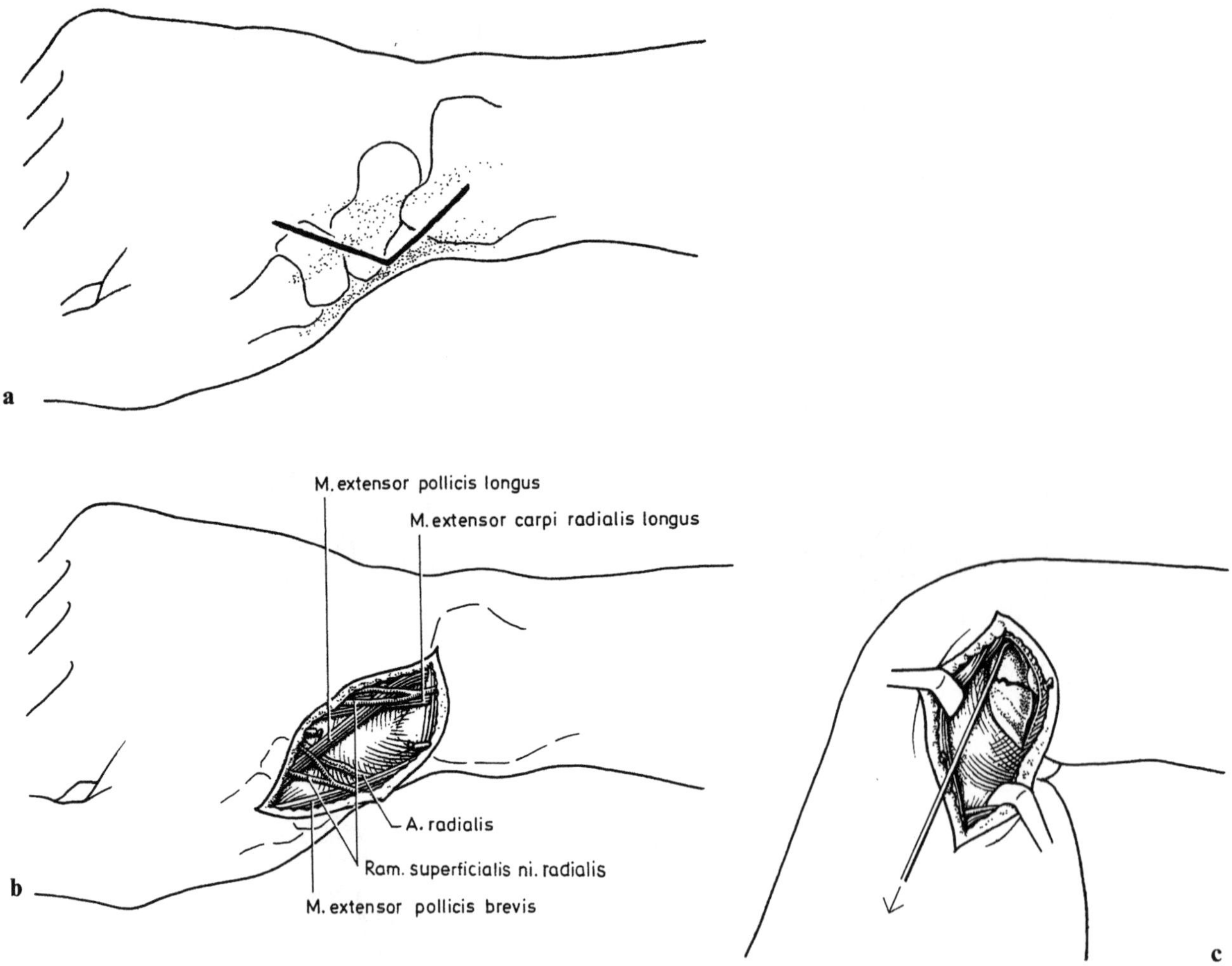

Fig. 97 a–c. Fracture of the scaphoid (incision and dorsoradial approach)

a Angled skin incision

b Topography: The extensor pollicis longus and extensor carpi radialis longus tendons are retracted dorsally along with superficial radial nerve branches. The radial artery and other superficial radial nerve branches are retracted to the volar side

c The radiocarpal joint is opened at the dorsal margin of the radial styloid. The fracture is reduced under vision by traction on a fine hook

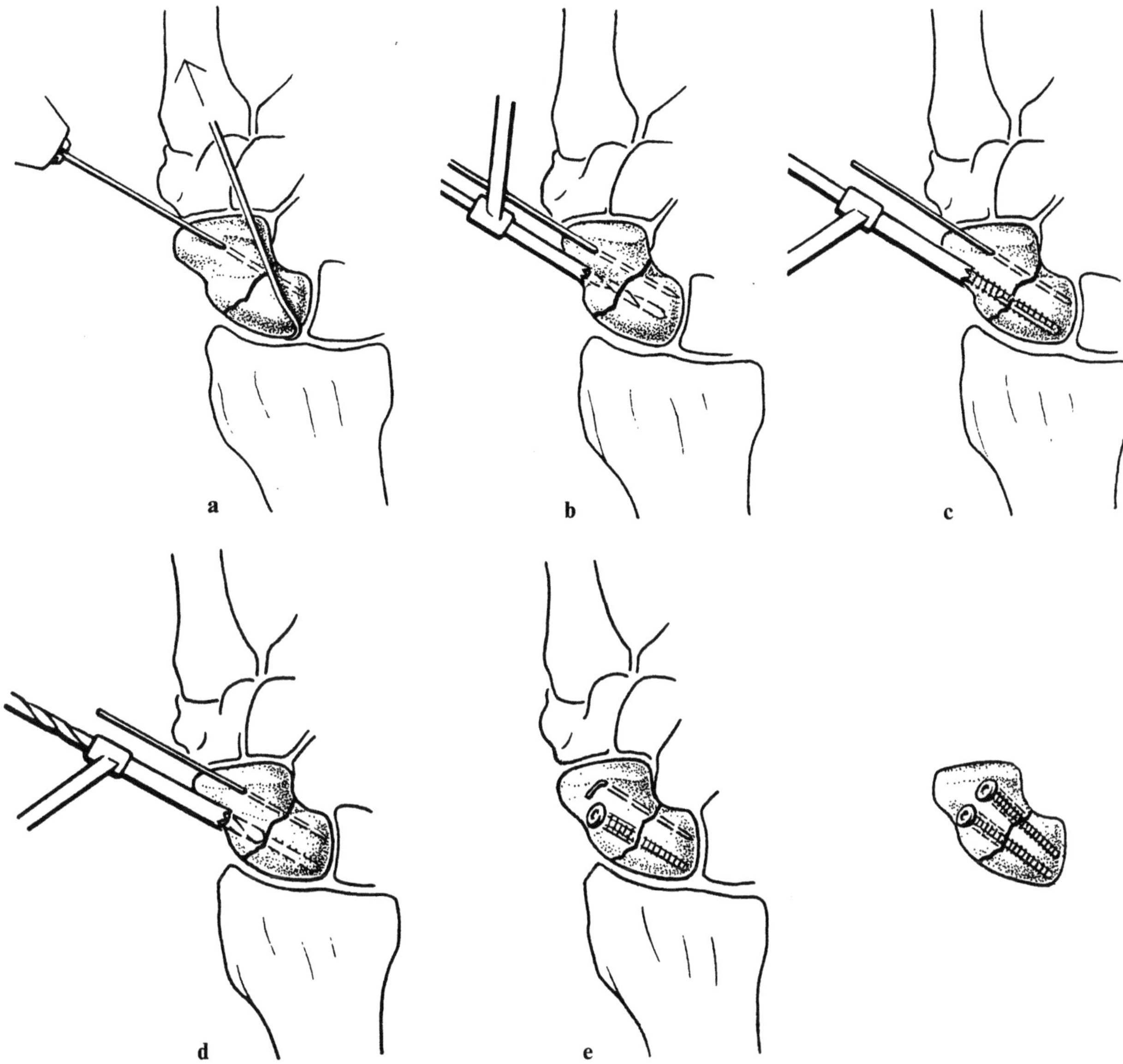

Fig. 98 a–e. Internal fixation of a scaphoid fracture through the dorsoradial approach

a The reduced fracture is transfixed with a thin Kirschner wire of predetermined length. Placement of the wire is checked by image intensifier or X-ray

b A hole (2.0 or 1.5 mm) is drilled parallel to the wire

c The drill hole is tapped (2.7 or 2.0 mm)

d The gliding hole is made (2.7 or 2.0 mm)

e The screw (2.7 or 2.0 mm) is inserted. The end of the guide wire may be bent over, leaving it in place to stabilize rotation, or it may be replaced with a second 2.0-mm screw

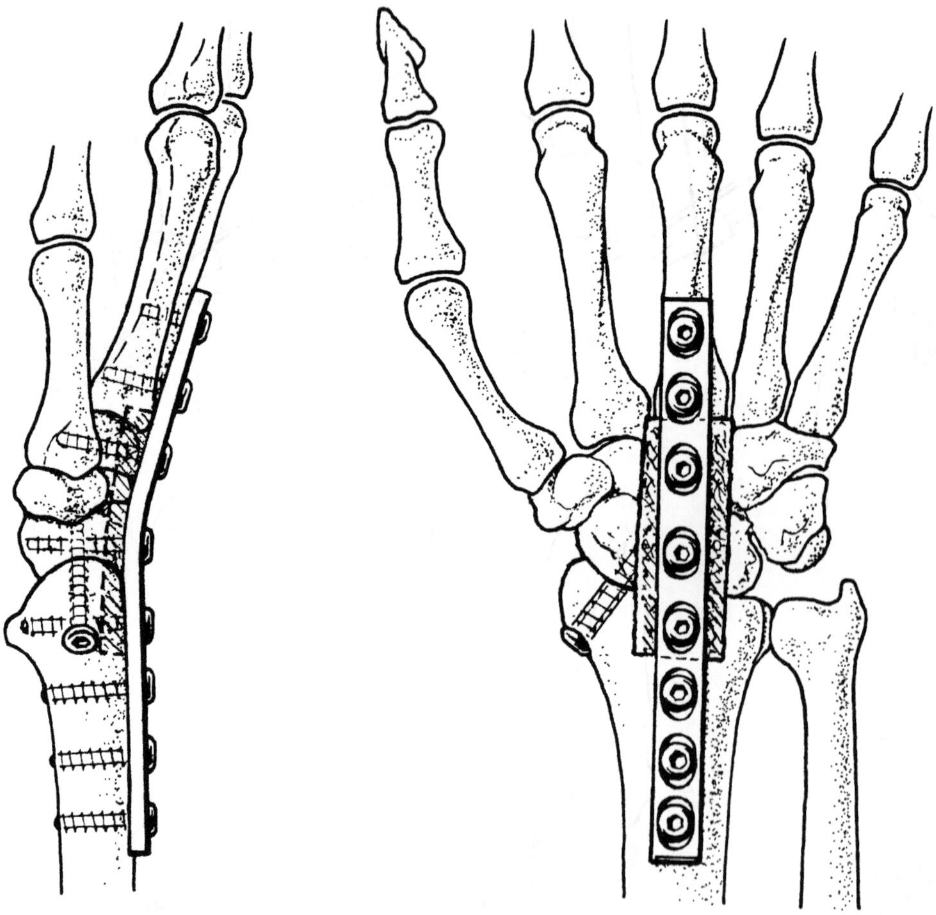

Fig. 99. Arthrodesis of the wrist with a 3.5-mm DCP

The radiocarpal and intercarpal joint surfaces are denuded of cartilage, and defects are grafted with cancellous bone. A 3.5-mm cortex lag screw is introduced through the radial styloid into the capitate bone. This pulls the carpus firmly against the radial styloid and keeps the distal radioulnar joint clear.

A flat, rectangular corticocancellous graft from the iliac fossa is inlaid into a prepared bed between the metacarpus and distal radius, and an 8-hole 3.5-mm DCP is secured over the graft. The radiocarpal joint is compressed with one screw in the capitate bone and one screw proximal to the bone graft in the radius. Adequate compression of the graft against the carpus is essential. The plate is attached to the 3rd metacarpal (or occasionally the 2nd metacarpal) with 2 or 3 screws, and to the radius with 3 or 4 screws

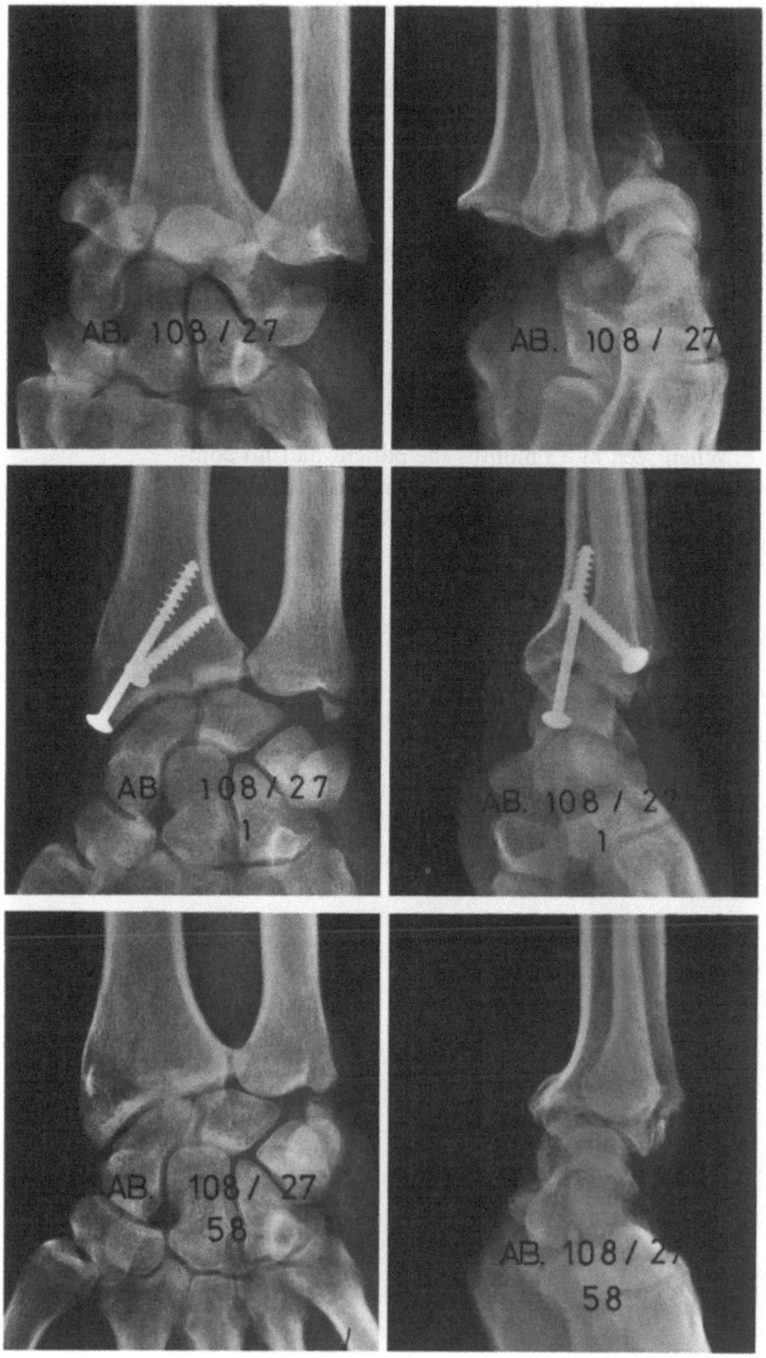

a

b

c

Fig. 100 a–c. Clinical example: screw fixation of a radiocarpal fracture-dislocation

Markus R., 33-year-old architectural draftsman, injured in a fall while playing soccer

a Fracture-dislocation of the left wrist with avulsion of the radial styloid

b Primary reduction and internal fixation were performed with 4.0- and 3.5-mm cancellous screws. A removal plaster wrist splint was worn for 4 weeks, and 100% work fitness was restored by 10 weeks. The screws were removed at $5^1/_2$ months

c On follow-up at $13^1/_2$ months the patient had no complaints, a 15° limitation of flexion, and an otherwise normal range of motion. Hand strength was normal. X-rays showed a small defect in the radial articular surface

Fig. 101 a–c. Clinical example: type B flexion fracture fixed with a volar T plate

Jose G., 40-year-old chemical plant worker, injured in a motorcycle accident

a Intra-articular radial fracture of the reverse Barton type. Primary closed reduction was unsuccessful

b Internal fixation was performed on day 10 with a volar T plate. A Kirschner wire used for provisional fixation was removed at the end of the procedure. A splint was worn until the wound healed. The postoperative course was uncomplicated, and the wrist was fully rehabilitated by 4 months

c When seen at 13 months the patient had no complaints and full function. X-rays showed a slight irregularity of the articular surface. Removal of the implants is not proposed

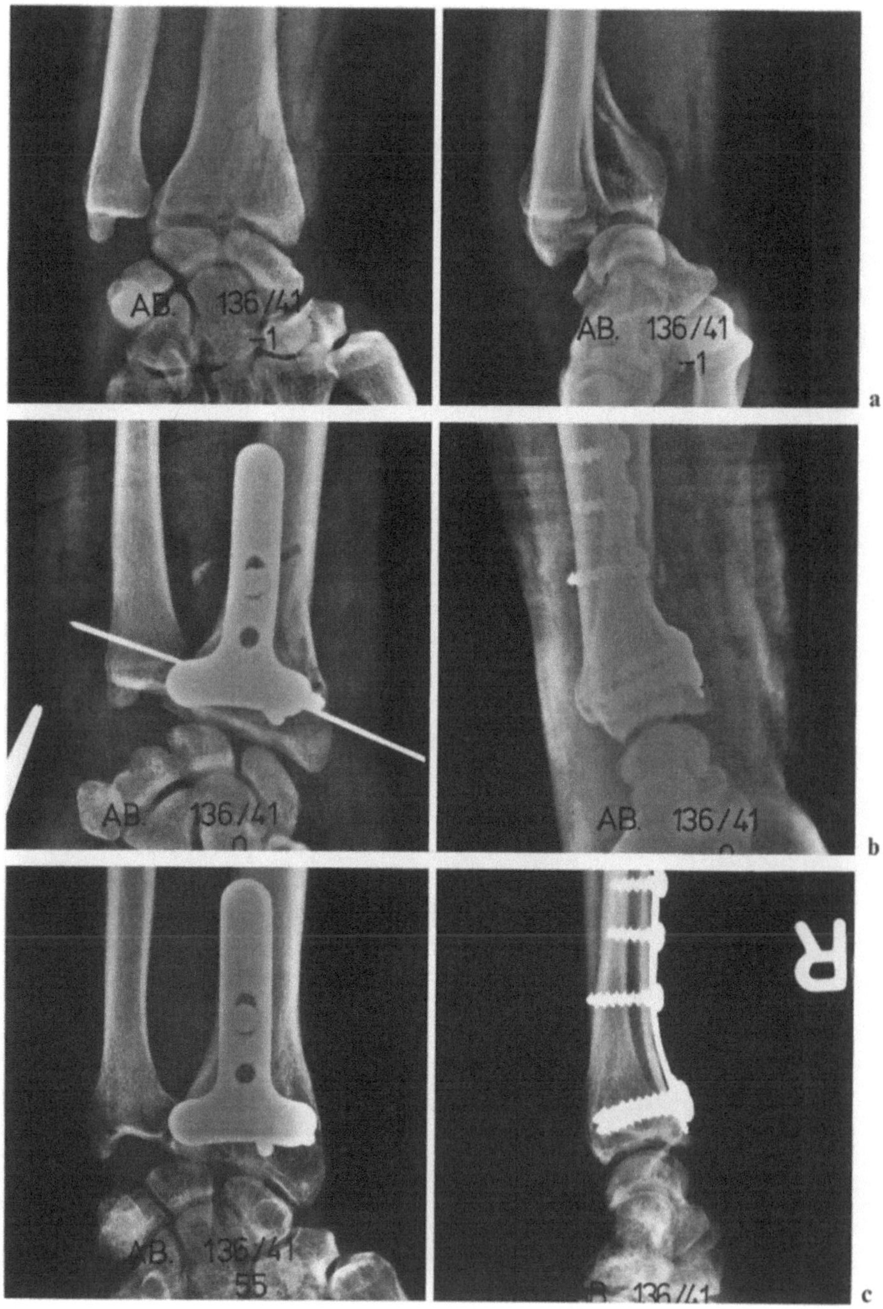
AB. 136/41
-1
AB. 136/41
-1
a
AB. 136/41
AB. 136/41
b
AB. 136/41
55
R
c

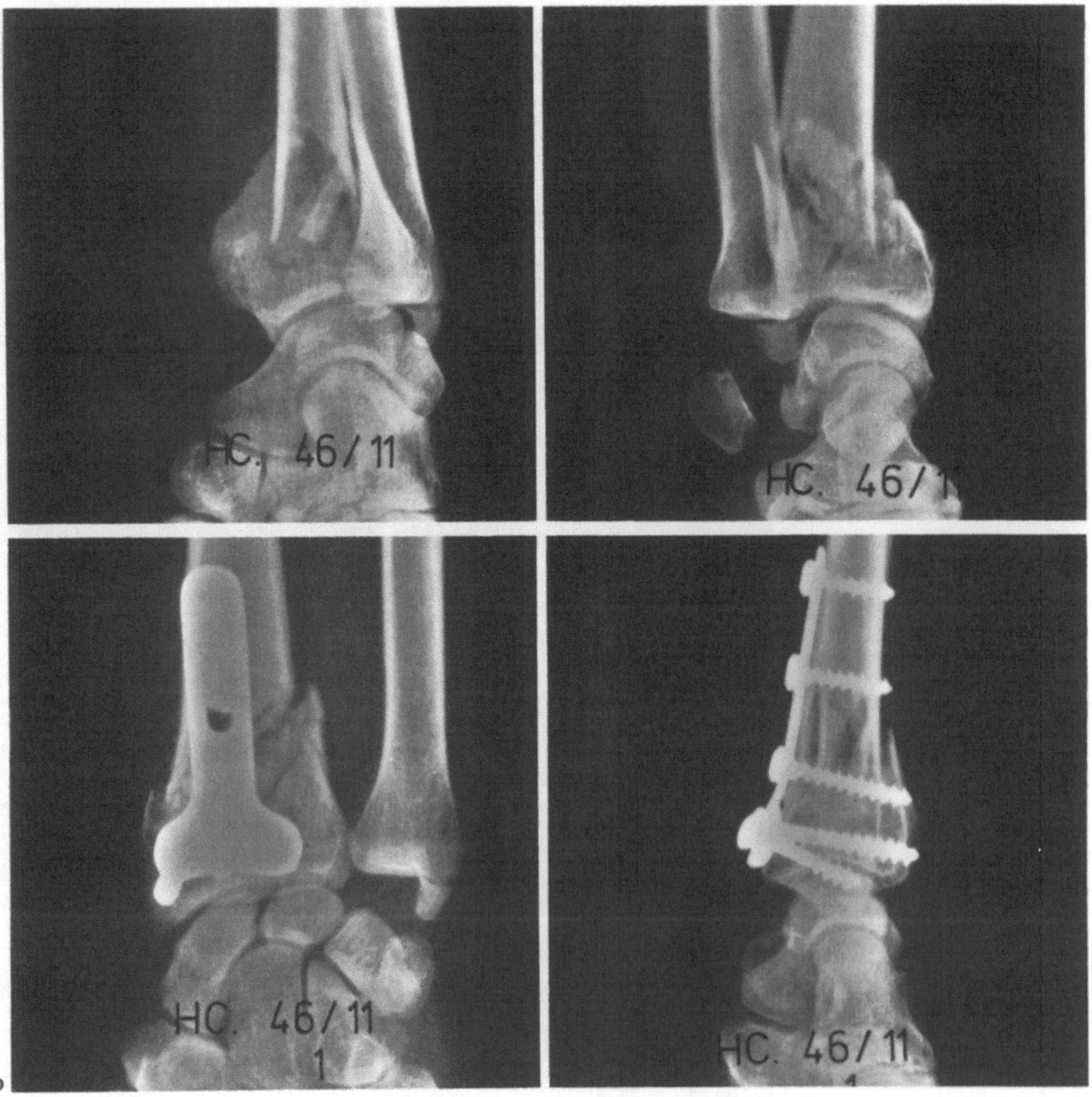

a

b

Fig. 102a–d. Clinical example: comminuted fracture of the distal radius with median nerve compression, fixed with a volar T plate

Gertrud M., 44-year-old secretary, fell on the outstretched left hand while skiing on 2/13/79. She noticed immediate hypesthesia of the index and middle fingers

a Displaced, comminuted fracture of the distal radius. The volar displacement is not easily appreciated on the postinjury films

b At operation the median nerve was found riding on a bone fragment that had displaced past the flexors toward the volar side. A standard internal fixation was performed using the T plate. Defects were grafted with iliac cancellous bone. The median nerve was decompressed by incising the retinaculum as far as the superficial volar arch.

Postoperative course was uneventful, and functional exercises were started from a removable volar splint. Full loading was possible at 8 weeks

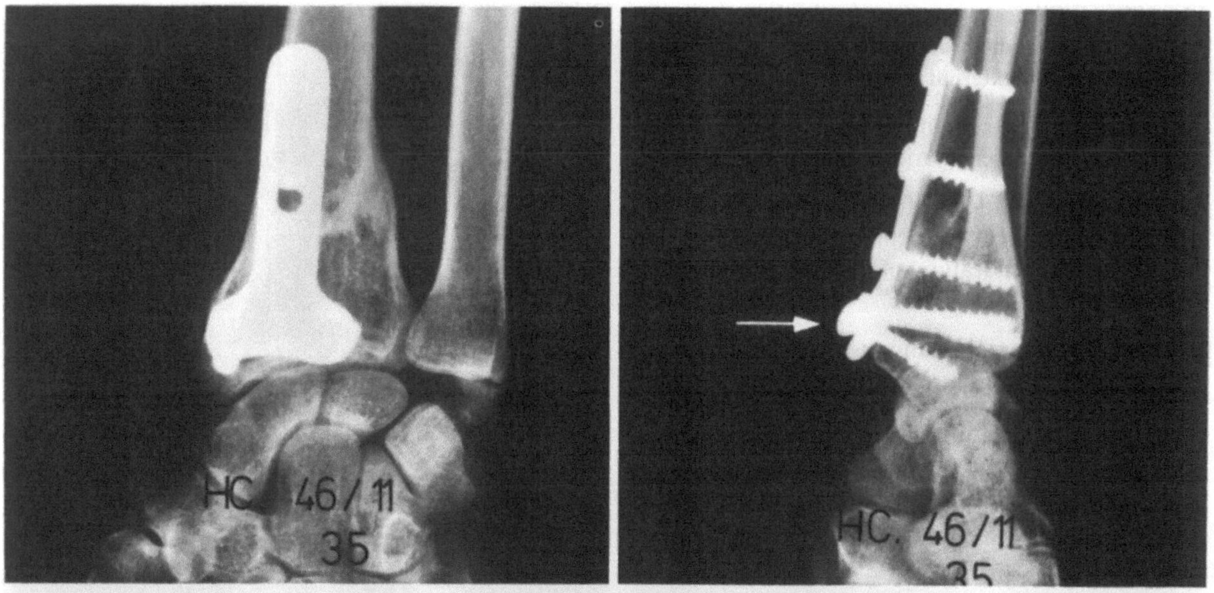

c

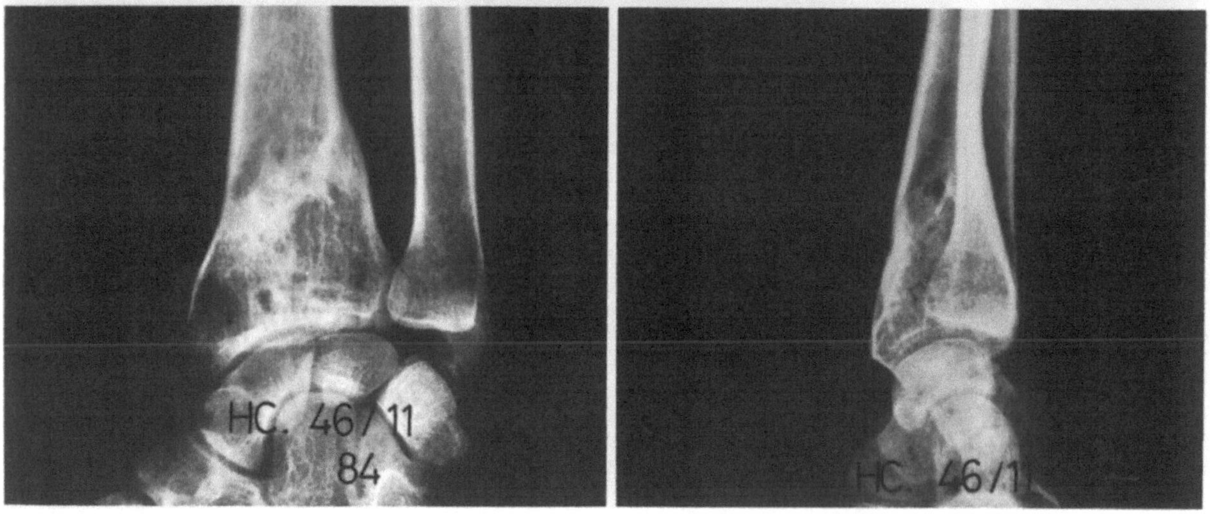

d

c Implants were removed at 8 months. A slightly loose plate screw had incited a synovitis with abrasion of the flexor pollicis longus

d On follow-up at $1^1/_2$ years, the patient had no complaints, full function, and had no difficulties performing her job. The fracture had united with a linear scar; there was no evidence of degenerative arthritis

Fig. 103 a–d. Clinical example: complex intra-articular fracture of the radius, managed by internal fixation combined with an external frame

Achmed W., 45-year-old diplomat, sustained a femoral fracture and other injuries in a traffic accident

a Complex intra-articular fracture of the distal radius with metaphyseal impaction and extension into the diaphysis; dislocation of the distal radioulnar joint

b Emergency internal fixation was performed, using the external fixator as a reduction aid.The main fracture was fixed with screws through a dorsoradial approach. The articular components were stabilized with Kirschner wires. Autogenous cancellous bone grafting was performed.
The Kirschner wires and external fixator were removed at 7 weeks

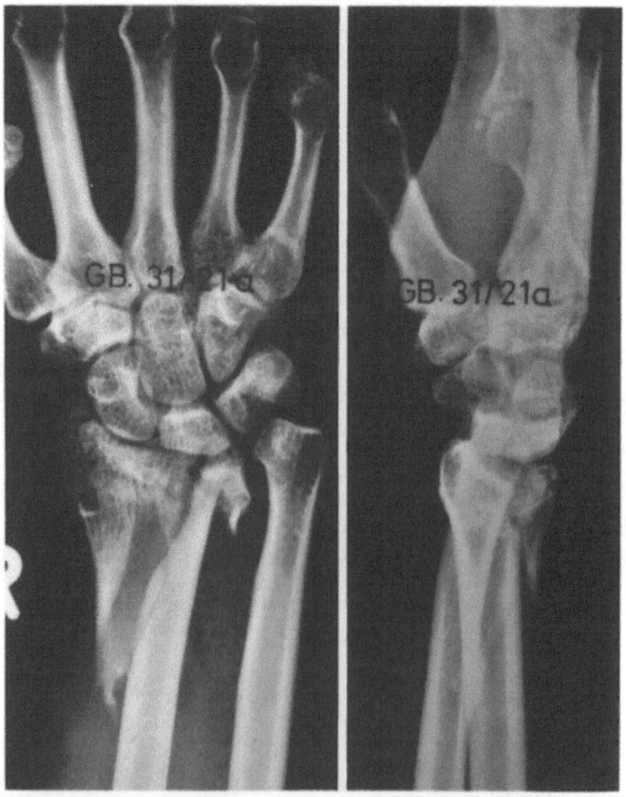

a

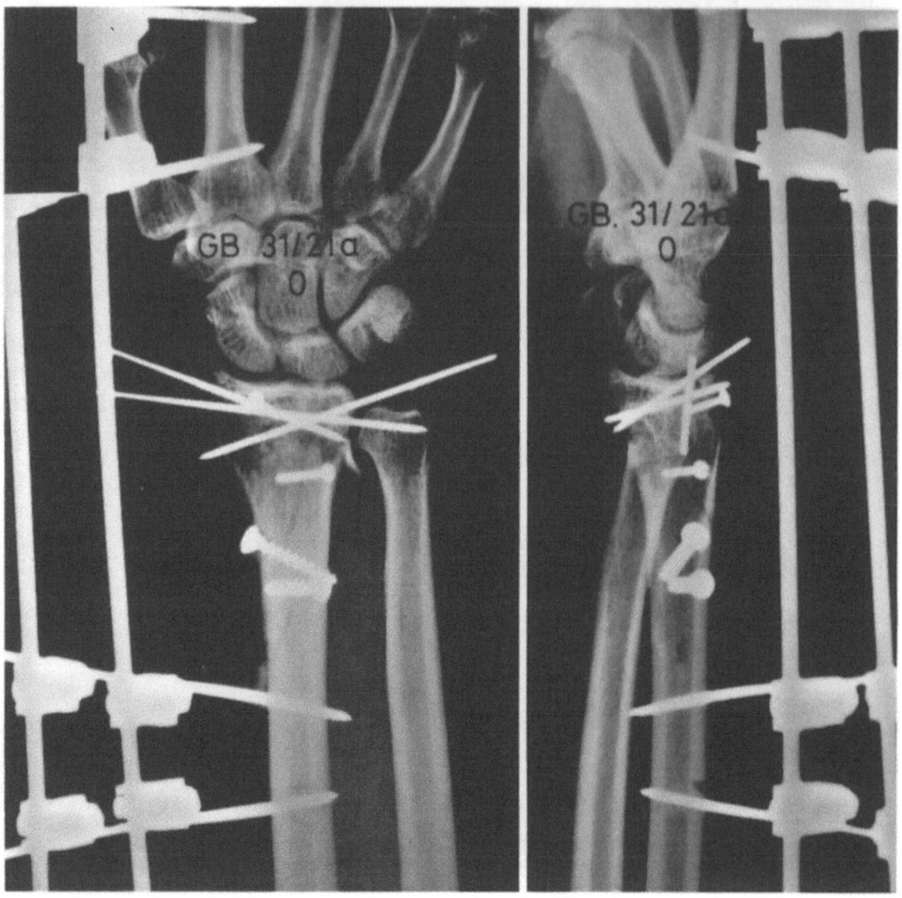

b

c Follow-up at $2^1/_2$ months confirmed union of the fractures

d At $1^1/_2$ years the patient had no complaints and full function. Removal of the screws is not proposed

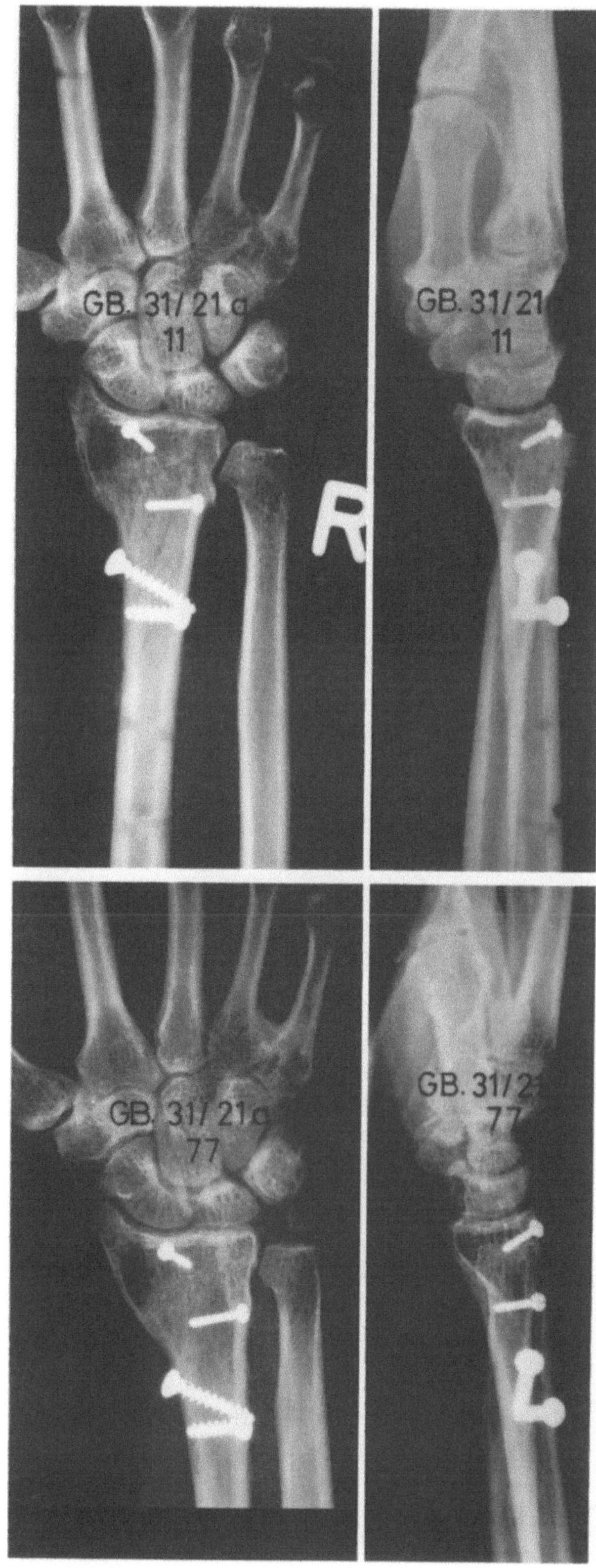

c

d

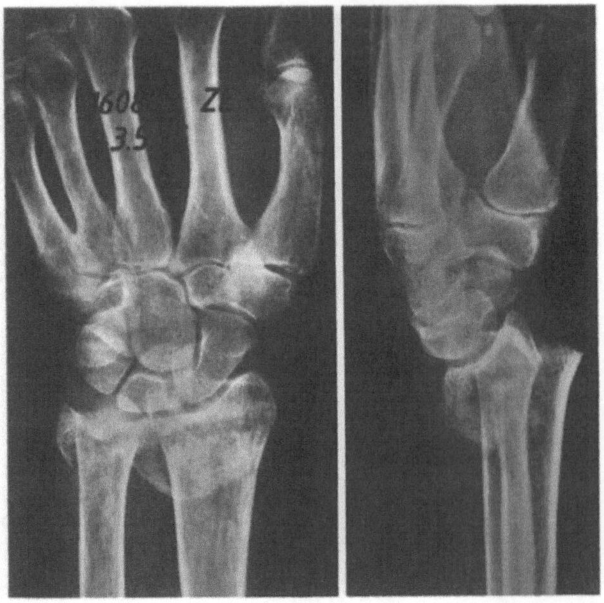

a

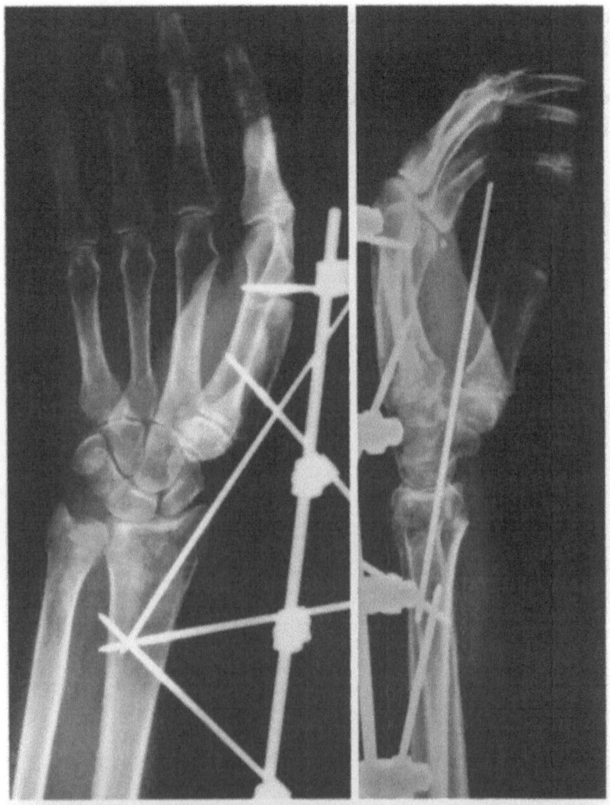

b

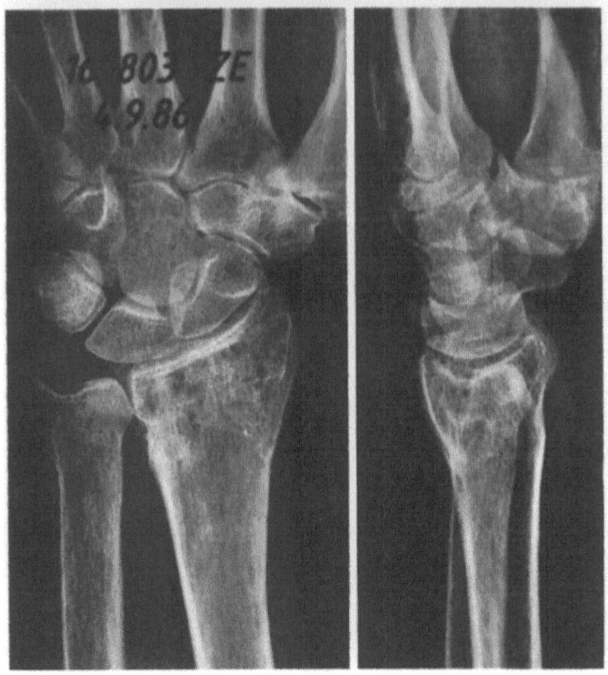

c

Fig. 104a–c. Clinical example: distal radial fracture immobilized with the external fixator

Emilie Z., an 82-year-old woman, fell onto the right hand

a Extra-articular extension fracture of the distal radius with dorsal impaction and a small accompanying fracture of the ulnar epiphysis

b Intraoperative postreduction film: The radial styloid has been fixed to the shaft with Kirschner wires, and the external fixator has been applied between the 2nd metacarpal and radial shaft to give adequate stability.
The Kirschner wires and external fixator were removed at 6 weeks

c Follow-up at 16 months confirmed fracture union. The patient had full function and no complaints

a

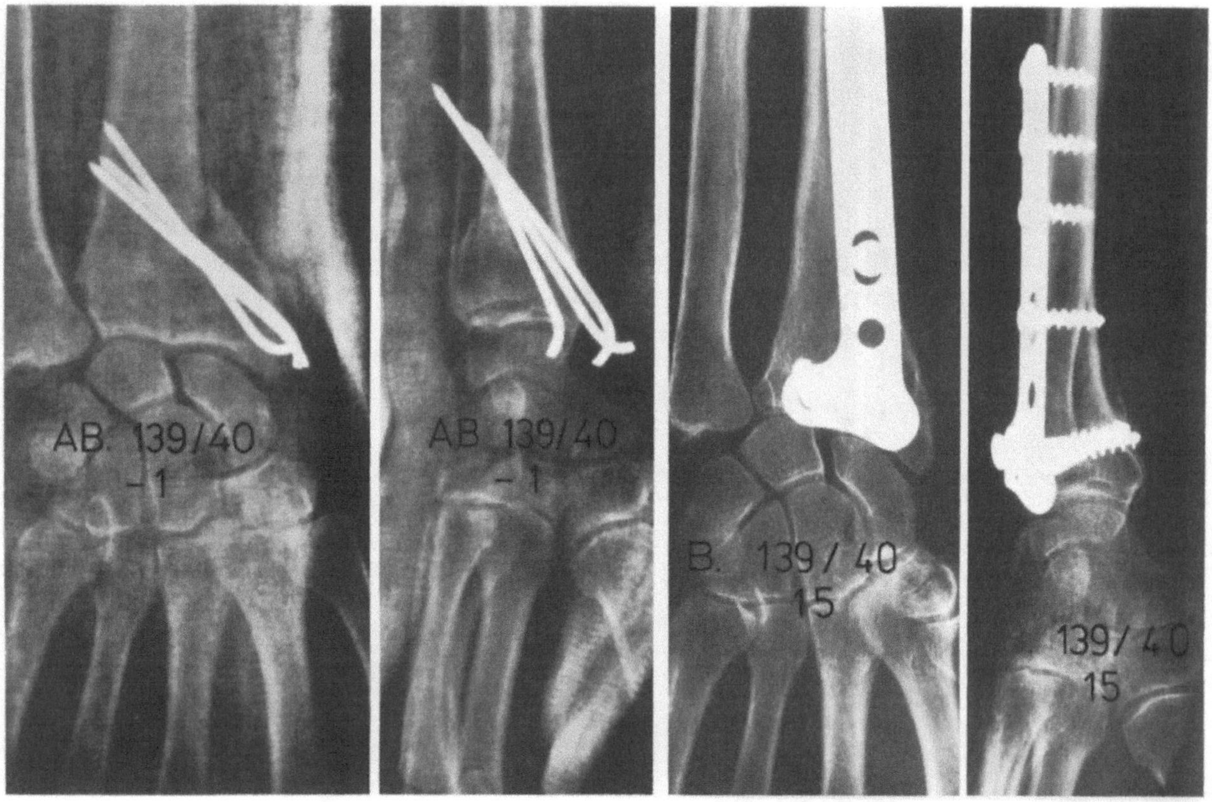

b

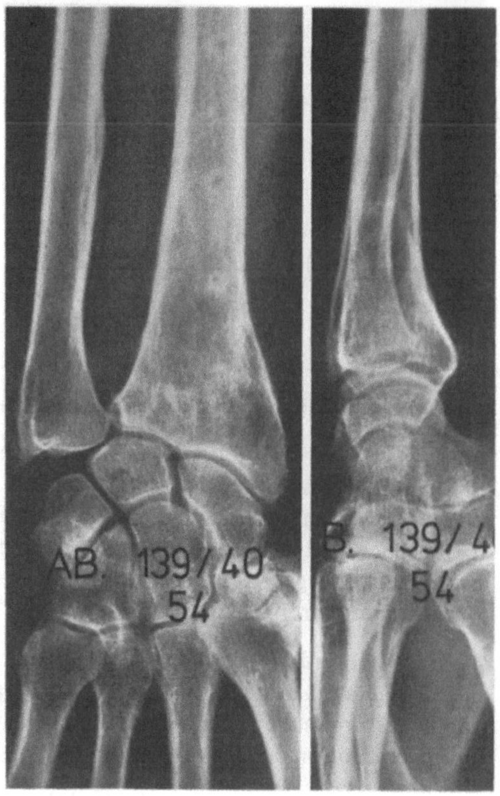

c

Fig. 105a–c. Clinical example: dorsal plating of an extension fracture

Regina H., 66-year-old retired school teacher, injured in a household accident

a Fracture of the distal radial metaphysis.Primary closed reduction and fixation with percutaneous Kirschner wires and plaster resulted in an inexact reduction with radial impaction and shortening

b Secondary internal fixation was performed 4 days later with a dorsal 120° T plate. A removable plaster wrist splint was worn for 2 weeks, followed by free mobilization.X-rays were taken 15 weeks after operation. Implants were removed at 8 months

c Follow-up at 1 year showed correct axial alignment with minimal shortening, no pain, and no degenerative arthritis. Patient had a 20° loss of flexion and extension; pronation and supination were unrestricted

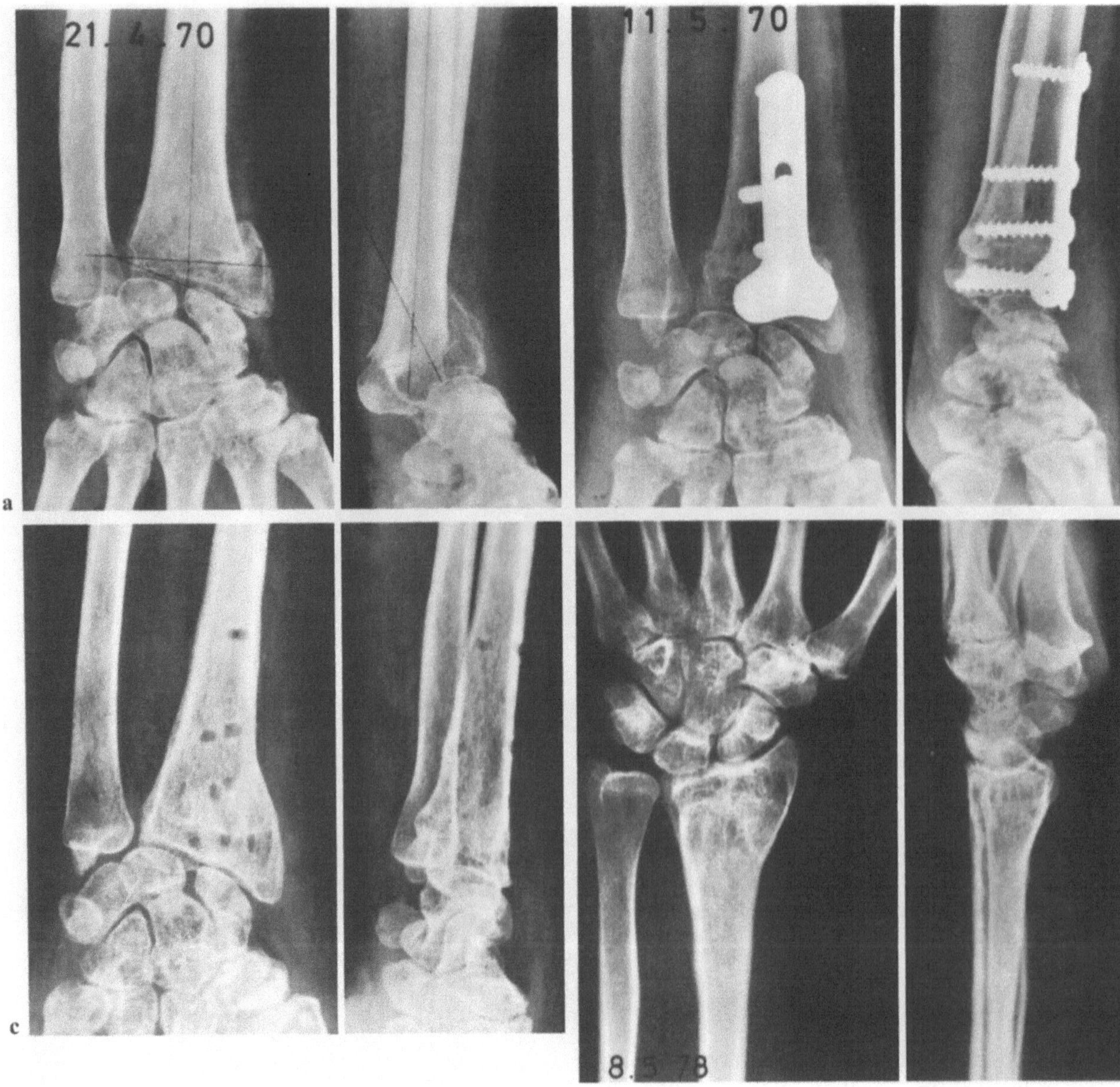

Fig. 106a–d. Clinical example: malunion of the distal radius treated by osteotomy and a dorsal T plate

Lena T., 41-year-old housewife, fell onto the hand on 2/5/70 sustaining a distal radial fracture. Closed reduction was performed and a cast applied. Secondary displacement ensued, and patient was referred for corrective surgery at 9 weeks. Patient had marked psychosomatic problems

a X-rays showed severe deformity with shortening and dorsal angulation of the radius, osteoporosis, trophic disturbances, and a general limitation of wrist and finger motion

b Corrective osteotomy was performed through a radiodorsal approach on 5/11/70. Autogenous cancellous bone grafts and a corticocancellous graft were applied and stabilized with a dorsal buttress T plate Postoperative course was uncomplicated, and functional exercises were initiated. Implants were removed at 6 months

c Follow-up at 17 months showed unrestricted finger motion and no trophic disturbances

d Follow-up at 8 years on 5/8/78 showed slight swelling of the wrist with a 25° limitation of volar flexion and 10° limitation of dorsiflexion. The ranges of abduction/adduction and pronation/supination were equal on both sides. The thumb and fingers functioned normally

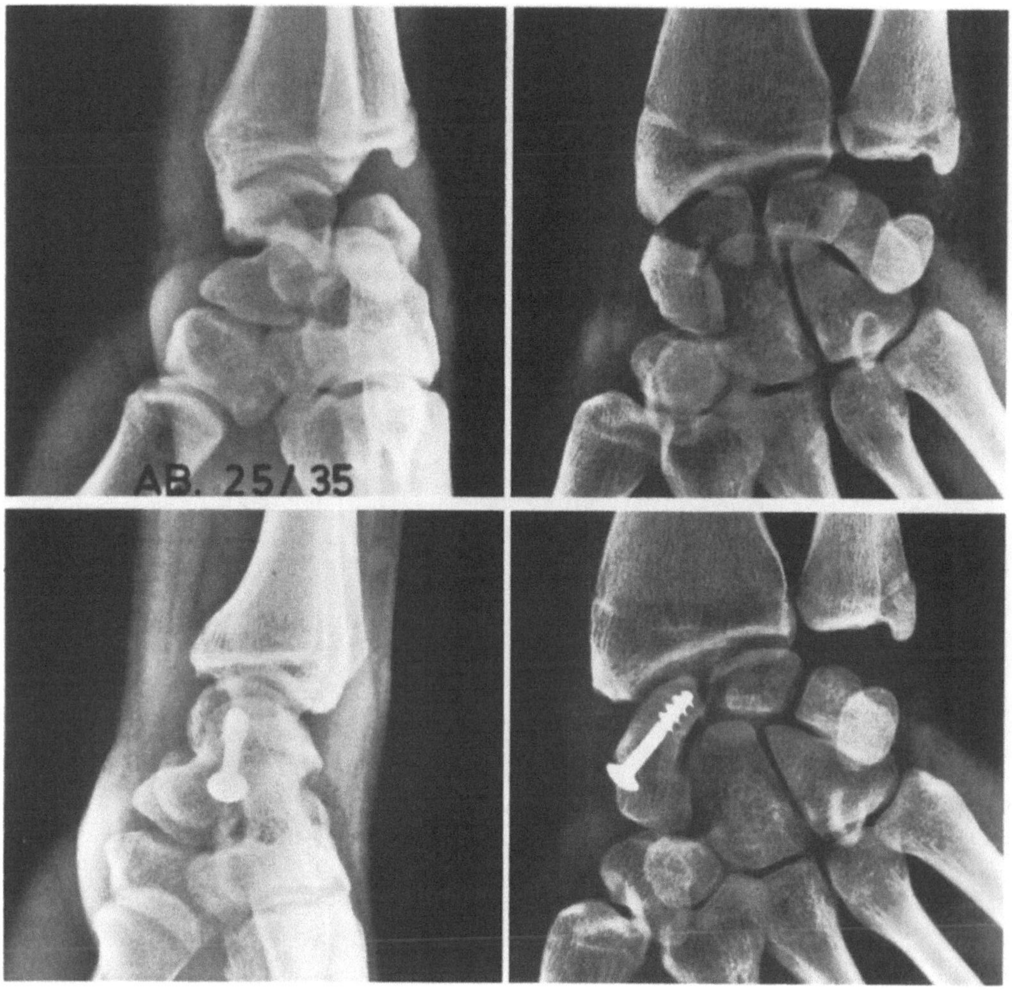

a

b

Fig. 107a, b. Clinical example: perilunar trans-scaphoid fracture-dislocation

Pierre W., 18-year-old student, injured in a fall on a moped

a De Quervain perilunar trans-scaphoid fracture-dislocation. The dislocation is reducible by closed manipulation; the scaphoid displacement is not

b At one week the scaphoid was openly reduced and fixed with a screw. Patient wore a cast for 4 weeks and was able to work and play sports at 8 weeks. Implants were removed at 11 months.
When seen at 1 year, the patient had no complaints. There was a 15° limitation of wrist flexion and extension, ulnar abduction, and pronation

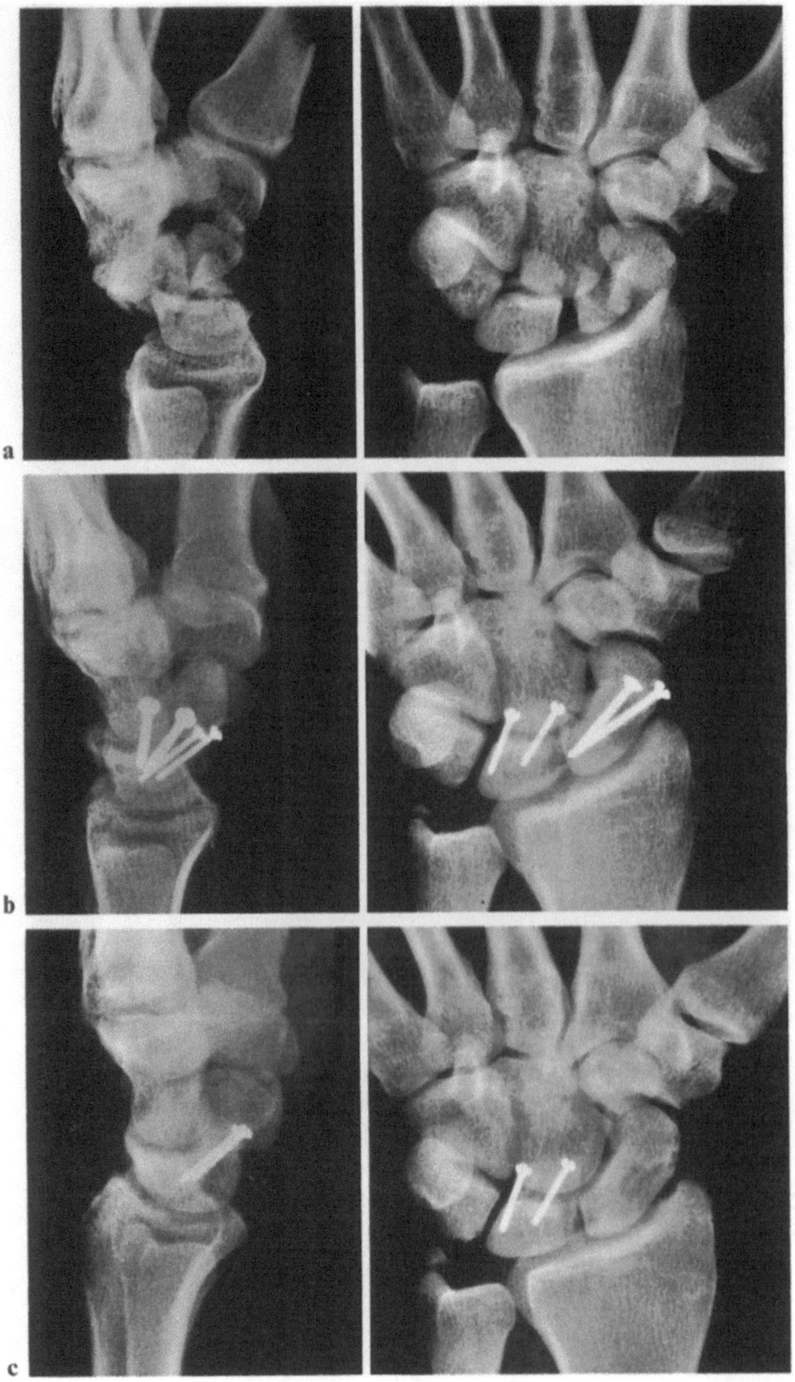

Fig. 108a–c. Clinical example: fracture-dislocation of the scaphoid and lunate

Daniel L., 21-year-old dispatcher, fell onto the extended hand while playing soccar on 9/11/85

a Perilunar trans-scaphoid fracture-dislocation with shearing of the volar end of the lunate

b Emergency internal fixation was performed through separate dorsoradial and volar incisions, stabilizing the scaphoid with two 2.0-mm mini screws and the lunate with two 1.5-mm mini screws. A forearm scaphoid cast was worn for 6 weeks. Work fitness was partially restored by 3 weeks and was complete at 11 weeks

c Follow-up at 9 months on 6/13/86 showed a 10° limitation of wrist flexion but otherwise equivalent motion ranges on both sides. Patient had no complaints. The screws were removed from the scaphoid, leaving the lunate screws in place

Fig. 109a–c. Clinical example: fracture of the trapezium

M. R., 30-year-old elevator installer, injured in a fall from a bicycle

a Longitudinal fracture of the trapezium

b Internal fixation was performed on day 7 with a small 4.0-mm cancellous screw. An external splint was not used, and functional exercises were started right away. Complete work fitness was achieved at 7 weeks. (Film taken at 40 weeks postinjury)

c The screw was removed at 11 months. The patient had no complaints, equivalent function on both sides, and no degenerative arthritis

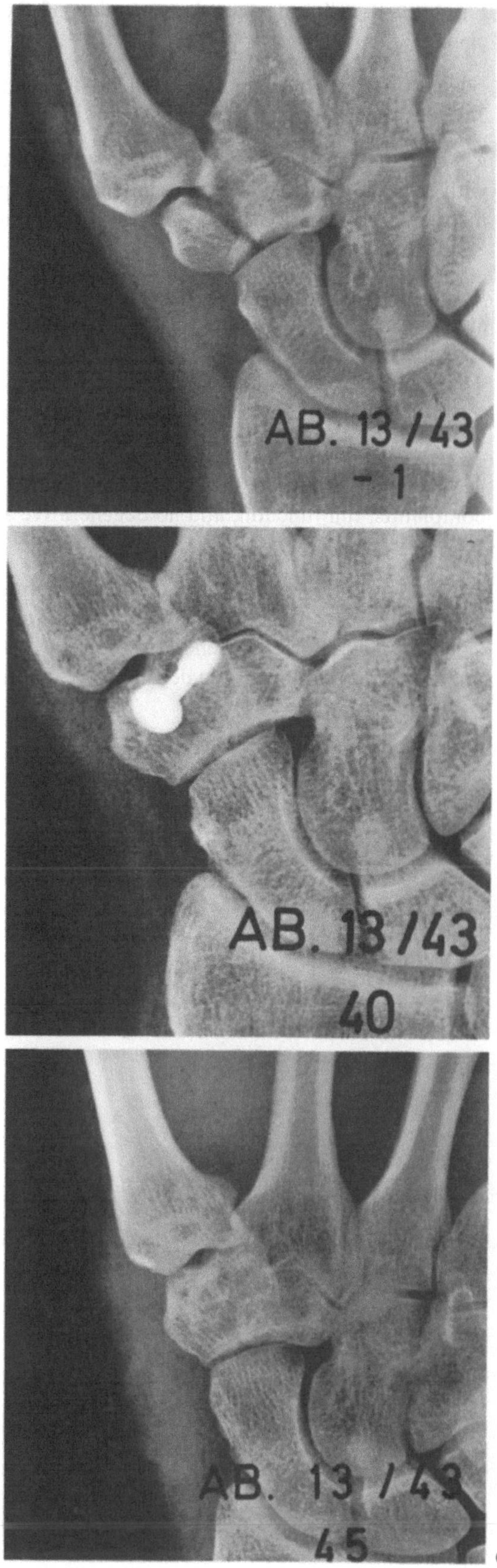

a

b

c

Fig. 110a–d. Clinical example: nonunion of the scaphoid

Luis B., 41-year-old merchant, fell on the hand on 3/29/69; the injury was treated as a sprain

a X-ray at 10 months postinjury shows a nonunion with a viable fragment and no evidence of displacement or cyst formation. Three months' cast immobilization was unsuccessful

b Internal screw fixation with osteotomy of the radial styloid was performed on 3/5/70, 13 months after the injury.
The postoperative course was uneventful, and a plaster cast was worn for 4 months. The screw was removed at 11 months

c When seen at 2 years the patient had no subjective complaints, full function, and no degenerative arthritis

d At 10 years the patient had no complaints and a minimal scar. Function was equivalent on both sides. X-rays showed regeneration of the osteotomized styloid and low-grade degenerative arthritis

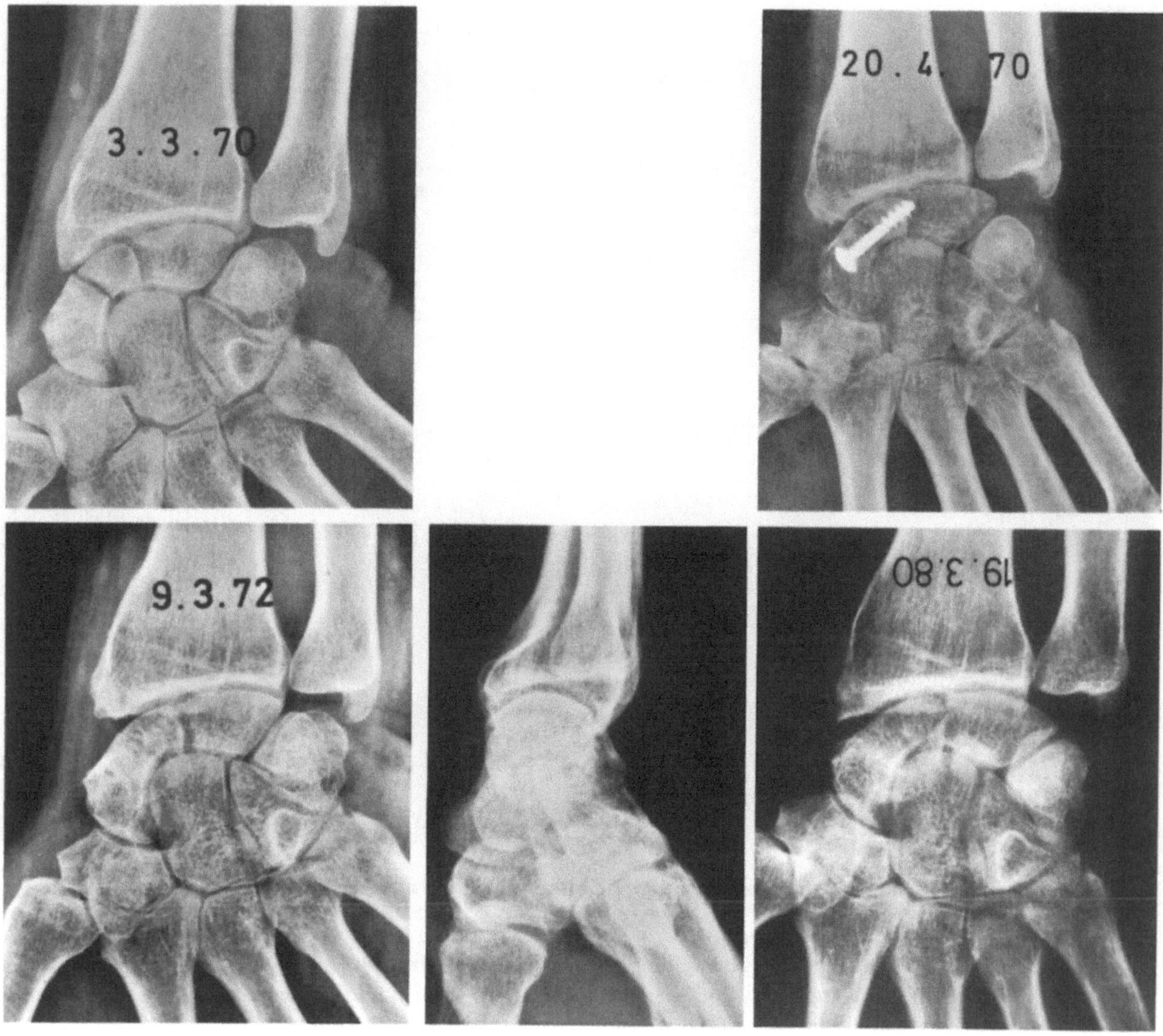

a b

c, d d′

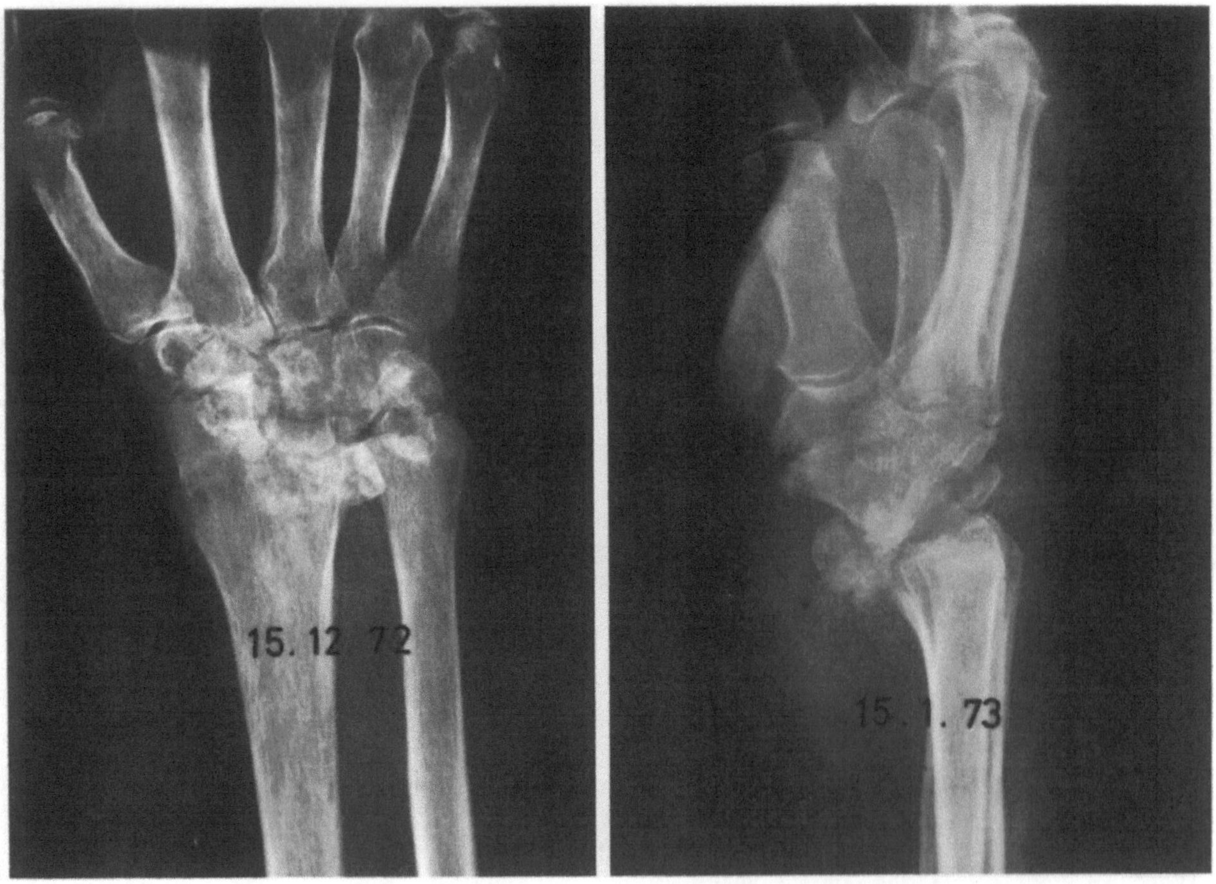

a

Fig. 111a–c. Clinical example: arthrodesis of the wrist with a plate and autogenous cancellous bone

Anna M., 76-year-old housewife, admitted with 2-year history of intermittent pain and swelling of various joints, especially the right wrist. Excisional biopsy in late 1972 indicated chronic synovitis, and *E. coli* were cultured from aspirated fluid

a X-ray taken in December 1972 showed a previously undiagnosed destructive osteitis involving the whole carpus

b Operation on 1/16/73 disclosed extreme osteoporosis with destruction of the proximal and distal carpal rows; the carpus was resected. The defect was grafted with autogenous iliac cancellous bone, accepting a slight loss of length, and was stabilized with a double one-third tubular plate (6-hole plate applied over an 8-hole plate) between the radius and 3rd metacarpal. The distal ulna was resected.
Histologic examination yielded a surprising diagnosis: tuberculosis of the bone.
The postoperative course was uneventful. Tuberculostatics were given after surgery, and the wrist was protected with a removable plaster splint. Patient convalesced in a sanatorium for several months.
The implants were removed at 16 months on 4/8/74. The nonunion was solid. Inflammation had resolved completely, and there was no corrosion. The hand was again useful

c Follow-up at 2 years showed no clinical or radiographic change in the operated area

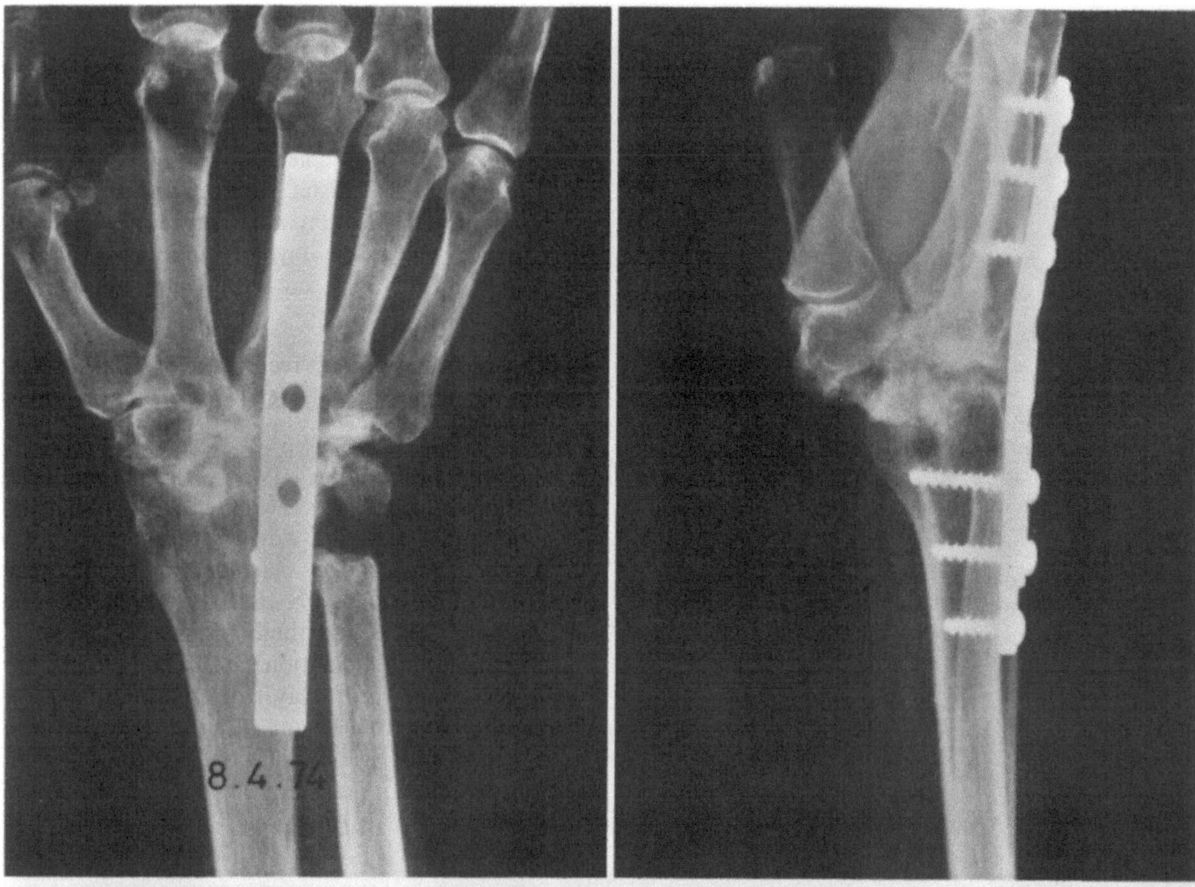

b

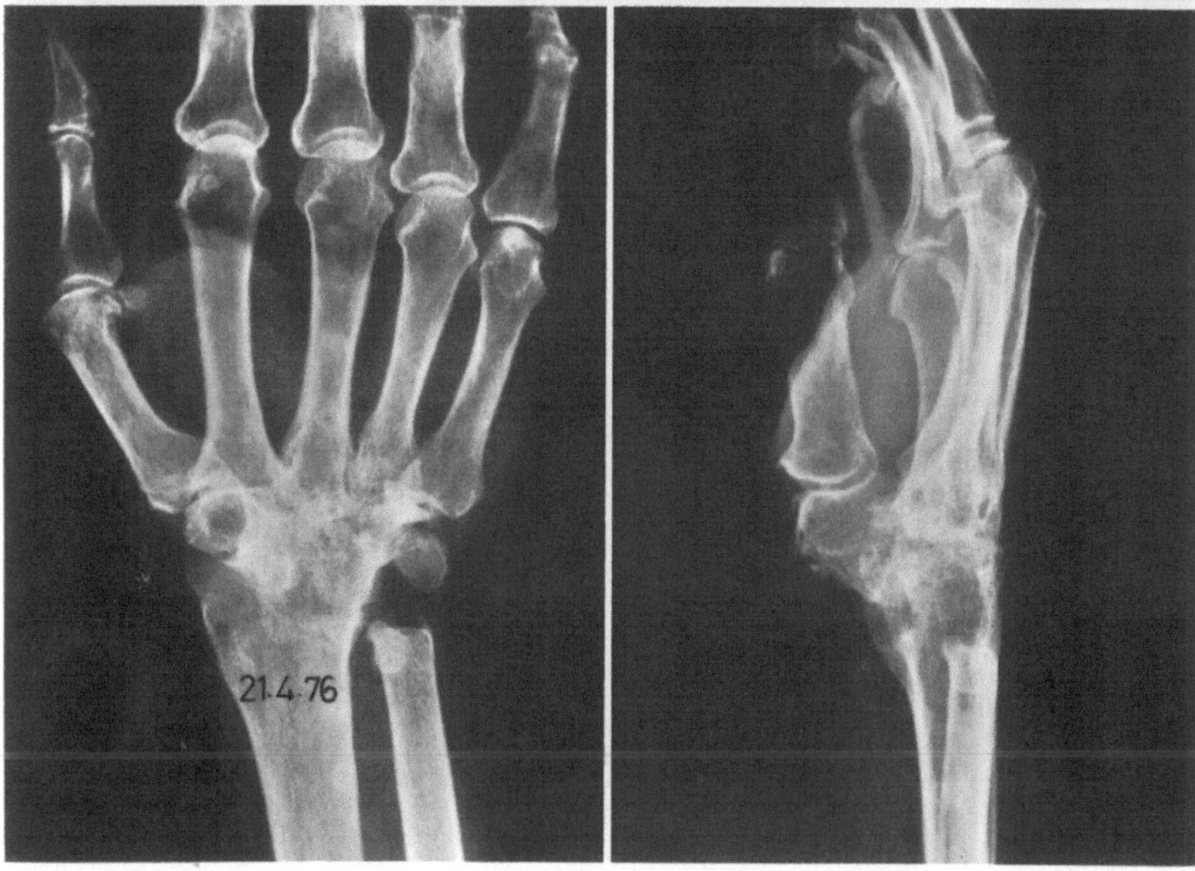

c

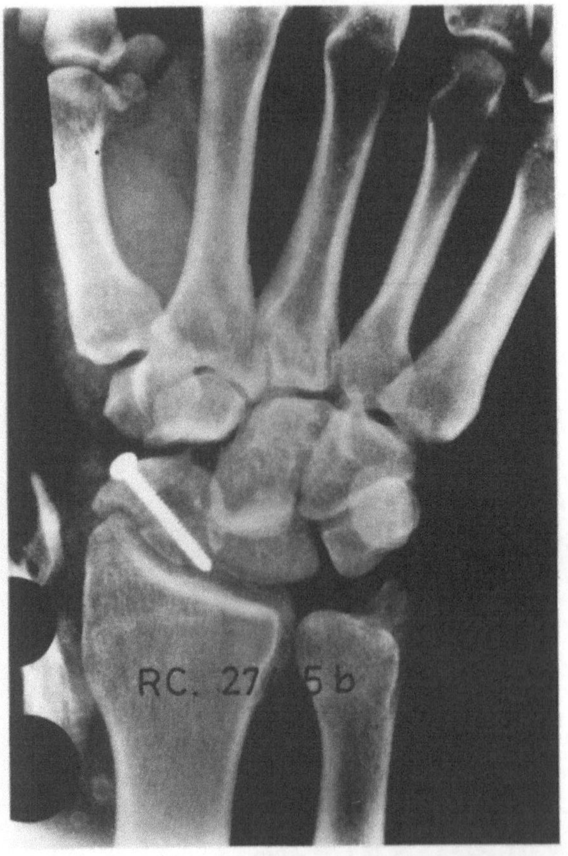

a

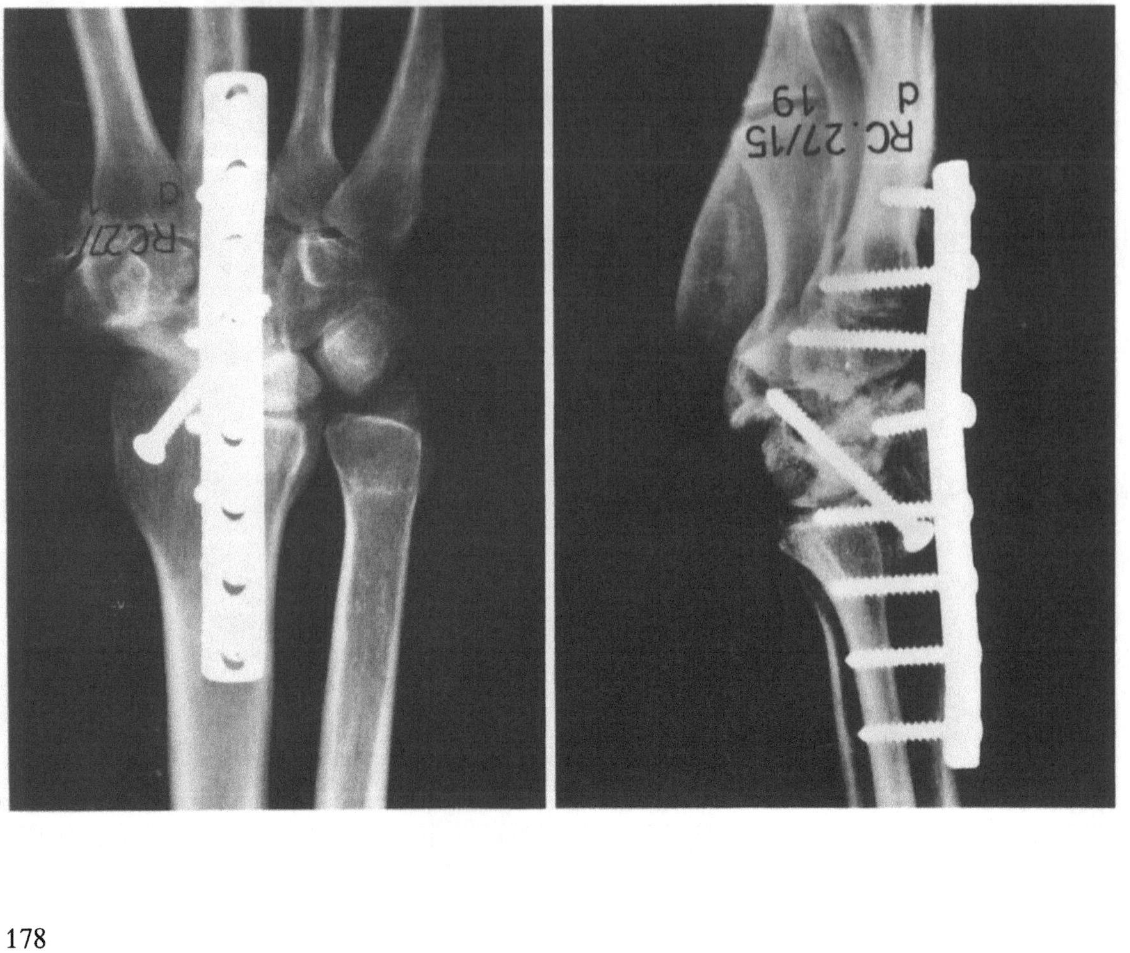

b

Fig. 112a, b. Clinical example: arthrodesis of the wrist with a DCP

Erich L., 40-year-old bricklayer, sustained multiple injuries in a fall from scaffolding on 6/19/84: cerebral concussion, ruptured spleen, fractures of the left proximal femur, left distal forearm, and right Quervain's fracture-dislocation. All fractures were operatively treated with a few days of the injury. The scaphoid was fixed with a screw following reduction of the dislocation

a Scaphoid necrosis with recurrence of volar dislocation of the lunate, producing a severe, painful limitation of wrist motion

b The wrist was fused on 4/19/85 with a 3.5-mm DCP and separate cortex lag screw between the radial styloid and capitate.
At 1 year the arthrodesis was solid, and the patient was fully active on the job. He had complete motion of the long fingers and thumb with normal ranges of pronation and supination. So far the patient has declined to take time away from work to have the implants removed

XIII. The Hand

A. Introduction

Internal fixations of the bones of the hand are technically demanding, and the surgeon undertaking these procedures assumes great responsibility. A thorough knowledge of the appropriate surgical instruments, proficiency in their use, and a sound grasp of the functional anatomy of the hand are essential to success. Atraumatic handling of the soft tissues during hand operations is crucial to the preservation of movement. Permanent motor impairment can result from improperly placed incisions and from damage to the peritendinous gliding layers and joint capsules. But when performed correctly, rigid internal fixation enables us to achieve better functional results than traditional treatment methods.

This particularly applies to open fractures of the hand with associated tendon, nerve, and vascular injury. Rigid internal fixation of the fragments with small implants makes it possible to gear the postoperative treatment program exclusively to the requirements of the soft tissues, and in many cases to achieve a primary reconstruction of all traumatized structures. Internal fixation also contributes to primary wound healing by reducing the need for splints and casts that can compromise blood flow.

At the same time, however, trauma-related circulatory disturbances (contusion, laceration), especially in the fingers, and constraints on tourniquet time set limits as to what can be achieved at primary intervention. In patients with multiple open fractures and associated tendon, vascular, and nerve lesions, and especially in patients with skin defects that require time-consuming grafting procedures, the surgeon should consider whether simple Kirschner wires inserted obliquely, axially, or in crossed fashion, possibly combined with hemicerclage wiring or an intraosseous wire suture, might be preferable to rigid internal fixation.

Very small fragments are unsuitable for screw fixation. Instead, we use small tension bands made of flexible wire or absorbable suture material. We fix some of these fractures with transosseous pull-out wire analogous to the Bunnell tendon suture.

Irreducible rotational deformities and steps in articular surfaces are considered absolute indications for operative fixation.

Owing to the widespread use of high-resolution image intensifiers, many surgeons reduce hand fractures by closed manipulation and insert percutaneous Kirschner wires when instability exists. A number of new techniques have been reported in recent years. In selected patients they are safe, simple, and effective, and their functional results are promising. The soft-tissue damage associated with these procedures is minimal and cannot be compared to that accompanying open reduction and rigid internal fixation with screws, plates, or tension bands. It should be noted, however, that the closed techniques can involve significant cumulative radiation exposure to the surgeon's hand, which, like the patient's hand, is necessarily situated within the primary beam. We feel that this effect is a potential cause for concern. Also, the heat generated by drilling a Kirschner wire through cortical bone is substantial and exceeds that produced by a high-quality drill bit. The cancellous bone, too, is extremely hard in the skeleton of the hand. One should not be misled by the fact that percutaneous drilling causes no visible thermal effects, as these may become manifest only later as foci of osteolytic necrosis.

B. Injuries of the First Ray

The first ray of the hand, called also the opposition or thumb ray, merits separate discussion for three reasons: 1) fractures of the base of the first metacarpal and its sequelae are clinically significant; 2) articular fractures are common in the metacarpophalangeal and interphalangeal joints of the thumb; and 3) almost all shaft fractures are made unstable by the pull of muscles and tendons and are resistant to reduction by closed methods.The surgical approaches to the first ray are fairly simple anatomically, except in Bennett's fracture-dislocation.

1. Fractures of the Base of the First Metacarpal

a) Approaches to the First Carpometacarpal Joint and Operative Technique

The main problem in achieving acceptable reduction and internal fixation of Bennett's fracture-dislocation is the difficulty of visualizing the small ulnovolar articular fragment.

Radiovolar Approach of Gedda and Moberg (Fig. 113). This approach definitely gives the best exposure. It begins with a curved, radiovolar incision at the level of the first carpometacarpal joint, which may be extended dorsally and distally. The fine radial nerve branches and the abductor pollicis longus tendon are snared and protected. The thenar muscles are retracted and if necessary are notched. The joint is then opened transversely on the volar side and also dorsally if required. The fracture is reduced under vision and temporarily fixed with a thin Kirschner wire inserted from the volar side, or with a small reduction forceps (Fig. 113).

Radiodorsal Approach (Fig. 114). An incision is made along the radial or ulnar border of the first metacarpal and extended proximally in Y fashion on the dorsal and radial sides. The periosteum is incised at the margin of the extensor apparatus, and the long extensor tendon is retracted, sparing the abductor pollicis longus insertion and the fine superficial radial nerve branch to the dorsum of the thumb (Fig. 118). The thenar muscles are sparingly stripped aside, and the joint is opened transversely on its radiodorsal or radiovolar aspect. The fracture is reduced and temporarily fixed. This approach gives a somewhat poorer exposure of the joint and articular fragments, but it is less traumatizing to the soft tissues and joint capsule.

Exposure of the joint can be markedly improved by dividing the abductor pollicis longus tendon in Z fashion and then repairing it at the end of the operation. Postoperative immobilization that includes the metacarpophalangeal joint of the thumb is maintained for 3–4 weeks.

b) Bennett's Fracture-Dislocation

This is a fracture-dislocation of the first carpometacarpal joint in which the metacarpal shaft fragment dislocates dorsoradially into an adducted position, while a small articular fragment remains attached to the carpus. Uncorrected, this injury will lead to a progressive traumatic arthritis with increasing pain and functional disability of the entire first ray. Acceptable hand function relies on preserving the abductability and opposability of the thumb and maintaining the width of the thumb web.

Many authors have sought reliable means of reducing Bennett's fracture and especially of maintaining the reduction.

Our experience has convinced us that for fractures with a large fragment, open reduction and rigid internal fixation with a screw is the most favorable option, despite the technical difficulties, and yields the best long-term results.

With a small fragment that cannot be solidly engaged with a screw, we advocate closed reduction and pinning according to the technique of Wagner or Iselin (Fig. 116).

Screw fixation of the fracture is done from the *dorsal* side in both the radiovolar and radiodorsal approaches (Fig. 115). In the rare cases where the fragments are large, fixation is accomplished with a 4.0-mm cancellous screw using standard technique.Smaller fragments are fixed with a fully threaded 2.0- or 2.7-mm screw. In a markedly displaced fracture whose surfaces are well exposed, a gliding hole can be drilled initially in the main fragment, and the thread hole drilled after the fracture is reduced. Excellent interfragmental compression is obtained with this technique. If the fracture must be reduced before drilling can be done, interfragmental compression can be a problem, because it is difficult to estimate the depth of the drill hole in the larger shaft fragment. The importance of this detail should not be exaggerated, however, and a review of our cases has shown that traumatic arthritis does not develop even when the reduction is less than perfect. The main concern is to correct the dislocation. A Kirschner wire used for provisional fixation may be left in place to stabilize against rotation.

If screw fixation is not appropriate for technical reasons due to the small fragment size or the presence of multiple fragments that were not detected preoperatively, we transfix the fracture with Kirschner wires under direct vision using Moberg's technique and secure the fixation with an additional Kirschner wire drilled from the first metacarpal into the trapezium or second metacarpal.

c) Rolando's Fracture

This term is applied to a Y-shaped intra-articular fracture of the base of the first metacarpal. Comminution is very often present. Internal fixation is technically difficult but is almost always necessary because of gross displacement and instability.

Operative Technique. The best exposure is obtained with a curved Gedda-Moberg incision, which we extend distally along the back of the first metacarpal (Fig. 113). Care is taken to spare the peritenon of the extensor tendons and the superficial radial nerve branches supplying the dorsum of the thumb.The first carpometacarpal joint is widely opened, dividing the abductor pollicis longus tendon as required (see above).

The dorsoradial approach may suffice when the articular component of the fracture is relatively simple (Fig. 114).

The first step of the internal fixation is restoration of the articular surface under vision. The articular fragments are temporarily fixed with small reduction forceps or Kirschner wires, which in suitable cases are replaced with an initial transverse screw (Fig. 117).

A reversed T plate for 2.7-mm screws is then applied as a neutralization plate to fix the reassembled articular fragments to the shaft. Stability can be greatly improved by driving an interfragmental lag screw through the plate into the main basal fragment (Fig. 117c).

Small areas of comminution or bone loss are frequent near the volar base and should be grafted with autogenous cancellous bone to shorten consolidation time.

If the fracture is still not absolutely stable, the thumb is held in abduction and opposition in a plaster splint for 4–6 weeks after surgery. The splint leaves the interphalangeal joint of the thumb free so that early active exercises can be performed. This is important for prophylaxis of tendon adhesions.

d) Extra-Articular Fracture of the First Metacarpal Base

This type of fracture is more common than Bennett's fracture. Typically there is medial angulation of the distal fragment with narrowing of the thumb web. Reduction is easily accomplished, but redisplacement very often occurs when the reduction is maintained in plaster, and pressure necrosis of the skin is not uncommon. Internal fixation is usually indicated, therefore. It provides excellent stability, permits early mobilization and partial loading of the thumb, and shortens rehabilitation.

Operative Technique. The fracture is exposed through a longitudinal radial or ulnar incision that may be extended proximally (Fig. 118). Usually the carpometacarpal joint does not have to be opened, but its position and inclination are marked by passing a hypodermic needle or thin Kirschner wire into the joint. A long oblique fracture is fixed with simple screws, and a transverse fracture is fixed with a reversed 2.7-mm T plate applied as a tension band. The plate should be bent upward slightly to secure abduction of the thumb. It is attached first to the proximal fragment, then the distal fragment is reduced against the plate with a forceps and definitively fixed (Fig. 117b). Again, stability is greatly improved by lagging a screw through the proximal shaft hole of the plate. With volar bone loss or comminution, primary cancellous bone grafting is indicated. A possible alternative to the T plate for slender bones is a radially applied 2.0-mm condylar plate. Usually the fracture is solid at six weeks and able to bear normal loads.

e) Implant Removal

The incisions are partly reopened for implant removal, taking care to preserve the sensory radial nerve branches to the dorsum of the thumb, which may be difficult to identify in the subcutaneous tissue. Because very persistent complaints can result if the sensory branches are injured, this procedure should be reserved for experienced surgeons.

2. Distal Fractures of the First Ray

a) Articular Fractures

Fractures are relatively common about the metacarpophalangeal and interphalangeal joints of the thumb. Many are open fractures that have associated injuries to tendons, nerves, and vessels.

Also common are small ligamentous avulsion fractures and chip fractures, which can be fixed with a single screw that is size-matched to the fragments (Fig. 118). The classic example is the avulsion fracture of the thumb during skiing. If the fragment is small, it is reduced and fixed with a Kirschner wire or with a Bunnell-type transosseous suture brought out through the radial skin.

b) Diaphyseal Fractures of the Metacarpus and Proximal Phalanx

Internal fixation is of recognized value in the treatment of these very unstable fractures, especially when combined injuries are present. It permits early mobilization without external fixation–a benefit of extreme importance for the first ray. We prefer to plate these fractures because of the excellent stability that is obtained (Fig. 118).

Approach: The fracture is approached through a dorsolateral incision, sparing the dorsal digital nerves. The extensor apparatus is carefully elevated, sparing the peritenon.

It is advantageous to plate the proximal phalanx on the lateral side. The mini condylar plate is excellent for fractures close to the joint (Fig. 118).

3. Secondary Operations on the First Ray

a) Carpometacarpal Joint

The major surgical disorder is osteoarthritis of the saddle joint, which may be degenerative or post-traumatic. Traumatic arthritis can result from an imperfectly reduced fracture-dislocation or from complex ligamentous injuries that cause joint instability. It is painful, is usually combined with varus, adduction, and flexion deformity, and seriously incapacitates the thumb ray. Several surgical options exist:

Excision of the trapezium is often performed for osteoarthritis, especially in females. The loss of thumb function is negligible, although it is common for some strength loss to occur.

For a long time it was recommended that the postexcision defect be grafted with autogenous tissue. Today the method of choice is to tether the thumb to the base of the second metacarpal with the distally pedicled half of the flexor carpi radialis tendon, reconstructing the intermetacarpal ligamentous connection.

Prosthetic replacement of the trapezium: Various plastic prostheses are available which are anchored in the shaft of the first metacarpal. Tendon transfers are necessary to keep the prosthesis from subluxating. Another method is to brace the joint cavity with Kirschner wires and pour in a semiliquid plastic compound. Total joint prostheses patterned after hip implants, in which a metallic head articulates with a plastic socket replacing the sellar surface of the trapezium, are rarely able to withstand the heavy loads that are placed upon this joint.

Arthrodesis is preferred in younger patients, in whom the first priority is maintenance of grip strength. This procedure relieves pain, however, only if the trapezioscaphoid joint is free of degenerative disease; this should be confirmed radiographically before operation. The functional losses from arthrodesis are often exaggerated, and in our experience they are of little real consequence. This may relate to our policy of early functional exercises with rapid mobilization of neighboring joints. The main concern for the patient is a pain-free power grip, especially in manual workers.

Operative Technique. The approach is similar to that for Rolando's fracture and employs a somewhat longer Y- or L-shaped proximal extension. The radial artery and its bifurcation are dissected free and snared with a tape (Fig. 120a). The carpometacarpal joint and the trapezium are exposed, and the joint is resected with a fine osteotome (Fig. 120b). The resulting defect must be completely filled with autogenous cancellous bone; otherwise consolidation is doubtful. Usually we take a corticocancellous graft from the ilium and slot it into the trapezium and first metacarpal base; we then apply a reversed T plate to compress the graft and hold it in place. The two proximal screws of the plate must occupy the exact center of the trapezium (Fig. 120c). Care is taken that the thumb is positioned correctly in opposition when the fixation is carried out.

An alternative to plating is a tension-band system employing Kirschner wires and a figure-of-eight wire loop (Fig. 120d).Again, autogenous cancellous bone grafting is necessary.

Even when very stable, the arthrodesis may take a number of months to consolidate, and removal of the implants should not be considered until after one year.

b) Metacarpophalangeal Joint of the Thumb
(Fig. 121)

This joint, with its relatively simple anatomy, has the smallest physiologic range of motion of any joint in the hand, although individual variations are large. The recommended position for arthrodesis of this joint is 5°–10° flexion, 5°–10° internal rotation, and 5°–10° abduction. The functional losses associated with arthrodesis are negligible. Either tension-band wiring or plating may be used. Cancellous bone grafts are rarely necessary.

c) Interphalangeal Joint of the Thumb

Arthrodesis of this joint may be indicated for post-traumatic or degenerative deformity or instability. The preferred position is the neutral position or very slight flexion. Functional losses are negligible when the neighboring joints are intact.

The joint is exposed through a Y- or H-shaped incision, as for all arthrodeses of the distal interphalangeal joints (Fig. 137). The joint may be fused with a distally inserted screw (Fig. 146) or with a tension-band wire. For the first technique, we use 3.5- or 2.7-mm extra-long cortex screws. The 4.0-mm cancellous screws are contraindicated because they cannot be removed later. The screw size is matched to the medullary cavity of the proximal phalanx, which must be carefully tapped before the screw is inserted.

d) Deformities of the First Ray

Significant adduction-flexion deformity or narrowing of the thumb web is correctible by a basal osteotomy of the first metacarpal. A tension-band plate or condylar plate combined with cancellous bone grafting has proved effective.The stability obtained is sufficient for early mobilization.

e) Thumb Reconstruction (Pollicization, Toe Transfer)

Small plates (condylar or H plates) have proved effective for stabilizing a finger transposition or free toe transfer for thumb reconstruction in adults.It allows postoperative care to be tailored to soft-tissue requirements. Generally these implants are too bulky for use in children, and these cases can be stabilized with Kirschner wires and wire sutures.

4. Illustrative Case Reports and X-Rays
(Figs. 122–133)

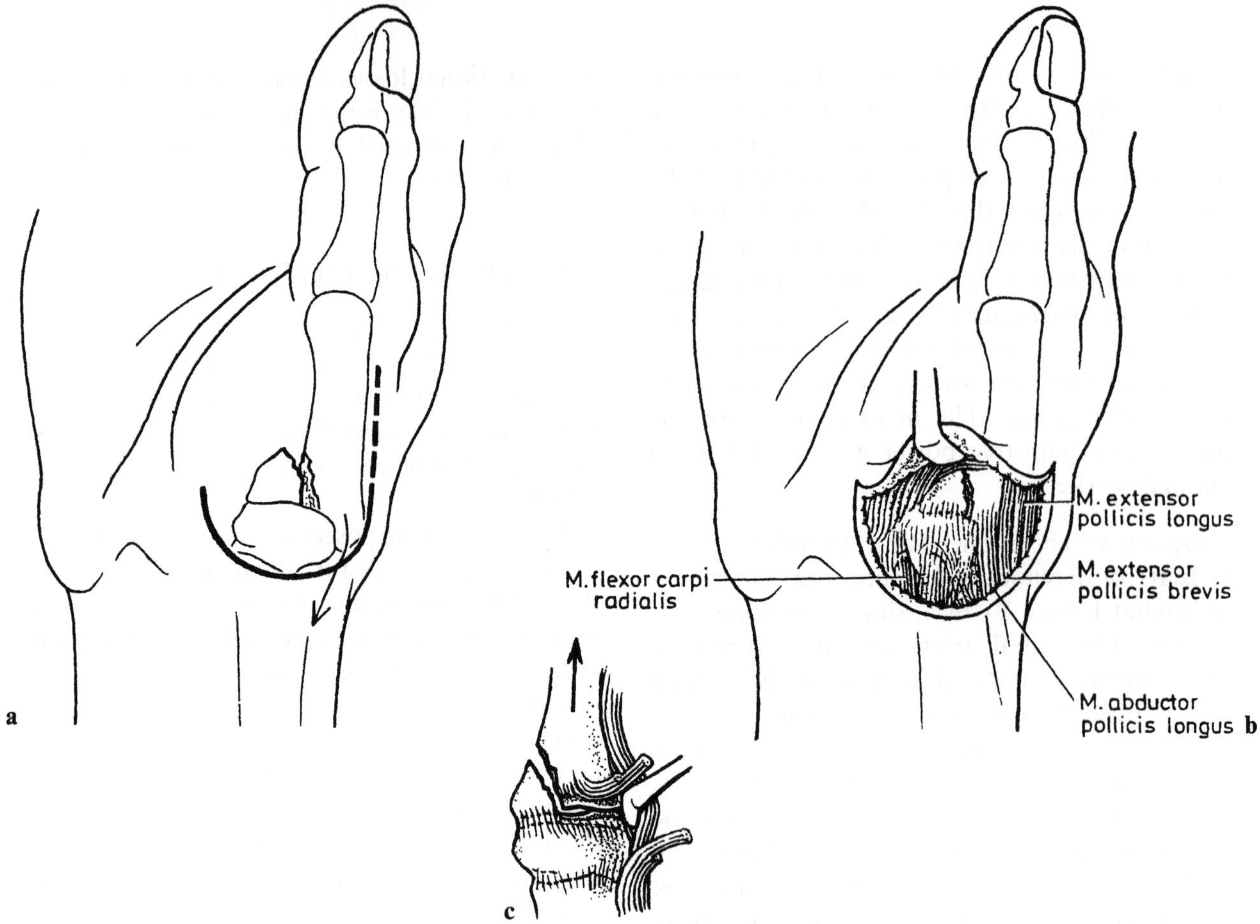

Fig. 113 a–c. Gedda-Moberg approach to the base of the first metacarpal

a Incision for Bennett's fracture, with possible extension

b Topography: view of the articular fragment from the volar side, with tendons

c Joint exposure is improved by dividing the abductor pollicis longus tendon in Z fashion

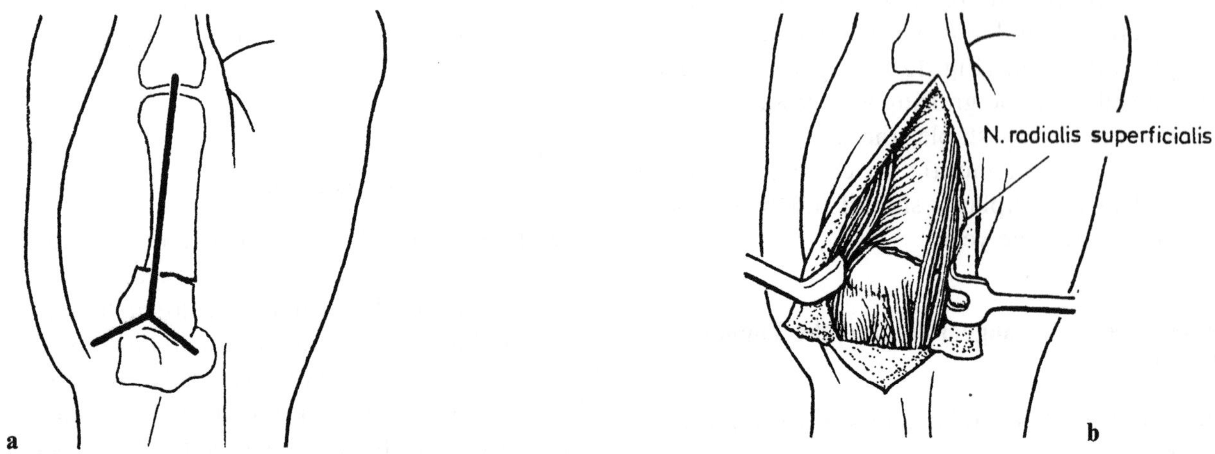

Fig. 114 a, b. Radiodorsal approach to the base of the first metacarpal

a Y-shaped proximal extension of the incision

b Topography of an extra-articular transverse fracture: The sensory branch of the radial nerve is retracted dorsally

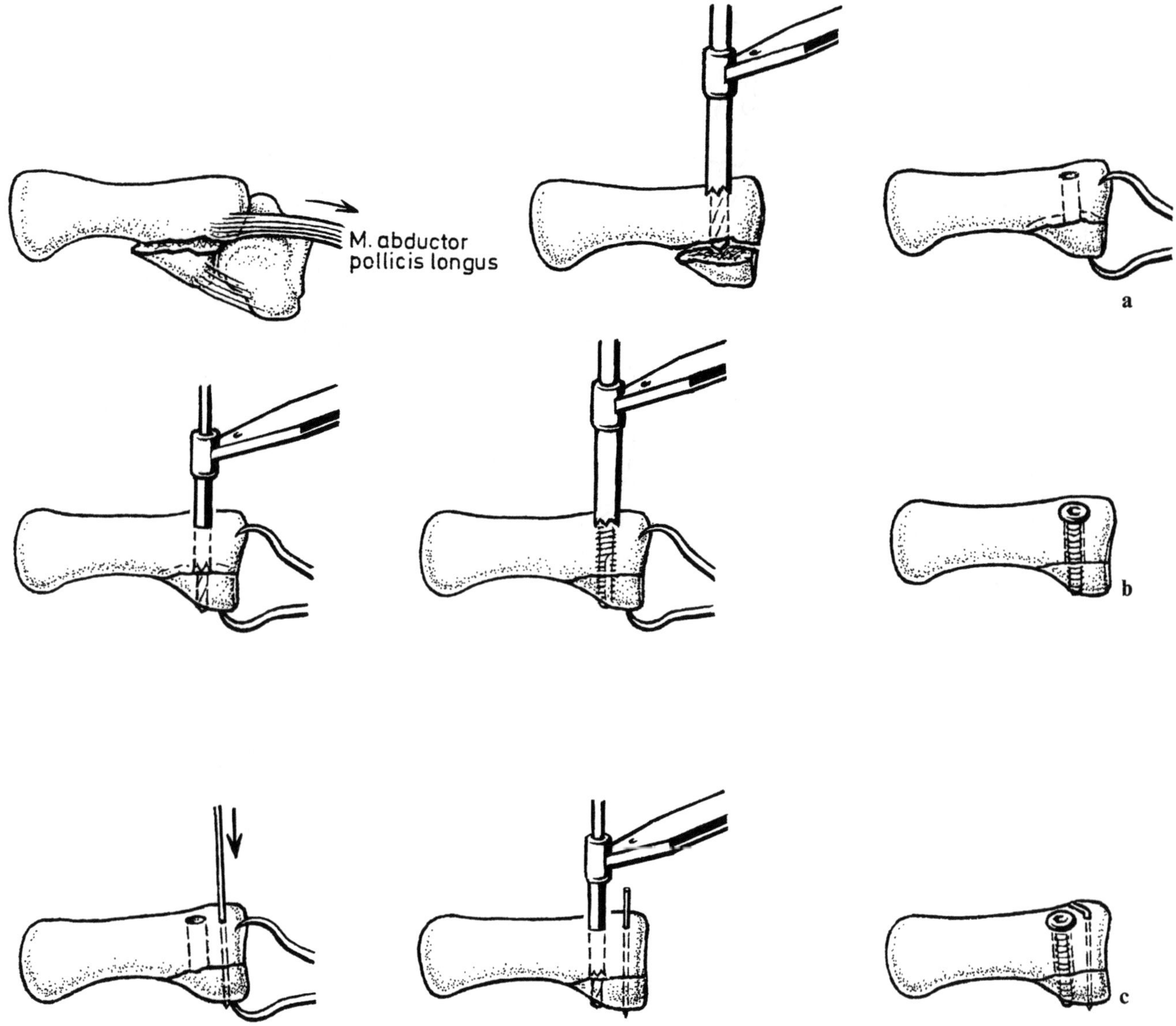

Fig. 115a–c. Screw fixation of Bennett's fracture

The size of the screw and drill hole is contingent upon the size of the fragment (2.7- or 2.0-mm cortex, less frequently the 4.0-mm cancellous)

a Prior to reduction, a gliding hole is drilled in the large fragment under vision.The fracture is reduced and held with a forceps

b The thread hole is drilled through the insert sleeve, tapped, and the screw inserted

c Variation: After completion of the gliding hole, the fracture is reduced and held with forceps, which is then replaced with a Kirschner wire. The thread hole s drilled through the insert sleeve. The lag screw is inserted, and the wire is left to check rotation. The end of the wire is bent close to the bone with the bending iron (see Fig. 25/9)

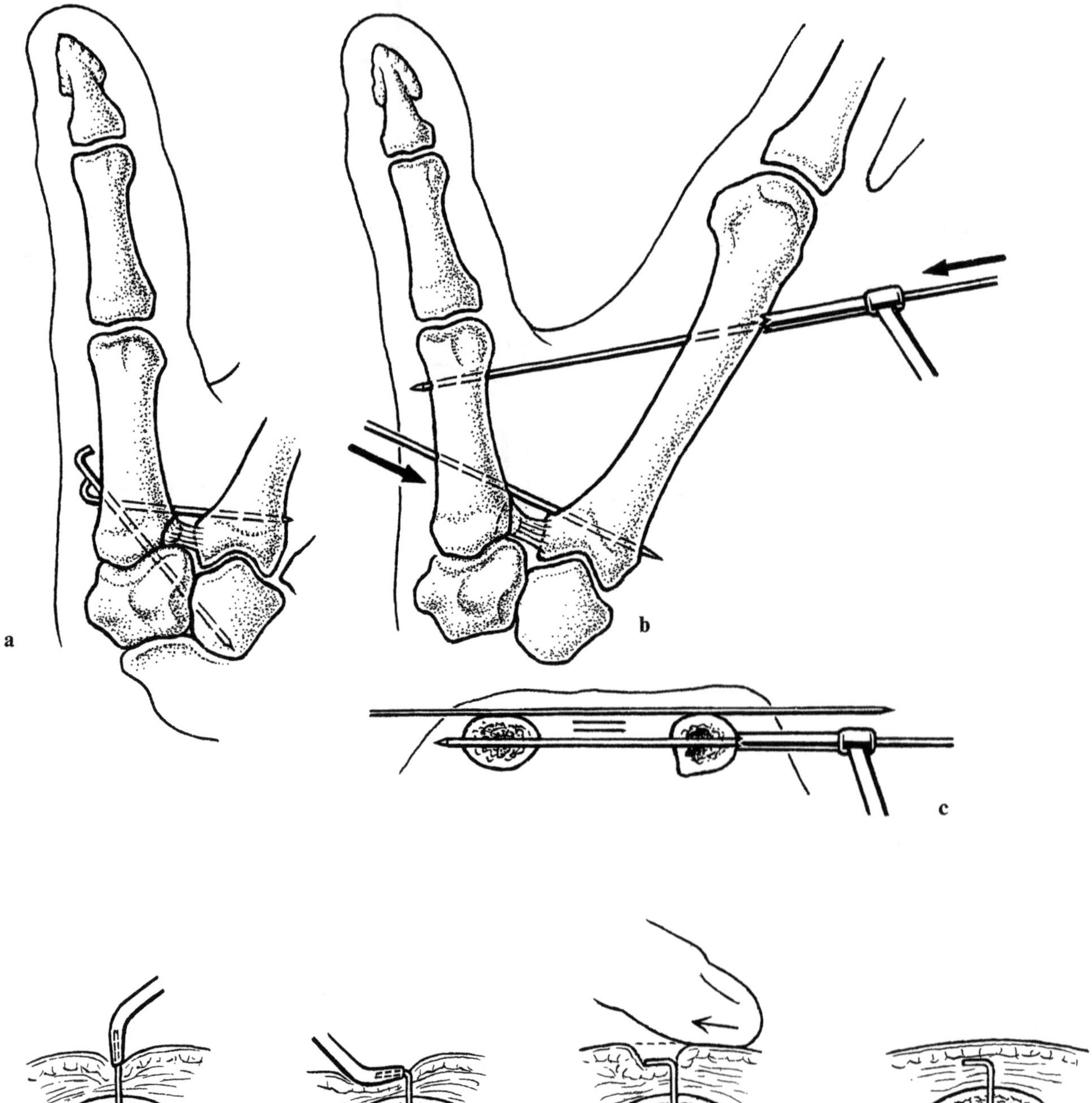

Fig. 116a–d. Bennett's fracture with a small fragment: percutaneous Kirschner wire fixation

a Wagner's technique (modified): After closed reduction by traction, a Kirschner wire is drilled percutaneously from the first metacarpal into the carpus under image intensifier control. A second wire is drilled through the first and second metacarpals

b Iselin's technique with a double Kirschner wire: The fracture is reduced by traction, and the thumb is abducted to open the thumb web. A first, distal Kirschner wire is drilled from the second metacarpal into the first. A second, proximal wire is drilled from the first metacarpal into the base of the second metacarpal

c The preliminary placement of a Kirschner wire along the dorsal edge of both metacarpals is helpful in guiding the wire insertion

d The end of the wire is bent close to the skin with the angled bending iron. The instrument is placed over the wire and should slightly indent the skin. The wire is bent down and is buried by stroking the finger toward the wire tip

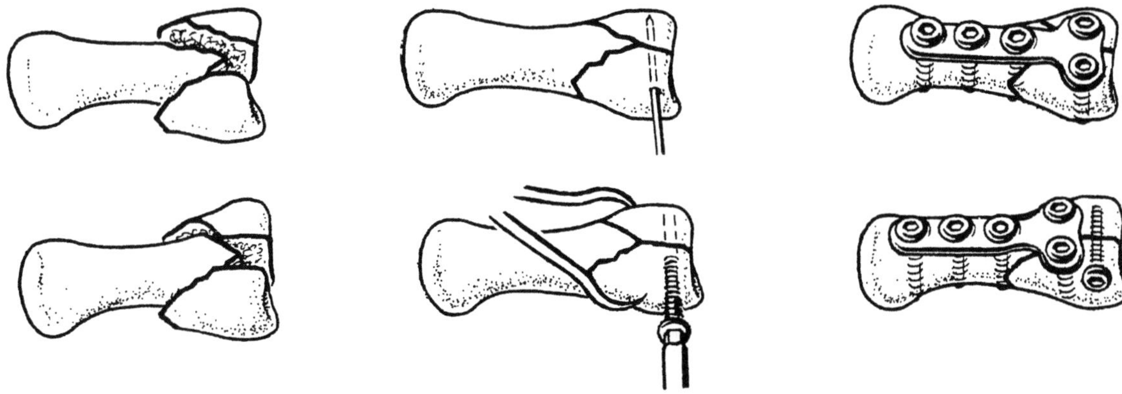

a

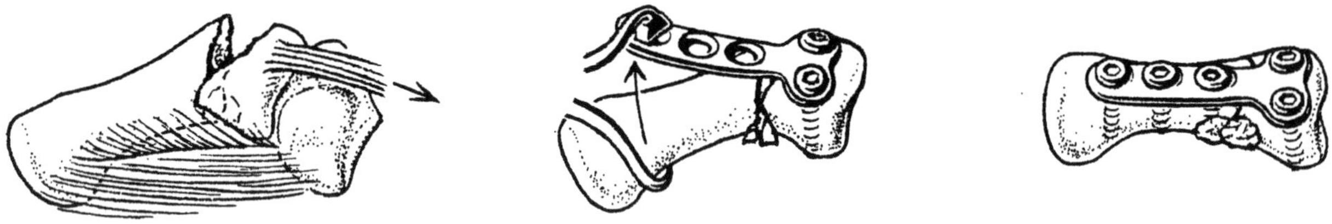

b

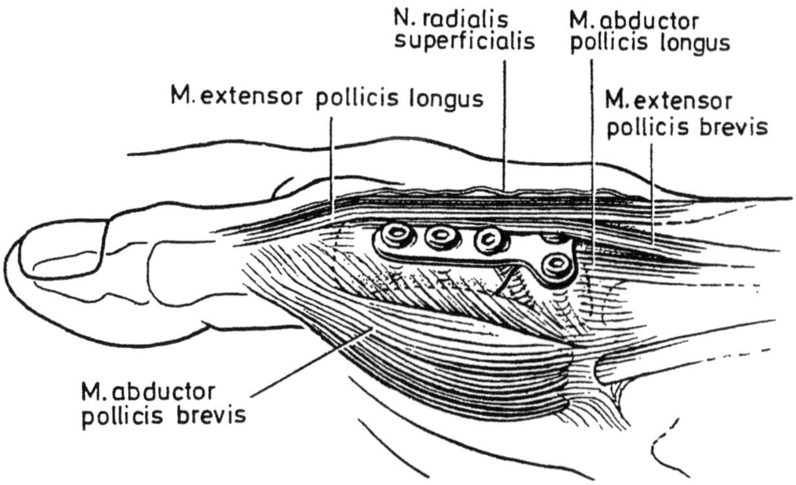

c

Fig. 117a–c. Internal fixation of Rolando's fracture and an extra-articular fracture of the first metacarpal base

a Rolando's fracture is fixed with a T plate alone or combined with preliminary screw fixation of the joint fragments, depending on the fracture type

b Extra-articular fracture: The T plate is first fixed to the proximal fragment and is used as a lever to aid reduction. Autogenous cancellous bone grafting is recommended for volar comminution

c General view: The plate for the extra-articular fracture incorporates an interfragmental lag screw. The extensor tendons overlie a portion of the plate. The sensory branch of the radial nerve is dissected and must be spared during implant removal

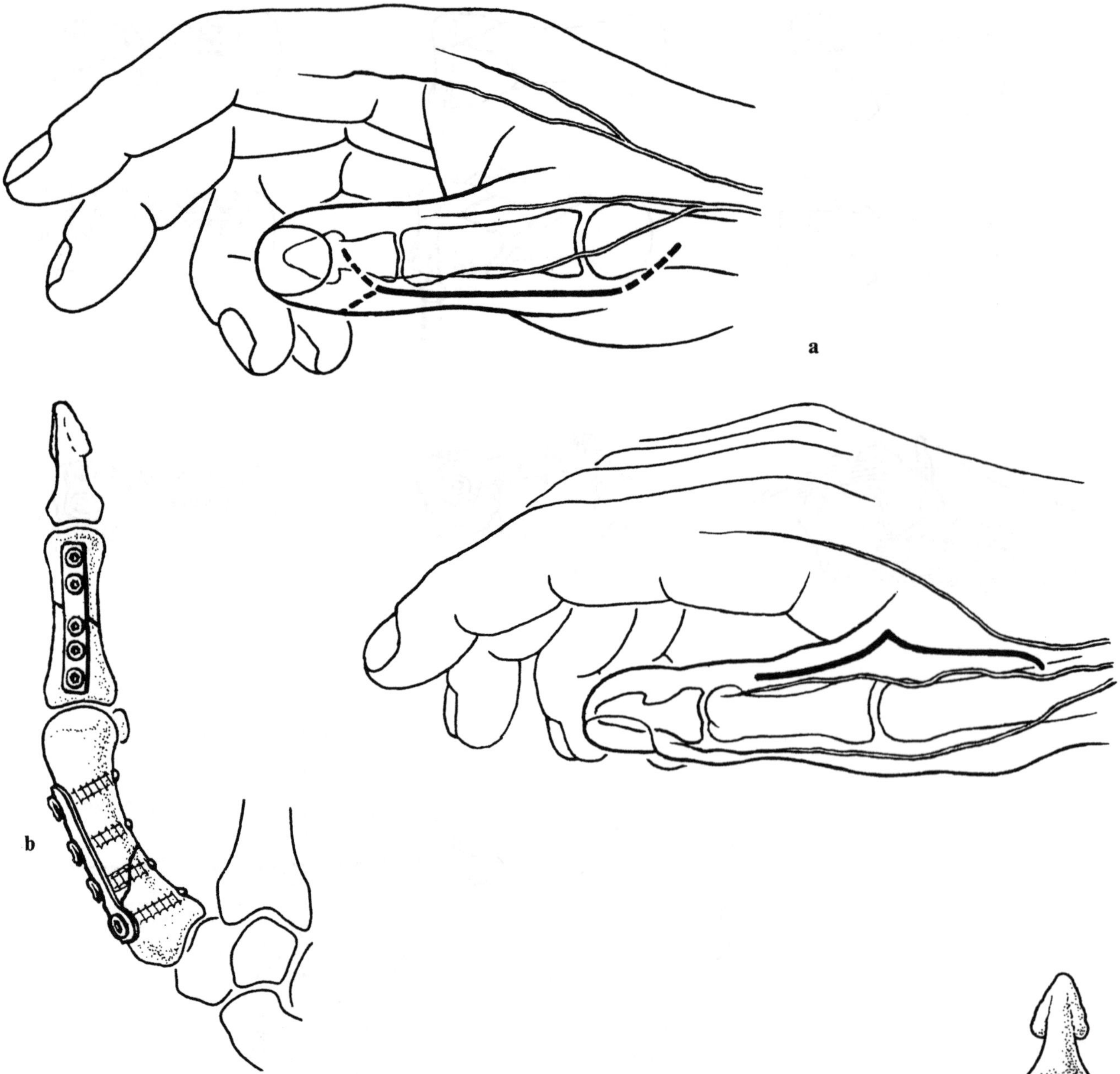

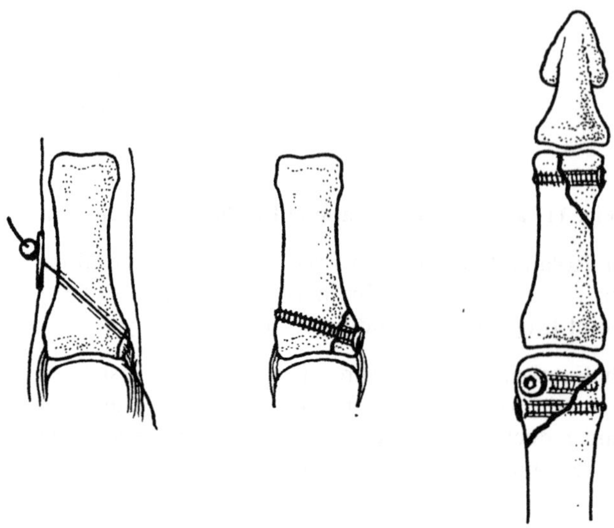

Fig. 118a–c. Internal fixations of the first ray

a Dorsoradial and dorsoulnar incisions, with extensions. Branches of the radial nerve

b Shaft fractures: A T-plate is used on the metacarpal shaft, and a lateral mini plate on the proximal phalanx

c Articular fractures: Screws are used to fix condylar fractures and to reattach larger avulsed fragments to the base of the proximal phalanx. A transosseous wire suture is used for small avulsed fragments

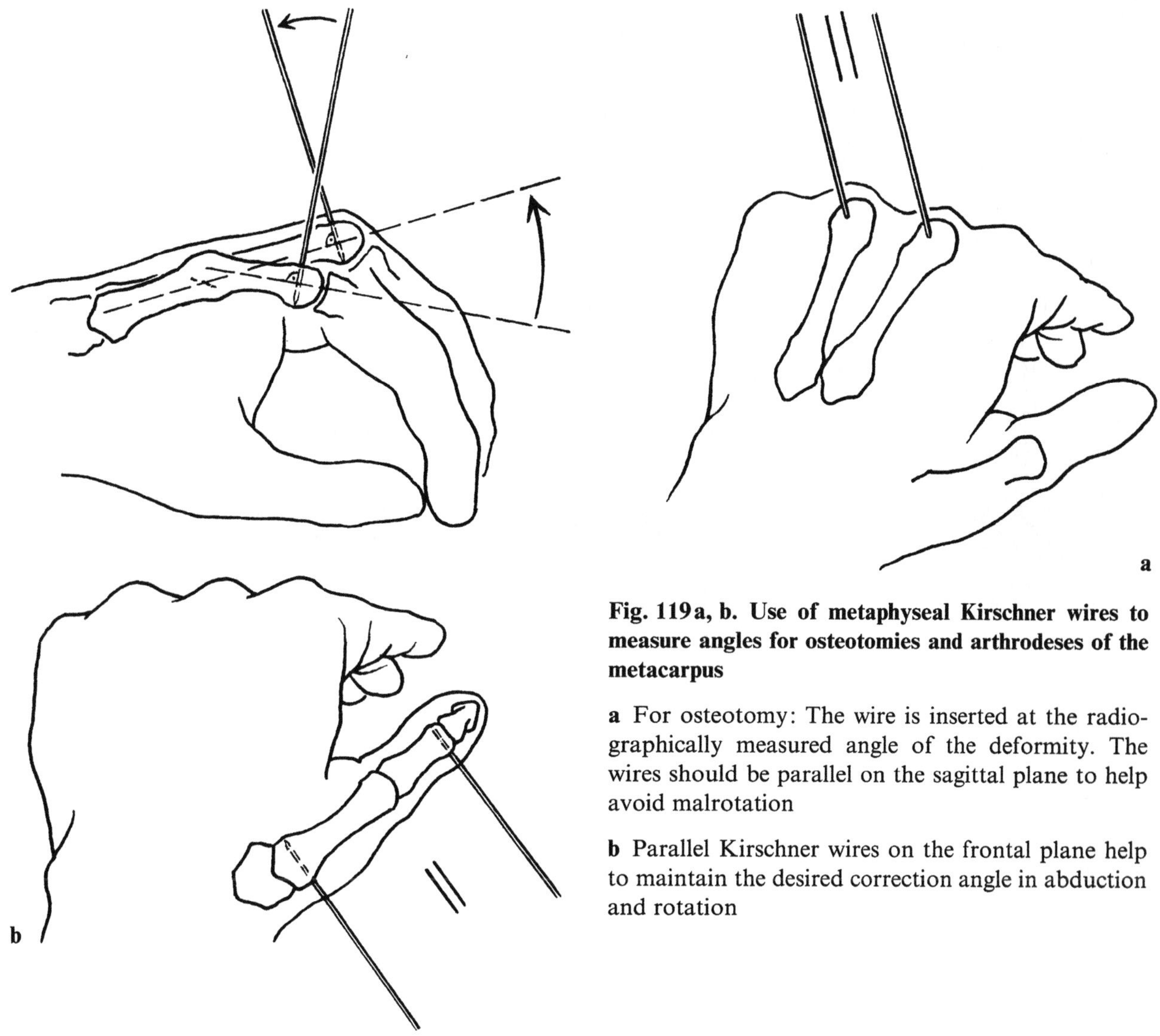

a

b

Fig. 119 a, b. Use of metaphyseal Kirschner wires to measure angles for osteotomies and arthrodeses of the metacarpus

a For osteotomy: The wire is inserted at the radiographically measured angle of the deformity. The wires should be parallel on the sagittal plane to help avoid malrotation

b Parallel Kirschner wires on the frontal plane help to maintain the desired correction angle in abduction and rotation

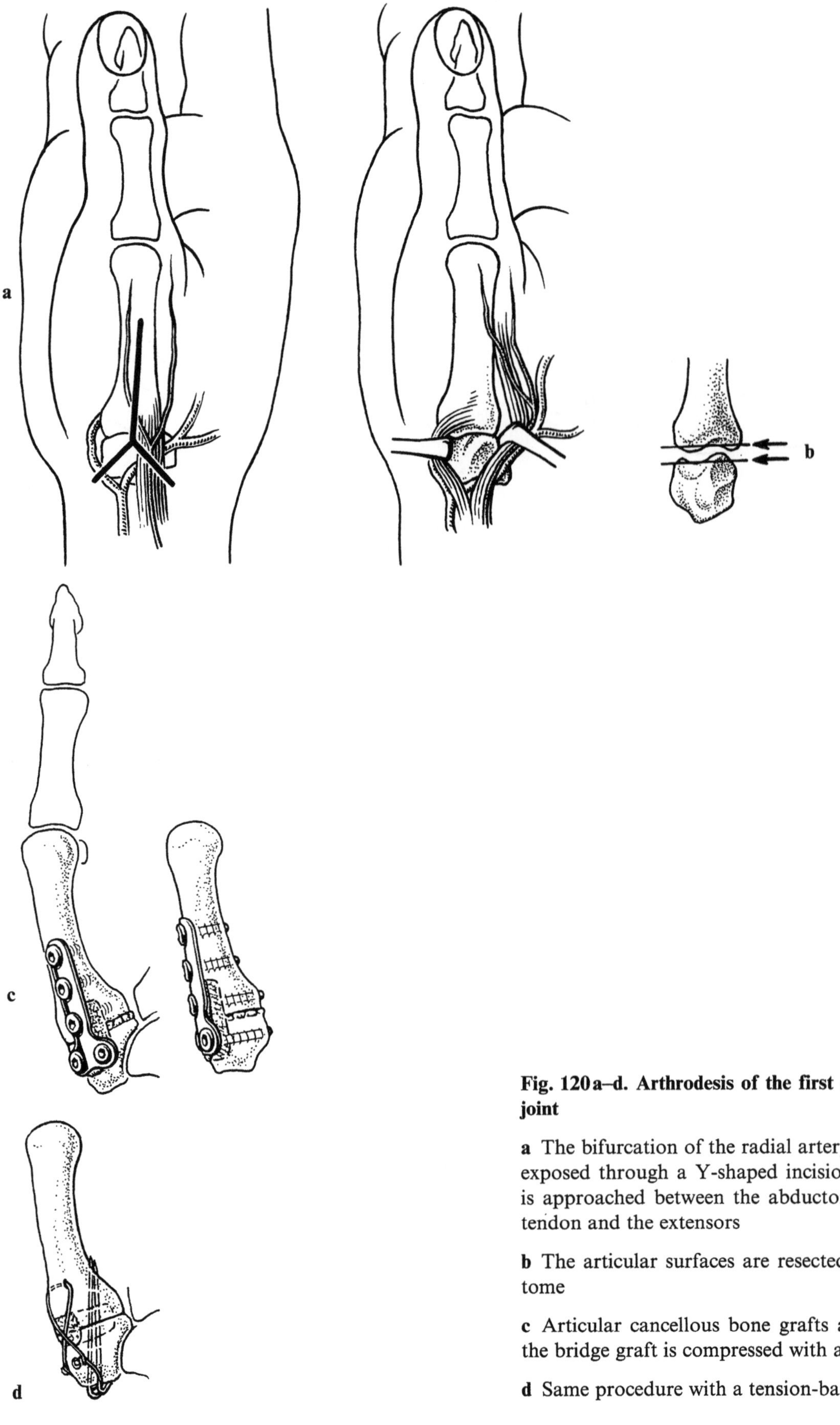

Fig. 120a–d. Arthrodesis of the first carpometacarpal joint

a The bifurcation of the radial artery and nerves are exposed through a Y-shaped incision, and the joint is approached between the abductor pollicis longus tendon and the extensors

b The articular surfaces are resected with an osteotome

c Articular cancellous bone grafts are applied, and the bridge graft is compressed with a T plate

d Same procedure with a tension-band assembly

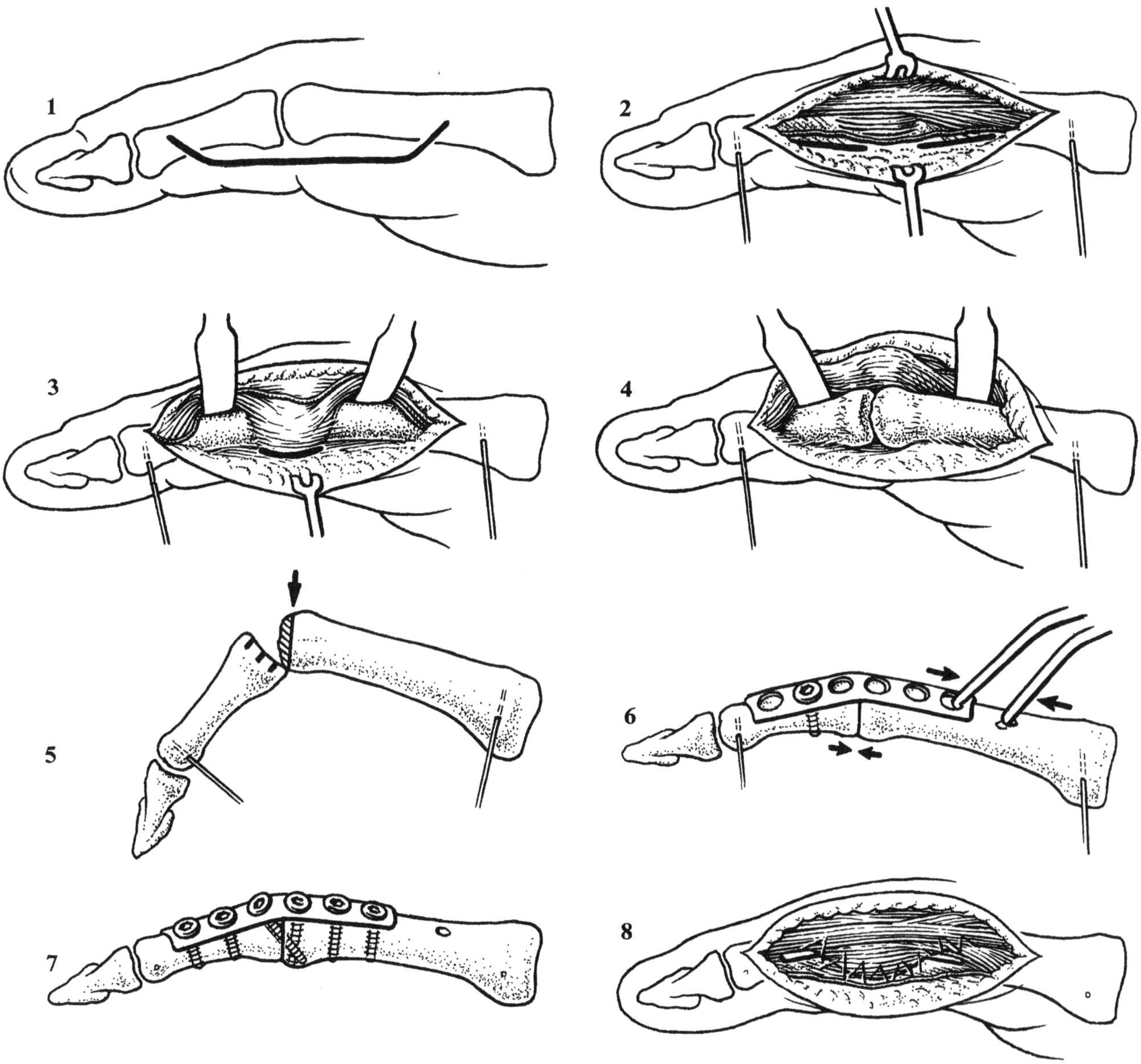

Fig. 121 1–8. Plate arthrodesis of the first carpometacarpal joint

1 Skin incision

2 Kirschner guide wires (angular alignment and rotation) are drilled into the metaphyses of the proximal phalanx and first metacarpal

3 Periosteum is incised adjacent to the extensor apparatus distally and proximally and is retracted with periosteal elevators

4 Joint is opened after division of the capsule and extensor apparatus; the collateral ligaments are incised

5 With the joint flexed, the metacarpal head is resected at a slightly oblique angle, and multiple drill holes are made in the concave articular surface of the proximal phalanx

6 A contoured 6-hole quarter tubular plate is tentatively attached to the distal fragment with screws. Axial compression is applied with the mini compression forceps, and the position of the arthrodesis is checked (flexion, abduction, rotation)

7 The plate is attached on both sides of the arthrodesis. A central interfragmental lag screw is inserted, avoiding screws already in place (see Fig. 38)

8 The joint capsule is closed with a continuous suture

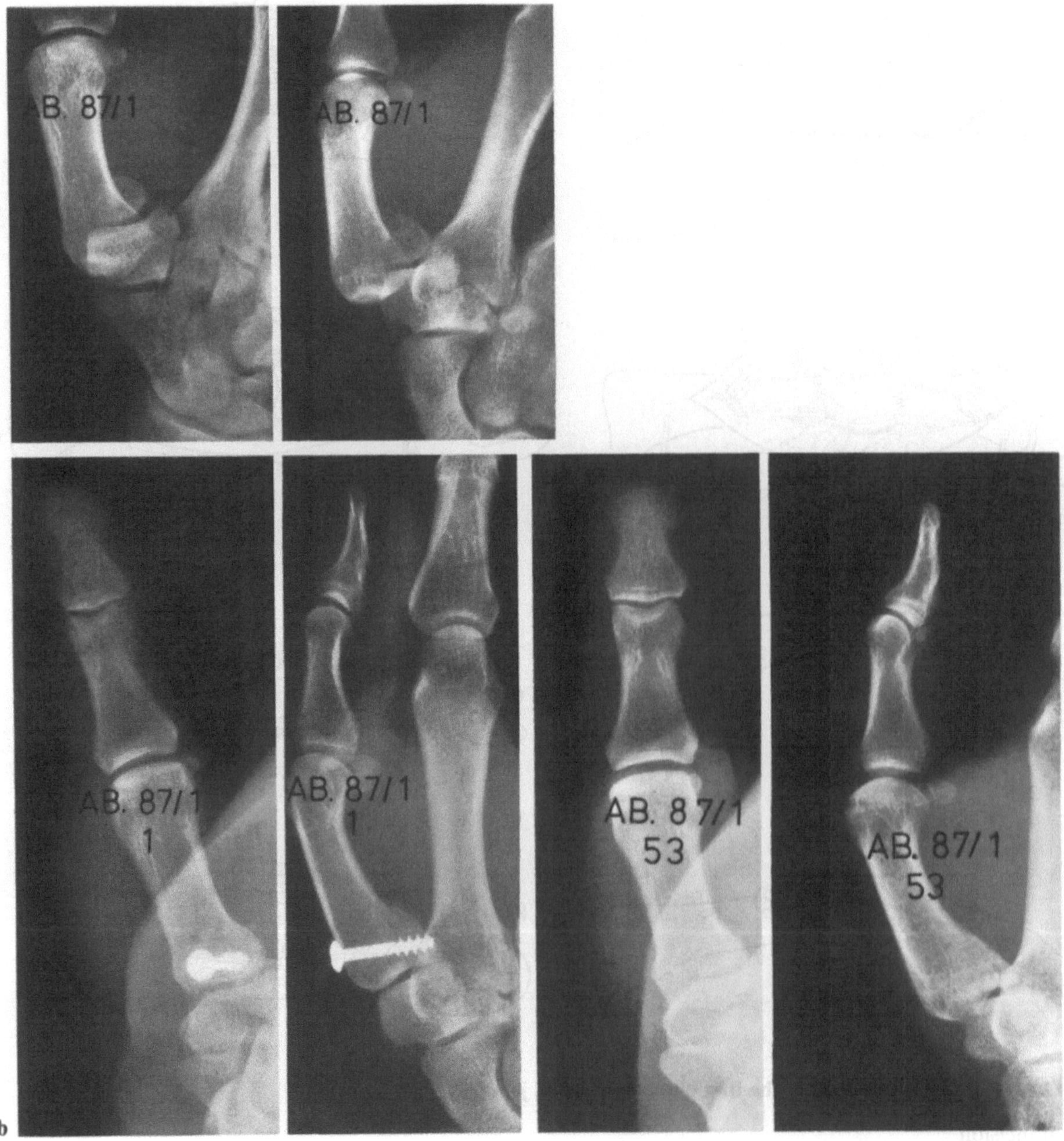

Fig. 122 a–c. Clinical example: screw fixation of Bennett's fracture

Beat W., 20-year-old auto mechanic, injured the right hand while playing handball

a Bennett's fracture-dislocation

b Internal fixation was performed 4 days postinjury using a 4.0-mm cancellous screw, and motion was started right away. Patient was 50% rehabilitated at 7 weeks and 100% at 9 weeks. Radiograph taken 1 year after operation

c Status after screw removal. Patient had equivalent strength and motion in both hands and no complaints. He resumed competitive handball 3 months after surgery

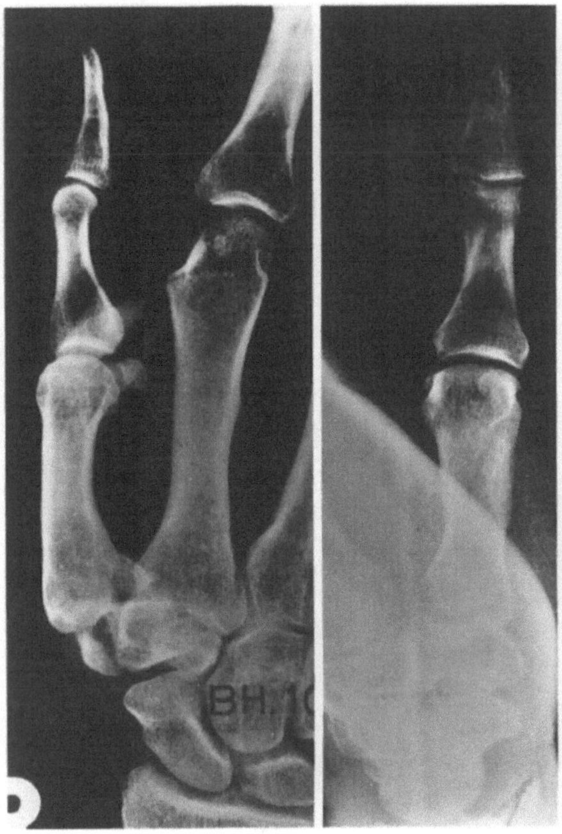

a

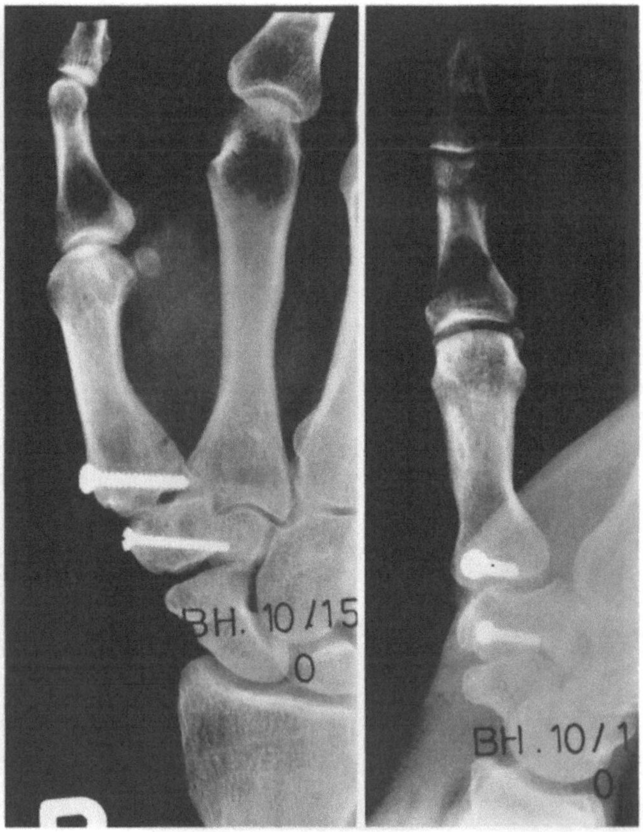

b

Fig. 123a–c. Clinical example: Bennett's fracture combined with trapezium fracture

Calogero T., 54-year-old doorman, underwent internal fixation of extra-articular oblique basal fracture of the right first metacarpal 15 years previously, fell onto the right hand on 5/11/84

a Bennett's fracture-dislocation of the first metacarpal and wedge fracture of the trapezium

b Four days later the first metacarpal was fixed with a 2.7-mm cortex screw and the trapezium with a 2.0-mm screw. A plaster splint was worn for 2 weeks; patient was able to resume work at 6 weeks

c At 4-month follow-up on 9/12/84, the patient had full function and no complaints.Both fractures were united. The screws were not removed

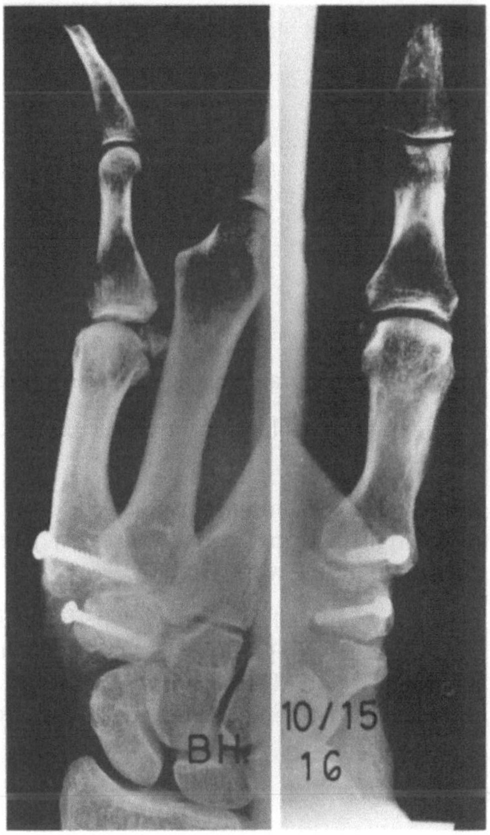

c

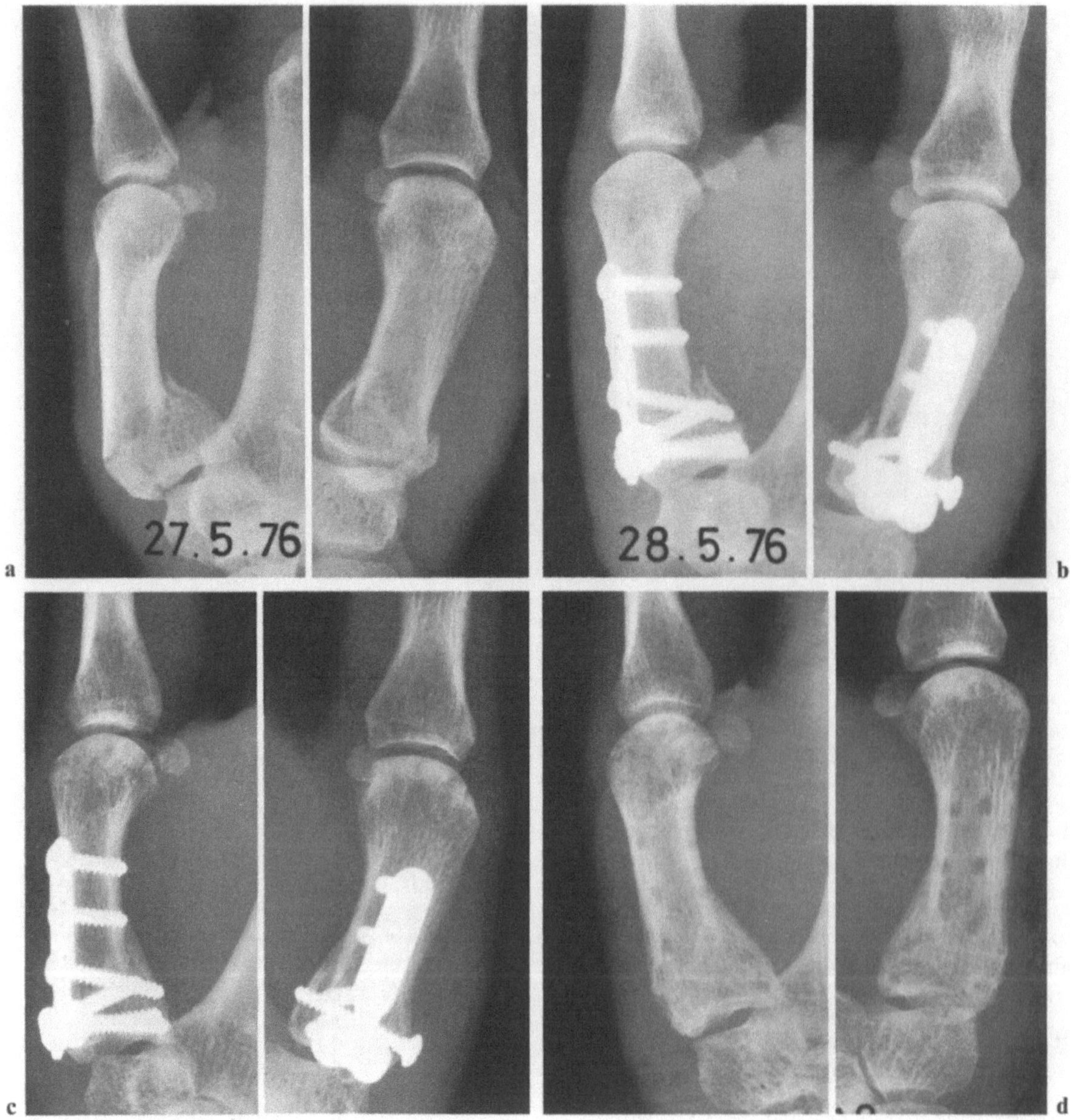

Fig. 124a–d. Clinical example: Rolando's fracture

Karl V., 46-year-old auto mechanic, injured on the job

a Rolando-type intra-articular fracture of the base of the right first metacarpal caused by jamming of the thumb during work

b Primary internal fixation was performed with a transverse, interfragmental 2.7-mm cortex lag screw and small T plate. The lag screw was inserted through the plate into the ulnar basal fragment. Reduction of the volar comminuted zone was not entirely satisfactory.Nevertheless, external fixation was not applied, and early motion was started.Rehabilitation was 50% at 8 weeks and 100% at 12 weeks

c By 17 weeks a solid fixation callus had formed on the volar comminuted zone

d Implants were removed at 23 weeks. Patient had no subjective complaints, unrestricted function, and no osteoarthritis

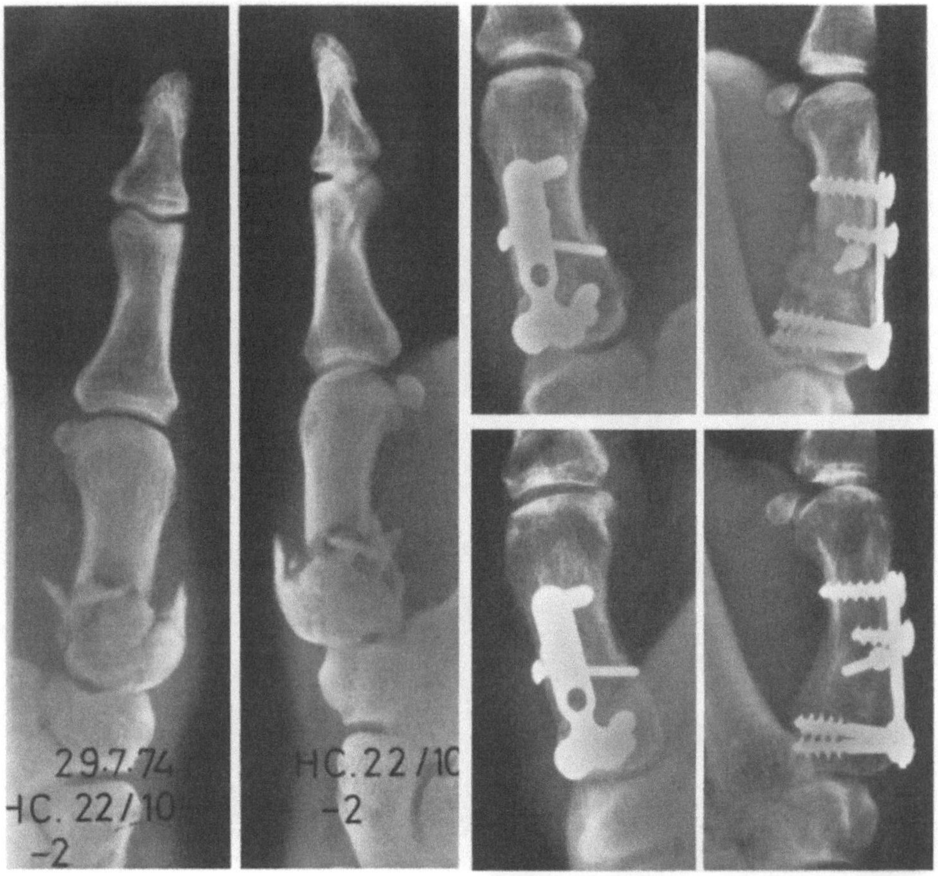

a b c

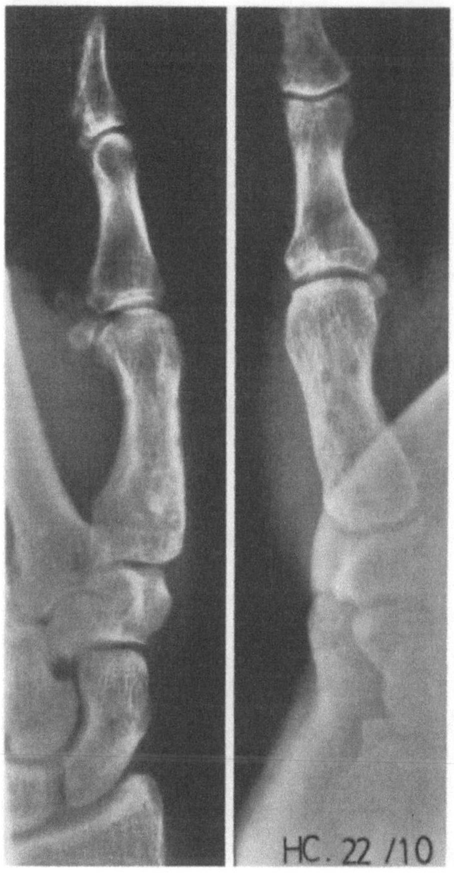

d

Fig. 125a–d. Clinical example: comminuted fracture of the base of the first metacarpal with bone loss

Matteo R., 46-year-old bricklayer, injured at work on 7/24/74; left hand was struck by a heavy metal fragment in an explosion

a Atypical comminuted Rolando's fracture with swelling and skin abrasions. The hand was elevated and immobilized

b The fracture was fixed at 3 weeks with a T plate and screw. The defect was grafted with iliac cancellous bone. Primary wound healing was achieved, and a dorsal plaster splint was worn for 4 weeks

c By 6 weeks the graft was healed, and partial rehabilitation was achieved.Implants were removed at 3 1/2 months

d When last seen at 5 months postoperatively, the patient had no complaints, slight loss of flexion in the MP joint, full extension, and a linear scar

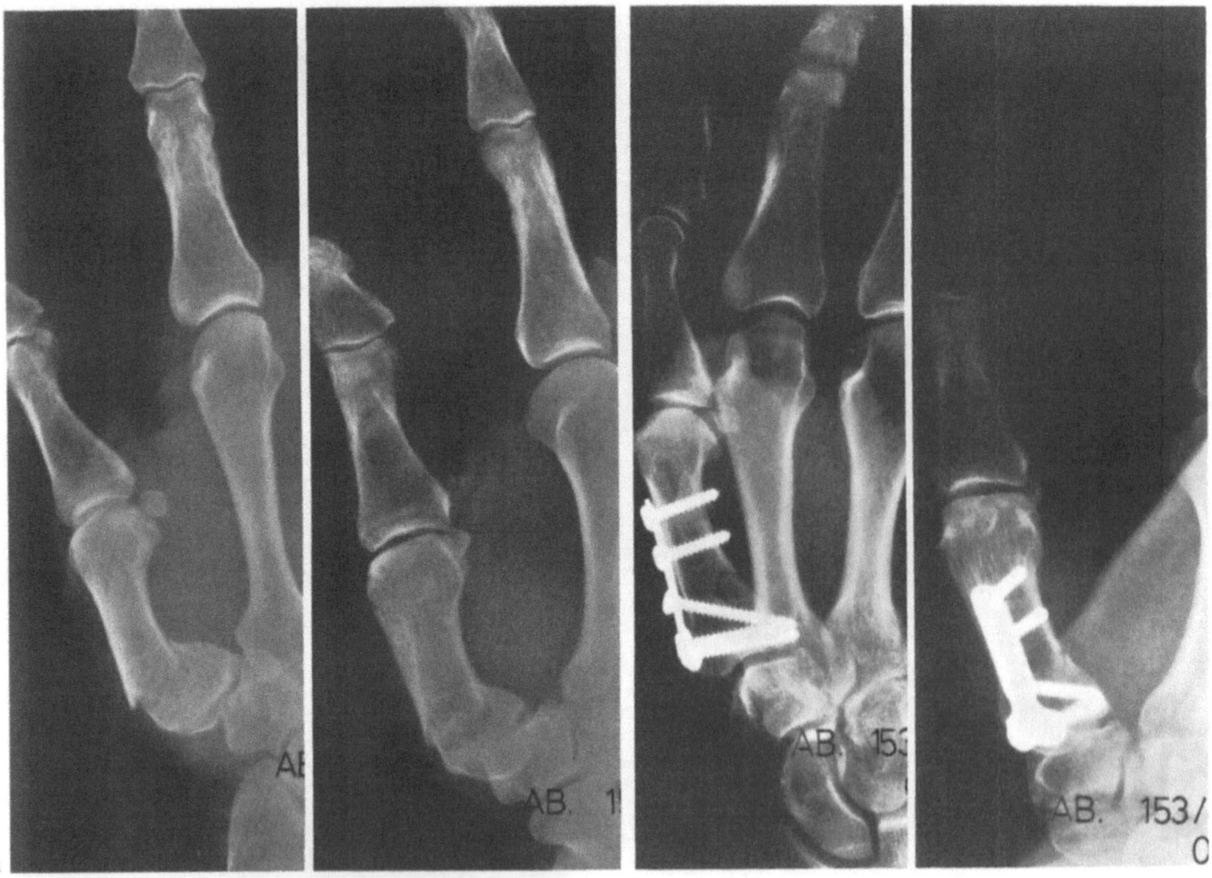

a b

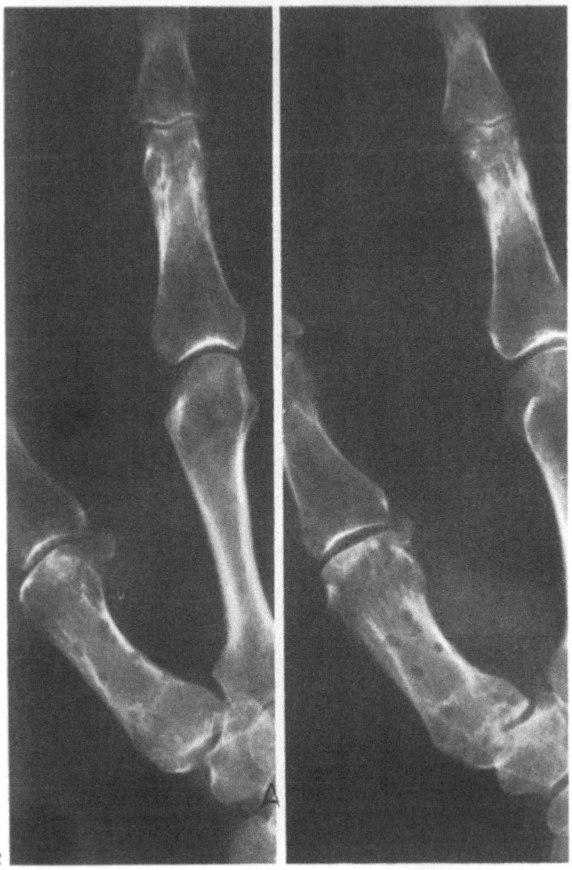

c

Fig. 126a–c. Clinical example: extra-articular fracture of the base of the first metacarpal

Walter K., 56-year-old postal worker, injured in a moped accident

a Transverse fracture of the base of the right first metacarpal

b Primary internal fixation was performed with a 2.7-mm small-fragment T plate. An interfragmental cortex lag screw was placed obliquely through the plate. Despite early mobilization, dystrophic symptoms developed due to preexisting severe carpal tunnel syndrome

c Implants were removed at 20 weeks, accompanied by median nerve decompression and neurolysis. Patient was fully rehabilitated by 5 months; he had no complaints and equivalent function in both hands

Fig. 127a–c. Clinical example: transverse fracture of the first metacarpal shaft

Jose R., 33-year-old carpenter, right hand struck by a falling piece of iron on 3/9/81

a Transverse fracture of the first metacarpal shaft with extensive crushing of the soft tissues

b Internal fixation was performed the next day with a 2.0-mm H plate. A low-grade infection ensued with prolonged fistulization. Implants were removed at 7 weeks, before infection had resolved

c Follow-up at 4 months on 7/13/81 showed equivalent thumb motion on both sides. The fracture was united, and the patient had no disability

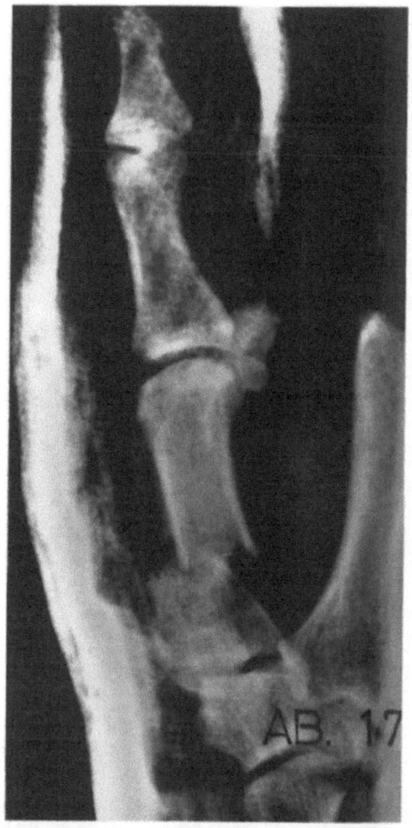

a

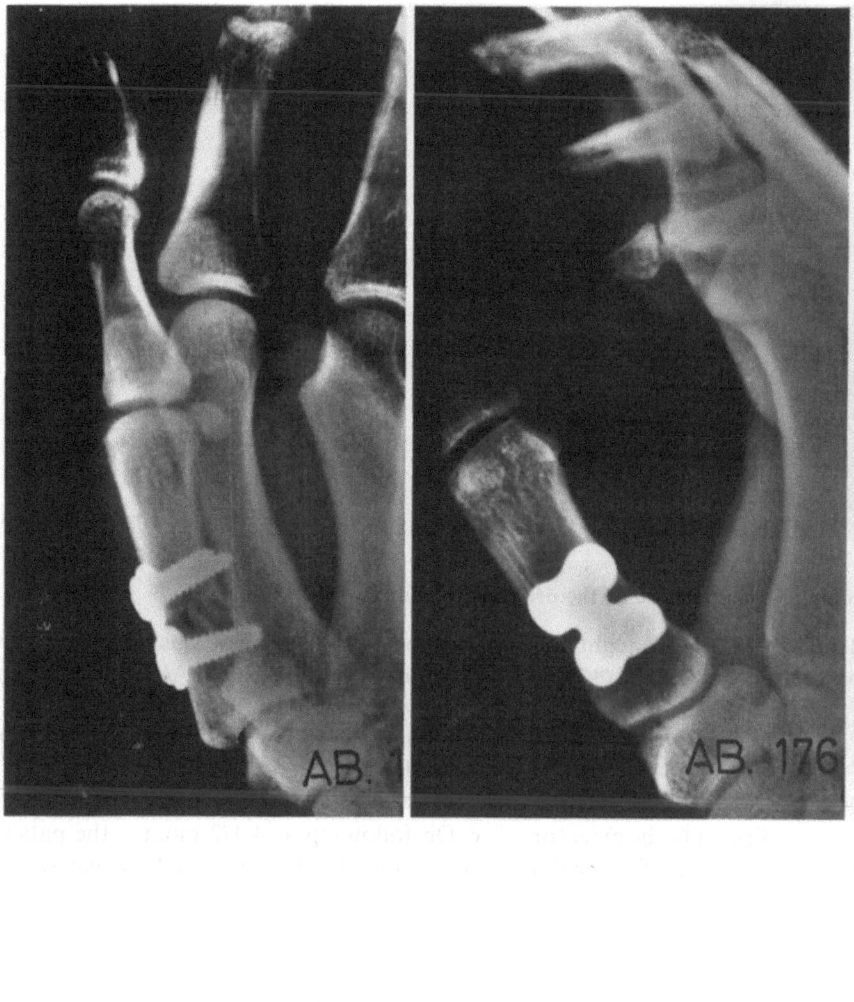

b

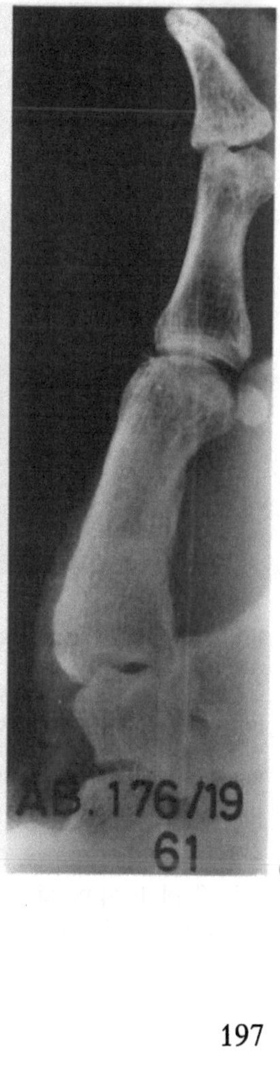

c

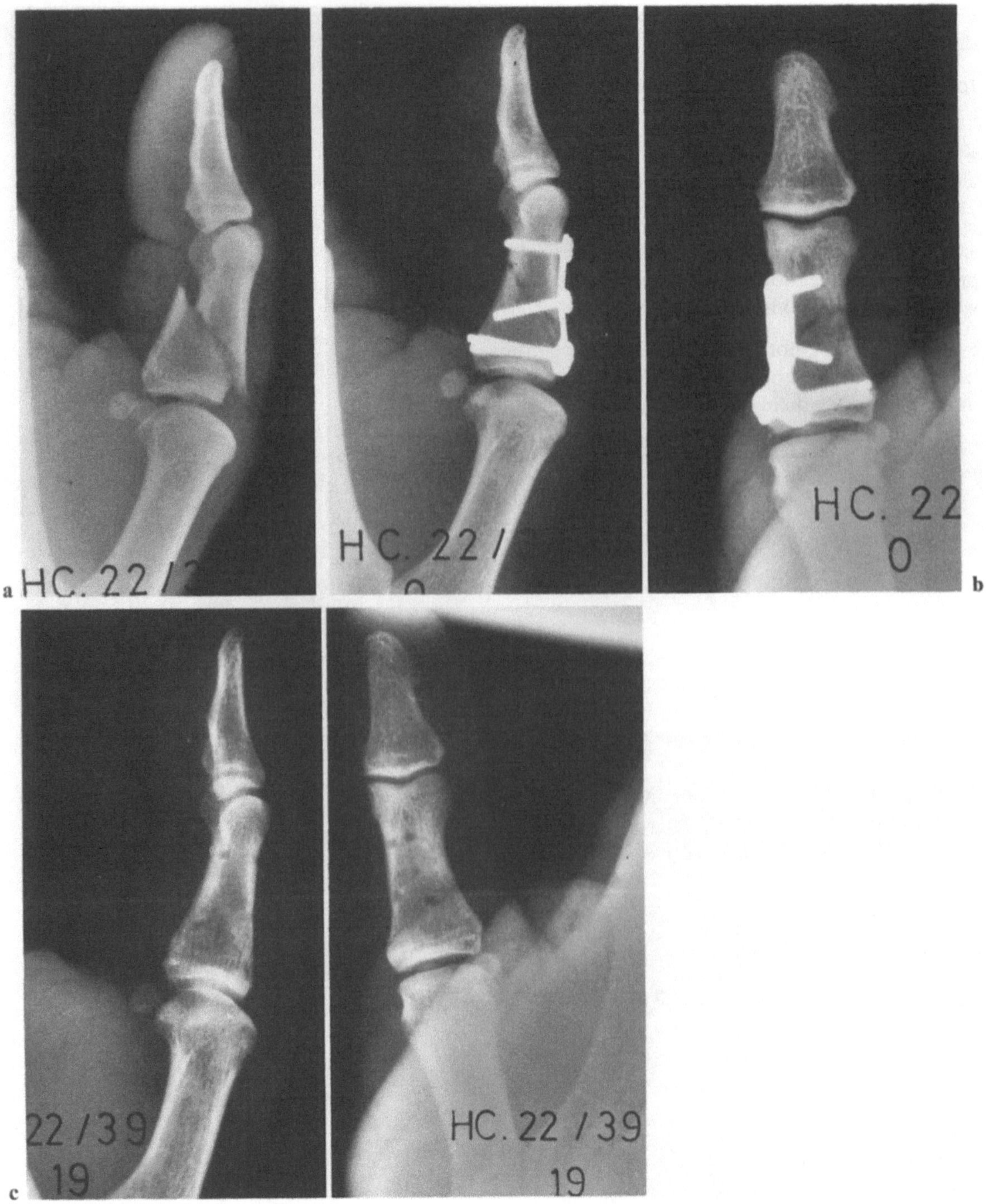

Fig. 128 a–c. Clinical example: open fracture of the proximal phalanx of the thumb

Caspar A., 27-year-old factory worker, caught the left thumb between a forklift and truck on 11/8/74

a Open grade 2 oblique fracture of the proximal phalanx of the left thumb

b Immediate internal fixation was performed with a mini T plate applied dorsally, adjacent to the extensor apparatus. The central screw is an interfragmental lag screw

The postoperative course was uneventful, and primary wound healing ensued. Active motion and weight lifting were commenced at 2 weeks. Patient was fully rehabilitated by 7 weeks; implants were removed at 4 months

c On follow-up at 4 1/2 months the patient had no complaints, full function, and a linear scar

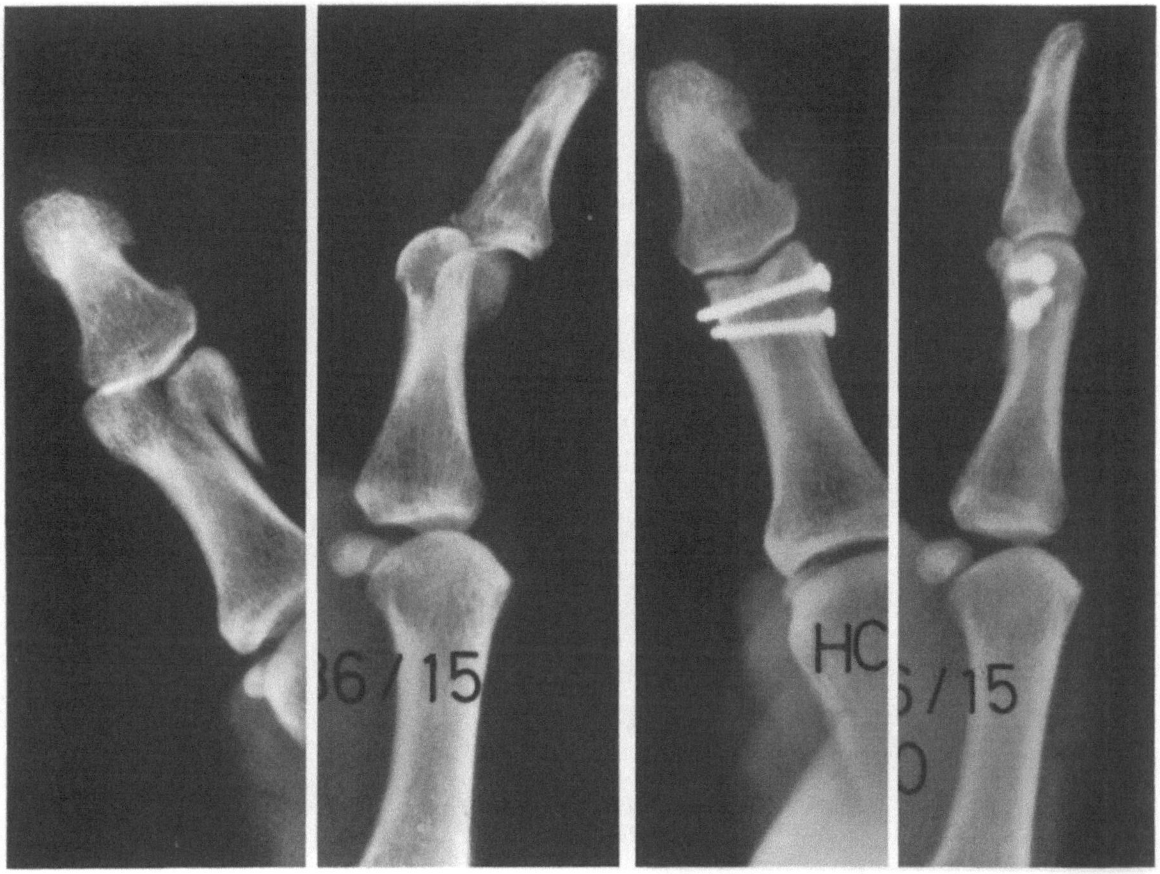

a b

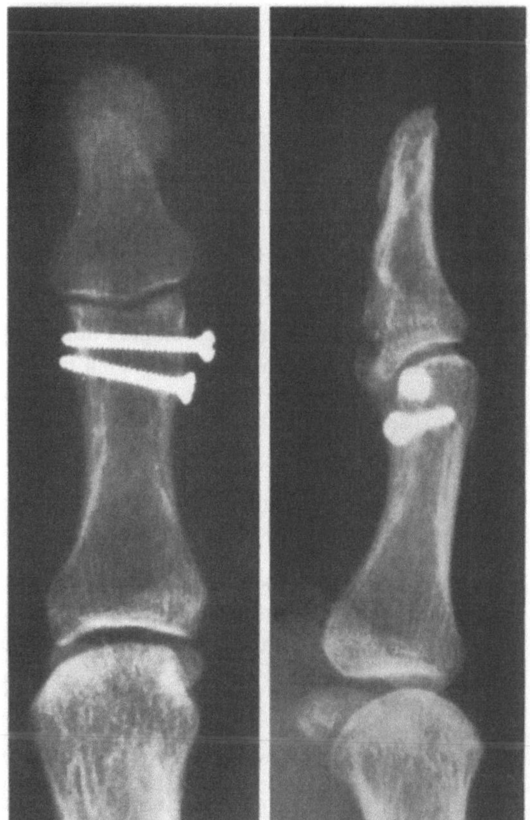

c

Fig. 129 a–c. Clinical example: monocondylar fracture of the proximal phalanx of the thumb

Margrit H., 50-year-old housewife, fell while skiing on 3/6/77

a Markedly displaced monocondylar fracture of the proximal phalanx of the thumb with an articular step

b The fracture was immediately fixed with two 1.5-mm mini screws
After an uneventful course, the patient was discharged with a protective splint

c At 2 1/2 years the distal screw was loose and was causing local complaints. Flexion and hyperextension were slightly decreased relative to the healthy side. The implants were removed shortly thereafter

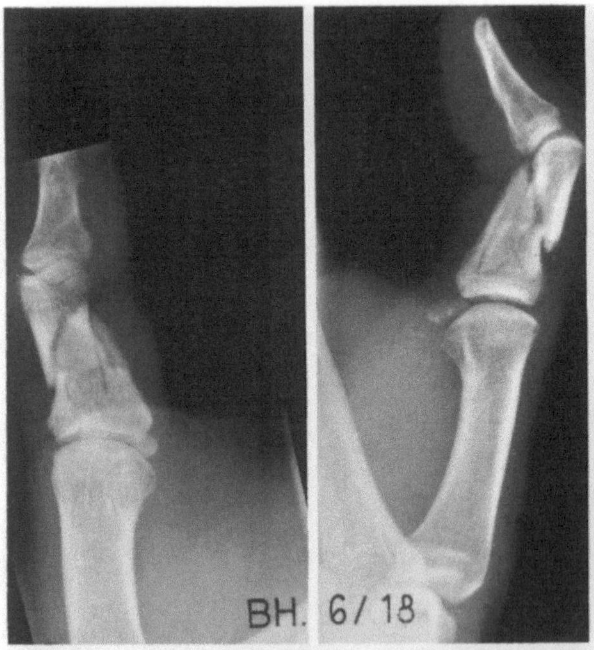

a

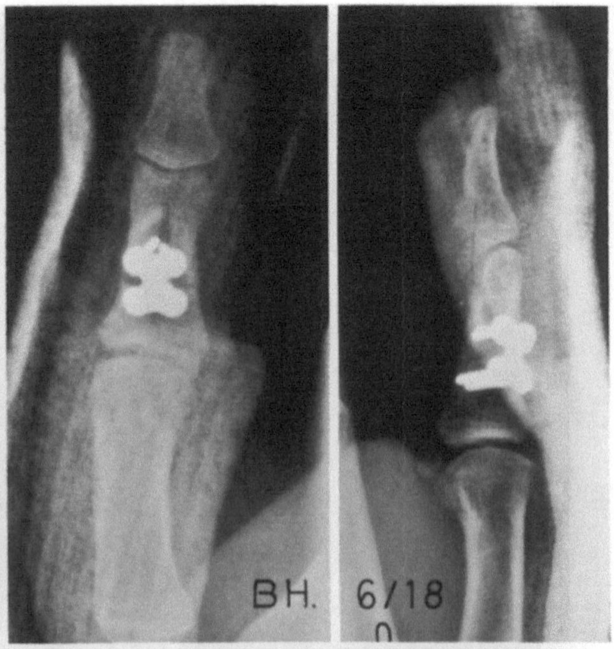

b

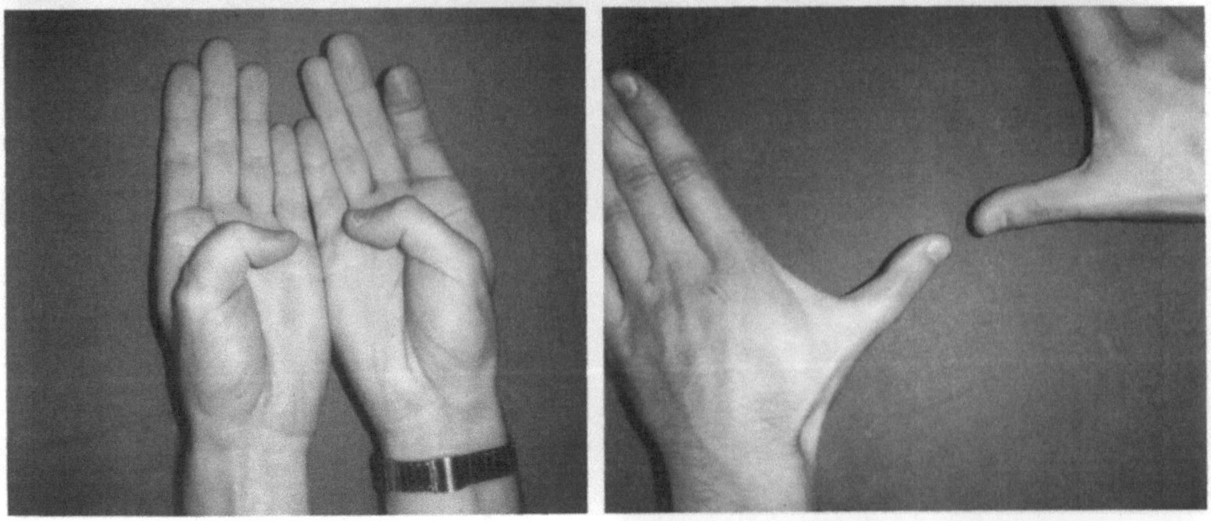

c

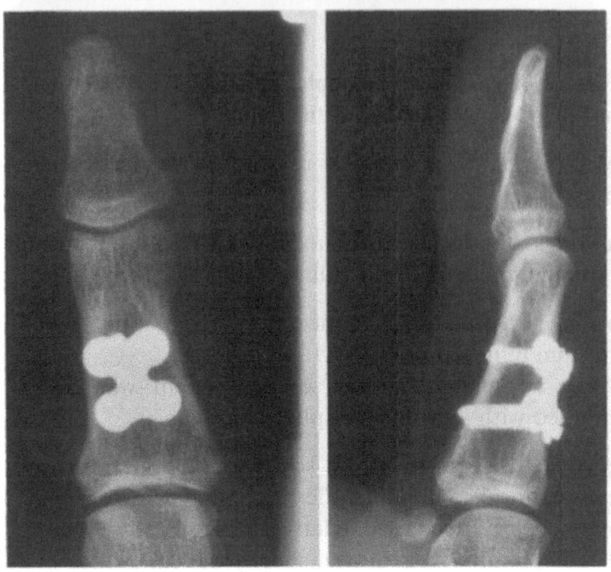

d

Fig. 130 a–d. Clinical example: Complex thumb injury. Mini H plate and primary extensor tendon plasty

Peter M., 23-year-old radio technician, caught left thumb in elevator doors on 10/25/83

a Complex open fracture of the proximal phalanx. Broad cutaneous wound and extensor tendon defect

b Emergency internal fixation: Mini H plate through the existing wound, tendon plasty, skin closure. Removable plaster splint. Active exercises without physiotherapy or ergotherapy. Patient returned to work at 4 weeks

c Function films at 12 months with implant in place

d Radiographs at 12 months. Later implant removal desired by the patient

Fig. 131 a–c. Clinical example: arthrodesis of the first carpometacarpal joint

Elisabeth A., 39-year-old laundry worker, fell on the hand sustaining a Bennett's fracture, which was treated conservatively in plaster

a Patient was referred to us 18 months later with a painful nonunion

b The carpometacarpal joint was arthrodesed by resecting the joint surfaces and applying a reversed T plate over a bridge graft
Postoperative course was uneventful, and no external fixation was applied. Consolidation of the arthrodesis and full rehabilitation were achieved by 3 months

c Final follow-up was at 8 months, and the implants were removed. Patient had mild complaints. The arthrodesis was solid, and the peripheral joints had complete function

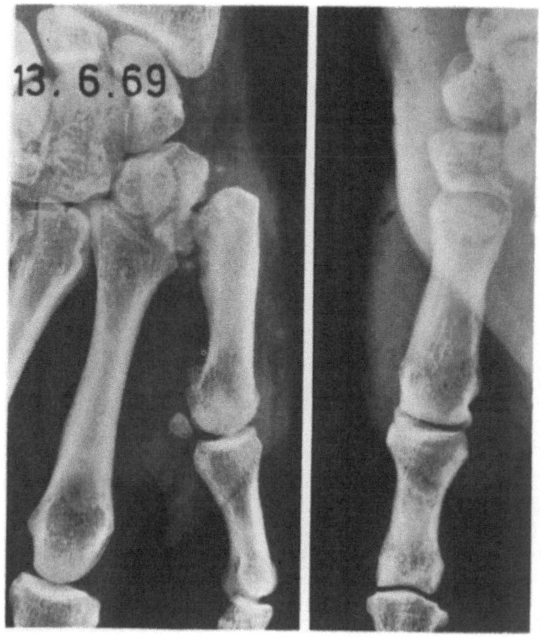

a

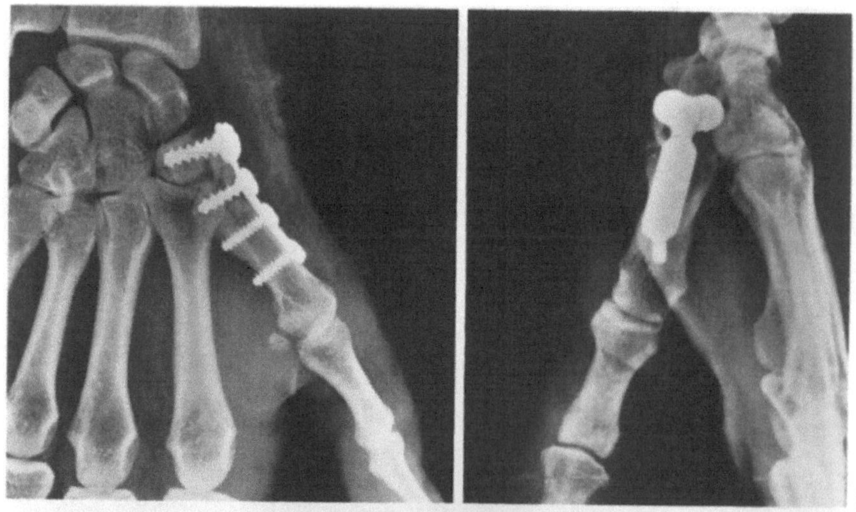

b

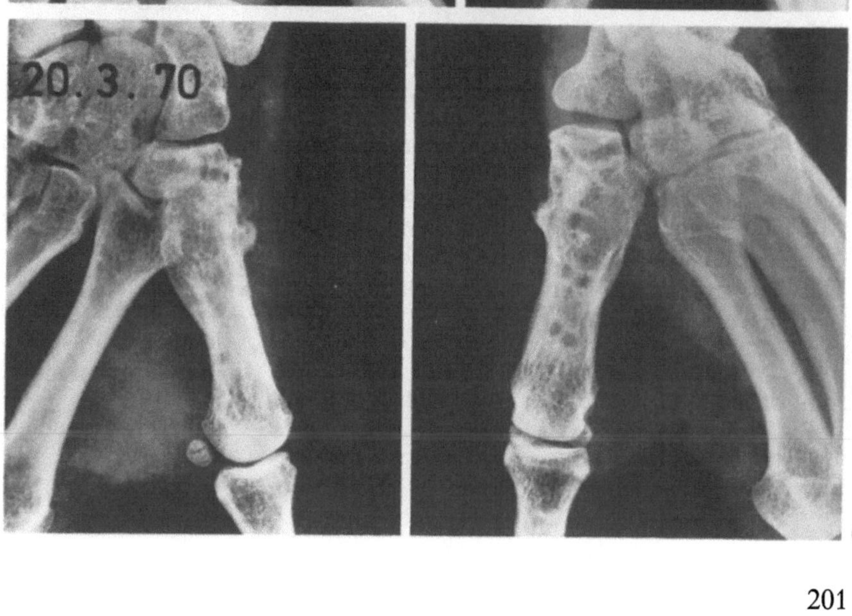

c

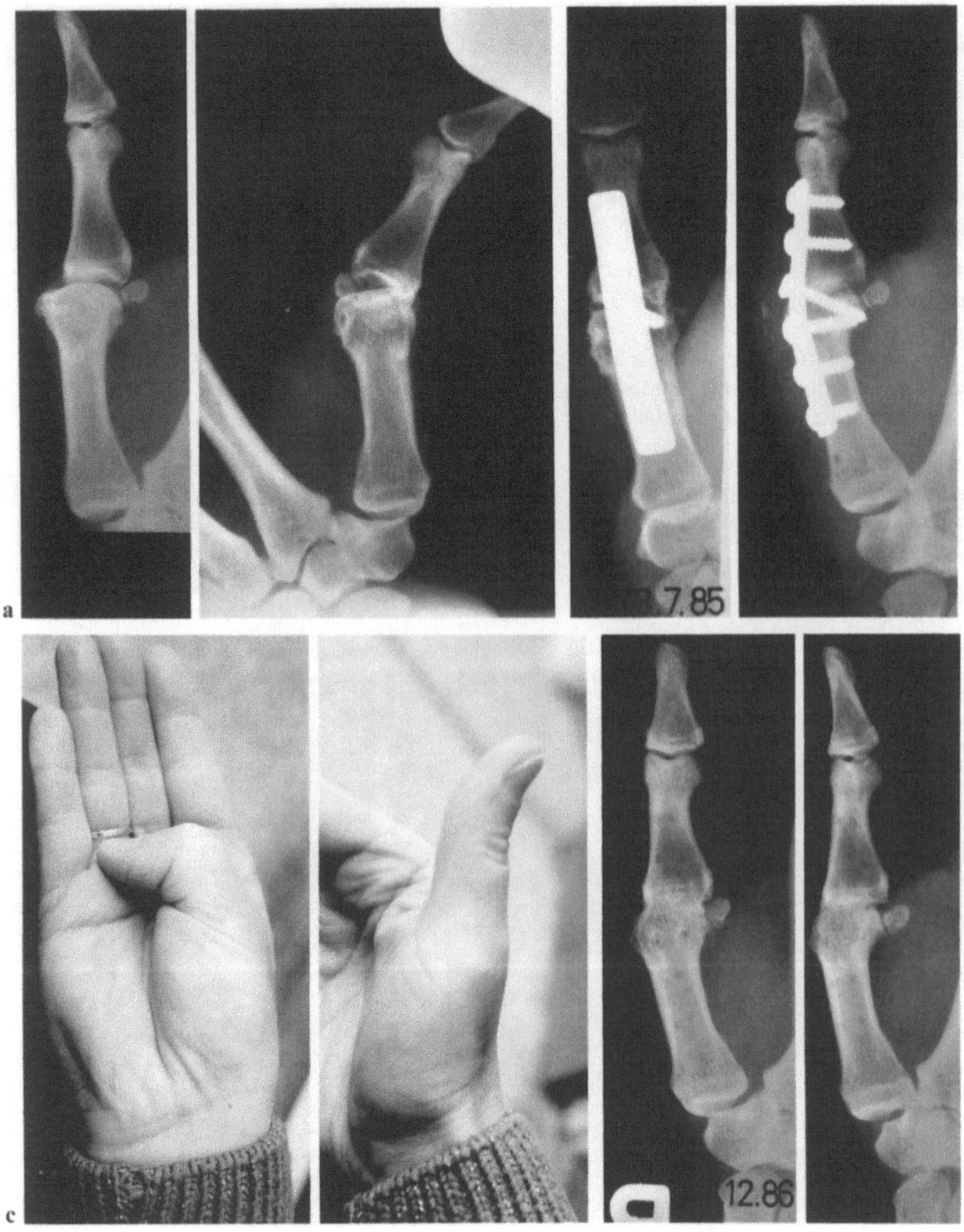

Fig. 132a–d. Clinical example: plate arthrodesis of the metacarpophalangeal joint of the thumb

Katharina K., 40-year-old housewife, sprained the MP joint of the right thumb in a bicycle accident 25 years previously. She had a long history of instability and experienced increasing complaints during part-time restaurant work

a X-ray showed marked osteoarthritis of the MP joint of the right thumb with volar subluxation and gross ulnar instability

b Arthrodesis was performed with a quarter tubular plate on 7/22/85. Motion was started early without a splint

c At 6 weeks patient had full mobility of neighboring joints and was able to lift weight. Implants were removed at 7 months

d Follow-up radiograph at 1 1/2 years

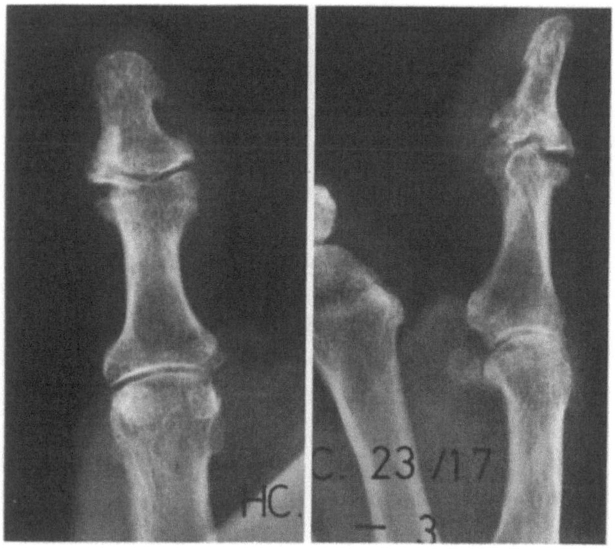

a

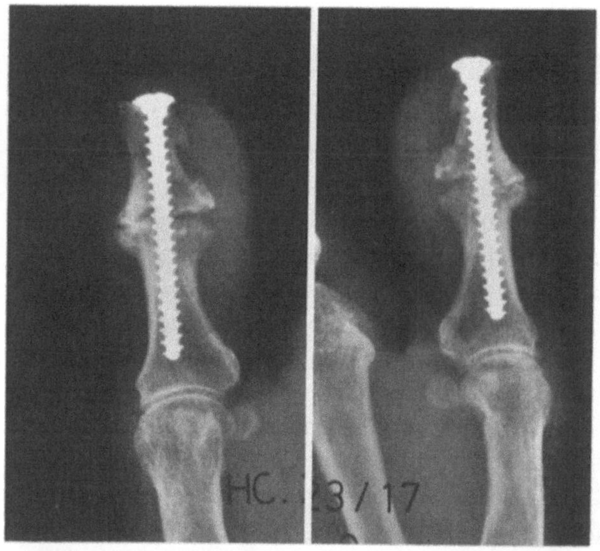

b

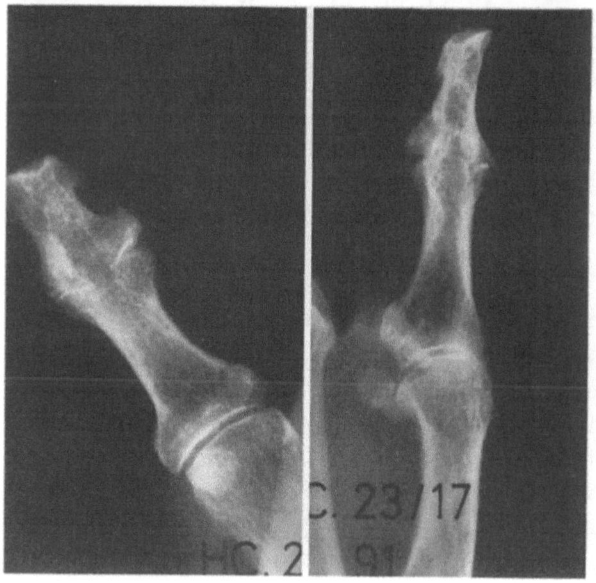

c

Fig. 133a–c. Clinical example: screw arthrodesis of the interphalangeal joint of the thumb

Klara M., 67-year-old housewife

a Painful traumatic arthritis of the IP joint of the left thumb 1 year after an intra-articular fracture

b Classic retrograde arthrodesis with a 3.5-mm screw was done on 12/18/74. Immediate motion and weight lifting were commenced. Implant was removed at 7 months

c Follow-up at 1 3/4 years showed a solid arthrodesis with a linear scar. The thumb tip was not painful

C. Injuries of the Second through Fifth Rays

The second through fifth rays of the hand, called also the volar rays, comprise a functional unit because they form the palm proximally and emerge from it distally. The second and especially the fifth rays occupy relatively exposed positions and display some individuality.

Displaced and unstable metacarpal fractures have proved to be an excellent indication for internal fixation with small implants. Exposure is relatively simple, owing partly to the fact that the extensor tendons converge proximally and do not directly overlie the implants. This decreases the likelihood of adhesion formation. The dorsal position of the implants corresponds to the tensionband position, which enhances the stability of the system. Generally the procedure itself is not too difficult technically, and excellent end results are obtained when internal fixation is followed by appropriate functional exercises.

In phalangeal fractures, there is greater diversity of opinion concerning the need for internal fixation. One danger is that the surgical exposure will cause additional trauma to the soft tissues. This particularly applies to the extensor tendons, which are prone to form adhesions with the underlying bone. In any case, postoperative exercises do not always lead to the desired result. Another problem is the high technical difficulty of the surgery. Optical magnification should be used to help limit soft-tissue trauma and improve reconstructive accuracy. Careful patient selection and an appreciation of one's limits as a surgeon are called for in this type of operation.

1. Approaches

One consequence of the soft-tissue problems is that implants used on the bones of the hand can be safely applied only at designated sites. We have had the best results with the following approaches:

a) Approach to the Second and Fifth Metacarpals

The skin is opened with a longitudinal dorsolateral incision that is angled at its proximal and/or distal ends. Fine nerve fibers are carefully identified and retracted. The periosteum is incised longitudinally with a scalpel a safe distance from the extensor apparatus and is carefully elevated for the length of the proposed implant. The extensor apparatus is retracted in its intact peritenon. The plate is attached dorsally. Best cosmetic results are obtained by placing the incisions between the second and third or between the fourth and fifth metacarpals, rather than on the borders of the hand.

b) Approach to the Third and Fourth Metacarpals

Longitudinal incisions have proved suitable for the central metacarpals and also for the fixation of multiple metacarpal bones. Usually the incisions are placed between the rays and may be extended proximally and/or distally in Y fashion (Fig. 134a). In this way it is possible to extend the exposure to a phalanx without crossing an interdigital fold. We find that the incision gives excellent exposure of two or even three metacarpals. We no longer use transverse incisions.

It is important to preserve the small dorsal nerves of the hand and especially the dorsal veins, which provide for almost all the venous return from the hand periphery. If transverse connections have to be divided, this should be done between fine ligatures; unipolar electrocoagulation leads to indeterminite necrosis. The extensor apparatus is carefully retracted to the side, sparing the peritenon. Rarely, a transverse slip between distal portions of the tendons (intertendinous connection, Fig. 134b) will have to be divided; it is reapproximated with sutures at the end of the procedure.

c) Periosteum and Interosseous Muscles

The periosteum is incised longitudinally only to the extent necessary to accommodate the implant and is held aside with a small periosteal elevator. This allows for minimal, less traumatizing stripping of the interossei. Reduction and provisional fixation are accomplished with small, atraumatic forceps. Finally the periosteum is reapproximated over the implant with a continuous row of fine, atraumatic sutures (Fig. 134c). This is easily done in secondary operations where the periosteum is thickened but usually can be done only partially in primary operations where the periosteum may be thin and torn. The periosteal suture can also reapproximate the interosseous muscles to their origins. It may be helpful to anchor some of the sutures to the implant itself.

d) Approach to the Metacarpal Heads (Fig. 136)

Special approaches are utilized for articular and subcapital fractures.

For the second and fifth metacarpals, the skin incision is extended past the joint and is angled at the end.

A Y-shaped interdigital extension of the incision, preserving the web, is very good for exposing two adjacent metacarpal heads.

For subcapital fractures, it may be necessary to notch the side of the extensor hood slightly. This is repaired with sutures at the end of the operation.

e) Opening the Metacarpophalangeal (MP) Joint (Fig. 136 b)

The skin is opened with a slightly curved, longitudinal paramedian incision, and the underlying MP joint capsule is dissected free and opened separately.It is closed separately with a fine continuous suture row at the end of the procedure. We use the same technique to close the extensor tendon as a second layer. Because this largely compensates for the lateral tension on the suture in flexion, functional exercises may be started right away.

f) Approaches to the Proximal and Middle Phalanges

We generally use long, dorsolateral skin incisions angled at the ends for operations on the fingers (Fig. 137). The incision should be long enough to avoid skin injury by instrument tension and pressure. The dorsal subcutaneous venous plexus is disturbed as little as possible. The volar neurovascular bundle is protected by maintaining its attachment to the volar skin flap. This basic incision gives access for various approaches to the bone, the choice of which depends on the type and location of the fracture:

- A longitudinal dorsal incision through the extensor tendon exposes the proximal one-fourth of the proximal phalanx. The approach is identical to that for the MP joint (Fig. 138a).
- Lateral approach to the distal part of the proximal phalanx (Fig. 138 b). The interosseous and lumbricalis lateral slips are mobilized and gently elevated; this may require division of the transverse retinacular ligament. The periosteum is directly incised and sparingly reflected dorsally. The yellowish gliding layer underlying the tendinous expansion is spared.
- Laterovolar approach for exposing certain fragments in the distal part of the proximal phalanx (Fig. 138c). The flexor tendon sheath is incised with the finger flexed, preserving the annular ligaments. The incised tendon sheath is repaired later if at all possible. Functional exercises are emphasized to avoid postoperative adhesions.

g) Approach to the Proximal Interphalangeal (PIP) Joint

Exposure of this joint or its fragments is often necessary for reduction of the articular surfaces, but it must not cause devascularization.

The following approaches may be used:

- Dorsal: by incising the central slip longitudinally to its insertion on the base of the middle phalanx (Fig. 138a).
- Dorsolateral: between the extensor tendon lateral slip and collateral ligament, with elevation of the lateral slip. The transverse retinacular ligament need to be divided, but often it cannot be separately identified in the traumatized area (Fig. 138c).

- Laterovolar: The collateral ligament is divided at its proximal insertion, and the joint is opened widely to expose both articular surfaces and the volar plate. At the end of the procedure the ligament is repaired with a direct or transosseous suture (Fig. 138d,e); absorbable material may be used for this if desired. The incised joint capsule is closed with very fine sutures.

h) Approach to the Distal Interphalangeal (DIP) Joint and the Interphalangeal (IP) Joint of the Thumb

The DIP joint is approached dorsally through a Y- or H-shaped incision (Fig. 137). Flap necrosis is not a problem with this incision owing to the excellent blood supply, and the cosmetic result is optimum. An oblique volarward extension may be made at the proximal or distal end of the incision.

The joint is opened by dividing the extensor aponeurosis transversely or in Z fashion. The aponeurosis is repaired at the end of the operation. Division of the collateral ligament is necessary for arthrodeses, and sometimes it can replace tenotomy in internal fixations.

The approach to the IP joint of the thumb is identical.

2. Fractures of the Second through Fifth Metacarpals

a) Basal Fractures

These injuries are seen with increasing frequency as a result of vehicular accidents, and they are especially common in motorcyclists. Some are multiple, and many are accompanied by dislocation. Injuries of this type can be difficult to appreciate on oblique radiographs.

Transverse and oblique fractures of the base of the fifth metacarpal are the most common. Given the unique position of the fifth ray, these fractures tend to be very unstable. Good results have been obtained by open reduction and internal fixation with the reversed T plate or mini condylar plate (Figs 135, 139). The rare avulsion fracture of the insertion of the extensor carpi radialis longus at the base of the second metacarpal can be fixed with a tension-band wire or screw.

Fracture-dislocations with small fragments are stabilized most effectively by closed reduction and percutaneous pinning to the adjacent, intact metacarpal and by temporary carpometacarpal arthrodesis. The open reduction of small comminuted fragments is extremely difficult because of the overlying insertion of the extensor carpi ulnaris tendon. Postoperative external immobilization is unavoidable in these cases.

b) Shaft Fractures

With a displaced spiral or oblique metacarpal shaft fracture, it is often impossible to correct shortening and maintain rotational alignment by conservative methods alone. Flexion deformity and shortening are considered relative indications for operative treatment, and rotational deformity is an absolute indication. When there is a long fracture line in a central metacarpal, screw fixation alone may be adequate depending on the strength of the hand and the cooperativeness of the patient. Increasingly, however, we prefer to reinforce the fixation with a neutralization plate, which will protect against bending and shear forces during mobilization. We always plate the second and fifth metacarpals, which are more exposed to uncontrolled external forces (Fig. 139).

In multiple fractures, the fixation should conform to the morphology of the individual lesions and to the presumptive stresses to which the lesions will be exposed after surgery (Fig. 41).

c) Subcapital Fractures

These fractures are especially common in the fifth metacarpal. Volar angulation and impaction of the neck are characteristic features. Many of these fractures are stable, and small marginal fragments and comminution are sometimes present. As a rule, fractures with minimal angulation may be treated conservatively with functional exercises.

A true lateral radiograph is needed to establish the degree of angulation; standard oblique views can be misleading. When significant flexion deformity exists, we realign the head by applying pressure between the shaft and flexed finger and secure it in correct rotational alignment with a percutaneous, transarticular medullary wire inserted from the distal side (Fig. 140). This simple procedure may be done under local anesthesia and does not require an image intensifier or power drill. Postoperatively the MP joint is held in flexion with a well-padded plaster splint applied over the projecting, bent end of the Kirschner wire. The wire is removed at three weeks. Because extraction of the wire creates a suction that may introduce microorganisms into the medullary cavity, the surrounding skin should be aseptically prepared before the wire is removed. Exercises are started right away.

The same technique is recommended for angulated subcapital fractures of the remaining metacarpals. Open reduction is mandatory, for, unlike the fifth metacarpal, the angulation cannot be compensated by extension at the carpometacarpal joint, and protrusion of the head into the palm causes pain when an object is grasped.

We have practically abandoned the internal plating of metacarpal neck fractures, although we still occasionally use a figure-of-eight tension band.

The impacted subcapital fracture–roughly comparable to an abduction fracture of the neck of the femur–should not be confused with a spiral or oblique fracture of the distal shaft of the fifth metacarpal. The latter is a common and unusually mobile fracture that results from "catching" of the little finger or from direct violence. We fix these fractures with an interfragmental screw combined with an L- or T-shaped neutralization plate or condylar plate (Fig. 131 a).

3. Articular Fractures

a) Fractures of the Metacarpophalangeal (MP) Joint

Intra-articular fractures of the metacarpal heads are usually open fractures with associated tendon lesions. The need for internal fixation is generally acknowledged, screw fixation being the preferred technique. Aftertreatment is geared toward the exigencies of soft-tissue healing (Fig. 139).

Displaced fractures of the base of the proximal phalanx are an indication for open reduction and internal fixation. Small cancellous bone grafts may be needed when there is depression of the articular surface. If screw fixation is inadequate, it should be supplemented with Kirschner wires. Postoperative mobilization may be deferred if stability is questionable.

Double fractures involving the base of a proximal phalanx and the head of the opposing metacarpal are usually the result of compressive trauma. Most are heavily fragmented but can be acceptably reduced by traction. Internal fixation is not advised if it cannot guarantee the stability necessary for early function. The best technique in such cases is to apply distraction with a transarticular external frame (the small external fixator).

In selected cases, an irreducible fracture of the MP joint may justify the primary insertion of a Swanson silastic prosthesis. This device is preferable to an arthrodesis.

b) Fractures of the Proximal Interphalangeal (PIP) Joint

Typical fractures of the PIP joint are:

Condylar fractures of the proximal phalanx are a classic indication for operative treatment. Devascularization must be avoided when the fracture is exposed. Internal fixation may be obtained with a simple screw, possibly combined with Kirschner wires, or with the mini condylar plate for 1.5-mm screws.

Dorsal dislocation fractures with avulsion of a volar fragment from the base of the middle phalanx. If the fragment is large, internal fixation with a screw is indicated. If possible the screw is inserted dorsally, from the area of attachment of the extensor tendon (Fig. 143 a). Small impacted areas are managed with a mini screw and washer inserted from the volar side.

If a marginal avulsion is not present and there is no tendency for the middle phalanx to displace dorsally, treatment may consist of brief immobilization followed by functional exercises. Scarring may lead to flexion contracture even after a period of months, and this must be countered by the use of dynamic extension splints–necessitating a corresponding period of management and follow-up.

With a true "pilon fracture" in which the dorsal rim of the middle phalanx remains intact, good results are obtained with the Agee dynamic splint: Two parallel Kirschner wires are drilled through the head of the first phalanx and base of the second phalanx and are used to construct a rocker mechanism that is linked distally by rubber band to a 2.0-mm screw driven percutaneously into the middle phalanx.

Flexion of the PIP joint tends to move the middle phalanx volarward, enabling exercises to be performed right away (Fig. 143b). Lateral radiographs must confirm, however, that the joint does not dislocate with extension of the digit. If this proves to be the case, the injury is not amenable to dynamic treatment, and the joint should be temporarily arthrodesed in slight flexion with a diagonal Kirschner wire.

Compression fractures of the base of the second phalanx with angular abduction deformity may necessitate open reduction and screw fixation.

c) Fractures of the Distal Interphalangeal (DIP) Joint and Interphalangeal Joint of the Thumb

Condylar fractures, avulsion fractures of the extensor tendon insertion or long flexor tendon insertion, and impacted fractures can all occur in the area of the DIP joint. Operative treatment is necessary for subluxated fractures with large dorsal fragments and for volar avulsion fractures (Fig. 144a).Various options have been presented for dorsal avulsion fractures: reattachment with a transfixing pull-out wire, a thin Kirschner wire, a small tensionband system of absorbable suture material, or a small screw.

None of these methods is sufficiently rigid, and we have seen instances of necrosis of the small fragment and of the extensor tendon insertion. We also have observed cracking of fragments during the attempt to insert a screw. As a precaution, then, we recommend that the fixation include temporary arthrodesis of the DIP joint with a thin Kirschner wire drilled obliquely across the joint (Fig. 144c, d).

d) Comminuted Articular Fractures

Comminuted PIP and DIP fractures justify arthrodesis, which should be performed secondarily if the condition of the soft tissues is poor.The basic technical options available for arthrodesis are screw fixation and tension-band wiring. When a large bony defect exists, the combination of tension-band wiring, screw fixation, and corticocancellous grafting should be considered.

In the rare cases where reconstruction of the extensor apparatus is possible and the collateral ligaments are intact, the Swanson silastic prosthesis may be implanted primarily, especially in the PIP joint. The lateral stability of this device is limited, however. Arthrodesis may eventually be necessary if the late result is poor.

4. Fractures of the Phalangeal Shafts

Operative treatment is indicated for phalangeal shaft fractures that cannot be reduced or maintained, and which are prone to secondary angular deformity or malrotation. Screw fixation is best in the proximal phalanx.Plating is rarely indicated, but it may occasionally be necessary for certain combined injuries and transverse fractures. For this reason mini plates for 1.5-mm screws have been designed and tested for use on the proximal phalanx (Fig. 139). The plate is attached to the lateral aspect of the bone.

For basal transverse fractures of the proximal phalanx and certain spiral fractures, excellent results have been obtained with a medullary wire inserted percutaneously across the MP joint (Fig. 142). Great care is taken to maintain axial alignment when the wire is introduced. The wire is inserted with a power drill under image intensifer control. Again, the bent end of the wire projecting from the skin must be shielded postoperatively with a well-padded splint. The wire is removed at three weeks.Today the the 2.0- or 1.5-mm condylar plate offers a good alternative for this type of fracture (Fig. 36).

Displaced shaft fractures of the middle phalanx are often difficult to reduce and maintain, as muscular forces tend to cause angulation. The 1.5-mm mini plate or condylar plate applied to the lateral side of the bone can be useful in this situation.

The oblique Kirschner wire or crossed Kirschner wires will probably continue to find use despite the tendency for distraction to occur. Care must be taken to avoid the concomitant fixation of neighboring joints. Excellent stability is provided by an oblique Kirschner wire combined with an intraosseous wire suture. This technique has become very popular because of its simplicity and low cost (Fig. 157).

In contrast to distal fractures of the ungual process, which can be reduced and splinted with the overlying fingernail, basal transverse fractures of the distal phalanx are often distracted and resistant to closed reduction. They are susceptible to nonunion. These fractures can be stabilized with an axial Kirschner wire introduced from the fingertip (Fig. 144d) and drilled through the DIP joint into the middle phalanx to create a temporary arthrodesis. Axial screw fixation has given good results in the treatment of nonunions (Fig. 144d).

5. Secondary Operations on the Second through Fifth Rays

a) Nonunions

Nonunions of the fifth metacarpal are more common than those of the third and fourth metacarpals.There is always volar angulation of the distal fragment, which is palpable on the palm and painful. Malrotation is also common. Following correction of the deformity, the nonunion is stabilized most effectively with a dowel graft and tension-band plate or with a compressed bridge graft. Functional recovery is rapid with early mobilization.

Nonunions of the phalanges are rare. The technique of internal fixation is the same as for the metacarpals, but smaller implants are used. Plates should be applied laterally where possible to avoid interference with the extensor apparatus.

b) Osteotomies

Osteotomies of the metacarpals or proximal phalanges are used chiefly to correct rotational deformity and occasionally to correct volar angulation and relative shortening following closed fracture therapy. The technique is similar to the operative treatment of nonunions. The functional results of osteotomy are excellent in the metacarpals but often are disappointing in the phalanges.

c) Transfer of Finger Rays

Amputations of the thumb, middle finger, or ring finger can profoundly affect the function of the entire hand. Loss of the thumb ray means a loss of opposition with the long digits, while a basal amputation of the middle or ring finger makes it impossible to hold small objects like coins or screws securely in the hand.Function can be improved dramatically in such cases by transfering the index finger to the first or third metacarpal, or the little finger to the fourth metacarpal. Internal fixation is best accomplished with a 2.7- or 2.0-mm DCP applied dorsally and an interfragmental lag screw.

d) Secondary Arthrodesis

Surgical fusion of the MP joints is avoided whenever possible because of its disabling effect on finger function.Implant arthroplasty is a possible alternative, although the standard prostheses used in rheumatoid surgery are not as successful in post-traumatic conditions because of the preexisting periarticular lesions. Nevertheless, prosthetic implants can be helpful in achieving a relatively stable, pain-free, and therefore useful level of residual function.

Arthrodeses of the PIP and DIP joints are performed with greater frequency. The proximal joint can be fixed with a screw or tension-band wire. The degree of flexion should conform to the patient's vocational demands and ranges from 20° to about 50°, increasing from the index finger to the little finger. Arthrodesis of the distal joint is generally accomplished with a screw inserted from the fingertip (Fig. 146). A position of extension or very slight flexion is most serviceable for this joint.

6. Fixation Techniques for Complex Injuries and Amputations of the Hand

For *complex injuries of the hand* involving combined bony and soft-tissue lesions or amputations, we must expand the aforementioned indications for skeletal fixation. *All* fractures in these injuries will require operative stabilization.

Conservative treatment methods no longer have a place in the management of these cases. Because the bones must provide support for the reconstructed soft tissues, bone fixation is a necessary preliminary to other restorative measures. Moreover, the extensive soft-tissue injuries create countless opportunities for adhesions to form during the healing period, resulting in impaired function.The only way to avoid this is through early active and passive mobilization of the injured hand–and this is possible only if appropriate skeletal fixation is maintained until fracture healing can occur.

The following fixation techniques are available:

Compression Plating

Compression plating is unquestionably the most stable internal fixation technique. It is relatively time-consuming, and some plates require extensive exposure of the bone. Use of the mini plates is preferred, therefore.

Indications: multiple or comminuted fractures, fractures with bone loss, intra-articular fractures

Disadvantage: implant removal is relatively difficult.

Screw Fixation

Screws provide high stability and are easily inserted in a minimum of time. Later removal is not essential.

Indications: longitudinal fractures, long oblique shaft fractures, intra-articular metaphyseal fractures, arthrodeses

Disadvantage: none

Kirschner Wires

This type of fixation is not very motion-stable, but the wires are quickly inserted and easily removed.

Indications: metaphyseal area, temporary fixations

Disadvantages: Kirschner wires usually interfere with soft structures and therefore limit movement; they are not stable enough for early mobilization.

Interfragmental Wire Suture with or without Kirschner Wire Reinforcement

This type of fixation provides excellent stability, especially when reinforced by a Kirschner wire. Subsequent removal is unnecessary (except for the Kirschner wire).

Indication: transverse shaft fractures

Disadvantage: interference with soft structures by Kirschner wire (see above).

External Skeletal Fixation

Often this is the only way to maintain apposition of fracture fragments when major soft-tissue injuries exist. This technique may be used temporarily in some instances until rigid internal fixation can be performed.

Indications: extensive soft-tissue injuries, fractures with bone loss

Disadvantages: The fracture fragments must be large enough to provide acceptable pin anchorage. Also, the external assembly is relatively uncomfortable for the patient.

Intramedullary Devices (Especially Bolts)

This type of fixation is very stable and is quickly installed.

Indication: transverse fractures

Disadvantages: Rotational alignment is difficult to establish and maintain. The intramedullary device cannot be removed and therefore precludes corrective osteotomy at a later time.It also interferes with vascularization of the bone through the medullary cavity.

Combination of Fixation Techniques

Some complex injuries of the hand require the combined application of several different skeletal fixation techniques. For example, in a shaft fracture having both a transverse and a longitudinal component, two cortex lag screws may be placed to reduce the longitudinal fracture, and then the transverse fracture may be fixed with a short plate or even an interfragmental wire suture.

The requirements of a *fixation technique for replantations* and complex injuries may be stated as follows: - Absolute stability, permitting immediate active or passive mobilization

- No interference with articular movement
- Rapid application or assembly, to avoid prolongation of operating time, which already is quite long (e.g., for replantations)
- Minimal additional bone exposure, as the blood supply is already compromised by the injury
- Implant removal (if necessary) should be possible without jeopardizing reconstructed soft structures.

Viewing these requirements in relation to the various options presented above, we must give preference whenever possible to techniques that offer the highest stability at the lowest cost in terms of technical difficulty and operating time. This would mean that simple screw fixation, where appropriate, is the most favorable option, while Kirschner wires and intramedullary devices are the least favorable.

Primary care is the goal for all injured structures. Even in the presence of bone defects, we perform bone grafting as a primary measure whenever possible. In the cases where optimum primary treatment is not possible, temporary bone fixation is carried out. The later, definitive fixation is planned at the time of primary care. As soon as the blood flow and soft-tissue status permit a second operation, the fractures are definitively stabilized.

Follow-up *radiographs* are taken at four-week intervals.With digital replantations, radiation absorption in the reimplanted bone may appear increased relative to the more proximal bones for about a three-month period. This reflects the poorer vascularity of the replanted bone and will disappear with passage of time.

One should be particularly alert for *signs of instability*. At the first sign of instability, the internal fixation should be revised, or the external load on the bone should be decreased. Usually this can be done only by immobilizing the extremity and accepting the attendant losses of function.

The techniques are illustrated by the case shown in Fig. 130.

Summary

Whereas conservative or operative fracture treatment may be appropriate for isolated fractures of the hand, stable operative fixation is essential for replantations and complex injuries. In selecting the technique that is optimum for a particular case, the surgeon must have a familiarity with and mastery of the various techniques of skeletal fixation that are available.

7. Illustrative Case Reports and X-Rays
(Figs. 147–167)

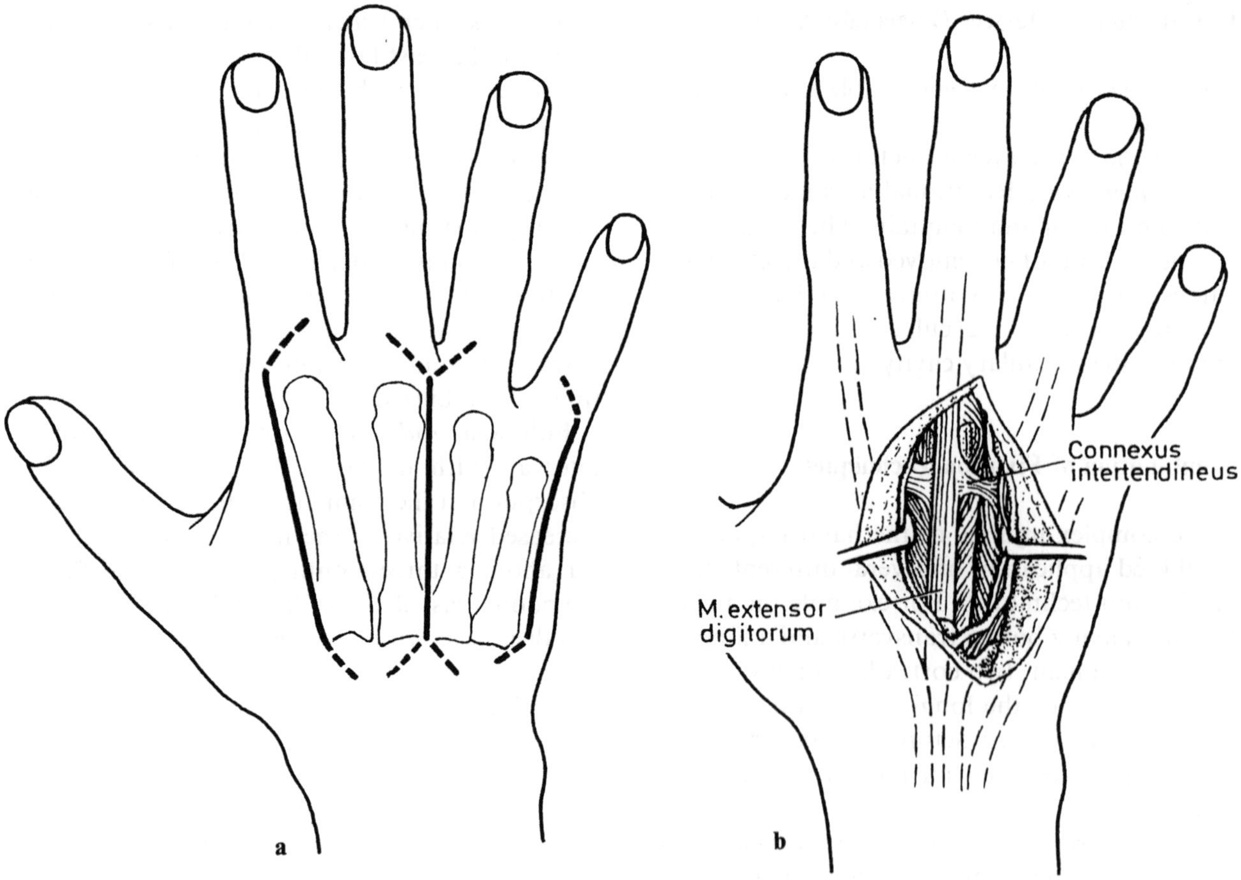

a

b

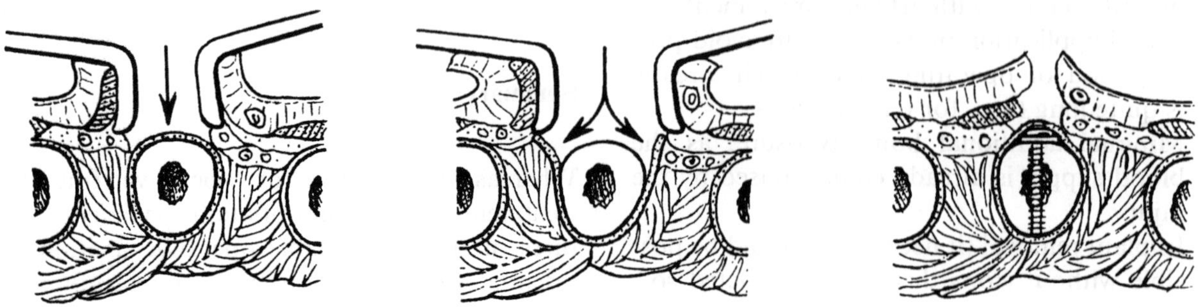

c

Fig. 134a–c. Approaches to the metacarpus

a Interosseous longitudinal incisions with angled or Y-shaped extensions

b Topography of the superficial layers, with veins and nerve fibers retracted. The extensor tendons form a proximal bundle in the retinaculum, and most do not run coaxially with the metacarpals

c Enlarged cross-section: The periosteum is incised longitudinally and sparingly reflected to expose the fracture. The implant is applied beneath the periosteum. The periosteal suture over the implant reapproximates the partially stripped interossei muscles and prevents adhesions with the overlying extensor tendons

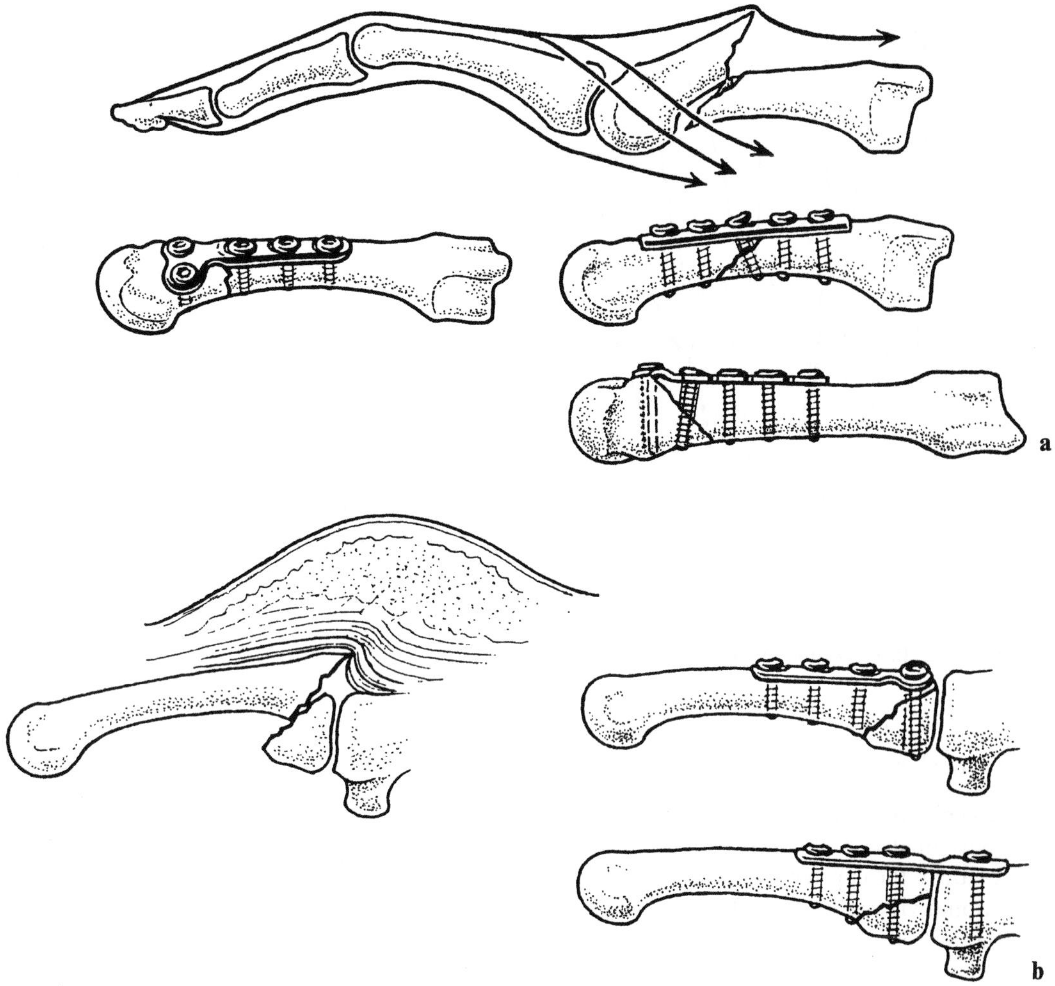

Fig. 135a–c. Implants for the stabilization of metacarpal fractures

a Spontaneous deformity after shaft fracture: volar angulation and shortening by the dominant pull of the flexors and intrinsic muscles. Implants for various fracture types: dorsal T plate for distal transverse fracture; quarter tubular plate with interfragmental lag screw for oblique shaft fracture; lateral mini condylar plate for oblique fracture close to the joint

b Basal fracture-dislocation: Displacement is masked by swelling. Perforation of the extensor bundle is a danger.Injury is fixed with a small T or L plate, which may be placed across the carpometacarpal joint

c Unstable fracture of the base of the fifth metacarpal with angulation and medial rotation; fixed with a dorsal T plate or mini condylar plate

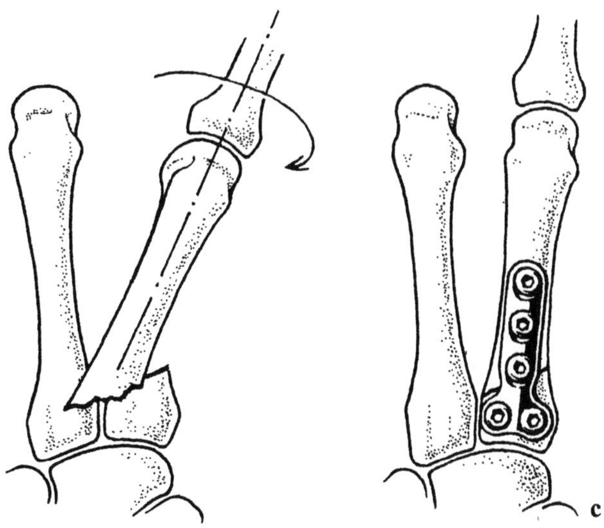

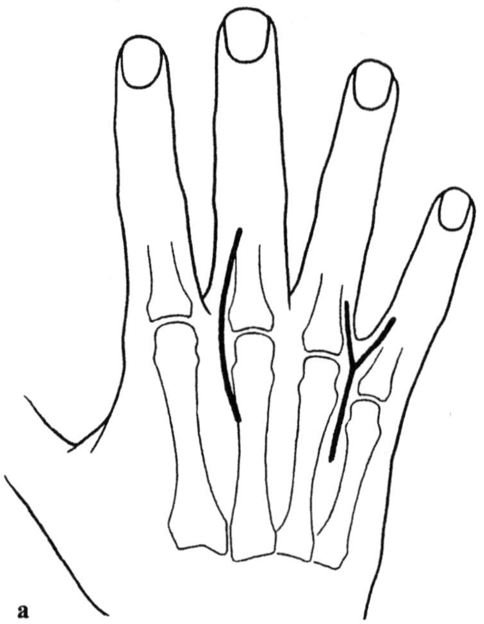

a

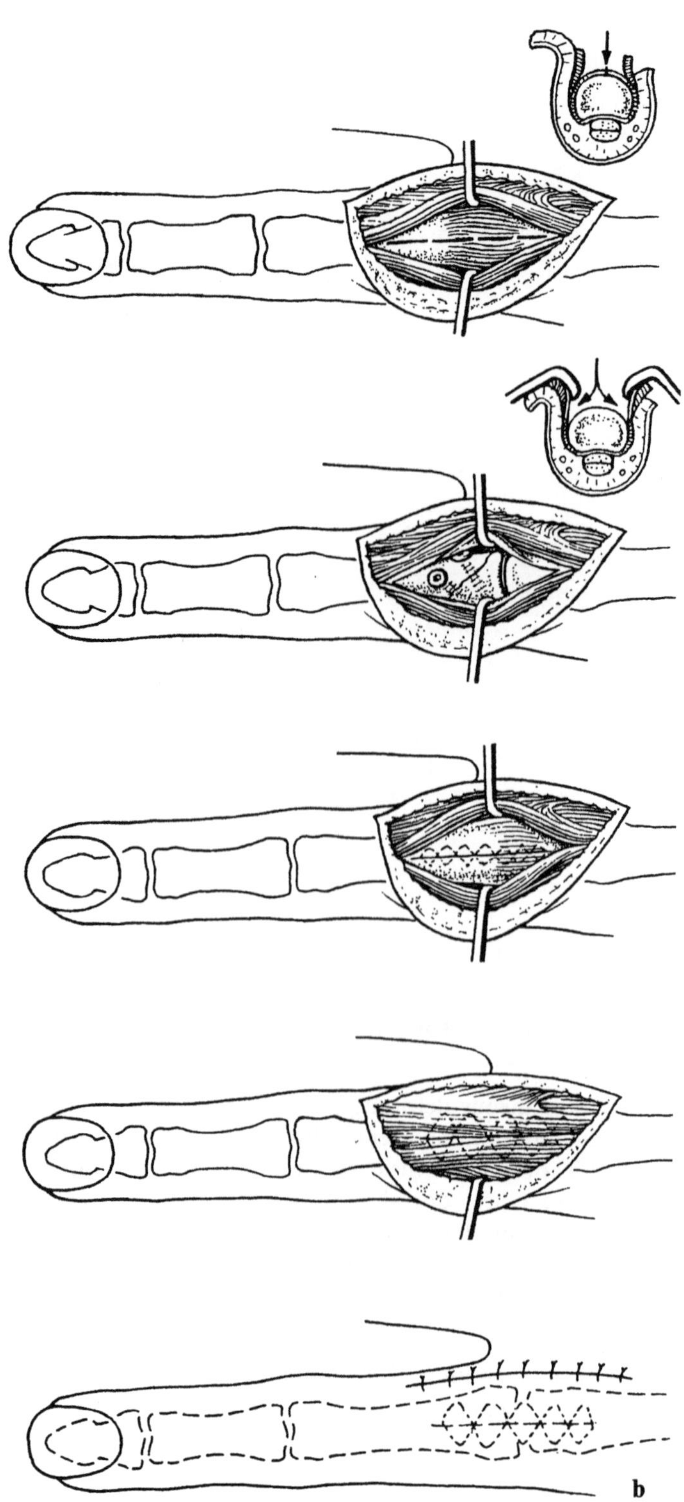

b

Fig. 136a, b. Exposure of the MP joints

a Skin incisions: curved, dorsolateral incision for exposing one MP joint, intermetacarpal incision with Y-shaped extension for exposing two joints

b Deep layers: The extensor aponeurosis is incised longitudinally, and a separate longitudinal incision is made in the capsule and periosteum (top and cross-sectional views). On completion of the fixation, both structures are closed separately with fine atraumatic sutures. We prefer a loose, double row of continuous sutures placed in shoelace fashion. The skin is closed with fine interrupted sutures

Fig. 137 a, b. Exposure of the phalanges (skin incisions)

a DIP joint is approached through a dorsal S-, H- or Y-shaped skin incision. A lateral Y-shaped incision is used for a volar approach

b Dorsolateral skin incision for the proximal phalanges and PIP joint, with simplified topography of the extensor apparatus

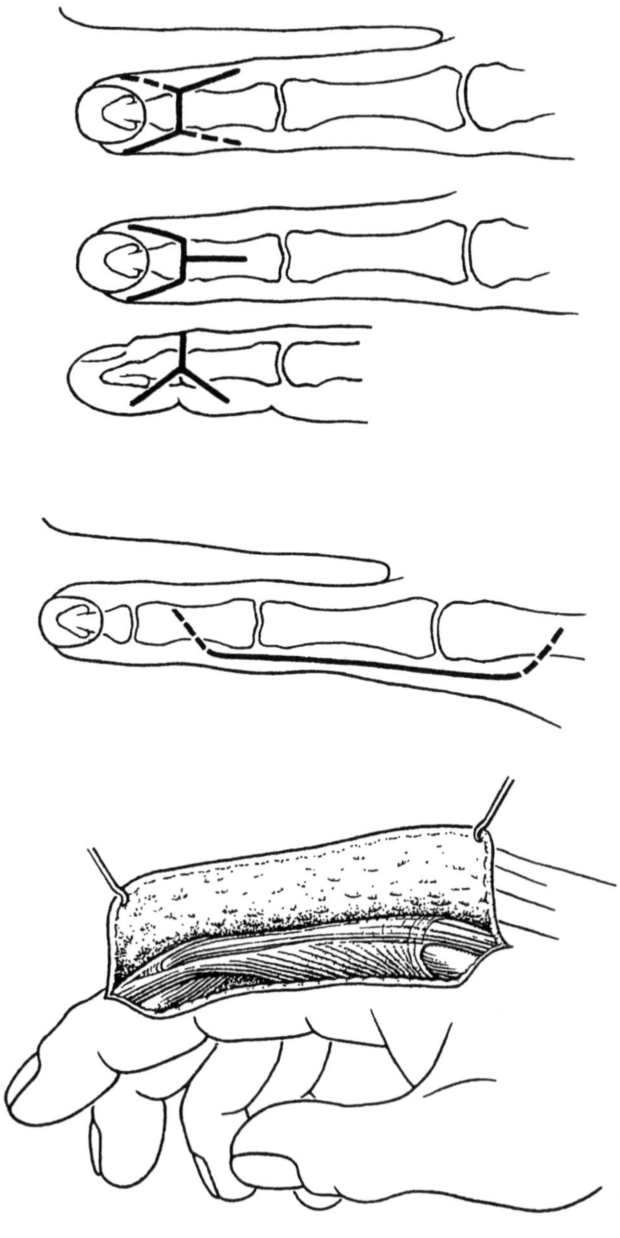

a

b

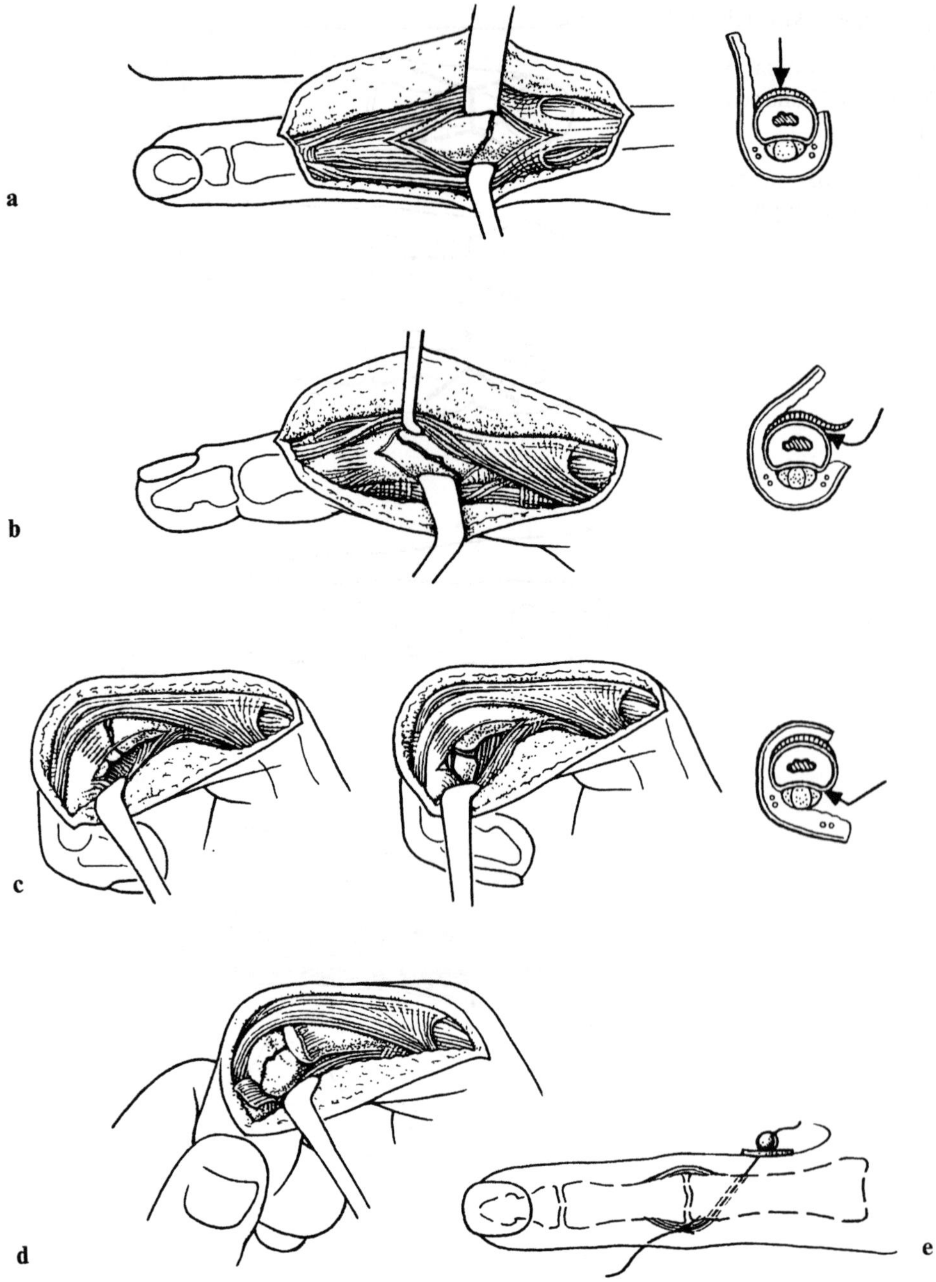

Fig. 138 a–e. Exposure of the phalanges (deep layer)

a Dorsal incision of the extensor aponeurosis – a distal extension of the approach to the MP joint

b Elevation of the interosseus aponeurosis for lateral exposure of the distal shaft of the proximal phalanx

c Approach to the distal metaphysis of the proximal phalanx and PIP joint with the finger flexed

d The base of the middle phalanx is widely exposed by dividing the collateral ligament and notching the volar plate

e The collateral ligament is reattached at the end of the procedure using a pull-out wire passed through an oblique drill hole in the bone

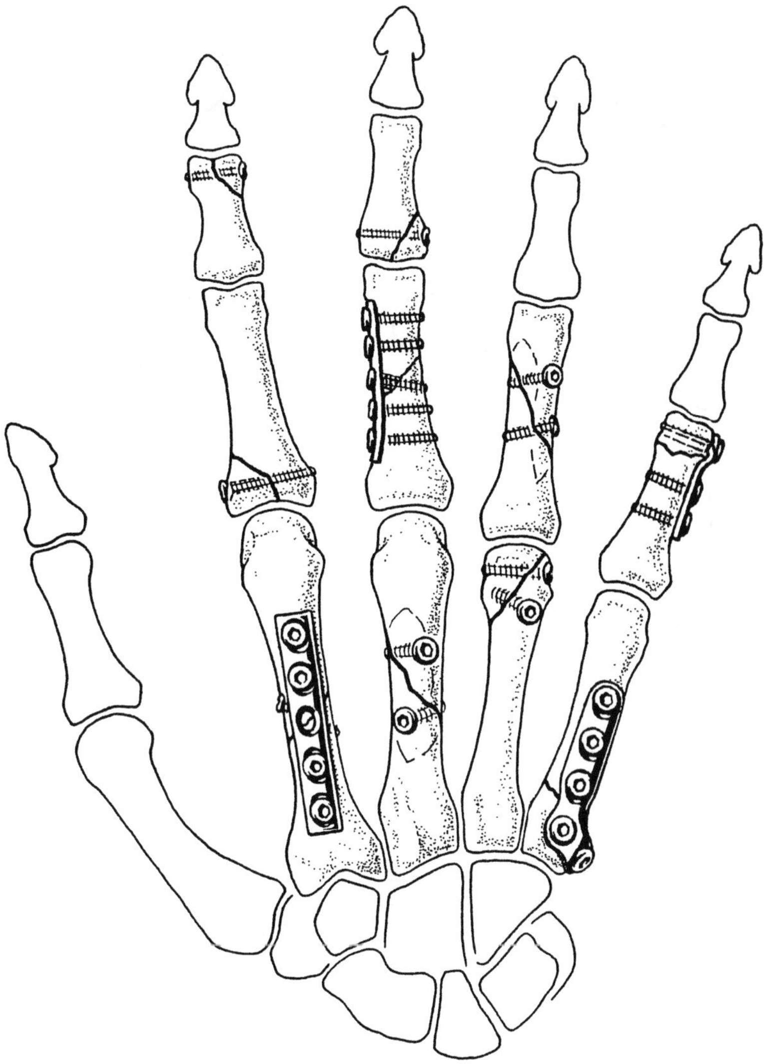

Fig. 139. Typical internal fixations of the metacarpals and phalanges

Fractures of the second and fifth metacarpals are fixed with a plate. Spiral fractures of the third and fourth metacarpals can be fixed with screws
Numerous types of phalangeal fracture are stabilized with small screws (2.0- or 1.5-mm). A subcapital fracture is fixed with a shortened mini condylar plate, and a short oblique fracture of the first phalanx is fixed with a straight mini plate applied laterally

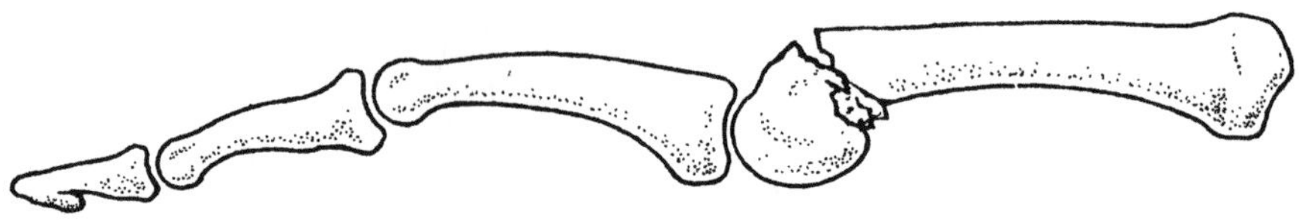

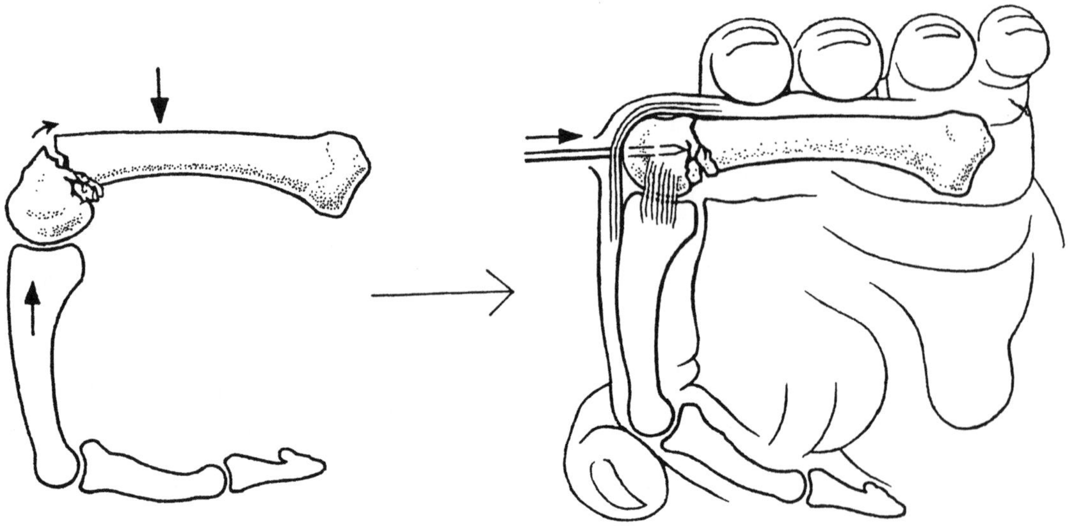

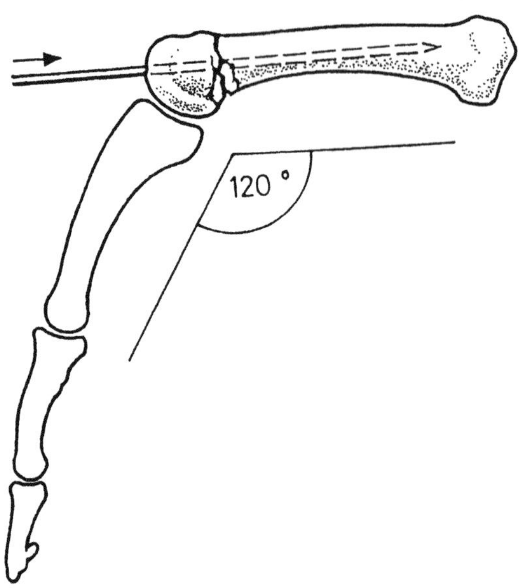

Fig. 140. Percutaneous medullary wire fixation of a subcapital metacarpal fracture

The metacarpal head is reduced and realigned under local anesthesia by exerting pressure between the metacarpus and flexed PIP joint. A 1.6-mm Kirschner wire is twisted into the medullary cavity of the metacarpal head with a hand chuck (not a power drill). The end is bent over, and a padded dorsal plaster splint is applied that also immobilizes an adjacent finger; the splint is worn for 3 weeks

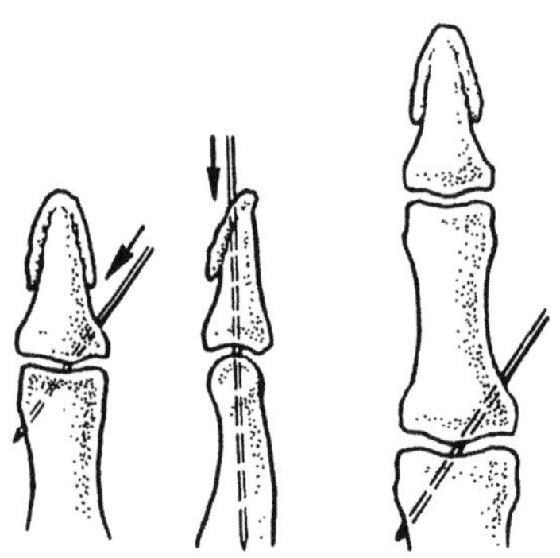

Fig. 141. Temporary arthrodeses of interphalangeal joints with a Kirschner wire

We prefer to drill the wire obliquely into the flared cancellous metaphyses

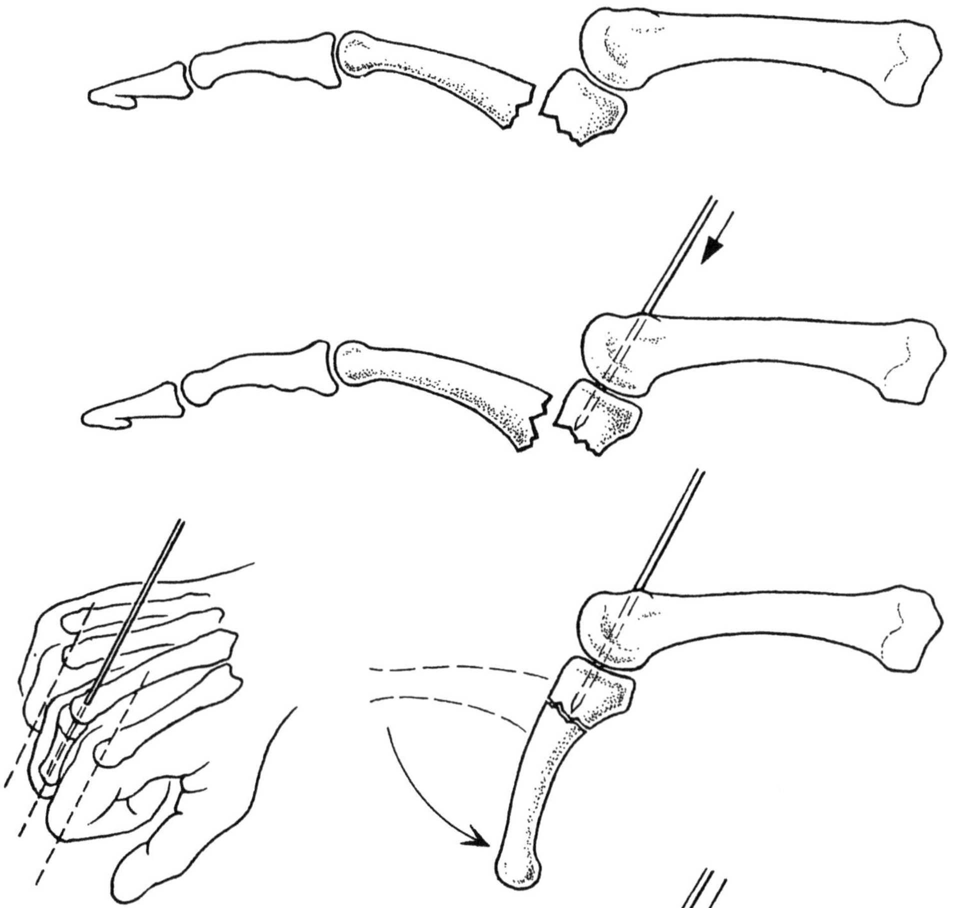

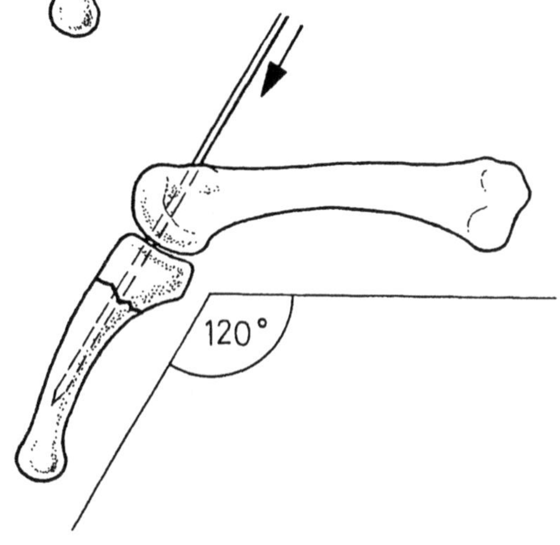

Fig. 142. Percutaneous medullary wire fixation of a basal fracture of the proximal phalanx

Typical angulation. A 1.6-mm Kirschner wire is drilled into the metacarpal head from the dorsal side at about a 60° angle. Axial alignment is checked in relation to the neighboring digits. The Kirschner wire is first drilled across the joint into the proximal fragment, the fragment is reduced by flexion, and the wire is drilled into the medullary cavity of the distal fragment.Alignment is checked, and the end of the wire is bent and clamped. A padded plaster splint is applied that immobilizes the operated finger and one adjacent finger; it is worn for 3 weeks

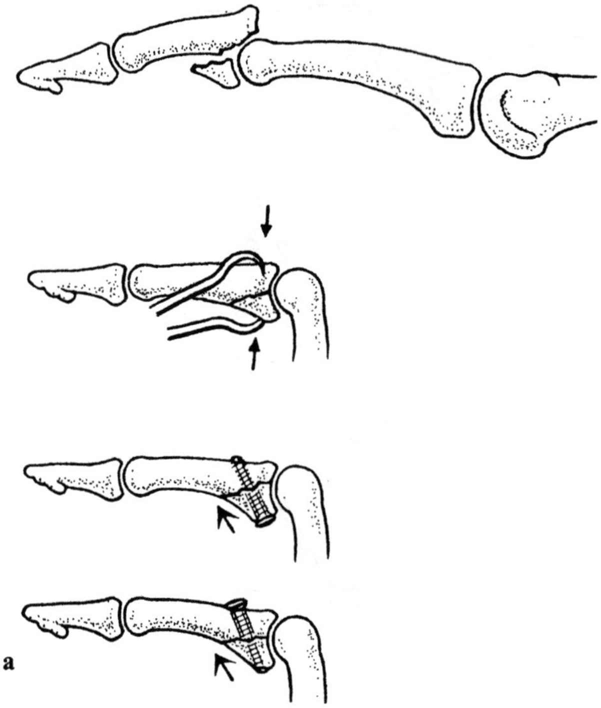

a

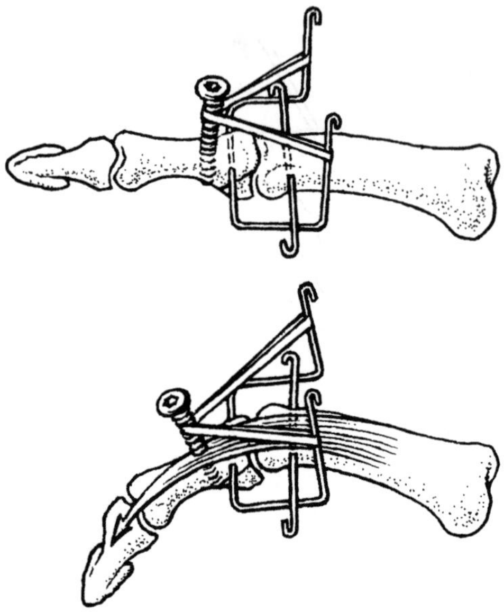

b

Fig. 143a, b. Stabilization of a fracture-dislocation of the middle phalanx (volar lip fracture)

a The displaced fracture is reduced and held in position with a small forceps. It is fixed with a screw inserted from the dorsal (middle slip) or volar side

b Agee's dynamic fixation technique: A transverse Kirschner wire through the base of the second phalanx is bent to form a frame that rotates about a second wire in the neck of the first phalanx. A rubber band connects the frame to a screw driven percutaneously into the second phalanx. The elastic tension keeps the joint reduced through the lever action of the frame and allows exercises to be performed. The function of the assembly must be checked on a lateral radiograph

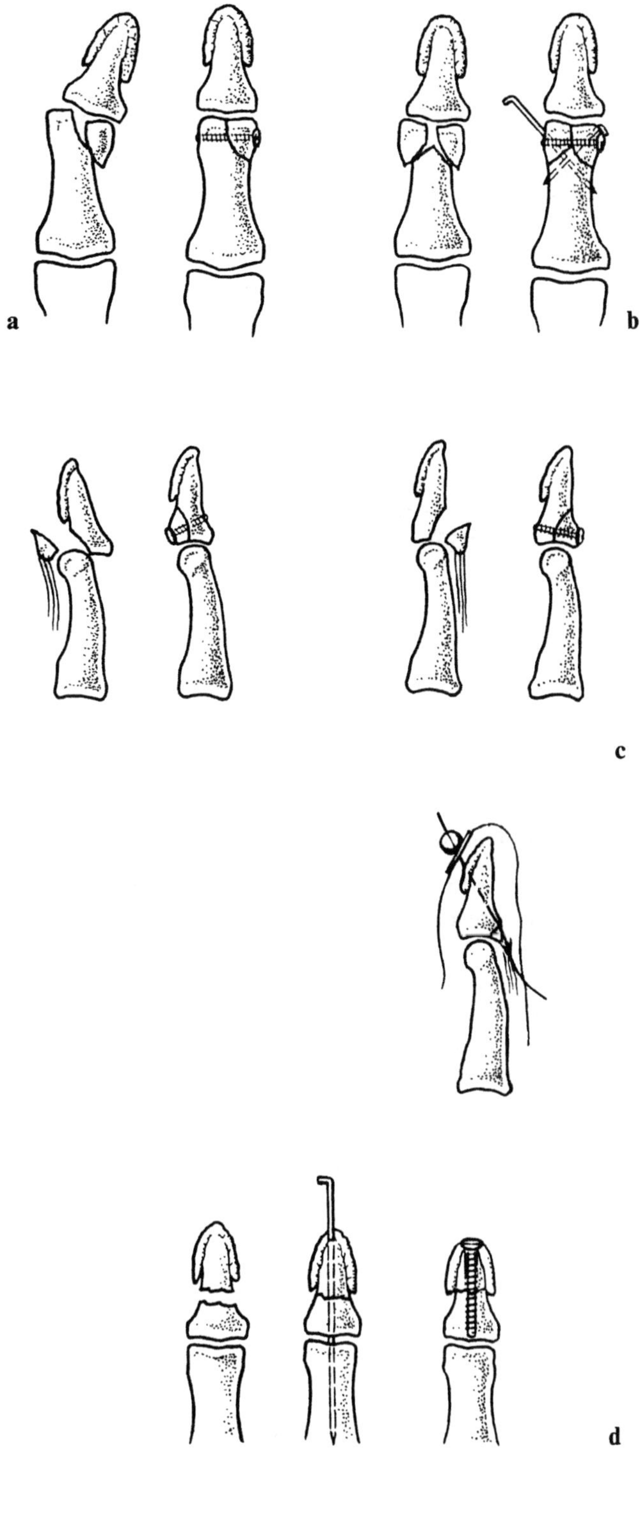

Fig. 144a–d. Internal fixations about the DIP joint and distal phalanx

a Screw fixation of a monocondylar fracture

b Bicondylar fracture managed by screw fixation combined with open or percutaneous pinning with a Kirschner wire. Alternative: mini condylar plate for 1.5-mm screws

c Screw fixation of a flexor or extensor tendon avulsion at the base of the distal phalanx.For a small dorsal fragment, we prefer transosseous pull-out wire fixation or a small tension-band wire

d Stabilization of a displaced transverse fracture of the distal phalanx with an axial Kirschner wire that temporarily immobilizes the DIP joint. Alternative: distal screw insertion, given a sufficiently large proximal fragment

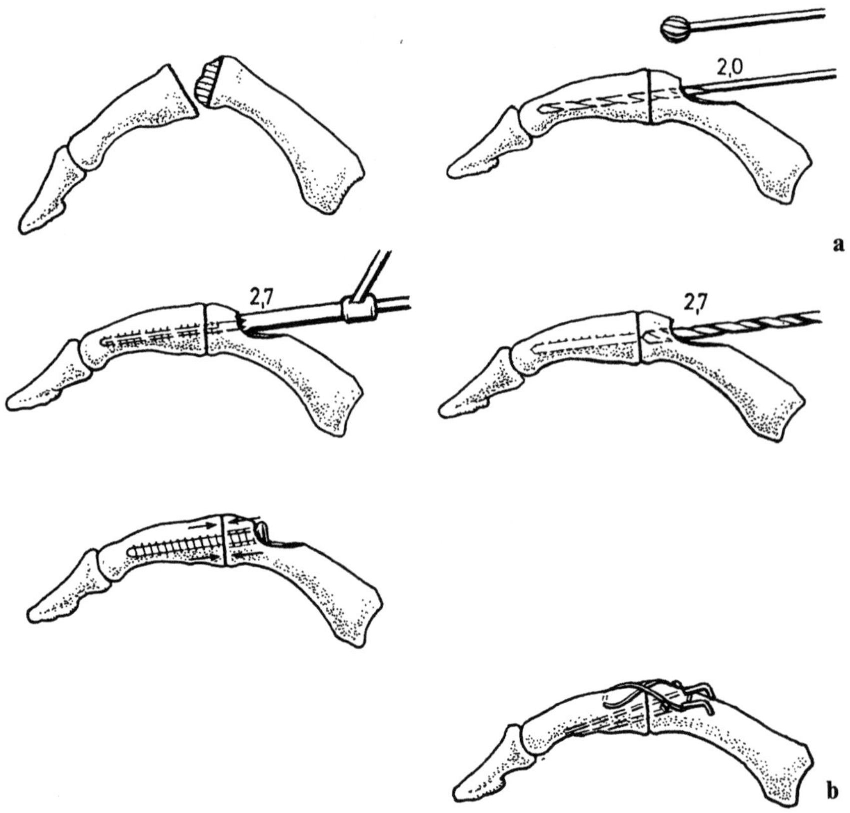

Fig. 145a, b. Arthrodesis of the PIP and DIP joints from the proximal side

a Screw arthrodesis of the PIP joint: The articular surfaces are resected to produce the desired degree of flexion. A wide dorsal slot is cut in the proximal phalanx with a spherical bur, and a 2.0-mm hole is drilled through the resected joint into the middle phalanx. The whole channel is tapped, a gliding hole is made in the proximal phalanx, and a 2.7-mm lag screw is inserted for compression. The screw head should abut against the volar cortex, as this helps to preserve the selected position

b Tension-band arthrodesis with a Kirschner wire and figure-of-eight wire loop. This is excellent for preserving the desired angle of flexion. The joint is resected as in **a**, and a Kirschner wire is drilled obliquely in the distal-volar direction. The angle and rotation are checked and corrected as needed. A second, parallel Kirschner wire is now inserted to control rotation. A transverse hole is drilled through the cortex of the middle phalanx, and a fine cerclage wire is pulled through and passed around the ends of the Kirschner wires in figure-of-eight fashion. The wire loop is tightened on each side. The alignment and strength of the arthrodesis is checked before closure

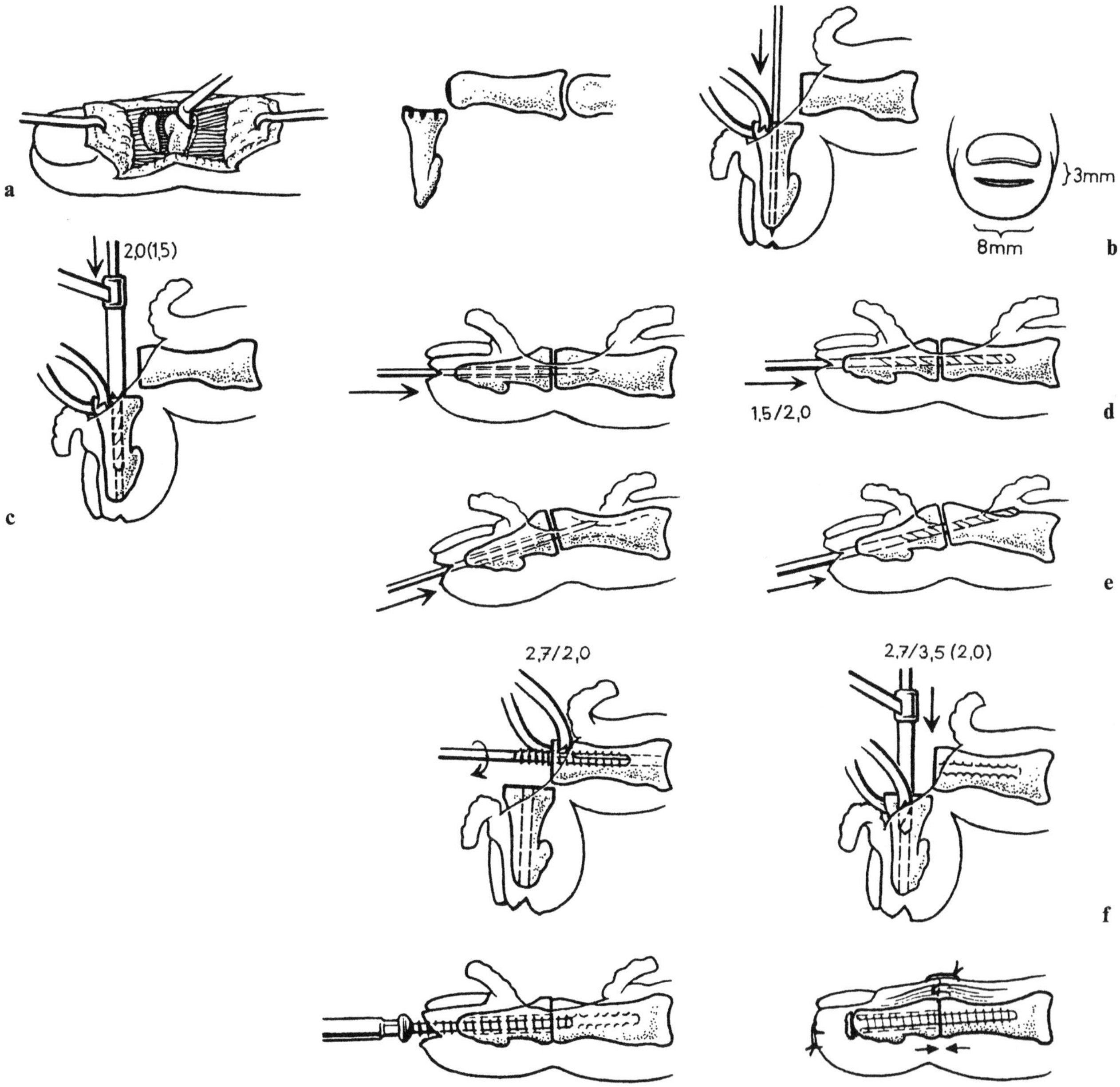

Fig. 146a–f. Screw arthrodesis of the DIP joint from the distal side

a An H- or Y-shaped incision is made, the extensor apparatus is transversely divided over the joint, and the collateral ligaments are incised. With the joint flexed, the proximal articular surface is sparingly resected. Multiple drill holes are made in the distal articular surface

b A 1.6-mm Kirschner wire is twisted manually into the medullary cavity of the distal phalanx and advanced through the ungual process until it tents the skin. A wide transverse incision is made over the wire tip, 3 mm from the nail, and is deepened to the bone

c The medullary canal is successively enlarged with drill bits, and a Kirschner wire is inserted retrograde to the joint. The bone ends are apposed, noting the contact area that is obtained

d The Kirschner wire is advanced into the medullary cavity of the middle phalanx and withdrawn. The channel is drilled open to the caliber of a thread hole and tapped

e Alternative for position of slight flexion: The Kirschner wire is drilled retrograde into the dorsal cortex, and the channel is enlarged with a drill

f The drill hole in the distal phalanx is enlarged to make a gliding hole, and the extra-long screw is inserted from the distal side. The extensor apparatus is repaired with sutures, and the skin is closed

a

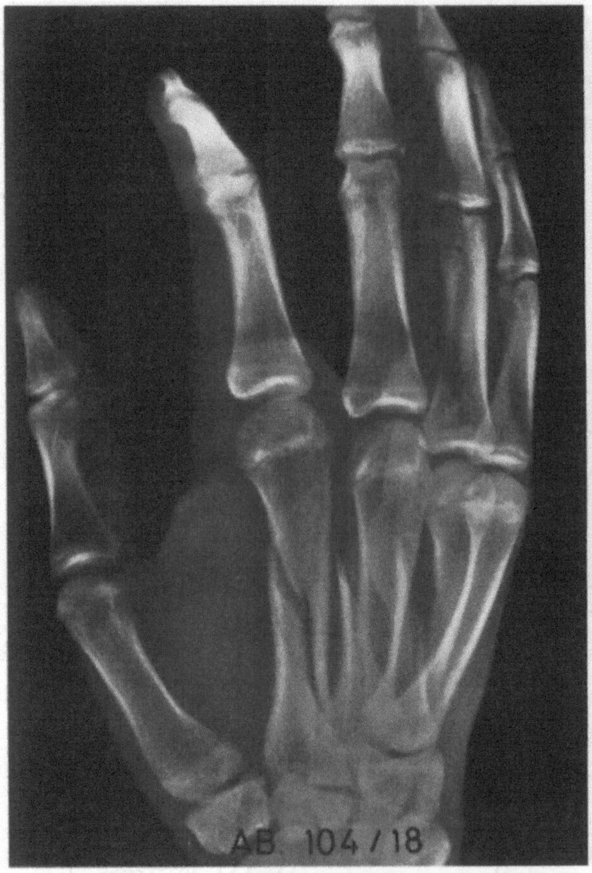

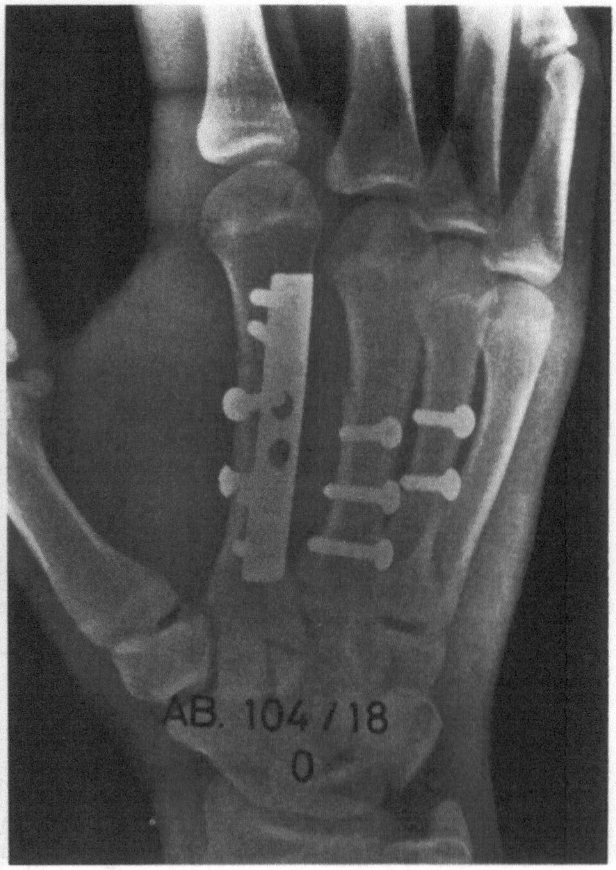

b

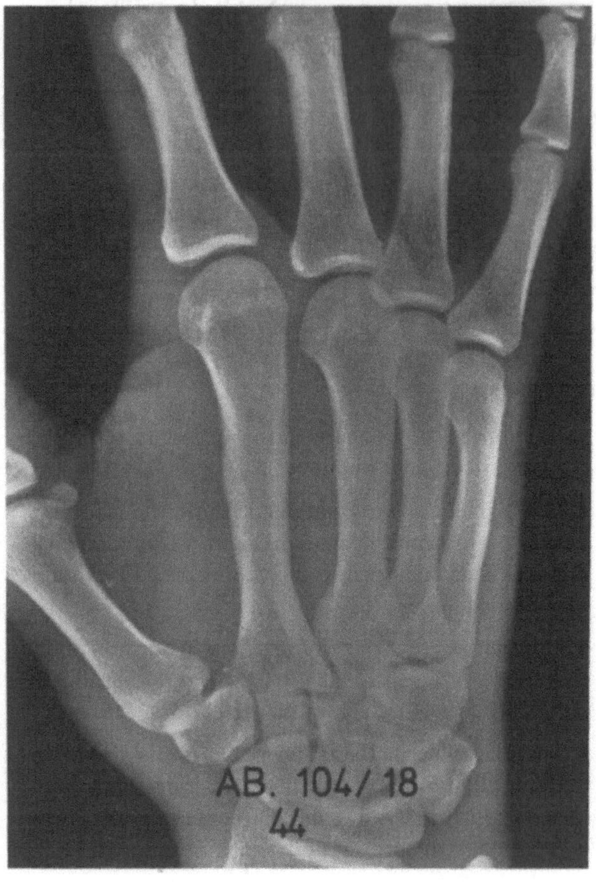

c

Fig. 147 a–c. Clinical example: multiple metacarpal fractures

Paul N., 17-year-old apprentice gardener, fell while playing soccer

a Spiral fracture of the 2nd metacarpal with a butterfly, simple spiral fractures of the 3rd and 4th metacarpals

b During primary internal fixation, the butterfly in the 2nd metacarpal was fixed with two 2.7-mm lag screws, and a 6-hole quarter tubular neutralization plate was applied with 4 screws. The 3rd and 4th metacarpals were fixed with 2.7-mm cortex lag screws. Distal-volar reduction of the 3rd metacarpal was incomplete (difficult to assess volar reduction without circumferential denudation of the bone!). Immediate functional exercises were started. Hand was fully rehabilitated at 8 weeks; the implants were removed at 5 1/2 months

c At 44 weeks postinjury the patient had no complaints and full function in all digits with equivalent strength in both hands

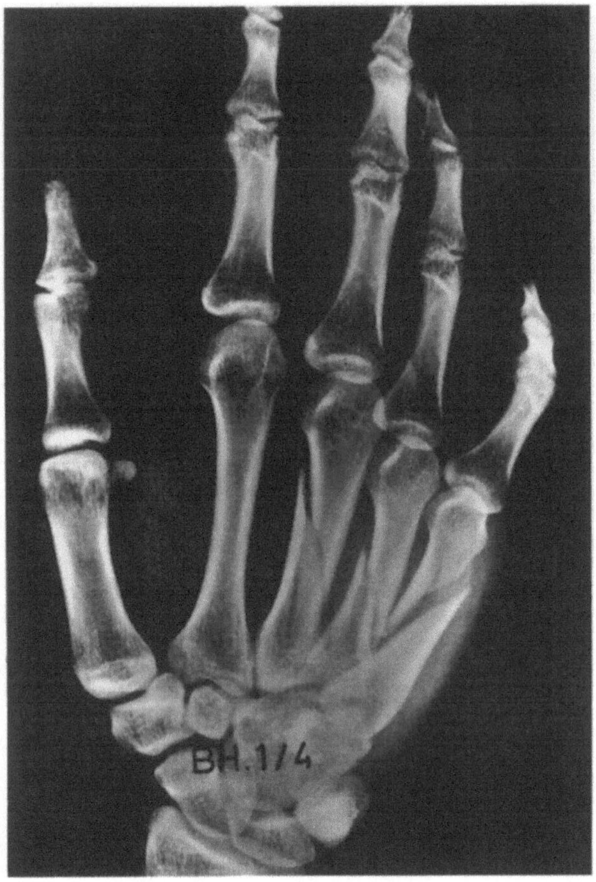

a

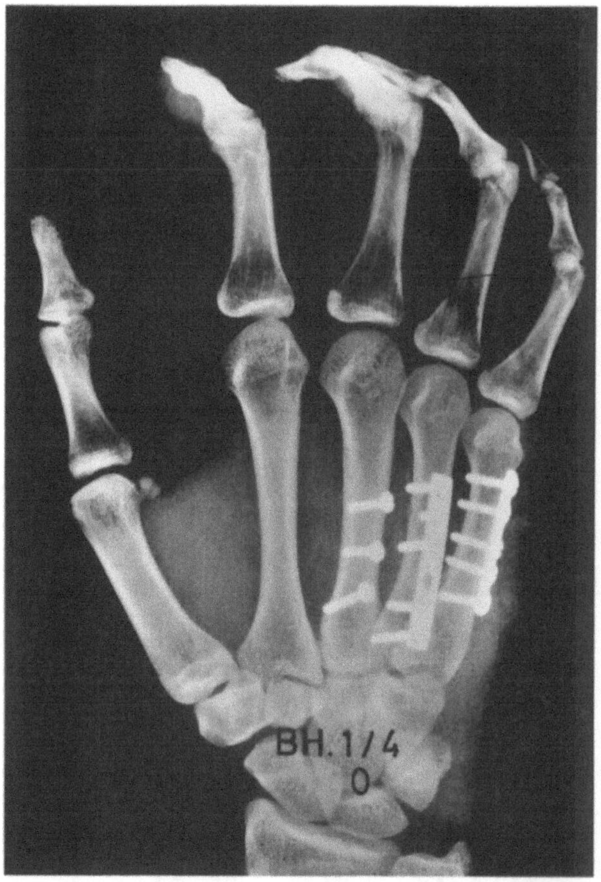

b

Fig. 148a–c. Clinical example: multiple metacarpal spiral fractures

Nicole F., 17-year-old salesclerk, fell on the right hand in a motorbike accident on 9/26/83

a Spiral fractures of the 3rd-5th metacarpals of the right hand, brain concussion

b Emergency internal fixation was performed through a longitudinal incision over the 4th ray. The 4th and 5th metacarpals were fixed with 2.0-mm DCPs (incorporating interfragmental lag screws), and the 3rd metacarpal with 2.0-mm screws alone. Despite functional exercises, extensor stiffness developed in the 4th and 5th MP joints. Patient returned to work at 7 weeks. Implant removal at 4 months was combined with extensor tendolysis and capsulectomy of the 4th and 5th MP joints

c At 16 months, on 1/8/85, the patient had no complaints and only a limitation of 20° extension in the MP joint of the ring finger. Full flexion

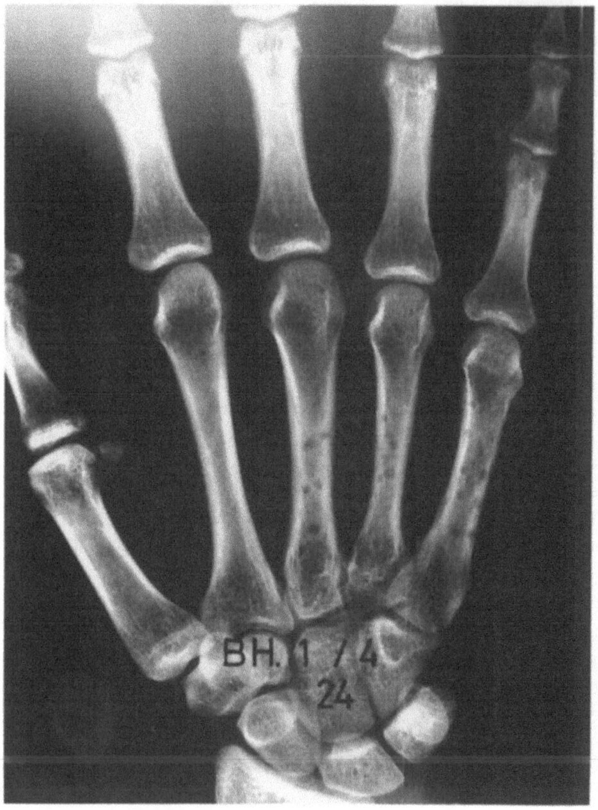

c

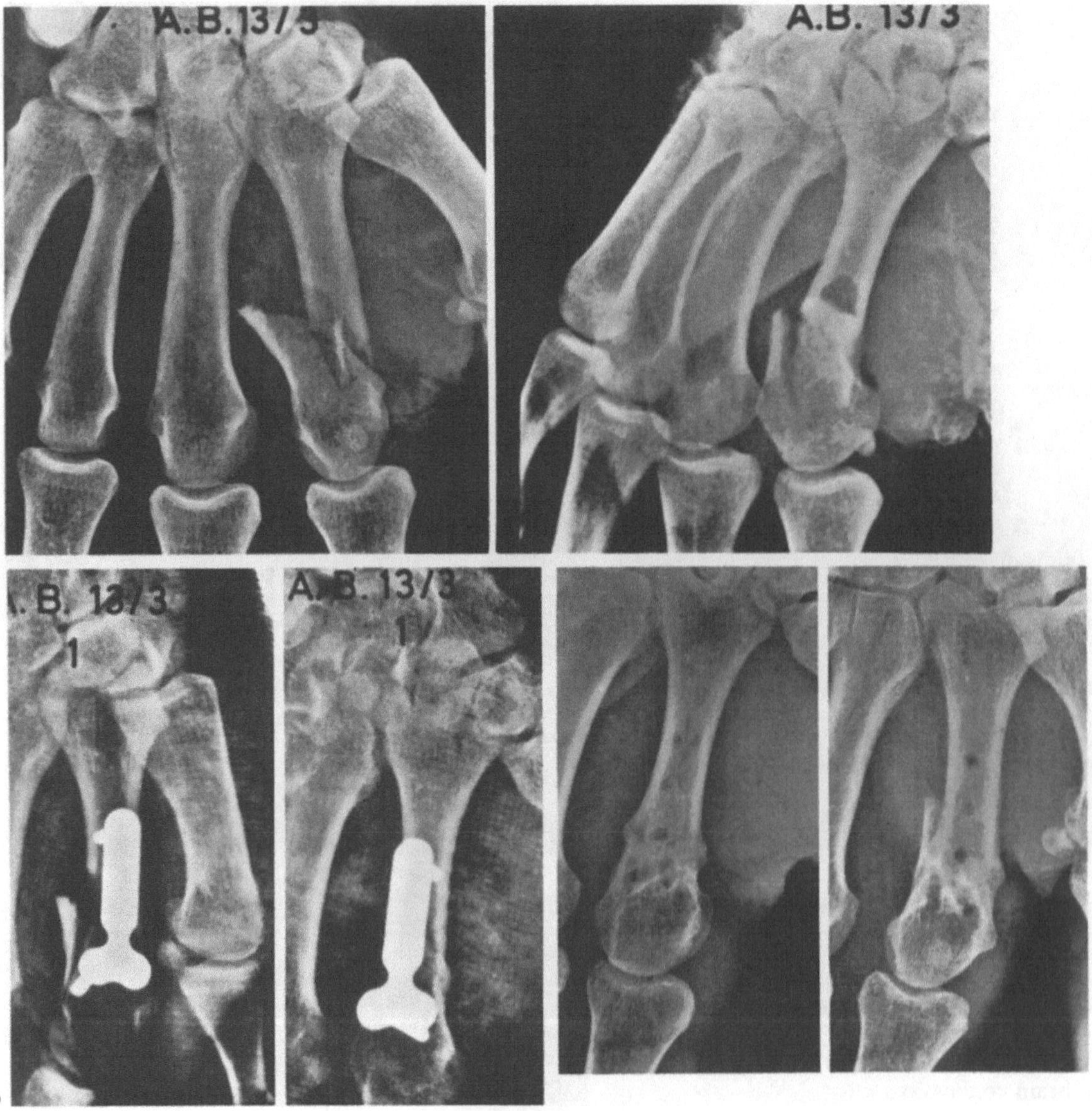

a b c

Fig. 149a–c. Clinical example: oblique subcapital fracture of the second metacarpal

Werner J., 36-year-old chemical plant worker, caught the right hand in a conveyor belt

a Open subcapital fracture of the 2nd metacarpal, fracture of the proximal phalanx of the thumb, extensor tendon injury of the middle finger

b The 2nd metacarpal was fixed with a small-fragment T plate, and a cast was worn for 4 weeks. Postoperative course was complicated by dystrophic symptoms. Hand was partially rehabilitated at 4 months and fully rehabilitated at 7 months

c Implants were removed after 6 months, and treatment was concluded at 7 months. Patient was fully rehabilitated and had no pain. The index and middle fingers could flex to 3 cm from the palm and showed slight strength loss

a
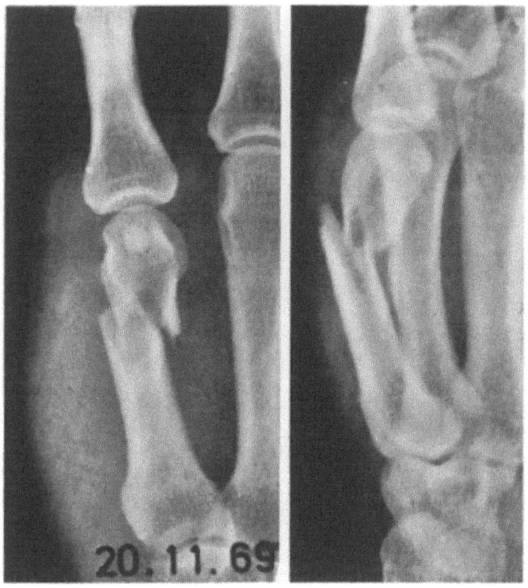

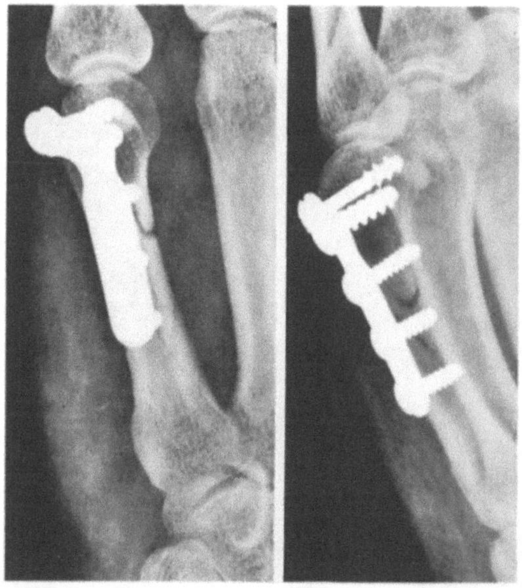
b

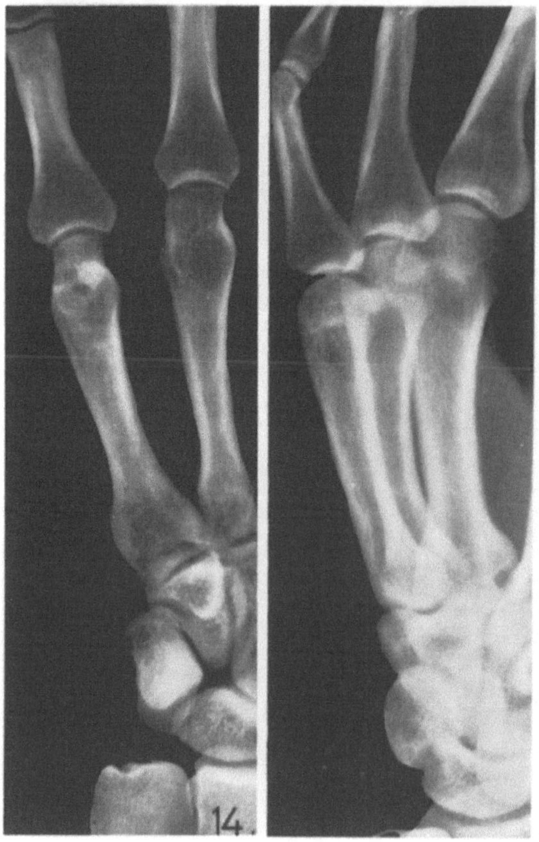

c

Fig. 150 a–c. Clinical example: open distal fracture of the fifth metacarpal

Ernst S., 39-year-old mechanic, sustained compression injury of the left hand on 11/20/69

a Open oblique fracture of the distal shaft of the 5th metacarpal with skin loss

b The fracture was fixed with an L plate after 4 days, and the skin defect was covered with a thick split-thickness skin graft. The postoperative course was uncomplicated, and functional exercises were started. At 7 months the implants were removed and the hand was fully functional

c Follow-up at 11 years on 7/14/80 showed a barely visible linear scar. Only a trace of the old fracture line is visible on the X-ray

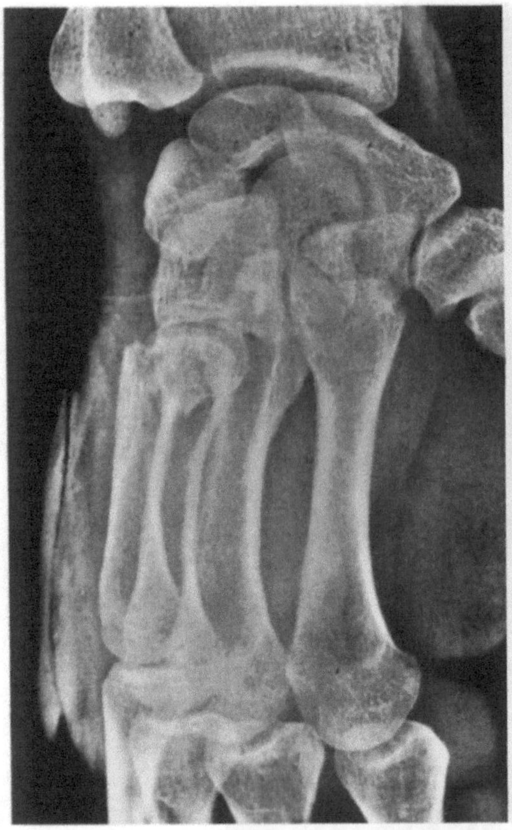

a

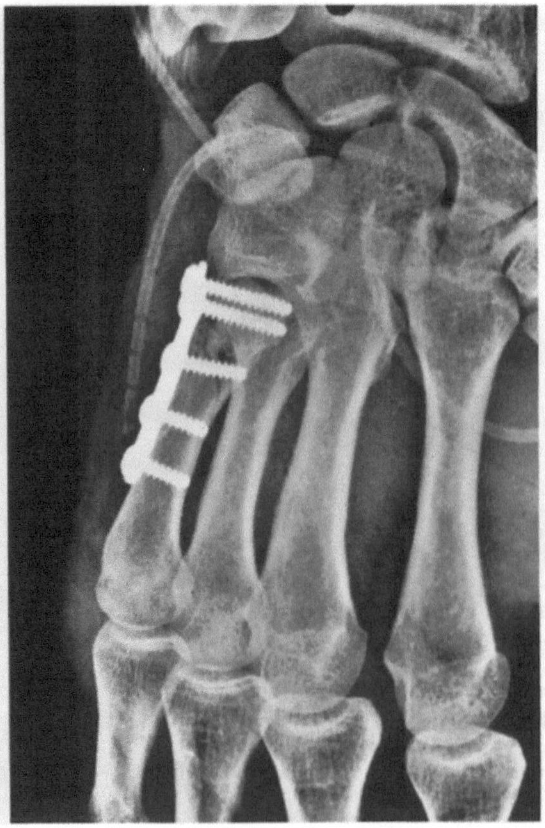

b

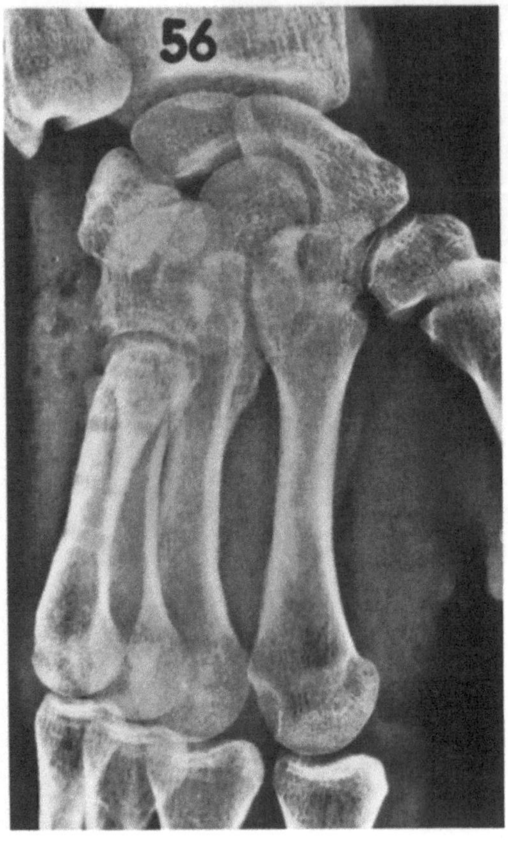

c

Fig. 151 a–c. Clinical example: fracture of the base of the fifth metacarpal

Ramon V., 36-year-old laborer, fell onto the hand

a Extra-articular oblique fracture of the base of the 5th metacarpal with shortening

b Primary internal fixation was performed with an articulated L plate.
The postoperative course was uneventful, and full rehabilitation was achieved by 40 days

c Implants were removed at 13 months. Patient had no complaints, full function, and equivalent strength in both hands

Fig. 152a–c. Clinical example: subcapital fracture of the fifth metacarpal

Angelo F., 40-year-old innkeeper, fell onto the right hand from a bicycle on 5/20/81

a Subcapital fracture of the 5th metacarpal. Nasal fracture and multiple contusions

b Fracture was fixed 5 days later with a 2.0-mm cortex lag screw and fine tension-band wire. Functional exercises were started after surgery. Fracture was united at 6 weeks, and hand was fully functional

c Radiograph taken at 9 months on 2/12/82, at time of implant removal, showed a slight widening of the metacarpal head. Patient had full function and no complaints

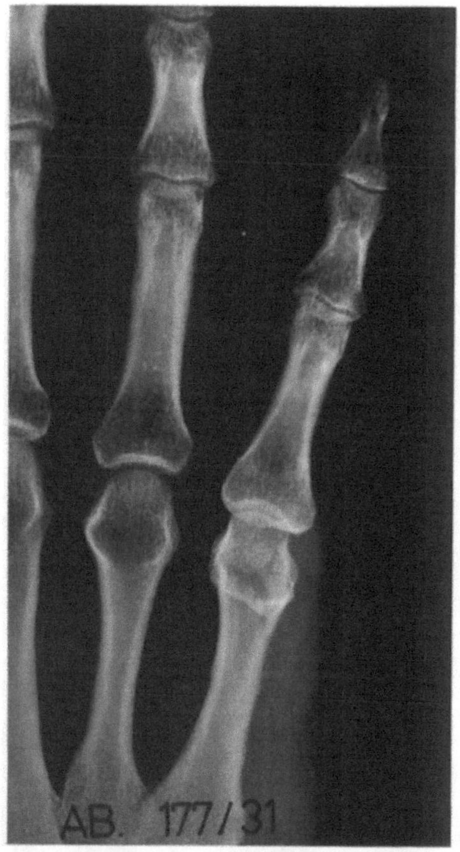

a

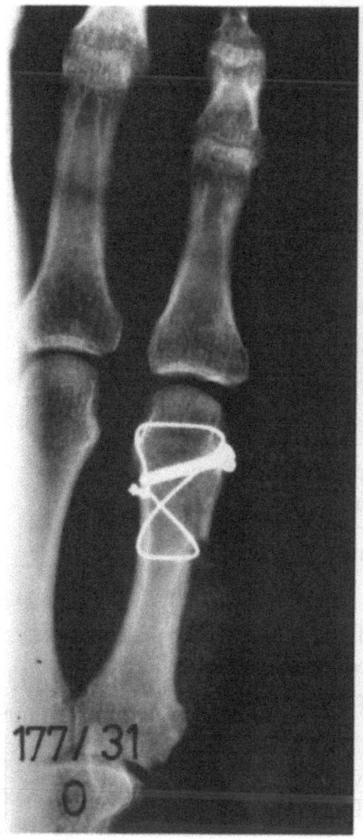

b

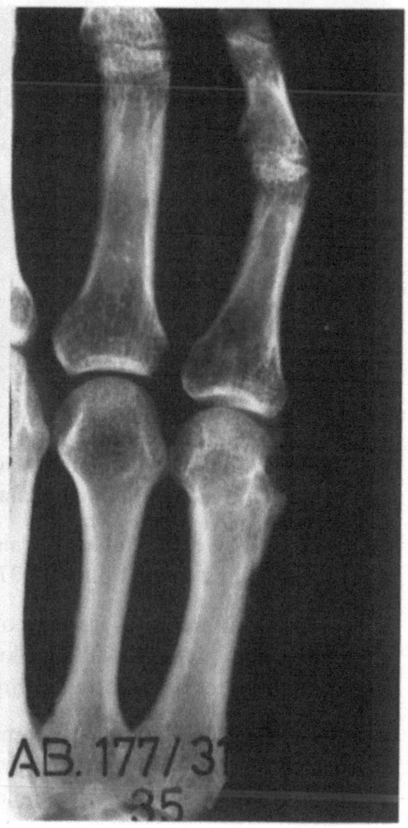

c

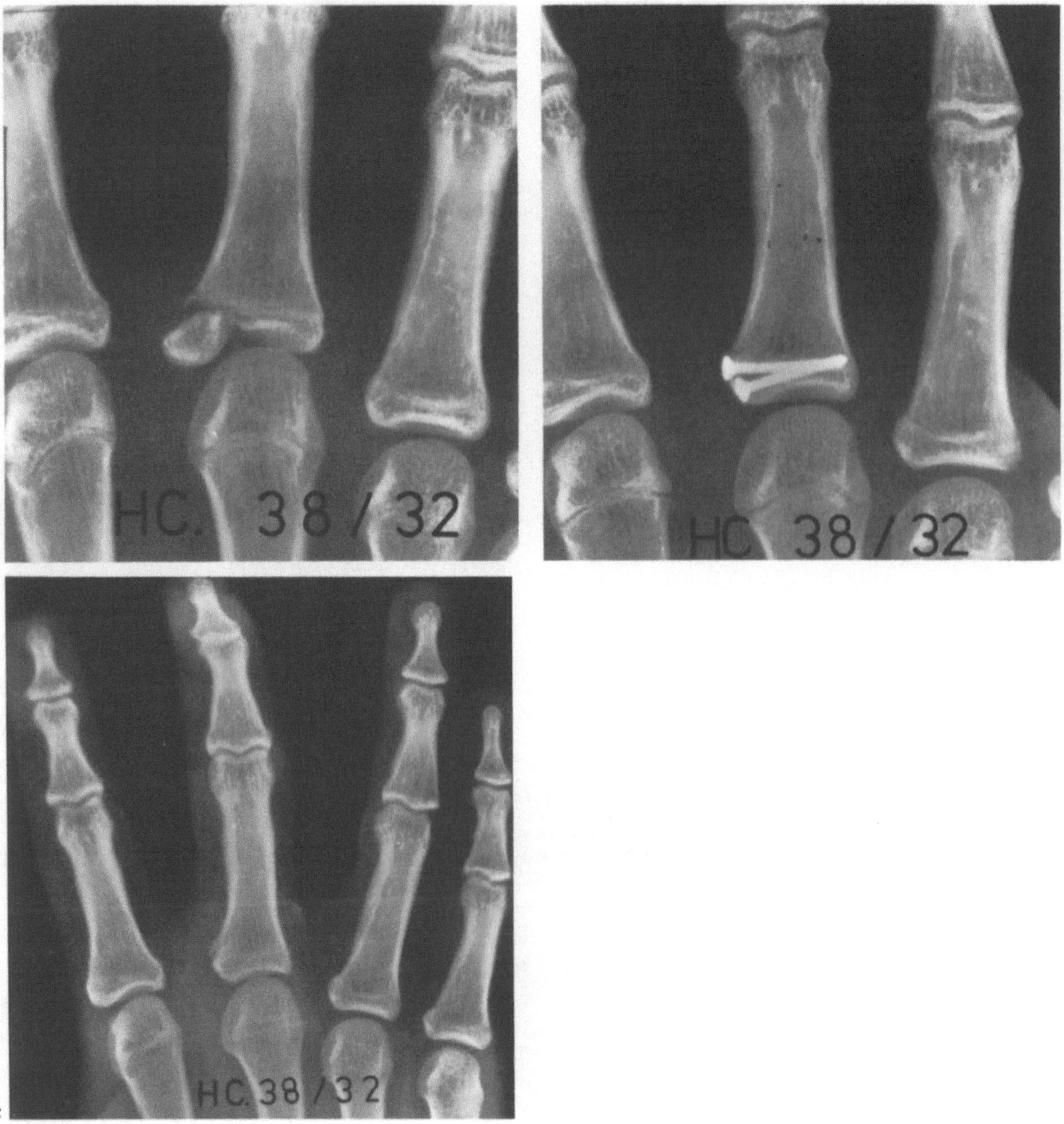

a b c

Fig. 153a–c. Clinical example: displaced avulsion fracture of the base of the proximal phalanx

Dominik B., 16-year-old clerical trainee, fell onto the right hand from a moped on 10/7/77

a Closed, radial avulsion fracture of the base of the third proximal phalanx with marked displacement. The growth plates have not yet completely fused

b Internal fixation with two 1.5-mm mini screws was performed on the day after the injury
Functional exercises, primary wound healing

c Follow-up and implant removal at 5 months: full function, no complaints, fracture union

▷

Fig. 154a–c. Clinical example: multiple phalangeal fractures

Roberto C., 20-year-old press operator, caught right hand in machinery on 9/19/83

a Complex hand injury with a closed oblique fracture of the proximal phalanx of the thumb, an open fracture of the proximal phalanx of the index finger with a torsion butterfly, and open oblique fractures of the distal index and middle fingers with nail avulsion

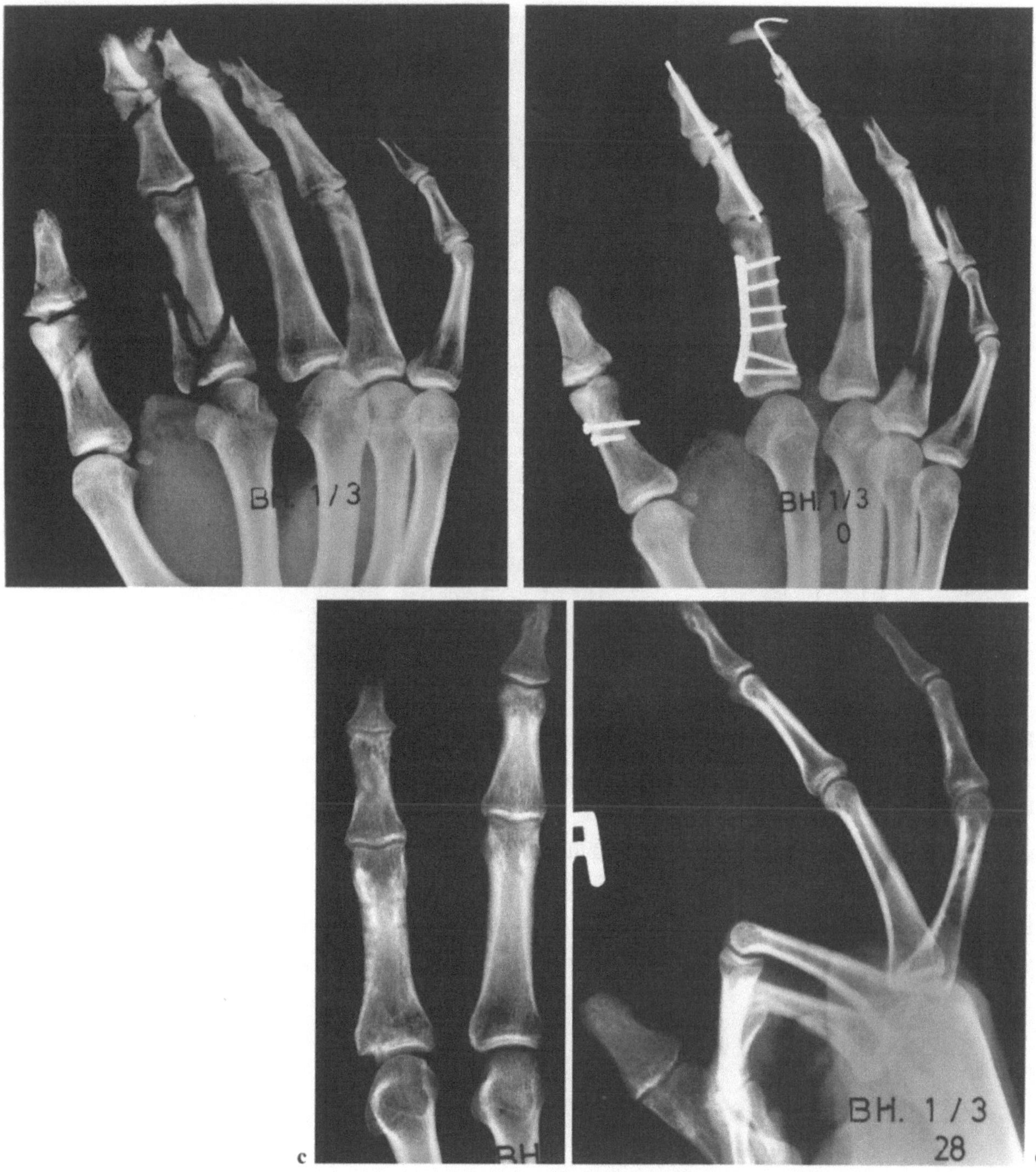

a b c c′

b At emergency internal fixation, the thumb was fixed with two 1.5-mm screws, and the proximal phalanx of the index finger with a 1.5-mm mini plate applied radially. The distal injuries were managed with percutaneous Kirschner wires, left in place for 4 and 8 weeks.
At 4 months the plate was removed, and the extensor apparatus of the index finger was freed of adhesions. Partial rehabilitation was achieved at 5 months

c Follow-up at 7 months on 4/17/84 showed a moderate trophic disturbance in the index finger, flexion to 4 cm from the palm, and 25° loss of extension in the PIP joint. Patient was fully rehabilitated and back at work

a, b

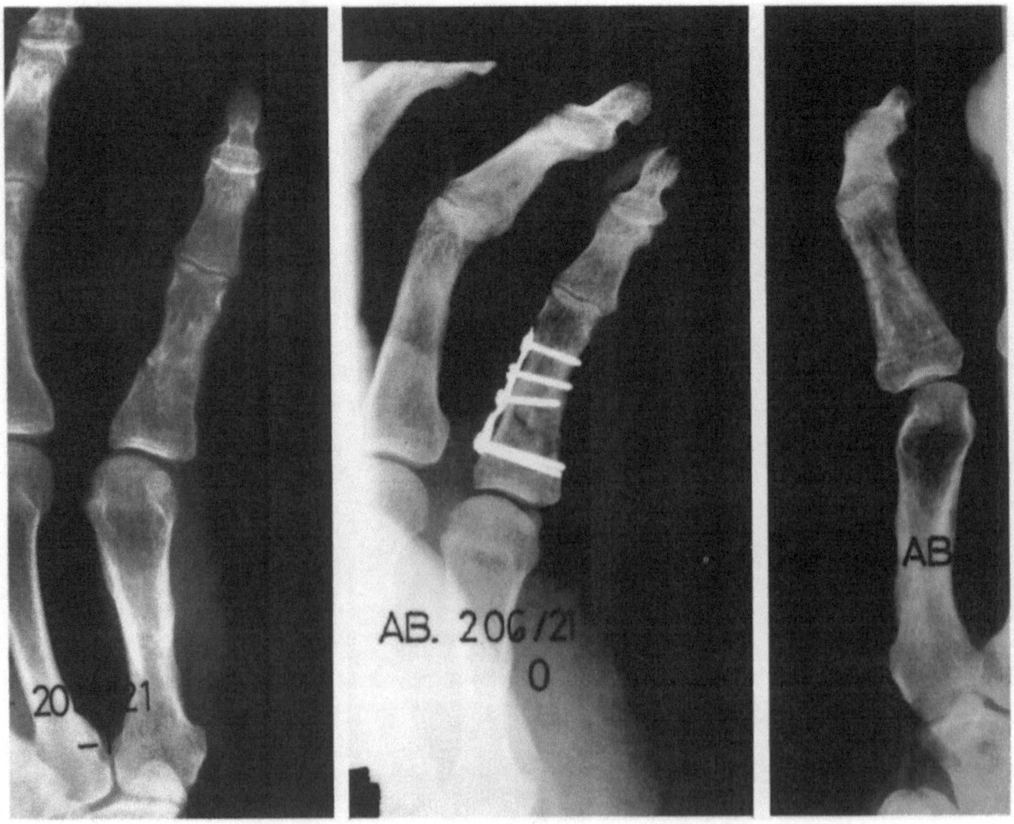

c

Fig. 155 a–c. Clinical example: transverse fracture of the proximal phalanx of the little finger

Josef R., 58-year-old dockworker, little finger of right hand struck by falling metal plate on 9/16/82

a Multi-part transverse fracture of the proximal fifth phalanx, close to the base. Severe swelling

b At 12 days postinjury the phalanx was fixed with a 1.5-mm condylar plate inserted from the radial side and was mobilized immediately after surgery. The hand was fully rehabilitated at 10 weeks

c Follow-up at 7 months confirmed fracture union. The implants were removed, and the extensor tendon freed. At 8 months there was a slight deficit of fist closure and a 50° extension loss in the PIP, which caused no subjective problems

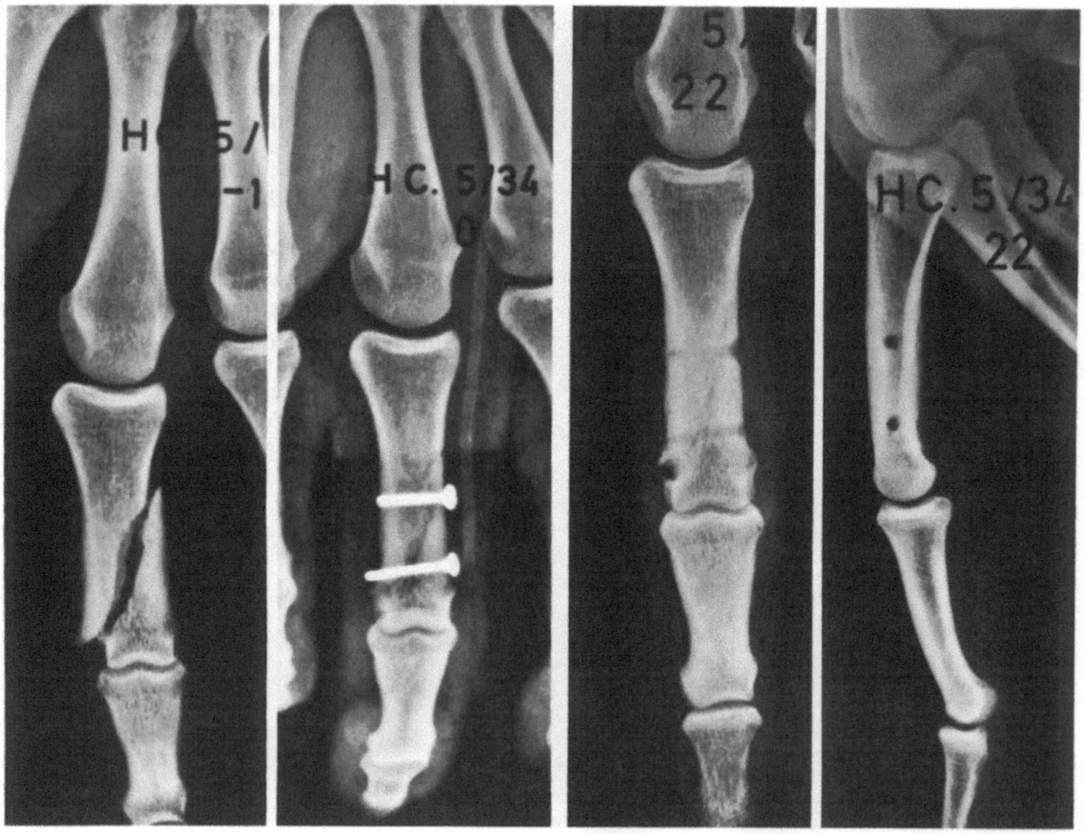

a b

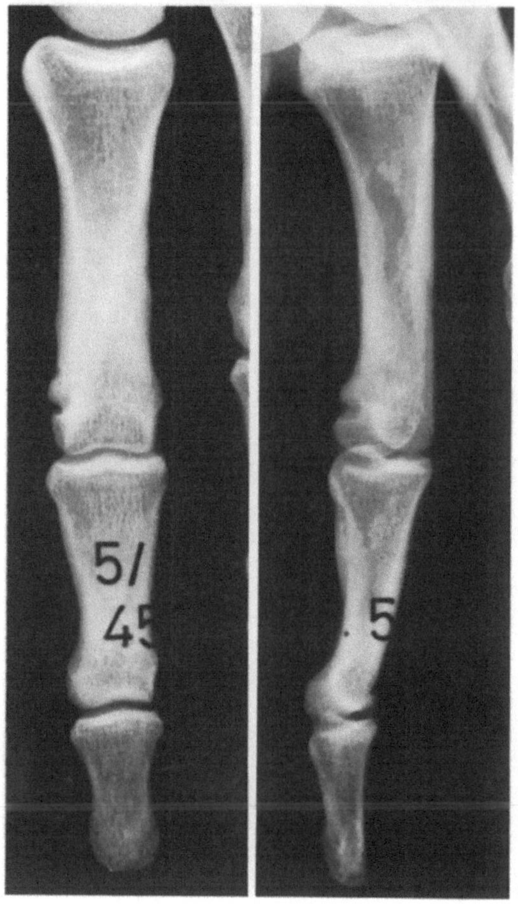

c

Fig. 156a–c. Clinical example: spiral fracture of the proximal phalanx

Christian C., 31-year-old postman, fell into a crevass on 7/28/71

a Spiral fracture of the proximal phalanx of the middle finger with rotational deformity. Closed treatment was unsuccessful

b Internal fixation with two 2.0-mm screws was performed one week postinjury. The postoperative course was uneventful, and functional exercises were started.
On implant removal at 5 months there was a slight flexion deficit and a linear scar. Necrosis of the fragment tip led to the development of a small metaphyseal cyst

c When seen in July of 1980, the patient had full function. A cystlike lesion was still visible in the distal metaphysis of the injured bone

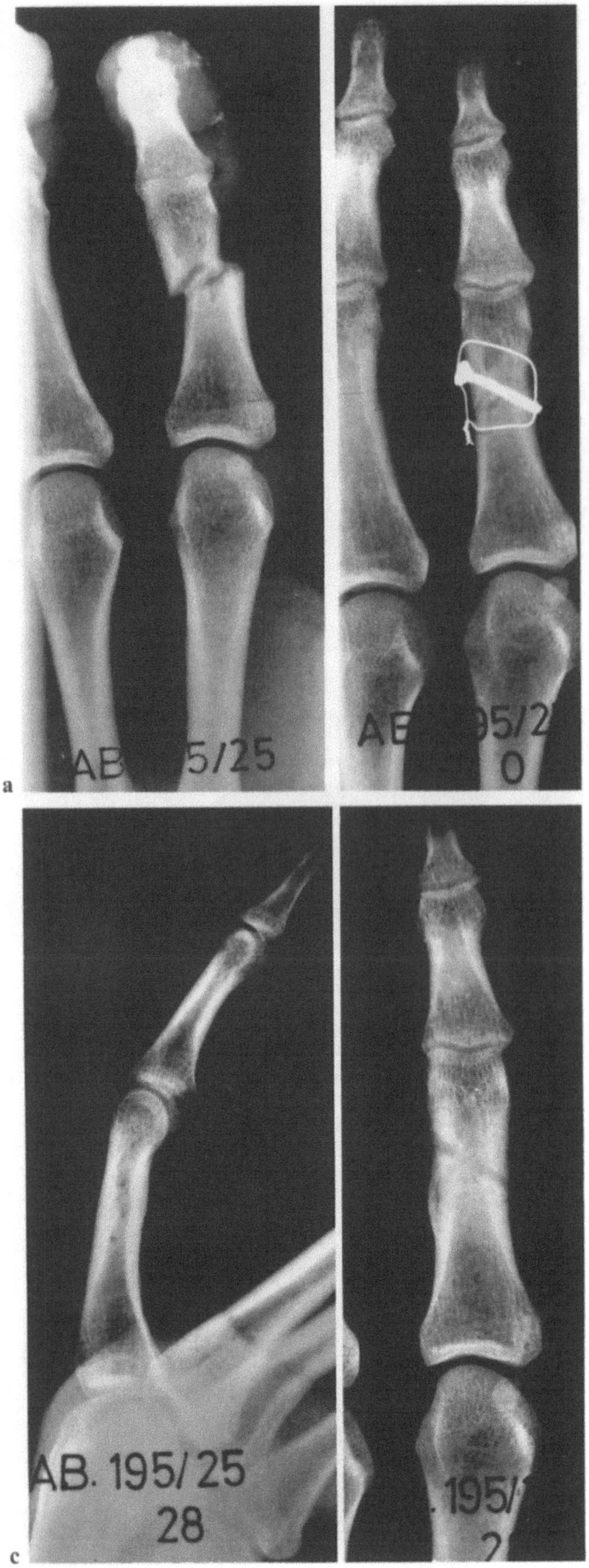

a b c

Fig. 157a–c. Clinical example: fracture of the proximal phalanx

Pierre G., 20-year-old salesclerk, fell on the hand during military training in early November, 1982

a Two-week-old short oblique fracture of the proximal phalanx of the left index finger

b The fracture was fixed with a 2.0-mm interfragmental lag screw and 0.6-mm intraosseous wire suture, followed by functional exercises. The hand was fully rehabilitated at 5 weeks

c Implants were removed at 7 months on 6/17/83. Patient had full function and no complaints. Fracture was united with fixation callus

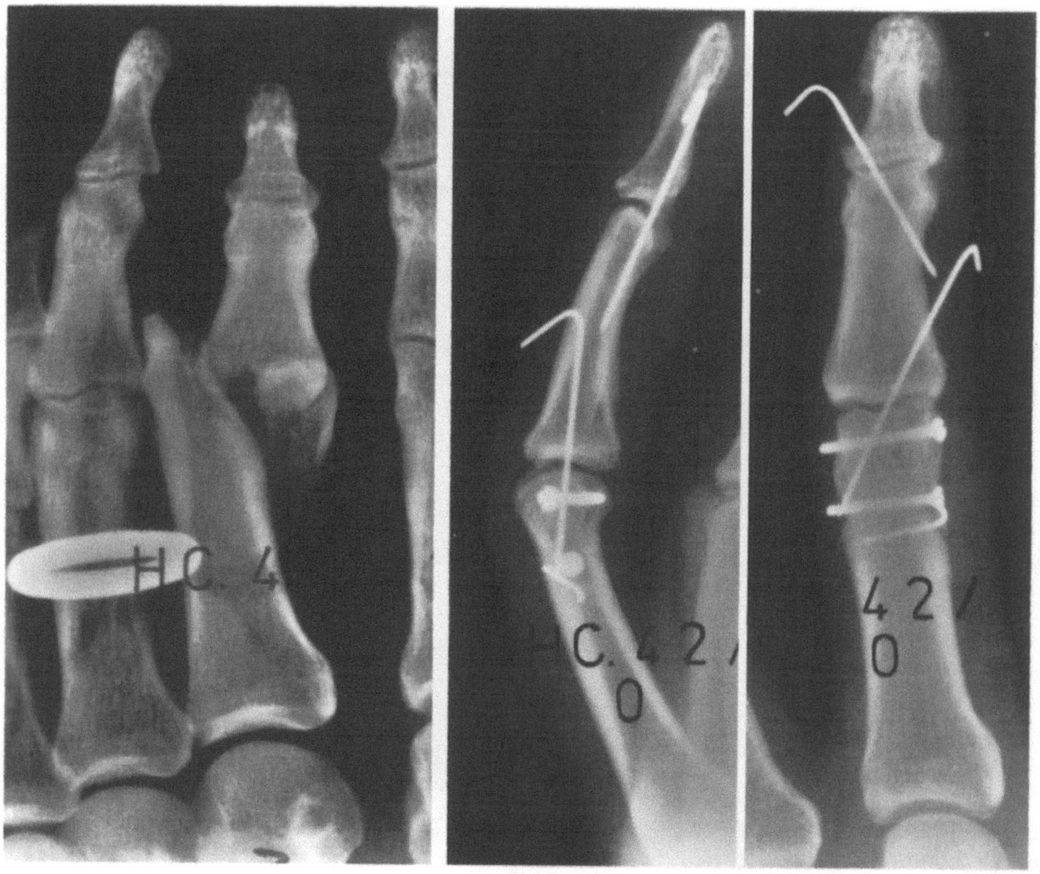

a b

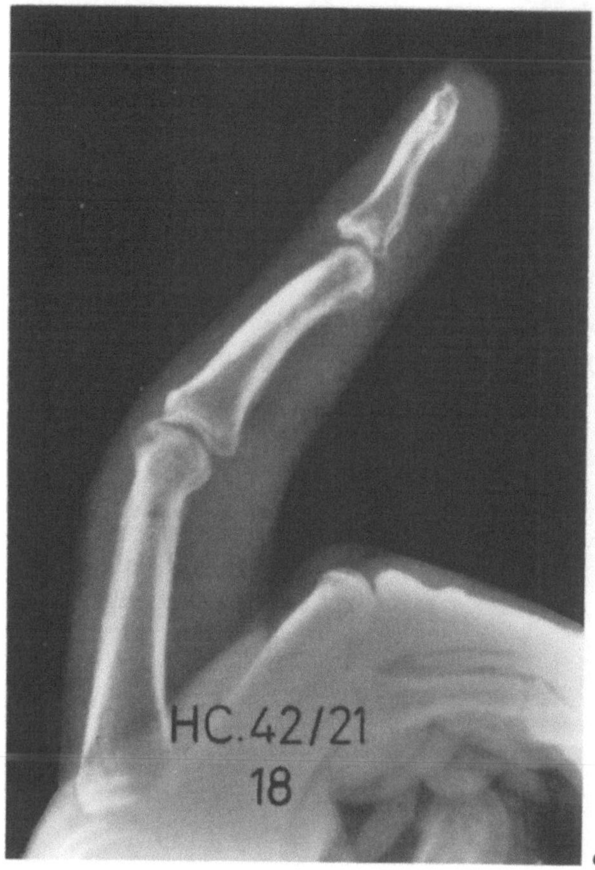

c

Fig. 158 a–c. Clinical example: open intra-articular fracture of the proximal phalanx

Bartholomäus L., 51-year-old civil servant, struck finger with axe while chopping wood on 4/21/78

a Partial traumatic amputation of the left middle finger with intra-articular fracture of the proximal phalanx and division of the extensor apparatus

b Emergency internal fixation was performed with two screws, and the extensors were repaired by direct suture. The PIP and DIP were temporarily immobilized with thin Kirschner wires for 3 weeks. The wounds healed without complications

c The screws were removed at $3^1/_2$ months. There was a 50° extension loss in the PIP joint but a free active flexion and no interference with the patient's work

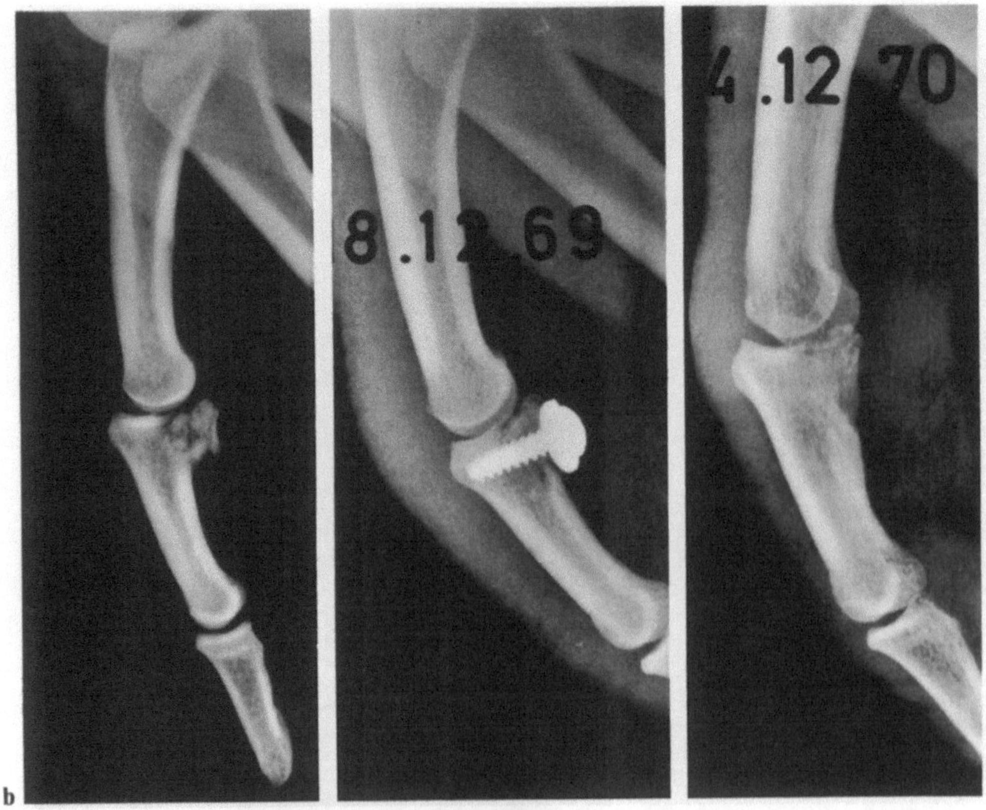

a, b c

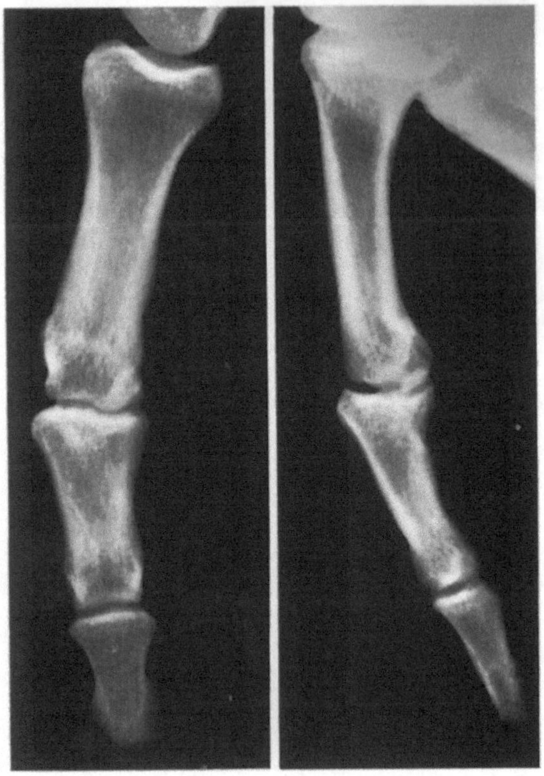

d

Fig. 159a–d. Clinical example: fracture-dislocation of the base of the middle phalanx

Peter M., 32-year-old farmer, index finger struck by engine crank on 12/2/69

a Intra-articular comminuted fracture of the base of the middle phalanx of the index finger with dorsal subluxation and ulnar deviation. Fracture was treated conservatively in plaster

b Secondary internal fixation was performed on 12/16/69. The comminuted area are compressed with a screw and washer inserted through a volar approach
Patient had good weight-lifting ability after an uncomplicated course.The implant was removed at 4 months

c By 12 months the patient had returned to farm work with moderate complaints. The subluxation was corrected, the deformity improved, and there was evidence of mild osteoarthritis

d When seen $10^1/_2$ years later on 7/7/80, the patient was fully rehabilitated and had no complaints. The ulnar deviation had not changed; active PIP joint flexion was 80°. There was no visible scar and no progression of osteoarthritis

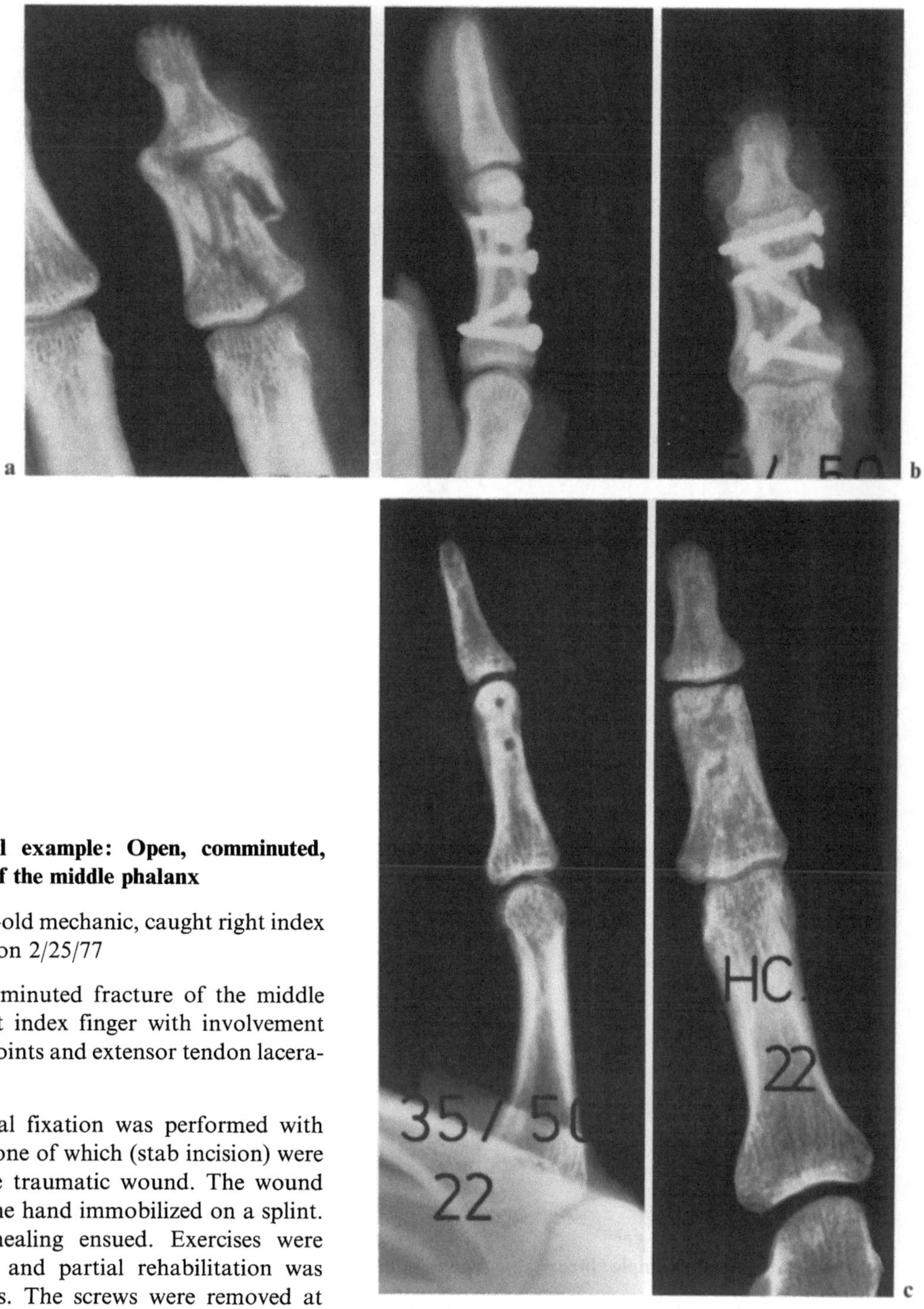

Fig. 160a–c. Clinical example: Open, comminuted, biarticular fracture of the middle phalanx

Giovanni I., 30-year-old mechanic, caught right index finger in machinery on 2/25/77

a Widely open comminuted fracture of the middle phalanx of the right index finger with involvement of the PIP and DIP joints and extensor tendon lacerations

b Emergency internal fixation was performed with mini screws, all but one of which (stab incision) were inserted through the traumatic wound. The wound was left open, and the hand immobilized on a splint. Partial secondary healing ensued. Exercises were started at 6 weeks, and partial rehabilitation was achieved by 7 weeks. The screws were removed at 3 months

c Follow-up at 8 months showed slight keloid scarring, decreased flexion in the DIP joint, and full function in the PIP joint

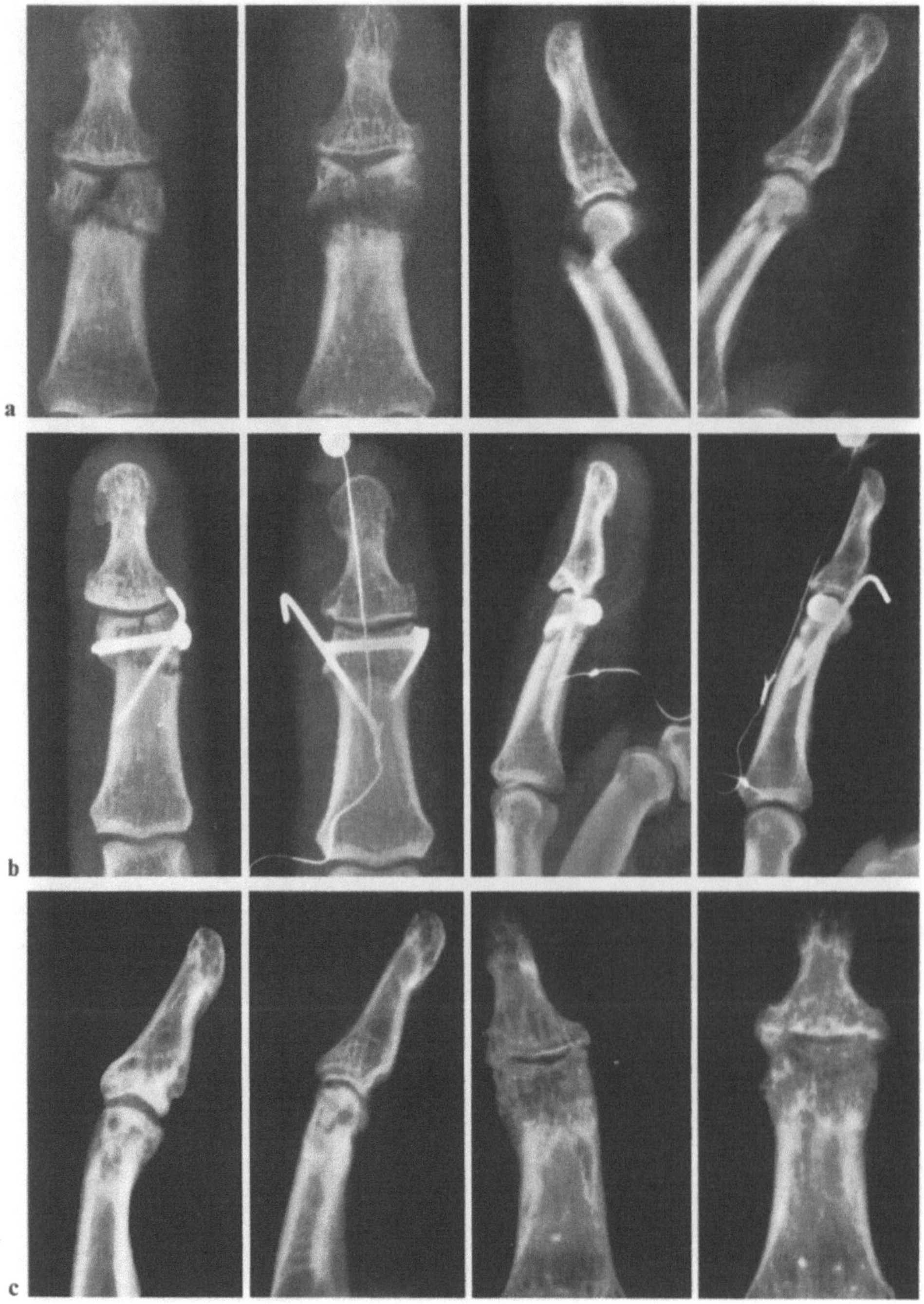

Fig. 161 a–c. Clinical example: bicondylar fractures of the middle phalanx

Anton S., 57-year-old bricklayer, caught left hand between two cement pipes on 10/17/74

a Displaced bicondylar Y fracture of the middle phalanx of the middle and ring fingers of the left hand with skin contusion

b Internal fixation was performed 4 days later using a combination of screws and Kirschner wires (buried and percutaneous). The extensor aponeurosis of the middle finger was divided and reapproximated. The hand was immobilized on a splint, and primary wound healing ensued. The pull-out wire and percutaneous Kirschner wire were removed at 5 weeks, the screws and buried Kirschner wire at 3 months. Patient returned to his former work at 6 months

c Follow-up at 6 years on 9/19/80 showed a linear scar, limitation of active motion in both distal joints, good grip strength, and incipient osteoarthritis in the middle finger

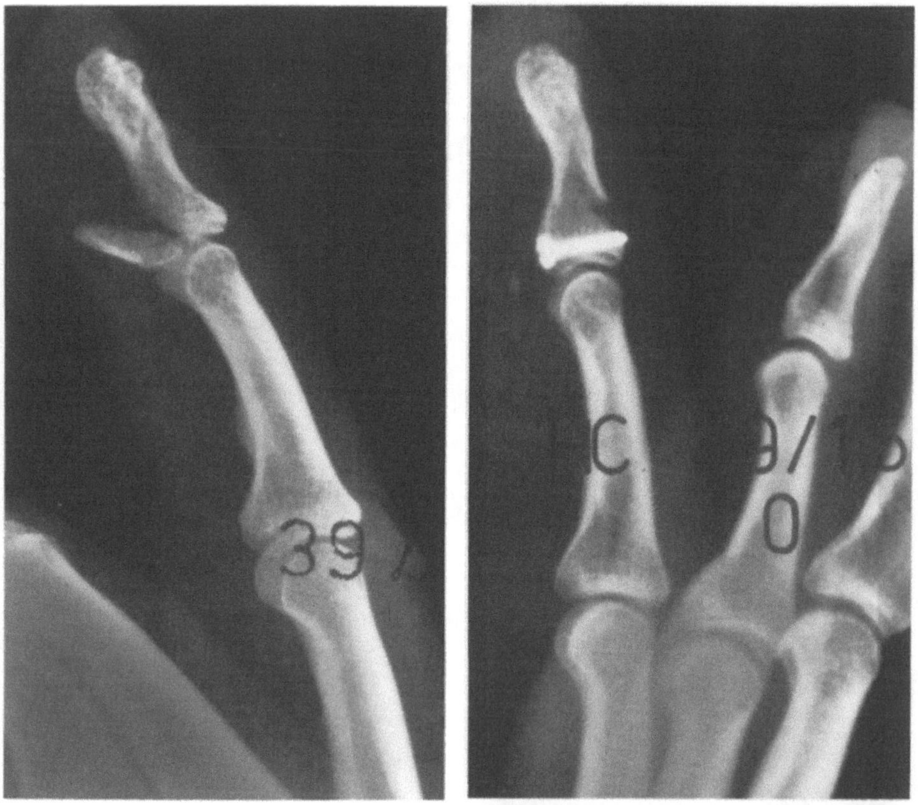

a b

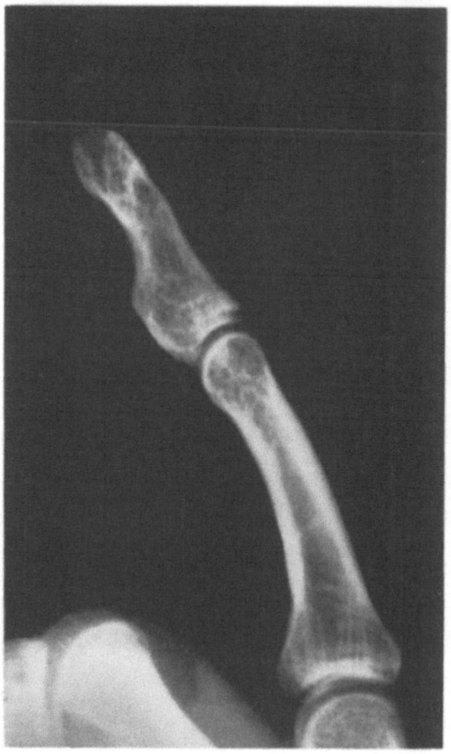

c

Fig. 162 a–c. Clinical example: avulsion fracture at the base of the distal phalanx

Heinz S., 44-year-old engineer, sustained ring-finger injury of the right hand from a tug on a dog leash on 9/24/79

a Markedly displaced avulsion fracture of the base of the distal phalanx

b The avulsed fragment bearing the flexor profundus insertion was reattached with a 1.5-mm mini screw inserted through an H-shaped radiopalmar incision with turn-down of a radial subcutaneous flap
The postoperative course was uneventful. The distal joint was immobilized in a plastic splint for 4 weeks, followed by active motion and resistance exercises. The screw was removed at 5 months as an office procedure

c Follow-up at 1 year on 9/20/80: Patient had no complaints, full function, a linear scar, and no evidence of osteoarthritis

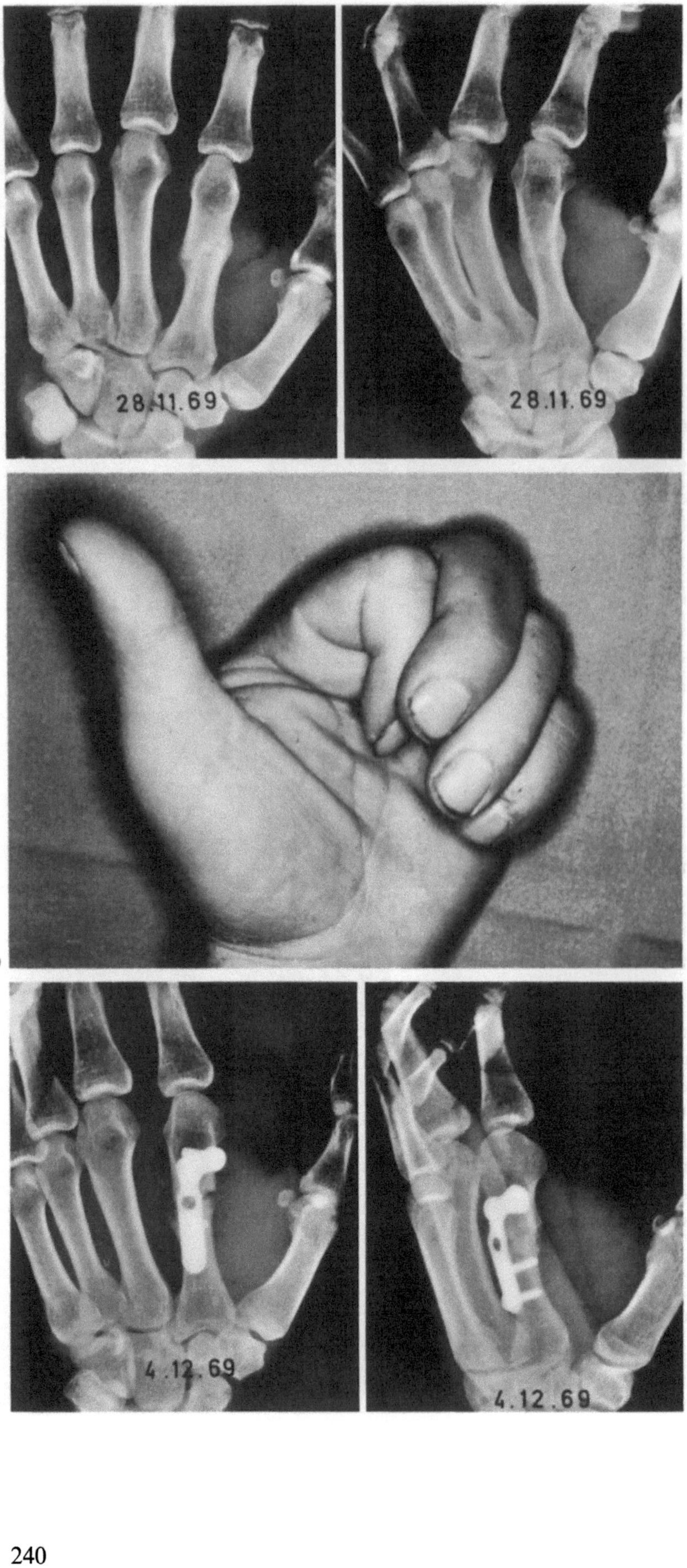

a
b
c

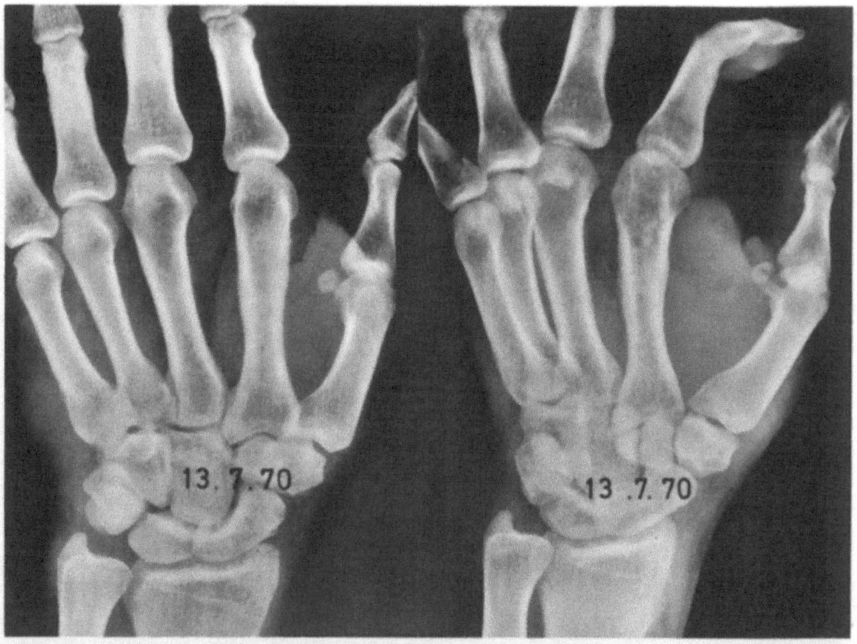

d

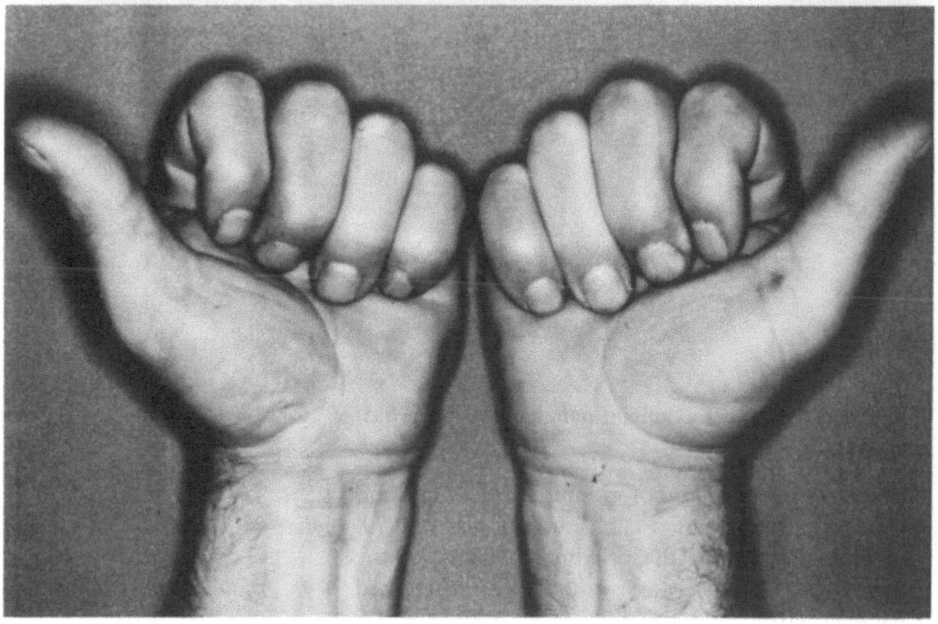

e

Fig. 163 a–e. Clinical example: osteotomy of the second metacarpal

Antonio C., 29-year-old iron bender, sustained open transverse fracture of the 2nd metacarpal shaft in a crush injury

a Fracture was treated conservatively by casting the index finger in subtotal extension; a rigid nonunion ensued

b Rotational deformity of the index finger

c Corrective osteotomy was performed 4 months postinjury; it was stabilized with a dowel graft and tension-band plate.

The postoperative course was uncomplicated, and functional exercises were performed without external fixation. The hand was fully rehabilitated by 3 months

d Implants were removed at 8 months

e On final follow-up at 10 months the patient had no complaints, full function, and no deformity relative to the uninjured side

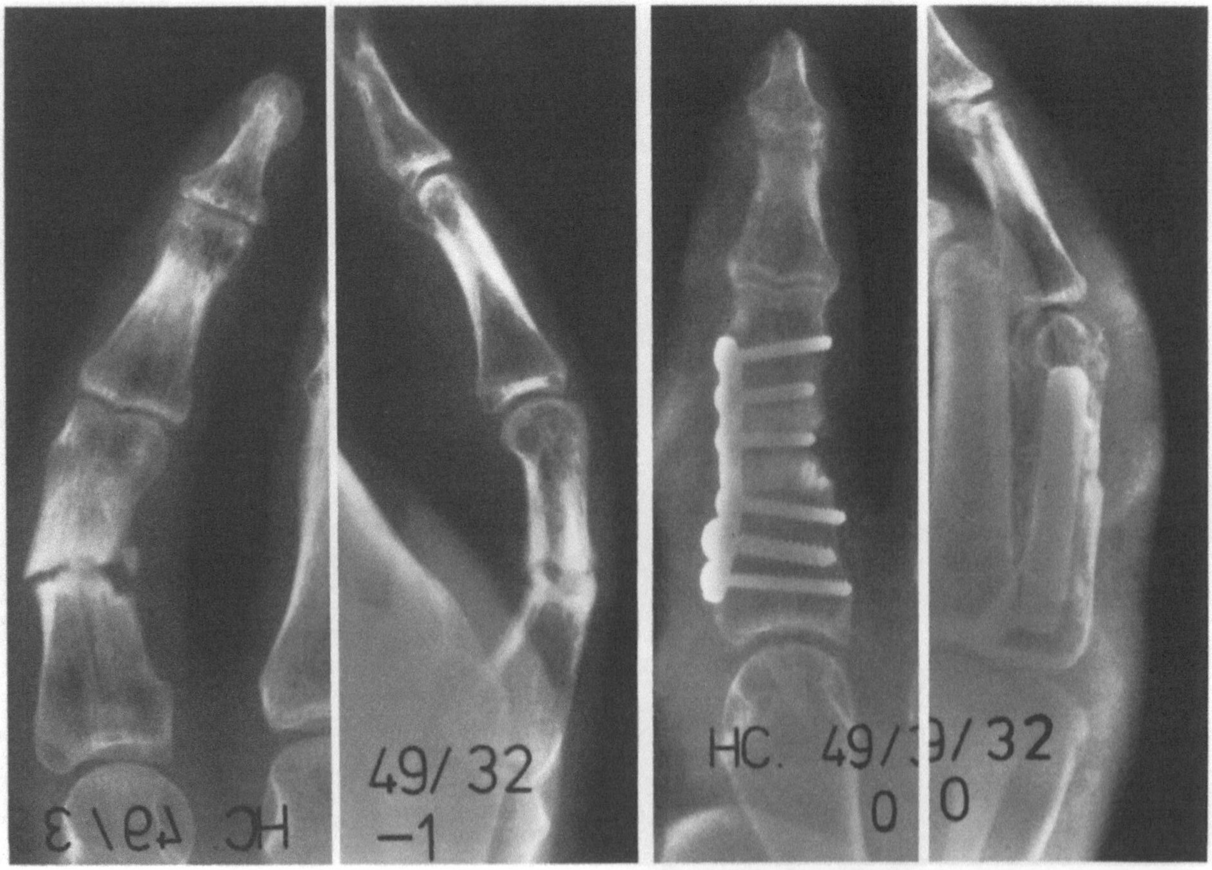

a b

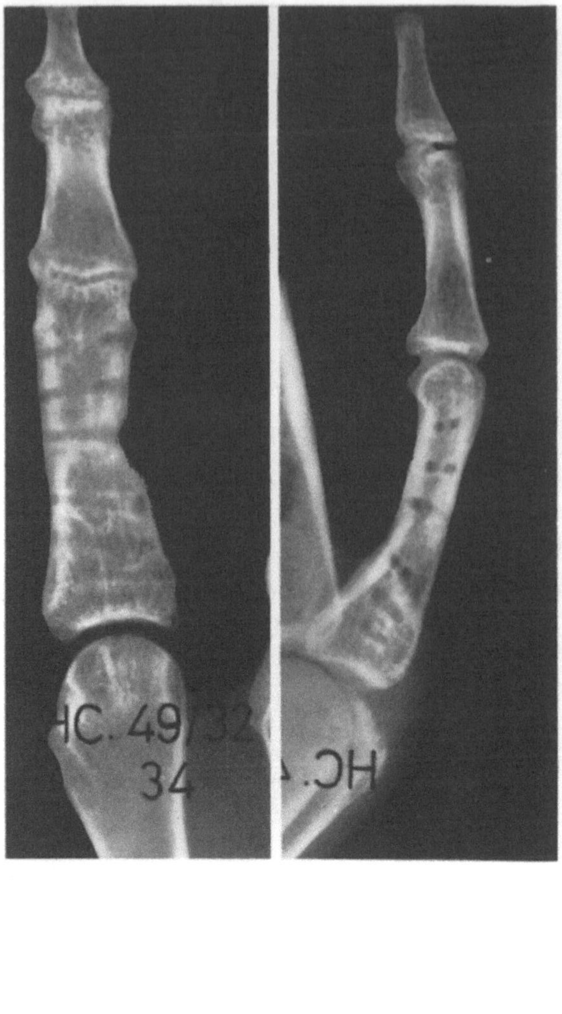

c

Fig. 164a–c. Clinical example: nonunion of the proximal phalanx

Hugo H., 20-year-old laborer, injured the right hand during construction of a cable railway on 6/20/79. The open fracture of the proximal phalanx of the index finger was treated initially with crossed Kirschner wires

a By 4 months the patient had a painful nonunion with ulnar deviation of the index finger, limited motion in all finger joints, and trophic disturbances

b Internal fixation was performed on 10/24/79 with a 6-hole 2.0-mm DCP applied laterally, and the nonunion was grafted with autogenous cancellous bone. Four months later the nonunion was solid. Plate removal and tendolysis were performed at 8 months

c When seen after 11 months on 9/26/80, the patient had resumed his former work. He had no complaints, a linear scar, free MP joint motion, a 35° range of active motion in the PIP and DIP joints, and a mild extension deficit

a, b

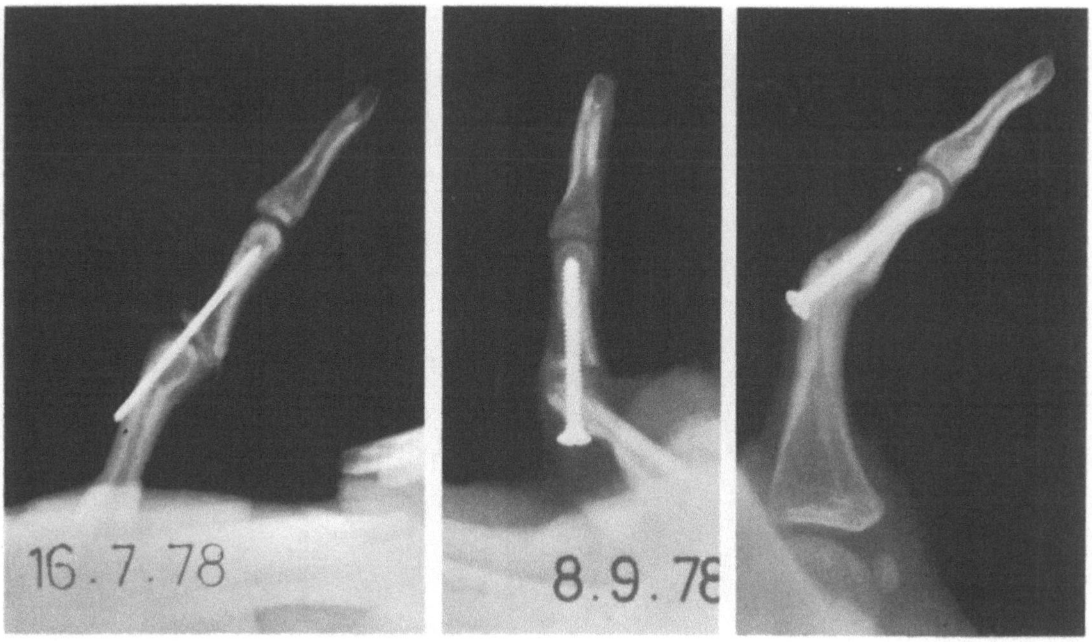

c

Fig. 165a–c. Clinical example: screw arthrodesis of the PIP joint

Ulrich Z., 20-year-old painter, collided with a car while riding a motorcycle

a Open fracture-dislocation of the base of the middle phalanx of the left little finger with bone loss, extensor tendon laceration and tendon defect. The wound was treated, the tendons reapproximated, and the fracture temporarily fixed with a Kirschner wire

b Definitive screw arthrodesis was performed at 6 weeks. The PIP was fused with a 2.0-mm cortex lag screw because of the very narrow medullary cavity of the middle phalanx. The bone defect was grafted with cancellous chips, and an aluminum splint was worn for 2 weeks. The hand was partially rehabilitated at 3 weeks after surgery and fully rehabilitated at 4 weeks

c Fifteen months after the arthrodesis, the screw head was causing some discomfort on the dorsal side of the finger. Patient had no other complaints, complete fist closure, and slight loss of DIP joint motion

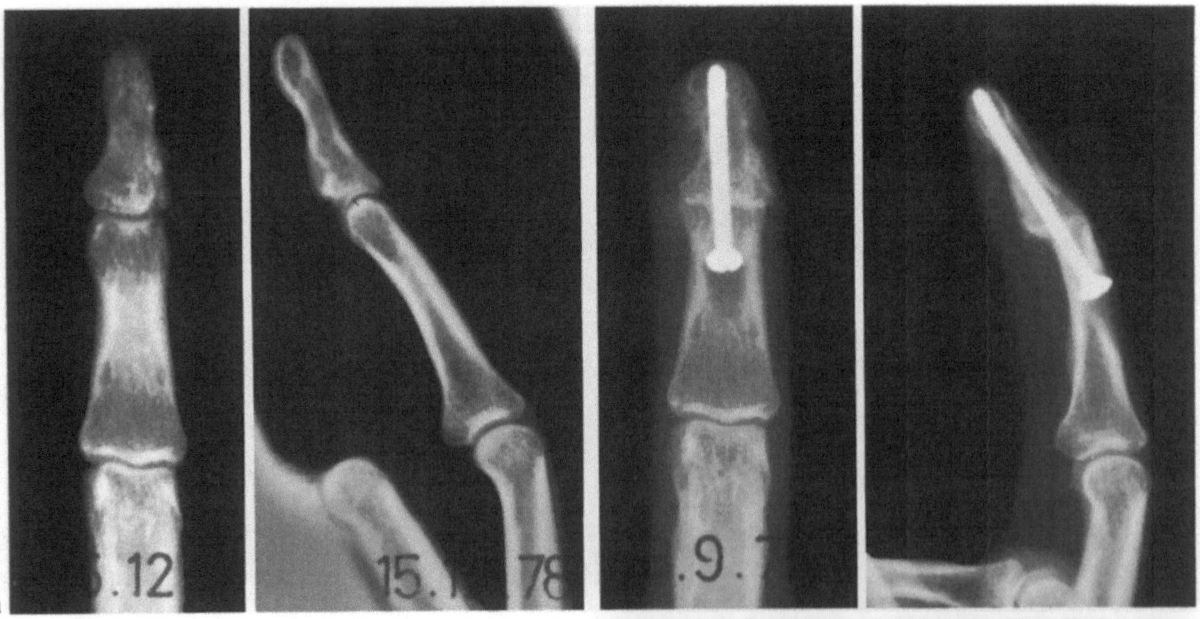

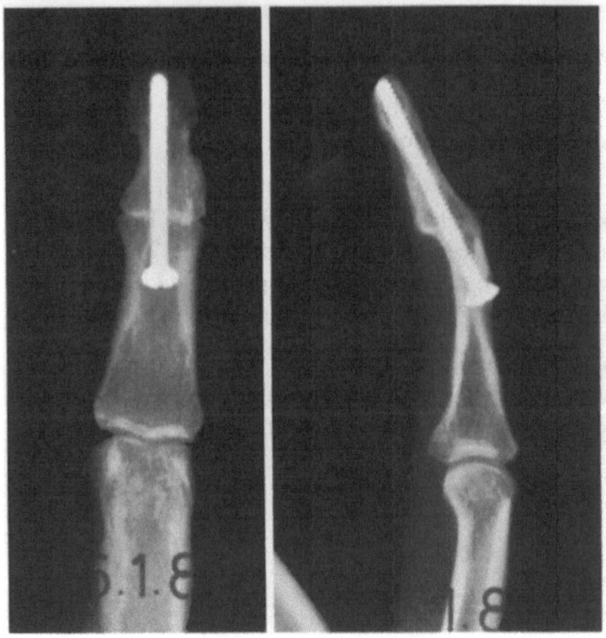

Fig. 166 a–c. Clinical example: screw arthrodesis of the DIP joint from the proximal side

Renee K., 36-year-old secretary
a Painful osteoarthritis of the DIP joint of the right ring finger following two operations elsewhere for a mucoid cyst

b Joint was fused with a 2.0-mm cortex lag screw inserted from the proximal side, and the hand was immediately mobilized. The patient was fully rehabilitated by 4 weeks

c The arthrodesis was solid at 16 weeks (X-ray). The screw head was causing some discomfort, so the screw was removed at 20 weeks. Thereafter the patient had no complaints and full function of the proximal joints

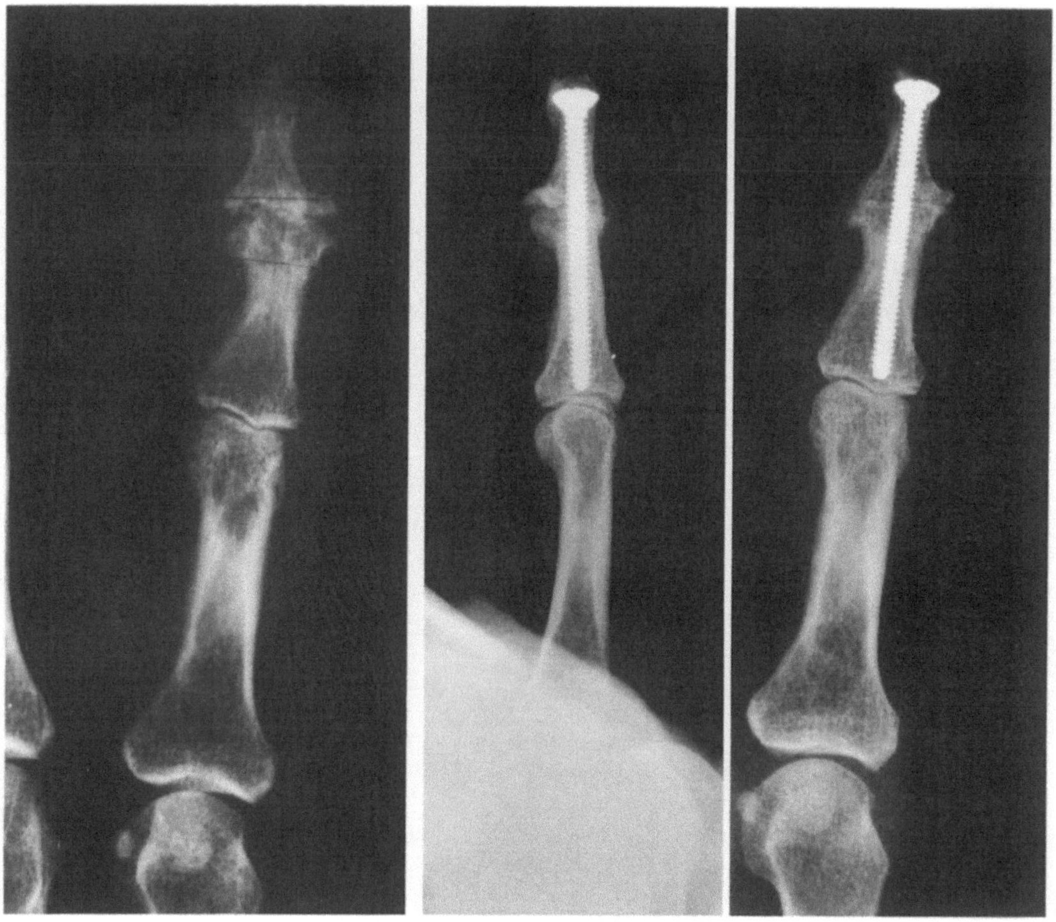

a b

Fig. 167a, b. Clinical example: screw arthrodesis of the DIP joint from the distal side

Georgina H., 53-year-old housewife, had long history of osteoarthritis of the DIP joint of the right little finger with Heberden's nodes, increasing deformity and pain

a Osteoarthritis of the distal joint of the little finger. Joint was fused with an extra-long 2.0-mm cortex lag screw inserted from the distal side on 5/5/84. A protective metal finger splint was worn for 2 weeks

b At 1-month follow-up on 6/7/84, the patient had unrestricted MP and PIP joint motion, no pain and no disability.

Two years later (on 5/5/86) the patient was not bothered by the screw, so it was not removed. She desires the same operation on the little finger of the other hand

XIV. The Knee

Major fractures of the complex knee joint that involve the femoral condyles and upper tibia are fixed with the larger implants of the ASIF standard set. Use of the SFS is limited to the smaller components of major fractures, ligamentous avulsions, and chip fractures. Given the very significant rise in the prevalence of knee joint injuries in recent years, it is appropriate to devote a separate chapter to them.

1. Patella

Transverse fractures of the patella are fixed by the classic technique of tension-band wiring as described in the *Manual of Internal Fixation*. Lately, increasing attention has been given to combining the wire loop with a Kirschner wire, since it is known that necrosis caused by wire tension can lead to shortening of the patellar ligament and upward displacement of the patella. Indications for small screws are limited to longitudinal fractures and to reconstructions of the distal pole.

a) Longitudinal Fracture

This fracture, which is not uncommon, can be difficult to diagnose on standard radiographs, and often it is visible only on tangential views. Fixation with small lag screws has proved effective as both a primary and secondary measure. We previously recommended 4.0-mm cancellous screws, but these are apt to break between the thread and shank when an attempt is made to remove them from the very hard cancellous bone. Thus, assuming it is possible to make a good preliminary gliding hole, it is better to use small, fully threaded screws that are size-matched to the fracture fragments (Fig. 168a). If the fragments are very small or split, washers should also be used.

b) Comminuted Fractures with Longitudinal Components

It is not unusual for longitudinal fracture lines to occur in a comminuted patellar fracture. These fractures should be fixed with screws before the tension-band wire is applied (Fig. 168b).

c) Fractures of the Distal Pole

Fractures and avulsions of the distal pole of the patella are seen with increasing frequency as a result of motor vehicle accidents. They correspond functionally to a rupture of the patellar ligament. The fracture pattern may be transverse or comminuted. If the proximal fragment is large, signifying an intact femoropatellar joint surface, partial patellectomy is contraindicated. The distal fragment can be broadly apposed to the proximal fragment and compressed with a lag screw, at which time smaller fragments are removed as required. This fixation is not strong enough to resist the pull of the quadriceps muscle, however (Fig. 168d, e).

d) Systems to Counteract Muscular Traction (Fig. 168 d, e)

It is necessary to augment and protect the screw fixation with a tension-band wire anchored in the tibial tuberosity. Various fixation techniques may be used proximally and distally:

– The wire is passed around the proximal pole

of the patella in the quadriceps tendon, as in the tension-band wiring of a patellar fracture.

- The wire is passed through a transverse drill hole in the upper patellar fragment.
- The wire is passed through a drill hole in the tibial tuberosity and crossed in front of the ligament. This ensures that symmetrical tension will act on both limbs of the wire.
- The wire loop is anchored on a screw placed transversely through the tibial tuberosity.

The choice of technique should be individualized because of the marked anatomic variations that are encountered. Care must be taken that the implants (wire loops, twist sites, screw heads) do not cause pressure necrosis of the skin, periosteum, or patellar ligament. The point where the wire crosses anterior to the ligament is another potential danger spot. The position of the implants, the length of the wire loop, and the amount of wire tension must be checked with the knee flexed before, during, and after twisting of the wire ends.

2. Tibia

a) Avulsion Fractures of the Intercondylar Eminence (Fig. 169)

These fractures correspond functionally to an avulsion of the tibial insertion of the anterior cruciate ligament of the knee. At one time they were mostly seen in children and adolescents, but today they are seen with increasing frequency as a result of winter sports accidents. Most are isolated, although some present as one component of a complex proximal tibial fracture or combined ligamentous rupture.The avulsed fragment must be accurately reimplanted into its bed and securely fixed in order to become revascularized.The extent of the injury is difficult to assess on roentgenograms, and so it is frequently underestimated in its size and displacement. Operative treatment is always indicated if the bony avulsion has ruptured the periosteal sheath, i.e., when significant displacement has occurred.

The fracture is approached through a longitudinal incision that exposes the anteromedial aspect of the upper tibia at the border of the pes anserinus insertion. The avulsed fragment is reduced with a hook and held firmly against the tibial plateau with a forceps. Most of these fractures can be stably fixed with two 4-mm cancellous screws, 35–45 mm long, slightly offset from each other and inserted with the help of an aiming device. The screws should be placed at approximately the same orientation as the anterior cruciate ligament; they may project slightly past the bony surface into the substance of the ligament. As the screw tips lie within the intercondylar fossa, they will not interfere with motion. The knee is immobilized postoperatively in a plaster cast. Occasionally, small avulsions can be adequately managed with a small cancellous screw driven into the eminence from above. While this screw does not align with the cruciate ligament, it nevertheless provides good interfragmental compression (Fig. 169d).

b) Avulsion Fracture of the Tibial Tuberosity

This rare injury is usually managed with a tension-band wire. Alternatively, a suitably contoured one-third tubular plate may be used to compress the fracture site and also perform a tension-band function (Fig. 170 c).

3. Ligament Repairs

Bony avulsions of the collateral ligaments of the knee can be repaired with screws and spiked washers instead of transosseous sutures. Plastic washers incorporating a radiopaque ring, which can be fixed with 3.5-mm cancellous or cortex screws, have proved excellent for this purpose (Fig. 170b).

The ligament is pulled taut in preparation for screw insertion.It is essential that the screw be placed precisely at the point of ligament insertion, which is easily recognized from the denuded bone and from the convergence of the fibers in a closely circumscribed area. Washers placed over the course of the ligament will cause adhesion of the gliding planes and interfere with free motion.

4. Lateral Avulsion Fractures (Femoral Condyle, Fibular Head)

These injuries correspond functionally to a rupture of the lateral collateral ligament of the knee. Since the powerful biceps muscle inserts on the head of the fibula, an anatomic reconstruction and fixation is necessary for a sound functional result. The avulsed fragment may be fixed with a Kirschner wire and tension-band loop or with screws. The peroneal nerve coursing nearby should be identified and protected. Generally these injuries are accompanied by tears of the joint capsule of the knee and other ligamentous injuries that will require suture repair (Fig. 170 a).

5. Osteochondral Fractures

Injuries that shear an osteochondral fragment from the femoral condyle or posterior patellar surface have been frequently reported in recent years. The loose fragment can remain viable for years, immersed in the nutrient synovial fluid. A sufficiently large fragment can be reimplanted and fixed with small screws whose heads are countersunk flush with the articular cartilage. The screws are removed at 5–6 months.

6. Secondary Operations

a) Nonunion of the Patella

True nonunions are rare and are stabilized with screws and cancellous bone grafts. More common is the traumatic separation of one fragment of a bipartite patella. Again, screw fixation combined with cancellous bone grafting may be appropriate for some of these injuries.

b) Osteochondritis Dissecans

The need to fix large osteochondritic fragments is generally acknowledged. The choice of technique depends on the stage of the disease at the time of diagnosis. A fragment still adherent to its bed is stabilized with screws. The immobilization and compression will promote reincorporation of the sequestered area. Small surface irregularities are of no consequence. The screw heads are countersunk somewhat deeper than usual to prevent abrasion of the opposing articular surface. Follow-up X-rays are taken monthly to monitor the progress of healing. Non-weight bearing is enforced for several months, and the screws generally are removed at one year.

If the osteochondritic area has separated and become a loose body, it is replaced in its bed and fixed with screws. In cases where the bed has undergone degenerative change or is partially filled with fibrous tissue, the bed should be freshened and lined with autogenous cancellous bone before replacing the fragment, which then projects slightly above the level of the joint surface. Screw fixation and aftertreatment are the same as described above (Fig. 171).

The surgeon should be cautioned that the screw heads are apt to be covered by newly formed cartilage at the time of removal and may be difficult to identify.

c) Osteotomy of the Tibial Tuberosity

Osteotomy to advance and medialize the tibial tuberosity is most commonly done to treat osteoarthritis of the femoropatellar joint or severe patellar chondromalacia in adults. Rarely, distal transfer of the tuberosity may be indicated in patients with a high-riding patella. The tuberosity can be advanced anteriorly by the interposition of a corticocancellous wedge (Fig. 172).

7. Illustrative Case Reports and X-Rays (Figs. 173–178)

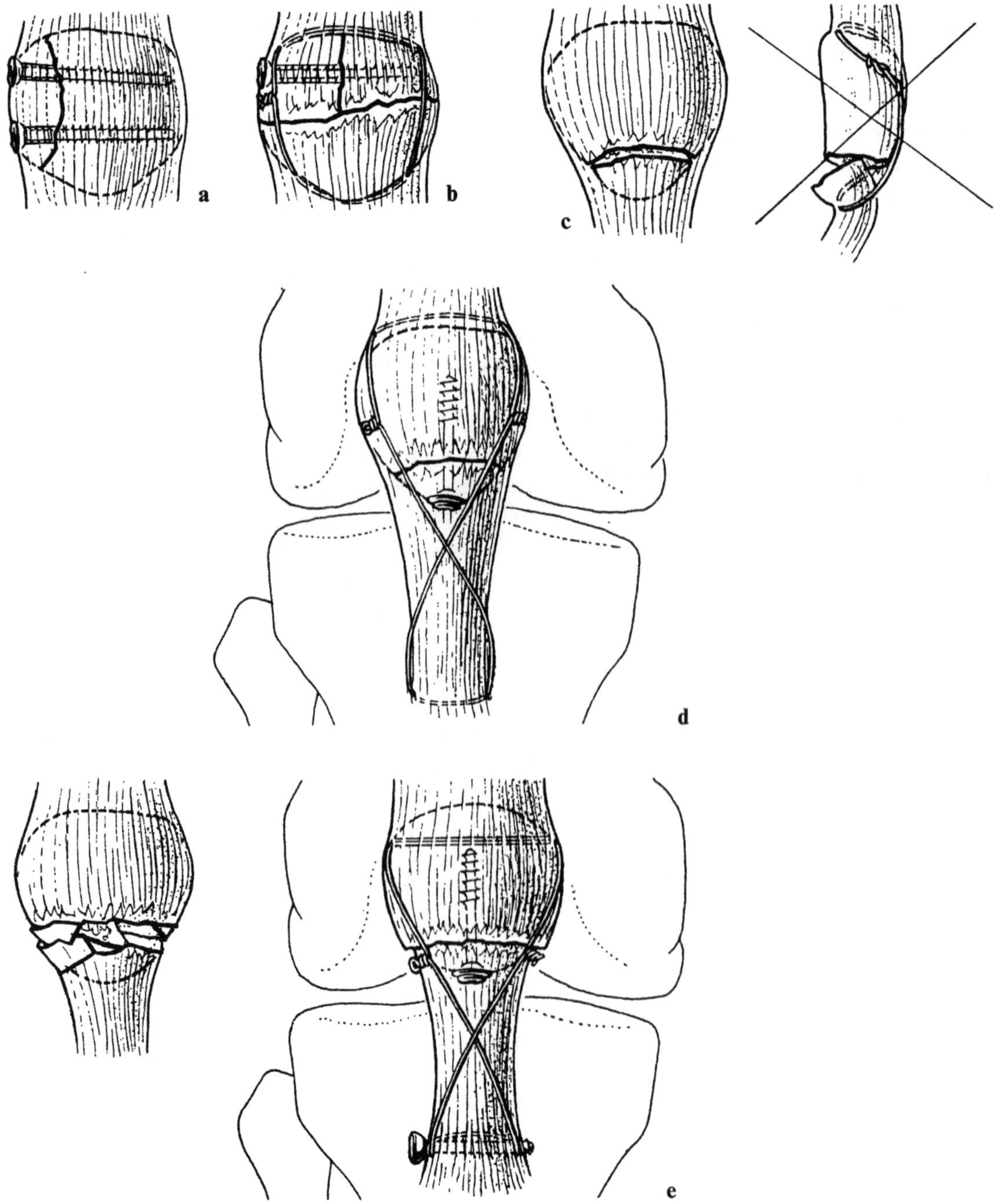

Fig. 168 a–e. Internal fixation of patellar fractures with small implants

a Screw fixation of a longitudinal fracture: 3.5-mm cortex lag screws are preferred, because their thread is easier to cut in the hard bone, and they are easier to remove than cancellous screws with an unthreaded shank

b Lag screw combined with circumferential wire loops for a transverse fracture with a longitudinal component

c A small distal fragment cannot be retained by a wire loop alone

d A simple distal pole fracture is fixed by an axial screw combined with a tension band anchored in the tibial tuberosity

e A comminuted distal pole fracture is managed by a partial patellectomy, followed by screw fixation of the remaining distal fragment to the main proximal fragment. This is reinforced by a wire loop anchored on a transverse screw in the tibial tuberosity. If a distal fragment is not present, the patellar ligament is sutured directly to the proximal main fragment

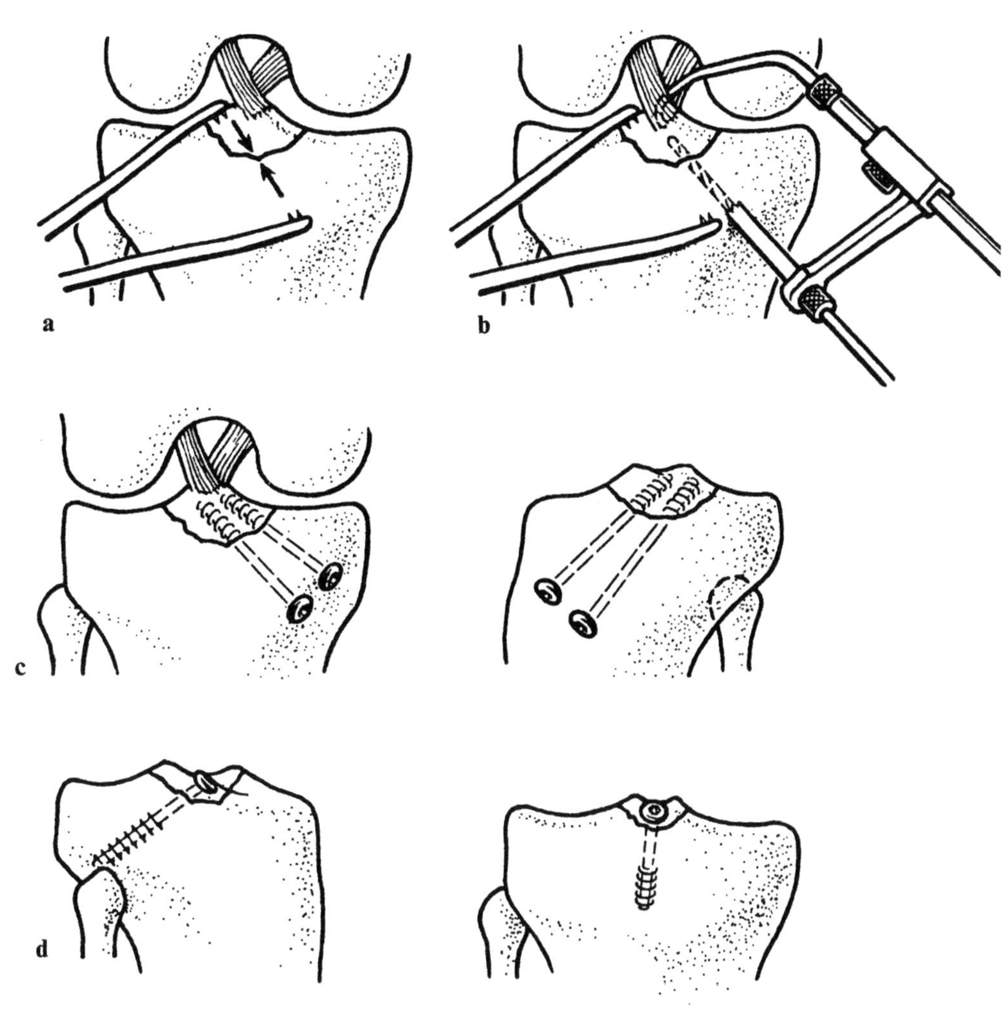

Fig. 169 a–d. Screw fixation of an avulsion fracture of the intercondylar eminence

a The fragment is reduced and held in place with forceps under vision

b The aiming device for the knee is used to drill 2.5-mm holes into the fragment from the medial side

c Cancellous screws with washers are inserted in offset fashion (anterior and lateral views)

d "Direct" screw fixation is suitable for a small fragment: With the patella retracted laterally, the screw is driven obliquely downward through the avulsion site. Caution: This may displace the fragment posteriorly, causing laxity of the anterior cruciate ligament

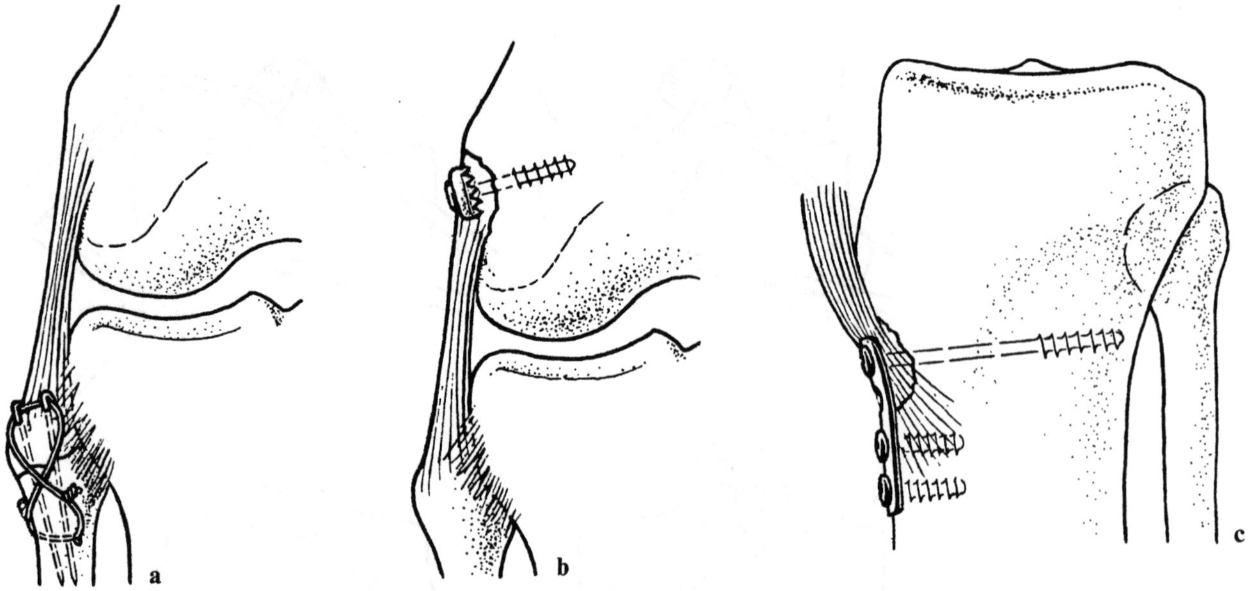

Fig. 170a–c. Fixation of small avulsed fragments about the knee

a Tension-band fixation of the head of the fibula

b Proximal bony avulsion of the lateral collateral ligament, reattached with a screw and plastic spiked washer

c Avulsion fracture of the tibial tuberosity can be fixed with a small tension-band plate or wire system

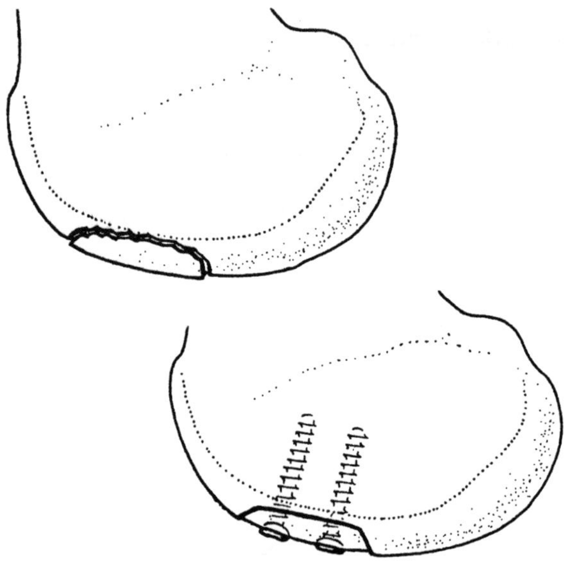

Fig. 171. Screw fixation of an osteochondritic fragment

A fragment that has not completely separated can be fixed in its bed with small cortex screws

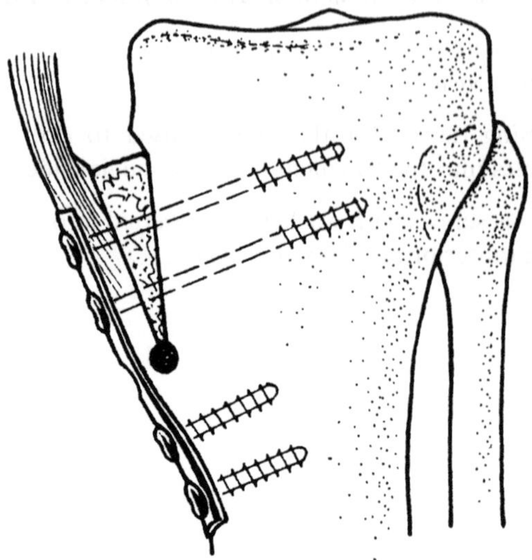

Fig. 172. Osteotomy of the tibial tuberosity

Combined medialization and anterior advancement of the tibial tuberosity by the Roux-Maquet-Bandi technique. The one-third tubular plate compresses the interposed wedge graft and fixes the tuberosity, which remains attached distally to the periosteum

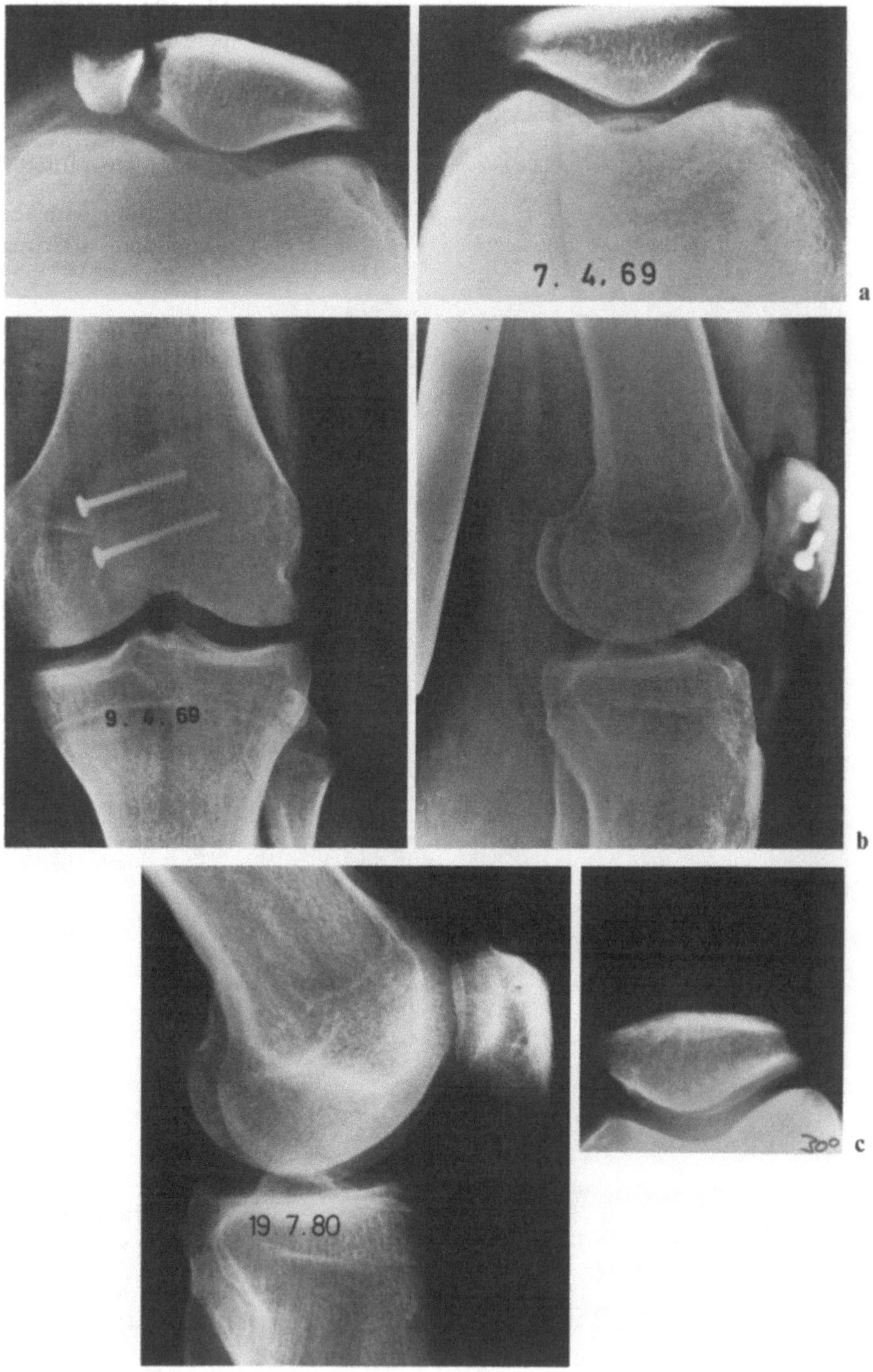

Fig. 173 a–c. Clinical example: screw fixation of a longitudinal fracture of the patella

Claus H., 38-year-old merchant, fell and struck the left knee on a stone on 4/5/69

a Longitudinal patellar fracture with 90° rotation of the fragment and severe swelling. The fracture is visible only on the sunrise view

b On day 4 the fracture was openly reduced and fixed with two small cancellous screws

The postoperative course was uneventful, and the knee was mobilized after wound healing was confirmed. Then a cast was applied for 4 weeks. Full weight bearing was started right away. The screws were removed at 1 year

c When seen 11 years later on 7/19/80, the patient had no complaints, full function, a linear scar, and no osteoarthritis. The screw tracks are still faintly visible on the lateral film

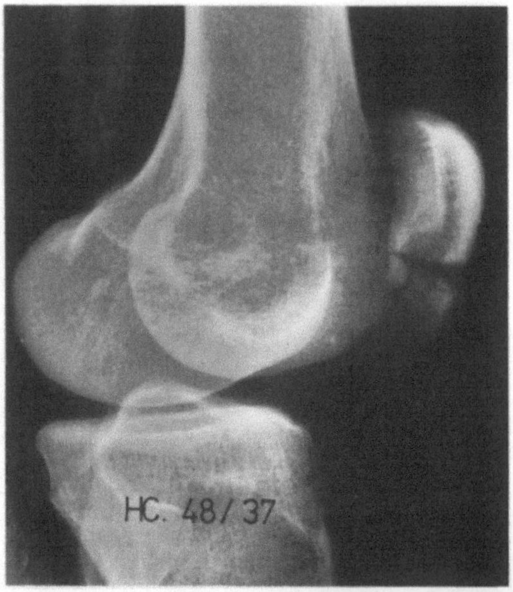

a

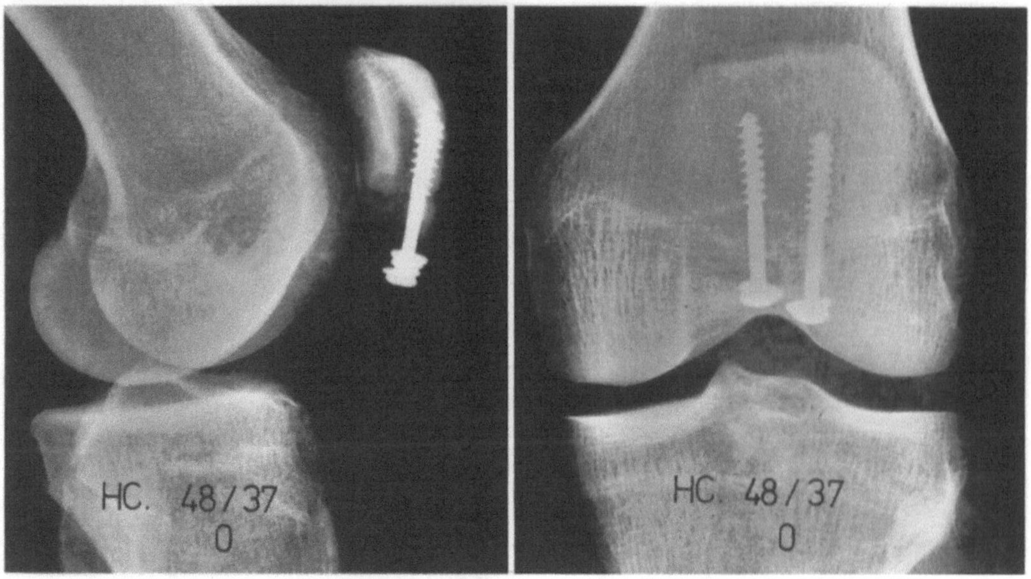

b

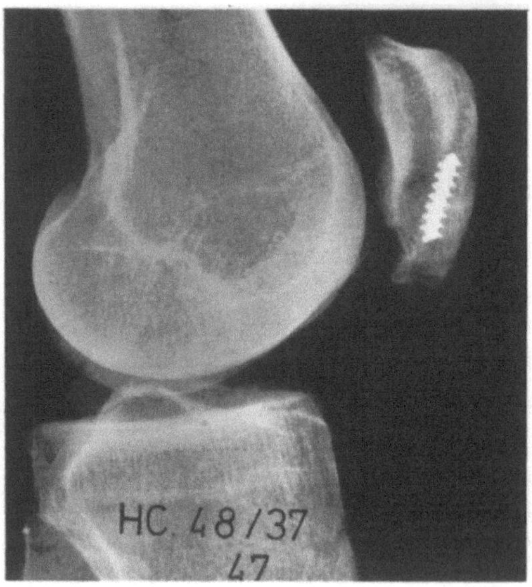

c

Fig. 174a–c. Clinical example: fracture of the distal pole of the patella

Jose D. S., 22-year-old kitchen worker, fell onto the left knee on 6/3/79

a Transverse fracture of the lower pole

b Fixation with cancellous screws and washers. Functional aftertreatment. Full weight bearing at 6 weeks

c At 10 months the Patient had full function, no complaints, no muscular atrophy. One screw broke during removal at the thread-shank junction

Fig. 175a–c. Clinical example: transverse patellar fracture with a longitudinal component ▷

Elsbeth M., 57-year-old housewife. Traffic accident on 10/14/70. Brain concussion

a Comminuted fracture of the lower pole of the patella with longitudinal fracture line

b Emergency surgery: partial patellectomy, proximally transverse screw. Reattachment of the patellar ligament to the proximal fragment. Reinforcement with a tension band wire, anchored in the tibial tuberosity. Cast immobilisation for 2 months. Implant removal at 8 months

c On 9/10/80, 9 years later, the patient had no complaints, full function and a linear scar. X rays without arthritis

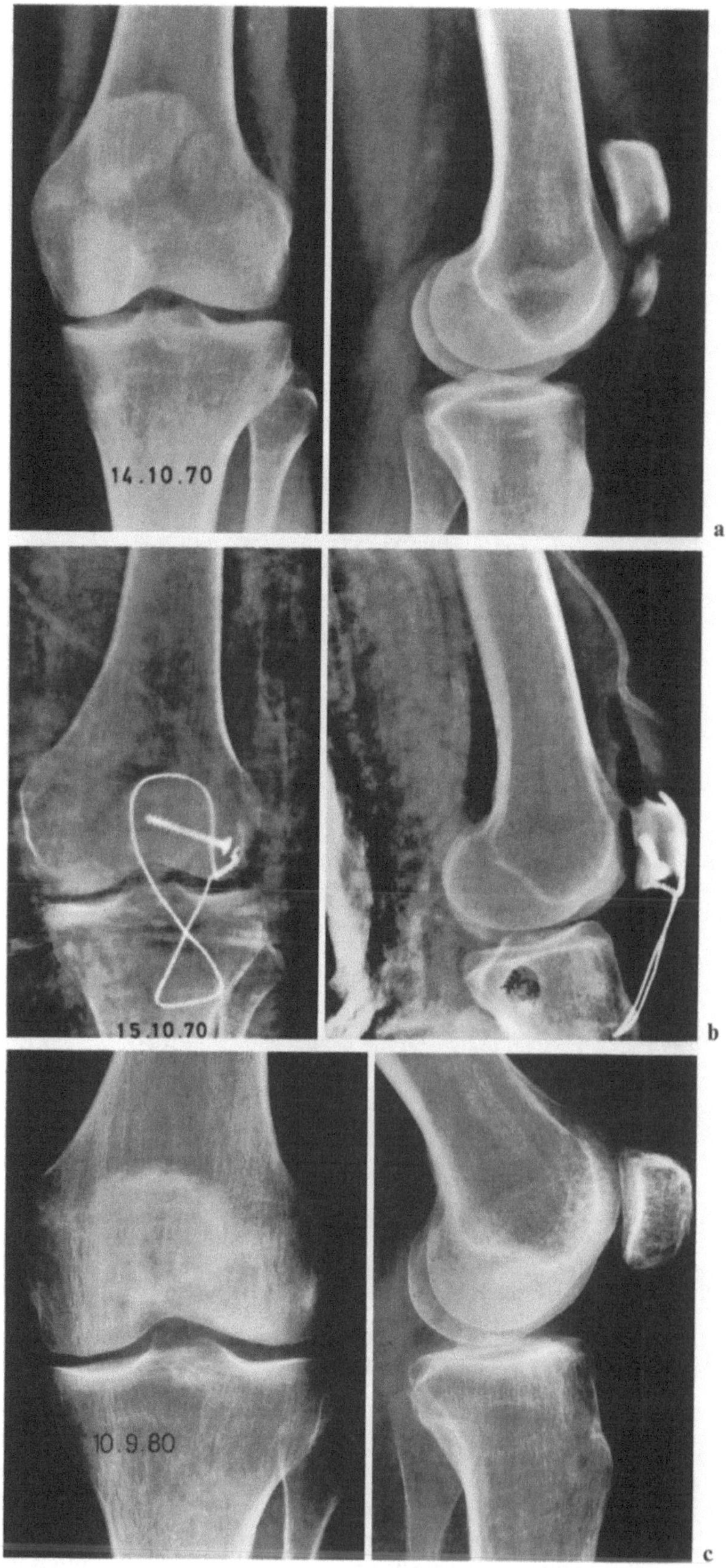
14.10.70
a
15.10.70
b
10.9.80
c

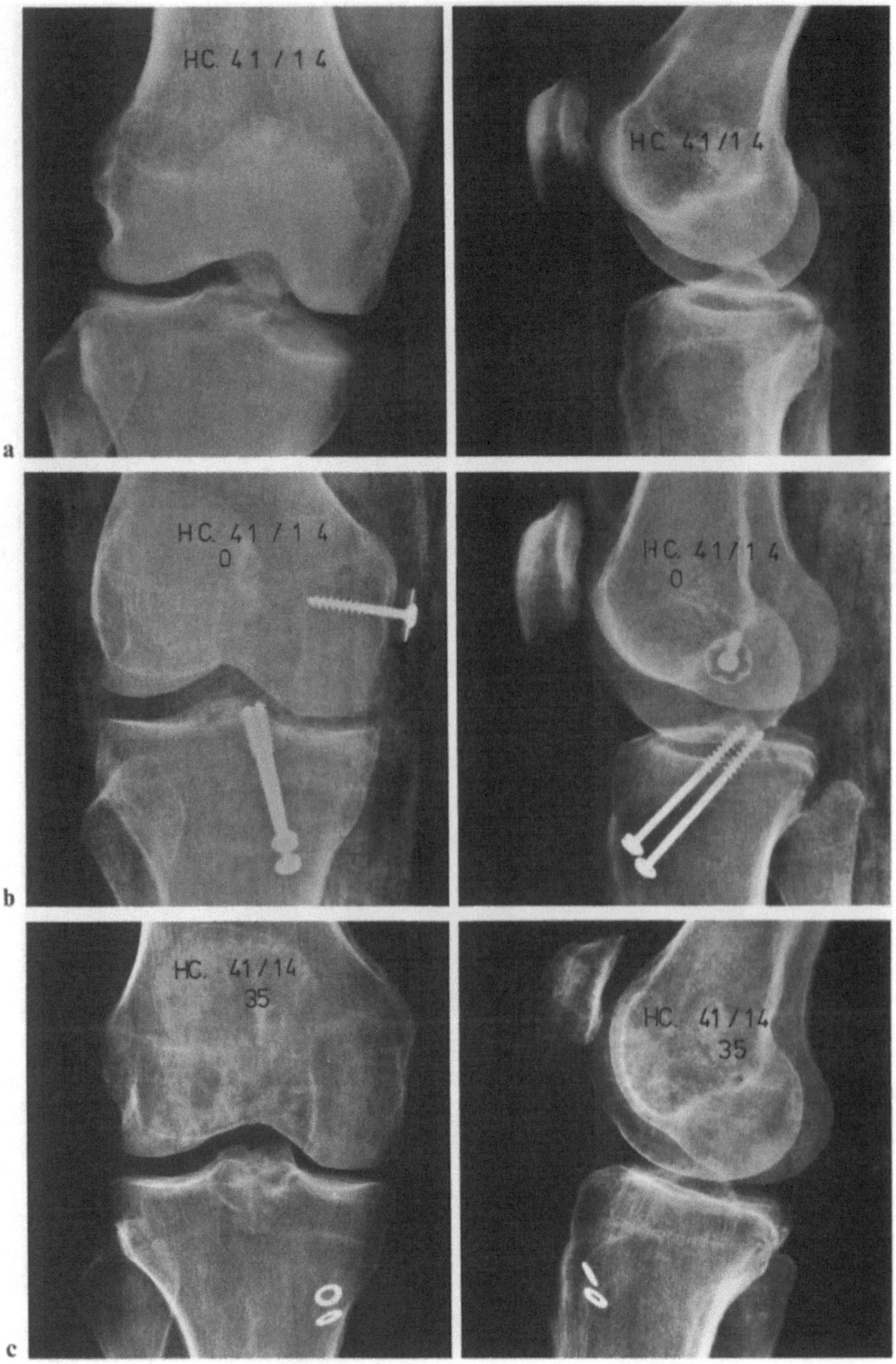

Fig. 176a–c. Clinical example: avulsion fracture of the intercondylar eminence accompanied by rupture of the medial collateral ligament of the knee

Jutta B., 44-year-old physician, fell while skiing on 2/16/78

a Avulsion fracture of the intercondylar eminence, anteromedial instability with femoral avulsion of the medial collateral ligament and partial femoral avulsion of the anterior cruciate ligament

b At emergency internal fixation the intercondylar eminence was fixed with screws, the medial collateral ligament was reattached to the femur with a screw and plastic spiked washer, and the capsule and cruciate ligament were repaired with sutures
The patient was discharged with a knee cast after an uneventful course. Mobilization and full weight bearing were started at 10 weeks

c Eight months later at implant removal, the knee was stable and painless and had full motion. Slight muscular atrophy was noted

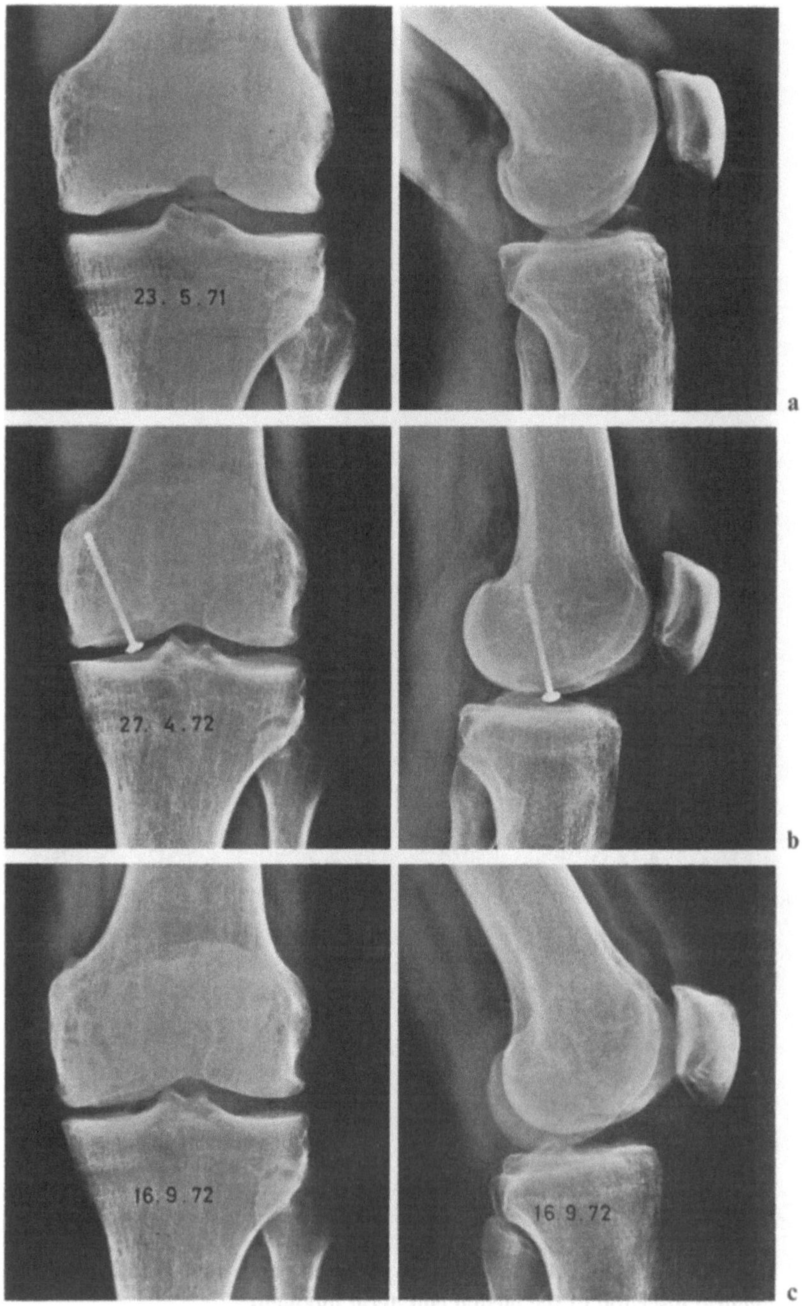

Fig. 177 a–c. Clinical example: screw fixation of an osteochondritic fragment in the knee joint

Constantino C., 25-year-old construction site worker, experienced locking of the knee joint after kicking a soccer ball with the left knee slightly twisted. Clinical examination showed a 30° extension deficit and mild effusion. X-rays showed a loose body avulsed from the medial femoral condyle and lying in the intercondylar fossa

a At arthrotomy 2 days later, the viable loose body was returned to its bed on the medial condyle and fixed with a small cancellous screw. One week later a non-weight-bearing cast was applied for 6 weeks, then the knee was exercised without weight bearing until week 10. Patient resumed full work load at 4 1/2 months

b At 11 months the patient had no complaints and equal knee function on both sides.X-rays confirmed incorporation of the fragment

c The screw was removed at 16 months

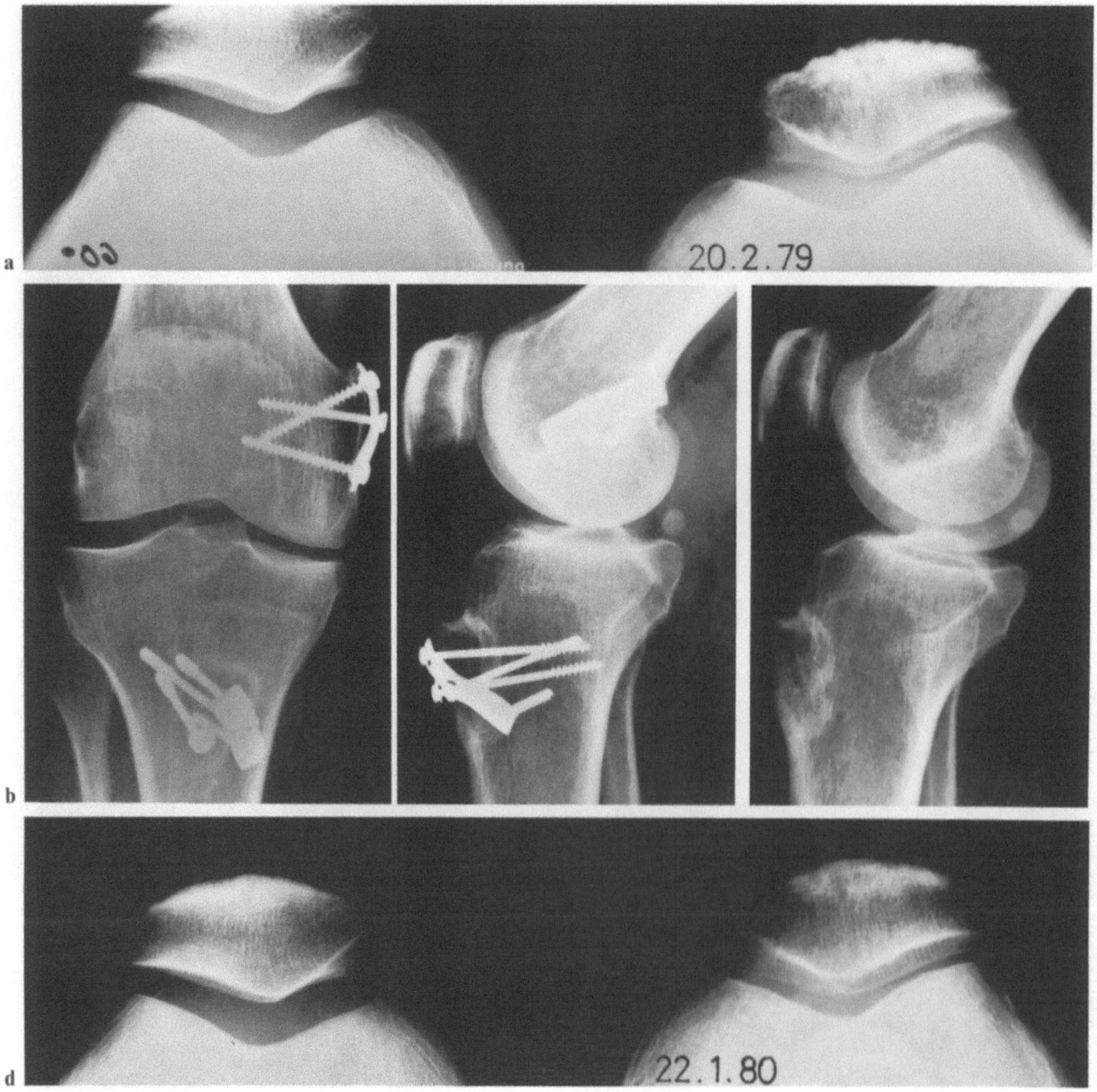

Fig. 178a–d. Clinical example: advancement and medialization of the tibial tuberosity and osteotomy of the femoral insertion of the medial collateral ligament

Caspar B., 34-year-old railway official, sprained knee while skiing in 1967. A slowly progressive patellar chondromalacia ensued, with medial instability of the knee and meniscus symptoms.Shaving of the patella, incision of the retinaculum, and medial meniscectomy were performed on 12/1/78 but were of no benefit

a Evidence of patellar lateralization and overload was noted in February, 1979. The tibial tuberosity was advanced and medialized (with an interposed graft) on 3/6/79, and the femoral insertion of the medial collateral ligament was osteotomized and advanced proximally. Quadriceps exercises were started, and a knee cast was worn for 8 weeks, followed by progressive weight bearing and mobilization. A gradual regression of osteoporosis was observed

b The implants were removed at 8 months

c Lateral radiograph following implant removal

d By 11 months patellar gliding was restored. At $1^1/_2$ years the patient had full function and showed marked quadriceps improvement. The knee was stable, and the patient was able to participate in sports

XV. The Tibial Shaft

Internal fixations of the tibial shaft in adults are ordinarily performed with standard-size implants. In the rare cases where internal fixation is indicated for tibial shaft fractures in children, the DCP for 3.5-mm screws has proved most useful owing to its strength and small size.

Individual small screws may be used in conjunction with standard implants for internal fixations of the adult tibia. The 3.5-mm cortex screws are recommended, following the technique shown in Figs. 23–24. Use of the separate insert drill sleeve is mandatory in the wide medullary cavity.Unguided, the 2.5-mm drill bit might easily bend or break if it had to penetrate two hard cortices in succession. The tap is subject to the same danger. Particular care must be exercised if the far cortex is thick.

There are basically three situations which justify the use of small screws in the tibial shaft (Fig. 179):

a) Narrow Bone Spikes

The small cortex screw is excellent for fixing bone fragments that terminate in narrow spikes. The danger of splitting the fragment is much less than if standard-size implants were used.

b) Small Butterfly Fragments

Similar considerations have led to the increasing use of small lag screws for the fixation of small butterfly fragments. The flat screw heads will not crack the cortex or damage the periosteum.

c) Detached Cortical Fragments

The accurate reassembly of small, detached cortical fragments is desirable in comminuted fractures. This makes it easier to reduce the remaining parts of the fracture, and it increases the overall stability of the assembly. Revascularization of the fragments may be anticipated if they are accurately fitted into place and fixed atraumatically with small cortex screws. The small, 4.0-mm cancellous screw is preferred in the more distal cancellous bone.

Very often it will not be possible to preserve the viability of small posterolateral fragments, and in these cases it is better to graft the defects primarily with autogenous cancellous bone than attempt an anatomic reduction.

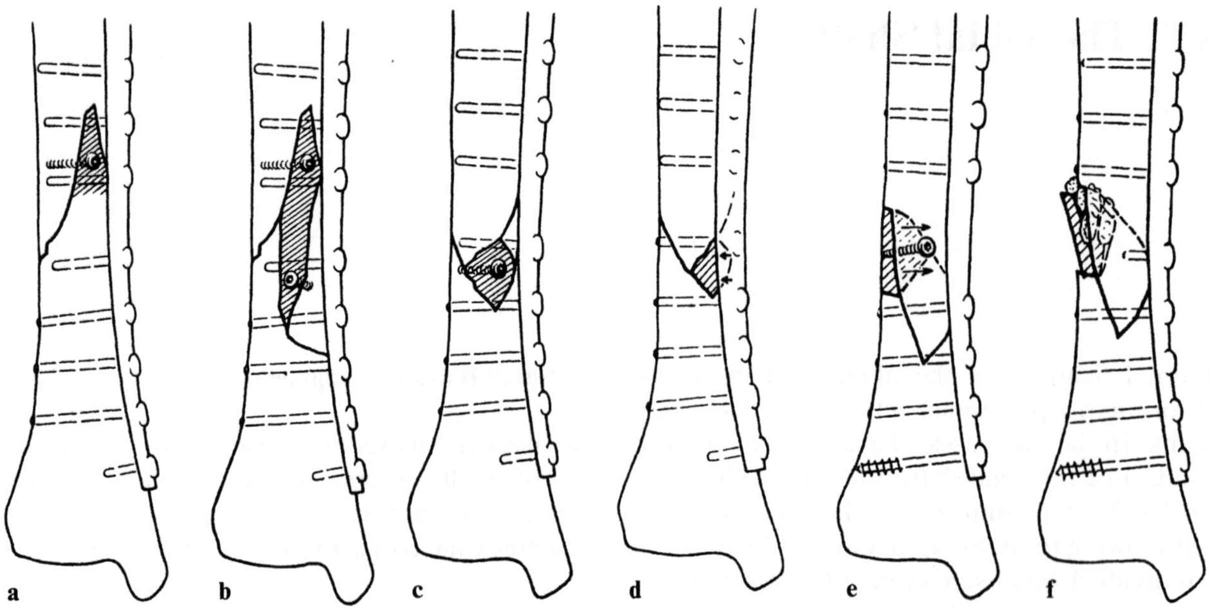

Fig. 179a–f. Applications of small cortex lag screws in the tibial shaft

a For fixing narrow bone spikes

b For fixing small anterior butterfly fragments

c For the stable fixation of anterior cortical fragments

d A small cortical fragment is stabilized by applying the main implant (plate) over it wherever possible

e A posterolateral butterfly fragment is anatomically reduced and fixed with a screw only if this can be done without devitalizing the fragment or sacrificing its periosteal attachment

f Here an anatomic reduction is avoided in the interest of fragment viability. The posterior cortex is grafted with autogenous cancellous bone

XVI. The Ankle Joint

Small implants have become a mainstay in the treatment of fractures about the ankle joint. This holds true for the various types of malleolar fracture as well as for distal articular fractures of the tibia and talus.

From the outset, the ASIF has considered most of these fractures to be an indication for operative treatment. But our techniques of skeletal fixation have evolved over time, owing to a growing understanding of concomitant soft-tissue injuries and surgical approaches and to an ongoing critical review of long-term results.

The small implants of the SFS have completely replaced the fibular medullary nail and large cancellous screws, and even malleolar screws have become largely obsolete. The small plates occupy little space, cause minimal tissue trauma, and are easily contoured to bony surface anatomy.

The present section is concerned more with the description of technical details than with questions of patient selection.

A. Distal Intra-Articular Fractures of the Tibia

Fractures of the distal, weight-bearing articular surface of the tibia are called "pilon fractures," a term coined by the French radiologist Destot in 1911. The noun *pilon* means "pestle" or "ram," and the verb *pilonner* means "to ram" or "to stamp." Thus, the French term graphically expresses both the morphology of the distal tibia and the mechanism of the injury.

Much has been written about the classification of these fractures. The most widely used classification, published by Gay and Evrard in 1963, is based on lesions in the frontal plane–the plane that is depicted on lateral radiographs. Three main groups are recognized: posterior marginal fractures, anterior marginal fractures, and "bimarginal fractures" affecting both sides of the articular surface. This classification assigns fractures of the posterolateral tibial margin to the pilon category, but ordinarily they are considered to be a type of malleolar fracture (fracture of the "posterior malleolus," known also as "Volkmann's triangle").

The morphologic differentiation of these complex fractures is difficult. A classification consistent with ASIF principles must take into account both the technical difficulty of the procedure and the prognosis of the injury.

After preliminary studies in 1979 and 1980, an ABC system for the classification of distal tibial fractures was developed in 1986 on the basis of extensive case data compiled at the ASIF documentation center in Bern (Fig. 180).

The major factors in terms of differentiation and prognosis are the condition of the weight-bearing articular surface and the degree of instability. Since the medial malleolus is non-weight-bearing and therefore not subject to osteoarthritis, we do not need to consider medial malleolar fractures in this context. Fractures of the lateral malleolus are considered only in terms of their potential for creating extra technical problems at operation. These would include multiple fractures and fractures that are associated with bone loss.

The articular injury may involve part or all of the joint.

- Type B fractures are partial articular fractures. One portion of the joint maintains its continuity with the shaft.
- Type C fractures affect the joint on all planes.

V, Y, and T fractures are the simple forms. In C2 fractures, a supramalleolar, metaphyseal cancellous bone impaction or comminution is combined with a split in the weight-bearing articular surface. These fractures are especially common in skiing injuries. Because the cancellous bone defect is often combined with angular deformity (usually posterior angulation), the postinjury radiograph can appear quite dramatic on one plane because of superimposition, and it can mimic a joint impaction. But a well-centered radiograph on a second plane will disclose fissures or possibly steps in the joint line, with no crushing of the articular surface. This type of fracture was first mentioned by Weber in 1966, and its features were analyzed and described in detail by Bandi in 1970. Its prognosis is relatively good (Fig. 180).

- A *depressed fracture* of the articular surface is caused by pure compression. The depressed segment may be central or peripheral, and its impaction precludes a closed reduction by ligamentotaxis.The segment must be pushed back into place from within (impactor, elevator, osteotome), creating a defect in the subchondral cancellous bone. This epiphyseal defect contrasts with the metaphyseal defect that is produced in C2 fractures (Fig. 180).

Depressed articular fractures almost always lead to osteoarthritis. In the more complex forms where depression and comminution coexist (type C3), it may be technically impossible to obtain an anatomic reduction. These injuries have the poorest prognosis of all the pilon fractures.

Operative treatment is indicated in these cases (soft tissues permitting) because of the need to reconstitute the articular surface and provide the stability needed for postperative functional exercises, which are important for cartilage regeneration.

Split fractures with associated metaphyseal cancellous bone impaction (type C2) and complex depressed fractures (types B3 and C3) are very challenging technically. In the former, an attempt must be made to reassemble the displaced metaphyseal fragments; in the latter, the main emphasis is on reconstructing the articular surface of the tibia. Since the technique of open reduction and internal fixation is similar for both types, we shall limit our description of surgical technique to three forms: the simple split fracture, the simple depressed articular fracture, and the complex fracture with a cancellous bone defect.

1. Split Fractures without a Cancellous Bone Defect (Fig. 182)

These fractures are usually approached through bilateral incisions. On the lateral side, attention is directed to fibular fractures, coexisting ligament tears, and anterolateral avulsions. Medially, the ankle joint is opened anterior to the medial malleolus so that reduction can be carried out under vision.

Simple screw fixation may be adequate in some cases, but medial plating is recommended when multiple fragments are found.A DCP or shaped plate may be preferred, depending on the fracture.

2. Simple Depressed Fracture (Fig. 180 B2)

This is a transitional form between the tibial pilon and malleolar fracture. Its main feature is a simple depression of the articular surface, usually combined with a split fracture extending upward from the joint. The latter may consist of an adduction fracture of the medial malleolus. Often there are associated lateral ligamentous tears, which must not be overlooked. This category would include marginal depression of the tibia with an associated fracture of the posterior malleolus. This injury is frequently missed on standard radiographs. The technique of operative treatment is described in the section on Malleolar Fractures (Fig. 215).

An anatomic reconstruction of the joint surface is crucial to postoperative mobilization and arthritis prophylaxis. A unilateral approach may suffice. Usually the cancellous defect is small and can be repaired with graft material taken from adjacent bone, such as the medial tibial metaphysis. An anterior fragment can be stabilized with a small T plate (3.5-mm or even 2.7-mm) pressed firmly against the bone with screws anchored in the intact posterior cancellous bone.

3. Complex Fractures with a Cancellous Bone Defect (Figs. 183ff.)

Two different mechanisms of injury are recognized in these fractures:

- Fracture caused by a skiing accident. Generally this is a closed fracture having multiple fragments and a complex structure. It is produced by a combination of compression, shear, and bending. A type C2 fracture morphology is present.
- Compression fracture. This is usually caused by a fall from a height or by sudden deceleration in an auto accident. The B3 and C3 morphologies prevail. A large percentage of these fractures are open, and many affect elderly or psychiatric patients whose ability to cooperate is limited. Thus, the soft-tissue problems and the patient's mental status are quite different than in sports-related injuries, and this will influence operative tactics, technique, and prognosis.

The operation for skiing-related pilon fractures is fairly standard and can serve as a model for the treatment of these complex injuries:

a) Operative Tactics

The basic tactical principles were defined by Rüedi, Matter, and Allgöwer in 1968 and have become well established:

- Internal fixation of the fibula
- Reconstruction of the tibial articular surface
- Autogenous cancellous bone grafting
- Medial buttressing with a plate

Internal fixation of the fibula is carried out first, because the length, angular alignment, and rotation of the fibula serve as indicators for the reduction of the tibial articular surface, and because a stable fibula will lend stability to the entire region.

After the fibula has been stabilized, the articular surface is reduced, followed next by reduction of the remaining fracture components. The epiphyseal and metaphyseal fragments, often scattered like the pieces of a jigsaw puzzle, must be reassembled and held in position with Kirschner wires. At this time the extent of the cancellous bone defect can be assessed. The defect is packed with autogenous graft material to create a solid epi- and metaphyseal block. The final step is to join this block to the tibial shaft with a medial plate. The plate not only serves as a buttress but also helps stabilize the articular fragments on the sagittal and frontal planes.

The choice of implant depends on the fracture type. The DCP, T plate, or cloverleaf plate is excellent for the medial side. A predominantly anterior impaction can be managed with a spoon plate or radial T plate (see Fig. 6).

In most open fractures the lesion is located on the medial side, and surgical tactics must be adapted accordingly. Primary internal fixation of the fibula is still recommended to facilitate subsequent measures. This may be combined with calcaneus traction or with three-point external fixation applied to the tibia, talus, and calcaneus. In suitable cases the medial reduction and cancellous bone grafting may be done primarily, leaving the preliminary Kirschner wires in place (Fig. 187). Medial plating is always contraindicated for open fractures, however.

b) Preparations

In most of these fractures there is considerable post-traumatic swelling whose extent cannot be predicted immediately after the injury.To avoid skin necrosis and other soft-tissue problems, we prefer to begin treatment by applying traction on the calcaneus with the leg elevated on a splint. The operation is performed as soon as swelling subsides, usually within 3–4 days. A longer delay makes reduction more difficult.

The preliminary traction will reduce angular deformities and diastases and will make it easy to recognize sites of articular compression.

The period before surgery should be utilized for preoperative planning. Usually additional radiologic studies (oblique X-rays, tomograms, possibly CT scans) are necessary to bring out all the details of the injury. The surgeon should study the films carefully so that he can identify special problems and adapt his technique accordingly. He must bear in mind that the presence of a tourniquet will limit operating time.

c) Approach

An accurate reconstruction demands complete exposure of all fracture elements and ligamentous injuries. Blood flow conditions in the tibial metaphysis are favorable. Long, bilateral incisions should be used to decrease instrument pressure on the skin and give sufficient access to deeper structures.

Lateral Incision (Fig. 181 b). A lazy S-shaped incision is made from the posterior border of the distal fibular shaft distally over the anterior border of the lateral malleolus. The superficial branch of the peroneal nerve coursing in that area is identified and spared. The approach must give access to the often complex lateral malleolar fracture and to anterolateral fragments of the tibia. Access may also be needed to lateral portions of the tibial articular surface, the superior surface of the talus, the anterior syndesmosis, and the fibulotalar ligaments. The latter are repaired if torn.

The bridge of skin between the lateral incision and medial incision (supplied by anterior tibial artery) should be at least 5 cm wide to maintain an adequate cutaneous blood supply (Fig. 181 a).

Medial Incision (Fig. 181 a). We prefer a slightly curved incision made from the distal anterior tibial border to the sole of the foot, passing anterior to the medial malleolus. The ankle joint is opened widely just anterior to the deltoid ligament, which is always intact. It is necessary to visualize the medial malleolus, the anteromedial parts of the joint, the adjacent metaphysis, the medial dome of the talus, and the posteromedial tibial border. Often there is a posteromedial fracture line (especially with posterior angulation) that needs to be reduced under vision; otherwise secondary displacement is a danger.

d) Reassembly of the Fragments

The reconstruction begins with *definitive fixation of the fibula.* We generally use a long one-third tubular plate (6- to 8-hole) for this purpose, as it gives adequate stability even in comminuted fractures. Technical details are discussed in the section on Malleolar Fractures (Figs. 202 ff.).

Reduction and reconstruction of the tibial articular surface can be very demanding technically. It is started on the lateral or medial side, depending on circumstances, and usually the operator will have to change his working site frequently while correcting and realigning any steps, depressions, or defects that are found. Sometimes the medial malleolar fragment will have to be turned forward and temporarily retracted to expose anterior joint incongruities (Fig. 184 a). Multiple Kirschner wires are inserted to hold the reassembled fragments temporarily in place.

e) Autogenous Cancellous Bone Grafting

Following restoration of the articular surface, the defects produced by compaction of the cancellous bone must be packed with autogenous cancellous chips to prevent subsequent collapse (supportive effect) and to accelerate fracture union (biologic effect).

Our preferred donor sites in elderly patients and in patients requiring large amounts of graft material are the iliac crest and iliac fossa (Fig. 185). In these cases the cancellous bone is harvested in a separate operation in order to shorten the tourniquet time for the main procedure.

In younger individuals who require less graft material, we take the cancellous bone from the upper tibia of the injured leg during the main operation. This is a very simple, safe, and time-saving procedure done on an area that is readily accessible in the sterile field. The proximal and distal tibia have separate blood supplies, so fracture healing is not affected. Also, non-weight bearing postoperatively protects both the donor site and the site of the reconstruction.

Technique: A skin incision 3–4 cm long is made over the medial aspect of the upper tibia. The periosteum is incised and reflected. The cortex is windowed with an osteotome, and the soft cancellous bone is harvested with a curette (Fig. 185). A considerable volume is available. At the end of the operation we measure the volume removed by filling the donor cavity with

Ringer's solution. The periosteum and skin are closed separately without a drain.

The finely textured cancellous bone is packed into the defect through a preexisting or specially created cortical opening in the anteromedial fracture area. This may be done after reduction and provisional fixation with Kirschner wires, or after the trial fitting of the medial plate, before screws have been inserted into the area of the defect. The cancellous bone is pressed firmly into place so that all cavities are filled.

f) Internal Fixation of the Tibia

Generally we begin by fixing the lateral tibial fragments with screws. We then contour the medial plate and attach it definitively. Rarely it is necessary to remove the posterior tab of the cloverleaf plate to avoid impingement on the tibialis posterior tendon. In complex comminuted fractures, screws must be placed on multiple planes to achieve a stable fixation.

When the cloverleaf plate is used, it is first attached distally, giving constant attention to the position and stability of the individual fracture elements and correcting any malalignments that are seen. A forceps holds the plate to the shaft temporarily while separate screws are placed as needed to secure remaining unstable fragments. It is not necessary to place screws into all the plate holes. However, it is necessary to anchor the implant solidly to the medial malleolus, as this will prevent secondary varus.

As the medial part of the fixation is carried out, the Kirschner wires placed initially are successively removed.The plate is attached to the proximal main fragment with 3.5-mm cortex screws (Fig. 186).

The operation is concluded by closing the joint capsule, partially suturing the periosteum, and inserting suction drains on each side. The soft tissues are easily reapproximated over the flat plate and screws. These do not significantly alter the normal ankle contour, and the patient is able to wear ordinary shoes.

g) Aftertreatment

We routinely elevate the foot on a right-angle plaster splint for several days postoperatively and start active exercises right away, avoiding excessive stress until the swelling has subsided. Thus, these patients will require a somewhat longer hospitalization than patients undergoing simpler internal fixations of the tibia. The surgeon should decide how to schedule and increment the resumption of weight bearing. Before the patient stands, the leg is placed in a rigid circumferential dressing and the wound checked for secondary hematomas. The primary functional goal is heel-to-toe rocking of the foot, and partial weight bearing of 10–15 kg may be allowed in suitable cases. Usually weight bearing is increased after 12–16 weeks, and full weight bearing is permitted at 16–20 weeks.

The medial plate is not removed until the 14th month. The large number of screws do not seem to be a problem, and corrosion is negligible because of the small areas of contact between the implants.

4. Secondary Operations

Secondary operations occasionally have to be performed on the distal tibia for nonunion or deformity. Most cases involve varus deformity, which often is associated with posterior angulation and malrotation. The combination of valgus and malrotation is less common. Osteotomy of the fibula is not always necessary. Double plates may be applied to the tibial metaphysis without concern. For anatomic reasons, the plate that will transmit the greater stress should be placed on the medial side, and it is advantageous to attach the end of the plate to the medial malleolus. The wide cloverleaf plate is sufficiently stable when applied under primary axial compression.

a) Varus Deformity

Operative correction is generally indicated for a symptomatic varus that exceeds about 8°. Fibular osteotomy usually is not required. In some cases we recommend the preliminary attachment of a short one-third tubular plate laterally between the main fragments to prevent splitting and gaping of the lateral cortex (Fig. 188 a).

Next the medial correction is carried out, which may involve opening a nonunion or performing an osteotomy. An open-wedge defect is filled with autogenous cancellous bone chips or with a corticocancellous graft. It is best to overcorrect the deformity slightly. The medial plate is applied and attached distally, and its upper end is pulled proximally with the tension device to compress the graft (Fig. 188c, d).

b) Valgus Deformity

Operative correction is indicated for a symptomatic valgus that exceeds about 12°. It is achieved by a simple wedge-resection osteotomy performed about 3 cm above the joint line and stabilized with a medial plate and axial compression. Osteotomy of the fibula is usually unnecessary (Fig. 189).

c) Malrotation

This frequently accompanies a varus or valgus deformity. Marked deformity of the fibula is often present, and correction requires osteotomy of both the tibia and fibula. The tibia is stabilized with a 3.5-mm DCP and one-third tubular plate or possibly with a cloverleaf plate (Fig. 190).

d) Aftertreatment

The stability achieved with these osteotomies allows early mobilization without plaster support in nearly all cases. Joint motion is regained quickly during bone healing–an advantage in terms of joint nutrition and blood supply. Generally the bone is solid enough for weight bearing by 8–12 weeks.

5. Illustrative Case Reports and X-Rays

(Figs. 191–195)

Fig. 180. Classification of distal tibial fractures

A = Extra-articular fracture
A1 = Simple fracture
A2 = Wedge fracture in which contact between the main fragments is preserved
A3 = Multi-part fracture with no contact between the main fragments

B = Intra-articular fracture involving only part of the articular surface
B1 = Simple split fracture
B2 = Depressed split fracture
B3 = Local comminution of the articular surface, preserving one wall

C = Circumferential articular injury
C1 = Split fracture involving the metaphysis (V, Y or T fracture)
C2 = Metaphyseal impaction without dissociation of the articular surface
C3 = Depressed, comminuted fracture of the articular surface

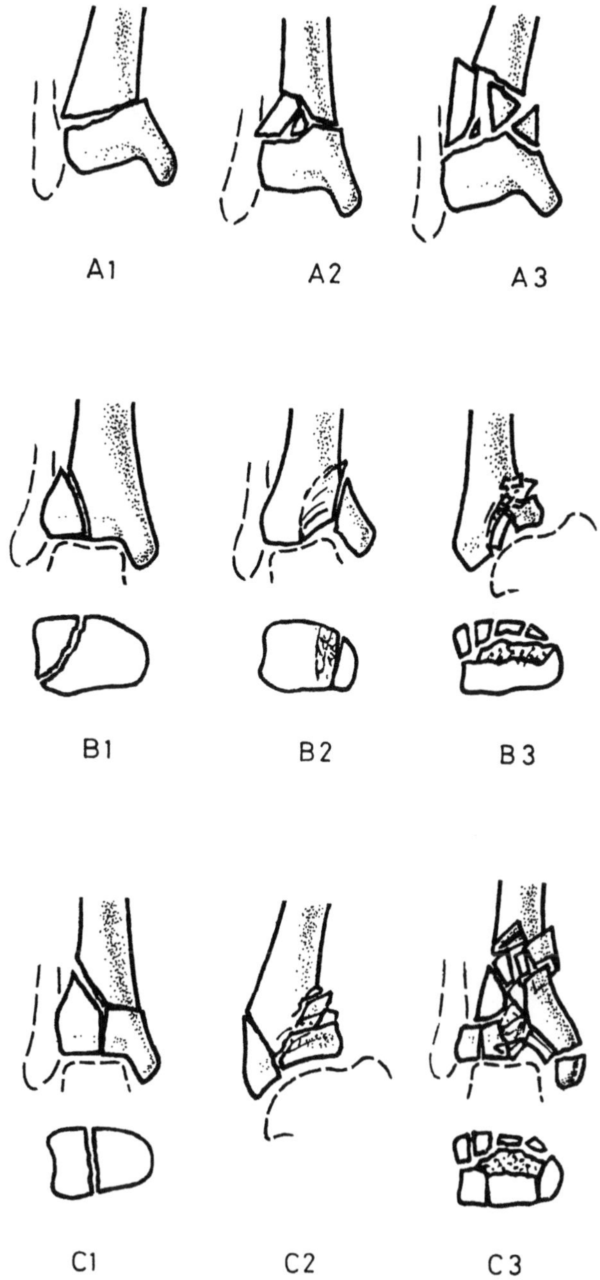

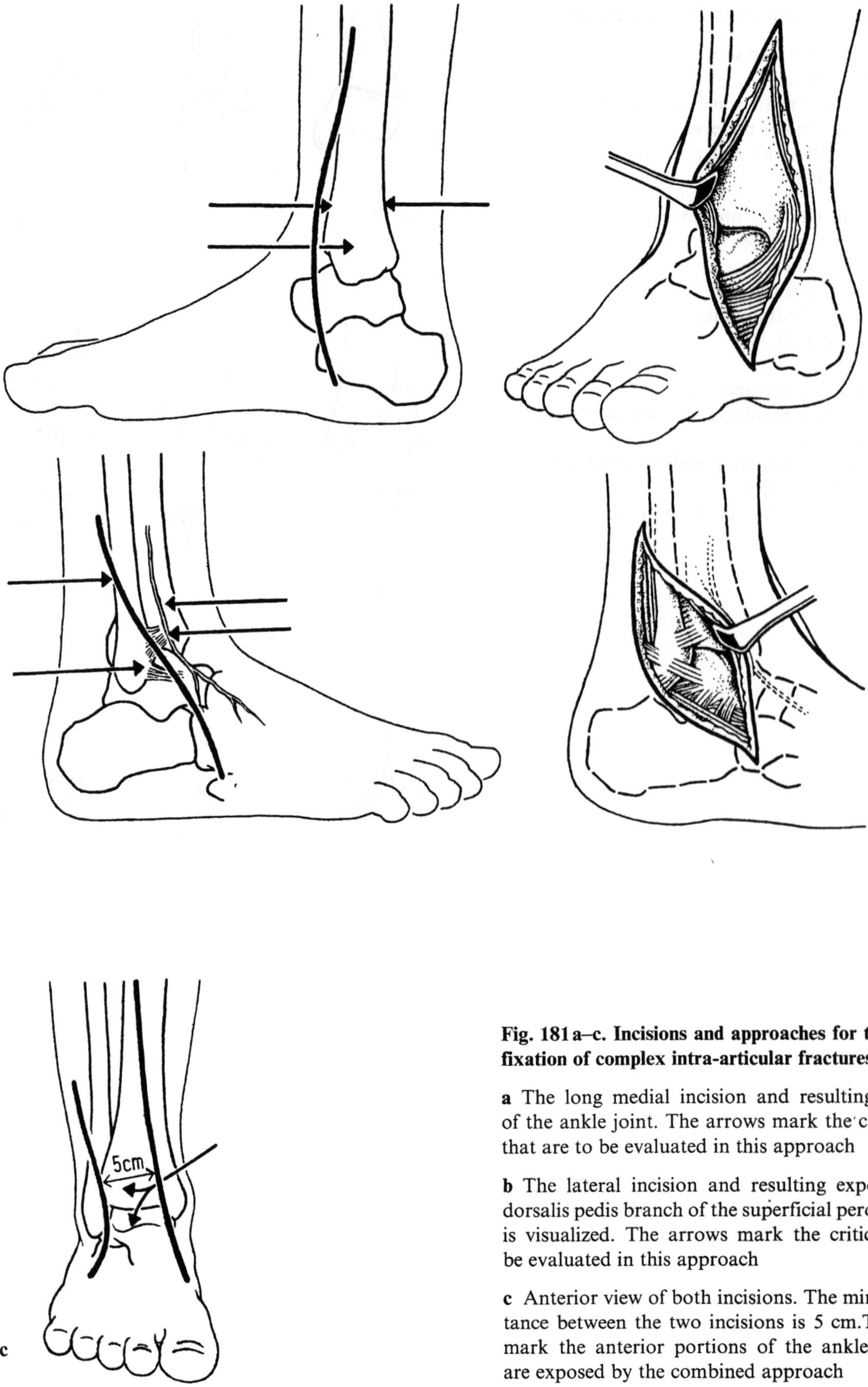

a

b

c

Fig. 181 a–c. Incisions and approaches for the internal fixation of complex intra-articular fractures

a The long medial incision and resulting exposure of the ankle joint. The arrows mark the critical sites that are to be evaluated in this approach

b The lateral incision and resulting exposure. The dorsalis pedis branch of the superficial peroneal nerve is visualized. The arrows mark the critical sites to be evaluated in this approach

c Anterior view of both incisions. The minimum distance between the two incisions is 5 cm.The arrows mark the anterior portions of the ankle joint that are exposed by the combined approach

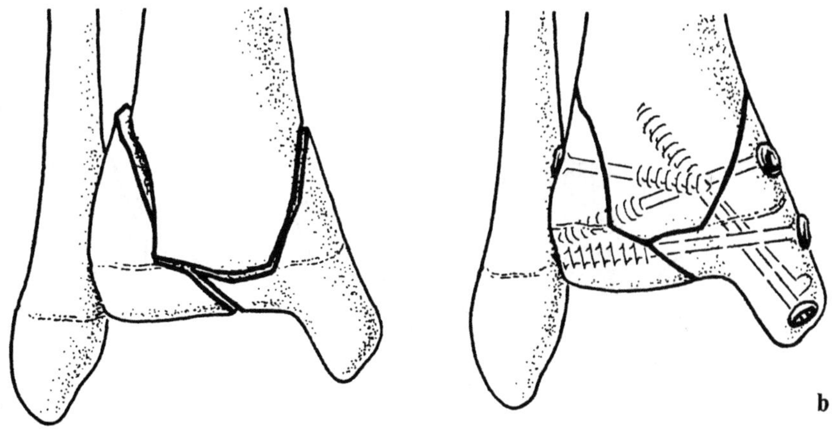

Fig. 182a, b. Split fracture of the tibial articular surface, fixed with cancellous screws through the bilateral approach

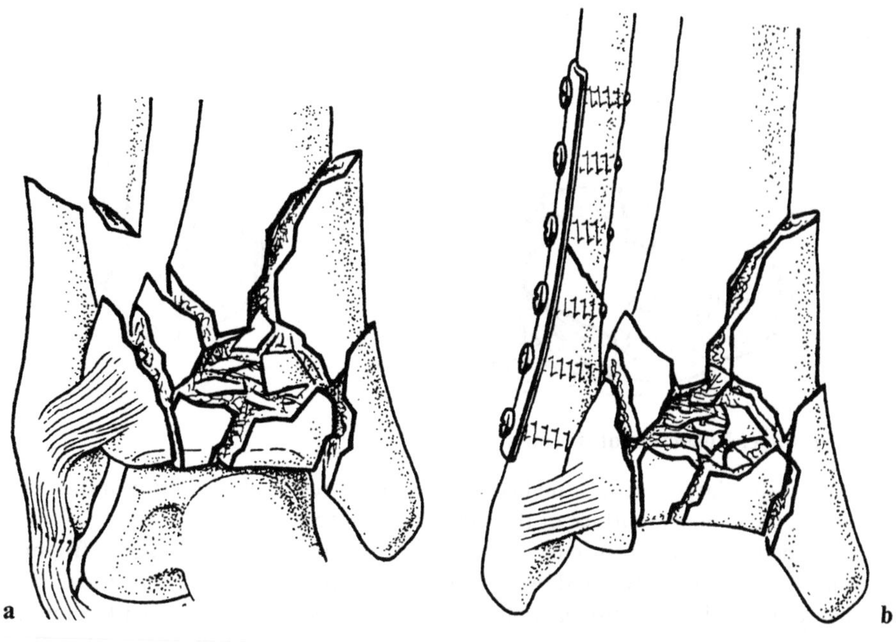

Fig. 183

a Comminuted fracture with impaction of the metaphysis and an oblique fracture of the fibula (type C2)

b Internal fixation of the fibular fracture (with a one-third tubular plate) is performed first to restore the length of the tibia and partially realign it

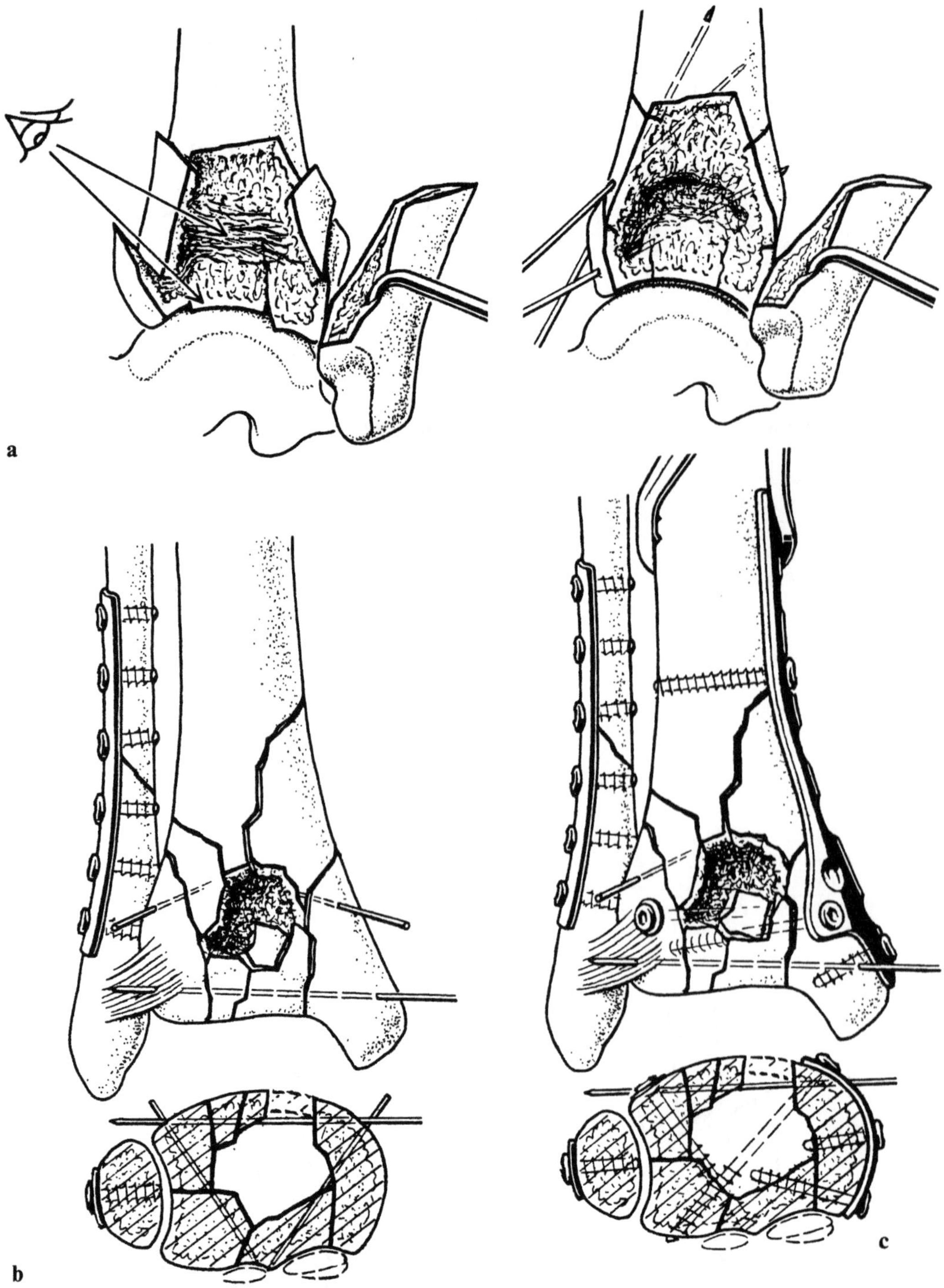

Fig. 184 a–c. Reduction of the tibial fracture

a With the large medial malleolar fragment retracted, the articular surface of the tibial is visualized anteromedially and is restored. The reassembled fragments are temporarily fixed with Kirschner wires. The extent of the metaphyseal defect can be assessed at this time

b Anterior and cross-sectional views

c The lateral fragments are fixed with screws. The medial cloverleaf plate is contoured and tentatively attached with screws. The Kirschner wires are successively removed as the definitive implants are applied

Fig. 185 a, b. Donor sites for autogenous cancellous bone grafts

a Grafts are obtained from the iliac crest and fossa in a separate, preliminary operation

b Cancellous bone may be taken from the upper tibia to supplement the iliac grafts (**a**) or if an unexpected defect is found. A small, medial longitudinal incision is made, the cortex is opened with a gouge, and the graft material is removed with a curette

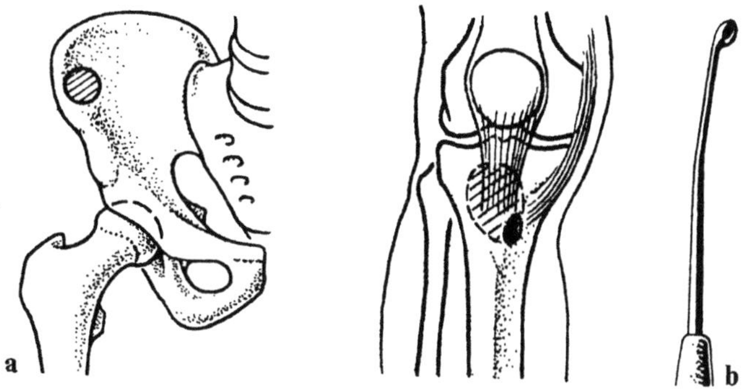

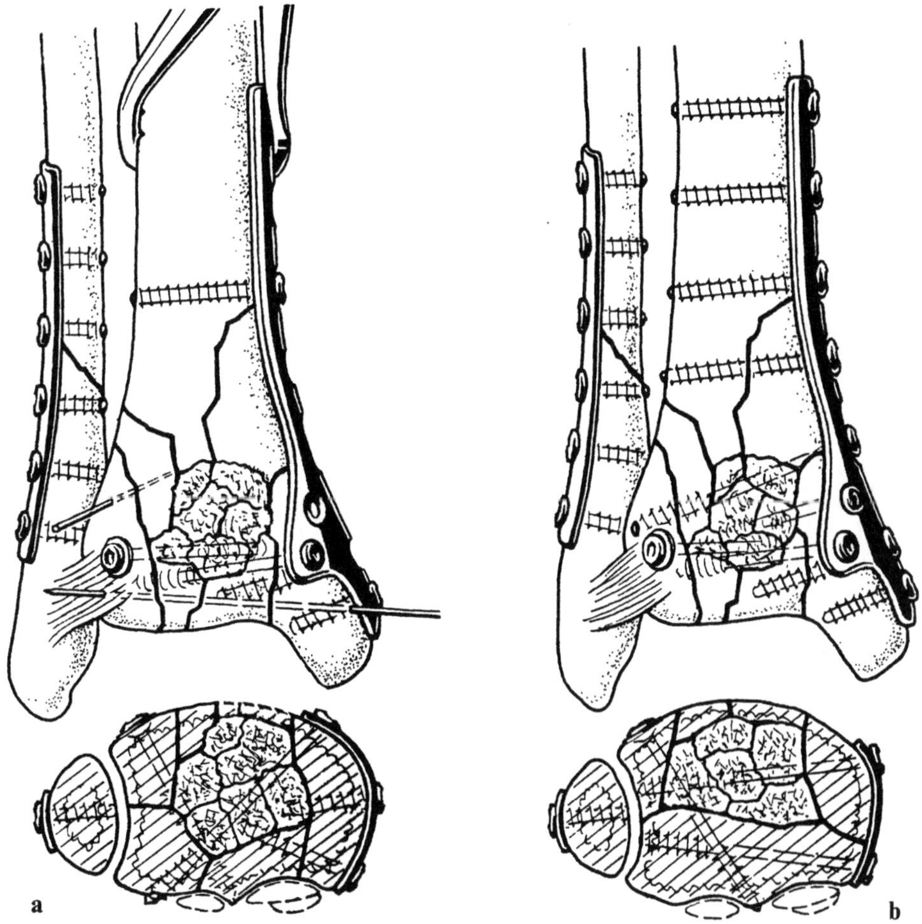

Fig. 186 a, b. Completing the internal fixation

a The defect is packed with cancellous chips, and the remaining plate screws are inserted (anterior view and cross-section). The full width of the plate is in contact with the bone, and the screws solidly engage the metaphyseal fragments

b Finished appearance of the internal fixation. Here the posterior tab of the cloverleaf plate has been removed to avoid encroachment on the tibialis posterior tendon canal

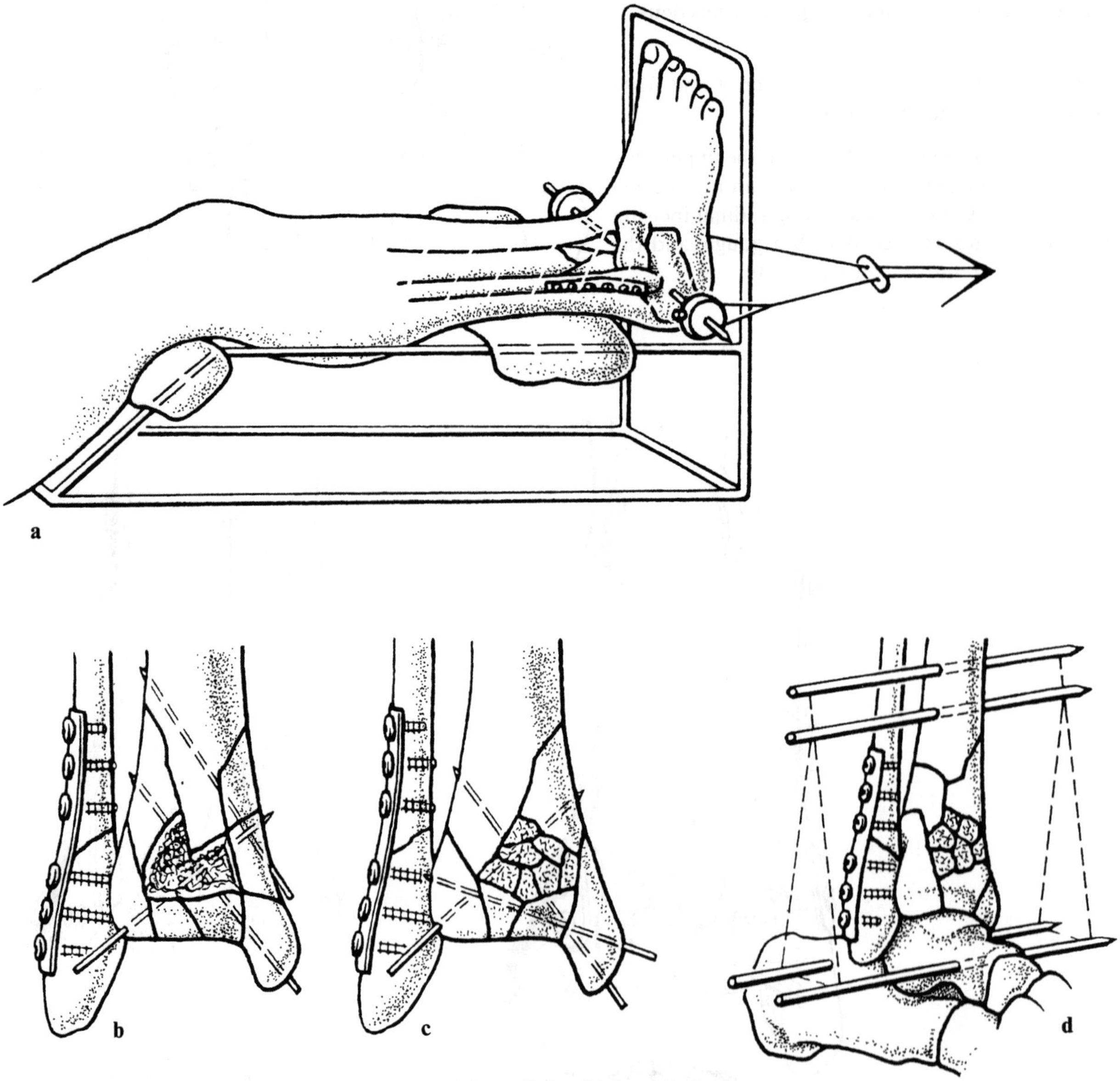

Fig. 187 a–d. Operative tactics in patients with medial soft-tissue lesions

a Primary internal fixation of the fibula combined with traction on the calcaneus

b Primary internal fixation of the fibula combined with temporarily reduction and fixation of the tibial fracture with Kirschner wires

c Primary grafting of the tibial defect with autogenous cancellous bone

d Internal fixation of the fibula combined with external skeletal fixation of the tibia. The example shows a triangular frame anchored in the tibia, the calcaneus, and the neck of the talus

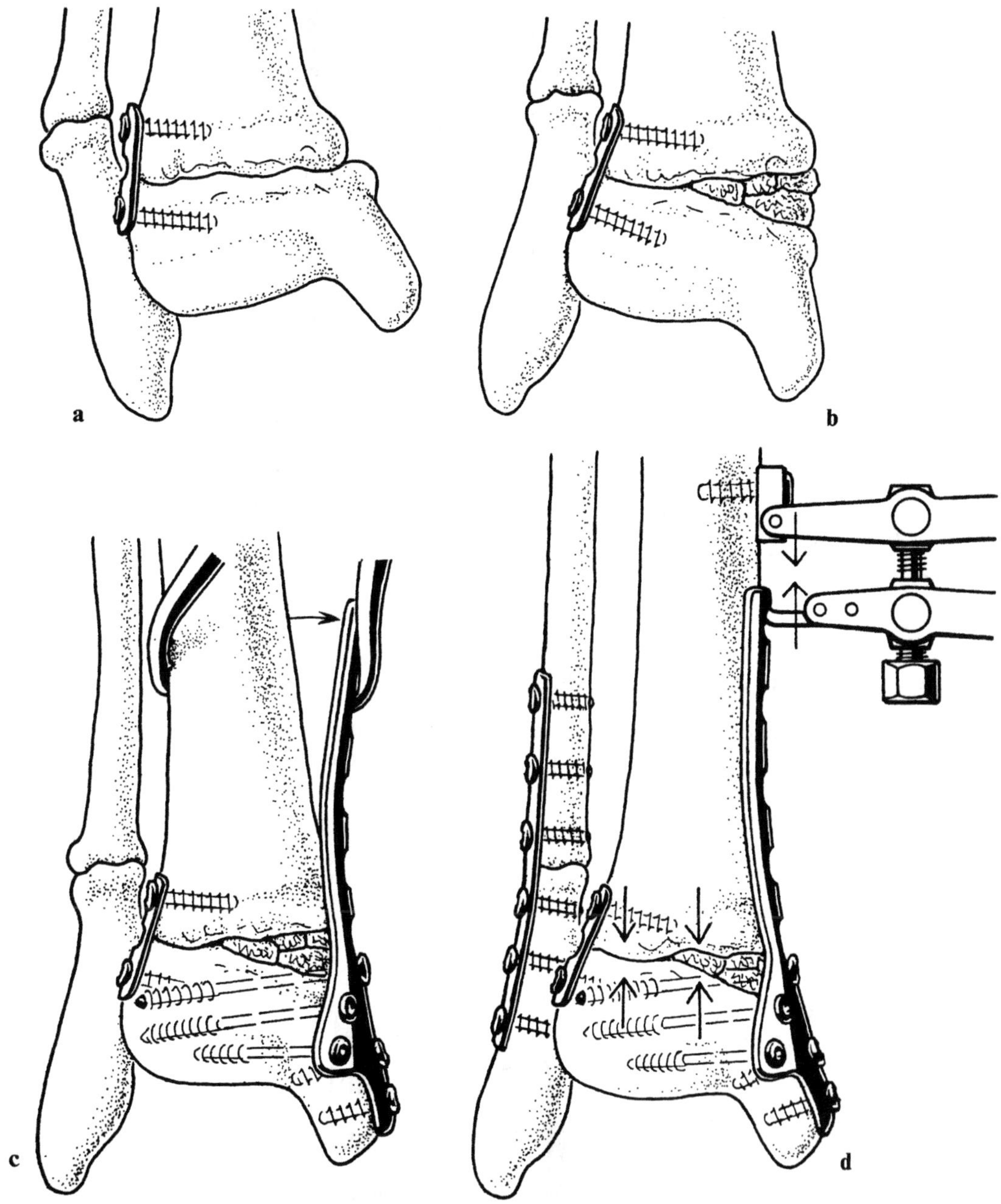

Fig. 188a–d. Correction of varus deformity

a A short plate is attached laterally to prevent distraction of the fragments

b Medial osteotomy is carried out, overcorrecting the varus, and the defect is supported with autogenous cancellous bone or a corticocancellous wedge

c The cloverleaf plate is applied and attached distally

d The plate is pulled proximally with the tension device to eliminate the overcorrection and compress the bone graft. The final step is internal fixation of the fibula

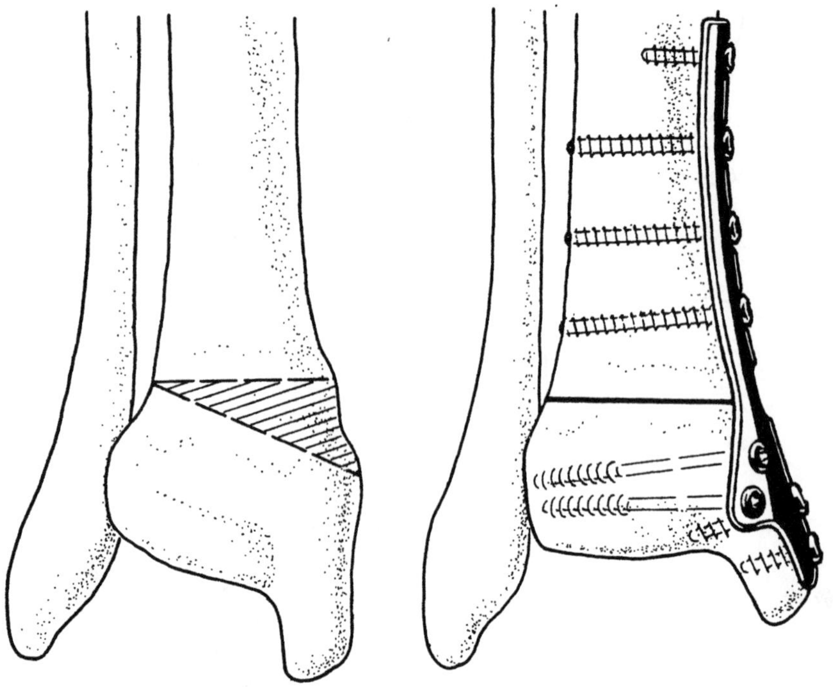

Fig. 189. Correction of valgus deformity with a cloverleaf plate

A medial wedge-resection osteotomy is performed, and the plate is attached. In some cases it is preferable to interpose an anterolateral bone wedge to avoid shortening. This may necessitate a fibular osteotomy

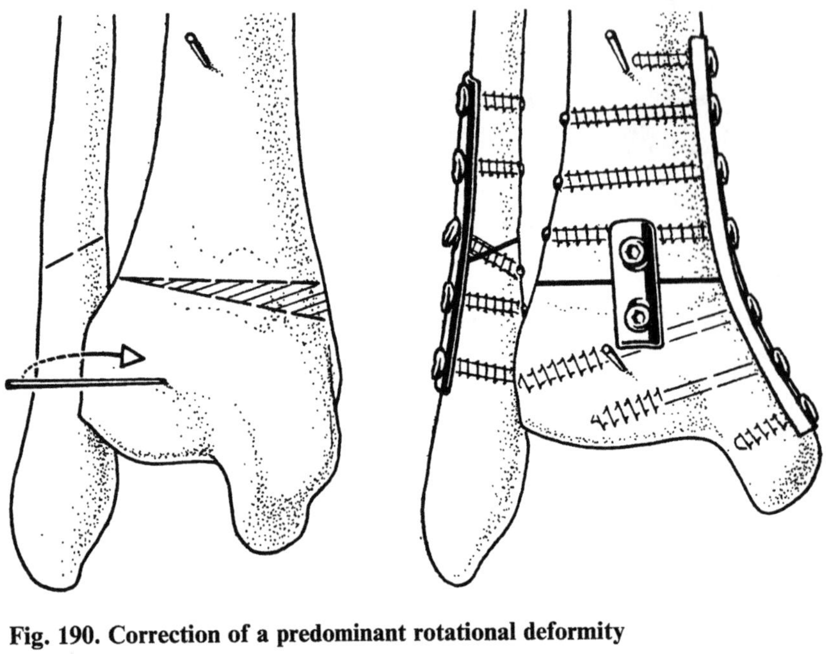

Fig. 190. Correction of a predominant rotational deformity

The osteotomized, derotated tibia is fixed with a 3.5-mm DCP and one-third tubular plate. A one-third tubular plate is also used on the osteotomized fibula

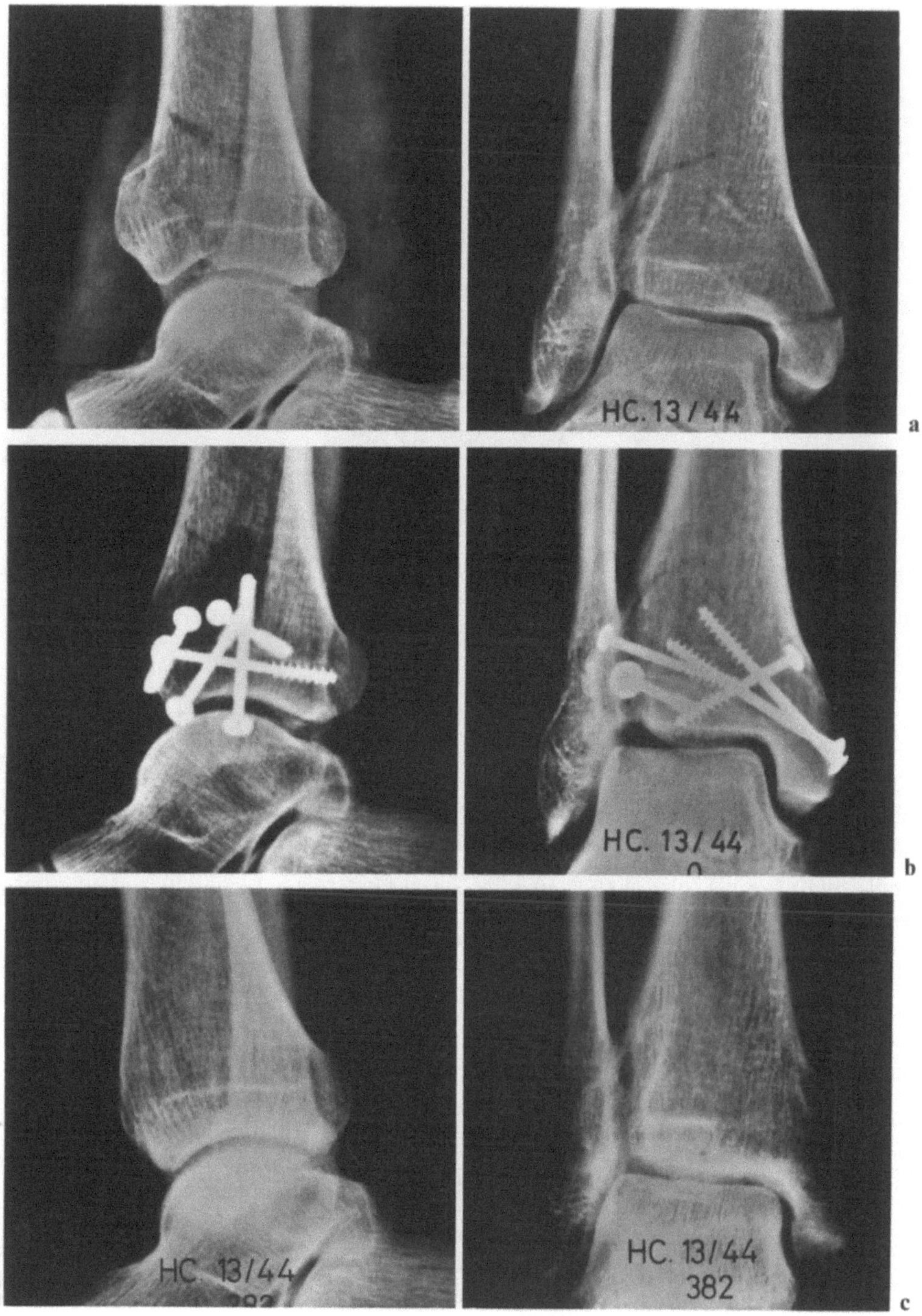

Fig. 191 a–c. Clinical example: tibial pilon fracture without a cancellous bone defect

Franz G., 47-year-old mechanic, fell while skiing on 2/15/73

a Tibial pilon fracture with multiple fragments, moderate anterior impaction, and no cancellous bone defect

b Emergency internal fixation was performed with five small lag screws. Weight bearing was commenced at 12 weeks after an uneventful course. The patient was fully rehabilitated at 4 months. The screws were removed at 8 months

c When seen 7 years later on 6/19/80, the patient had no complaints, linear scars, full function of the ankle and subtalar joints, and no muscular atrophy. X-rays showed no evidence of osteoarthritis

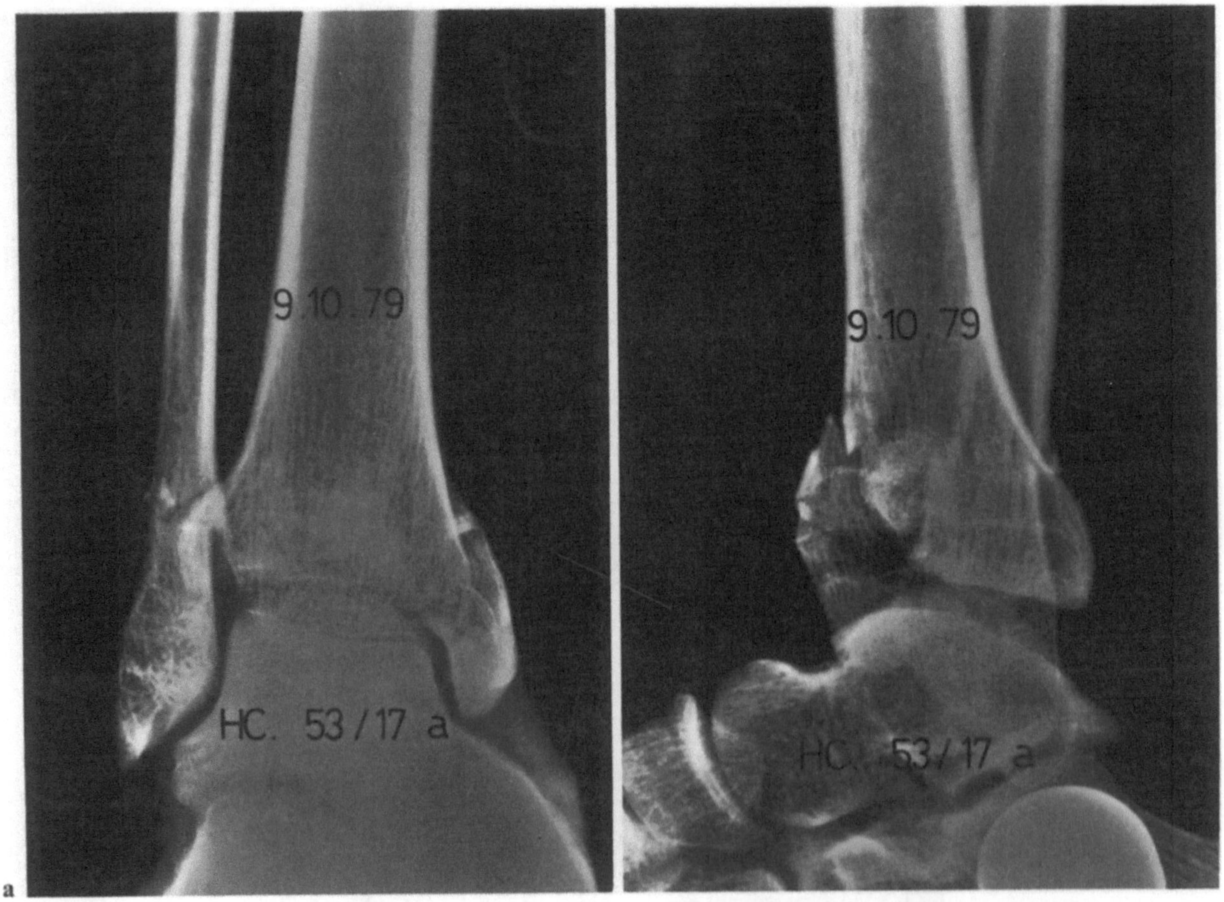

a

Fig. 192 a–c. Clinical example: anterior depressed tibial pilon fracture in a multiply injured patient

Klara J. E., 25-year-old guest worker, collided with a motorcycle while driving a car on 10/3/79; sustained a brain concussion and bilateral fractures of the upper tibia

a Right tibial pilon fracture with anterior depression of the articular surface, treated initially by traction because of the precarious condition of the soft tissues

b Internal fixation was performed on 10/12/79, using plates to stabilize both upper tibial fractures and the right tibial pilon fracture. Since the posterior cortex was intact, a radial T plate was applied anteriorly. Large pieces of cartilage had been sheared from the talus.

The postoperative course was uncomplicated. The bilateral injuries made mobilization difficult, and walking-pool exercises were started at 8 weeks. Partial rehabilitation was achieved by 6 months and full rehabilitation by 8 months

c On follow-up 7 years later the patient had no complaints, unlimited walking distance, linear scars, and no muscular atrophy. X-rays showed moderate osteoarthritis

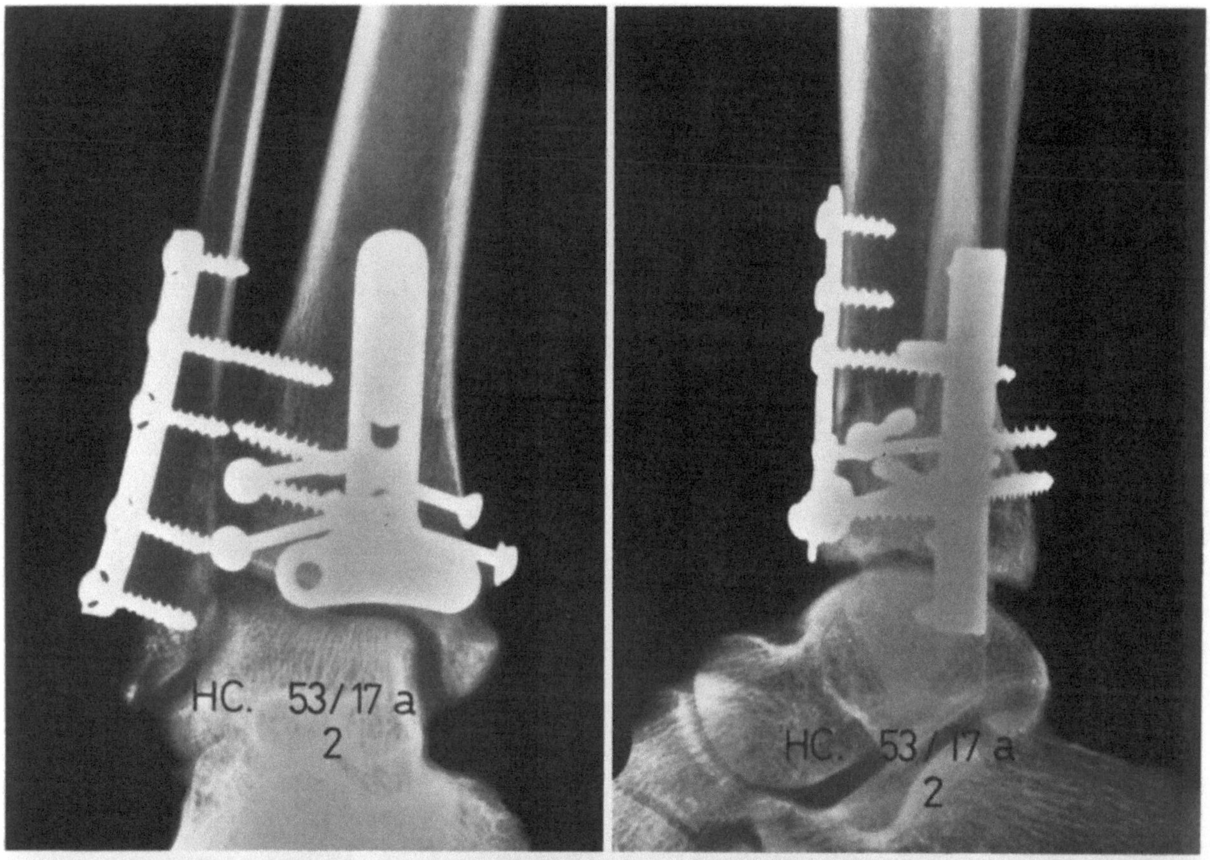

b

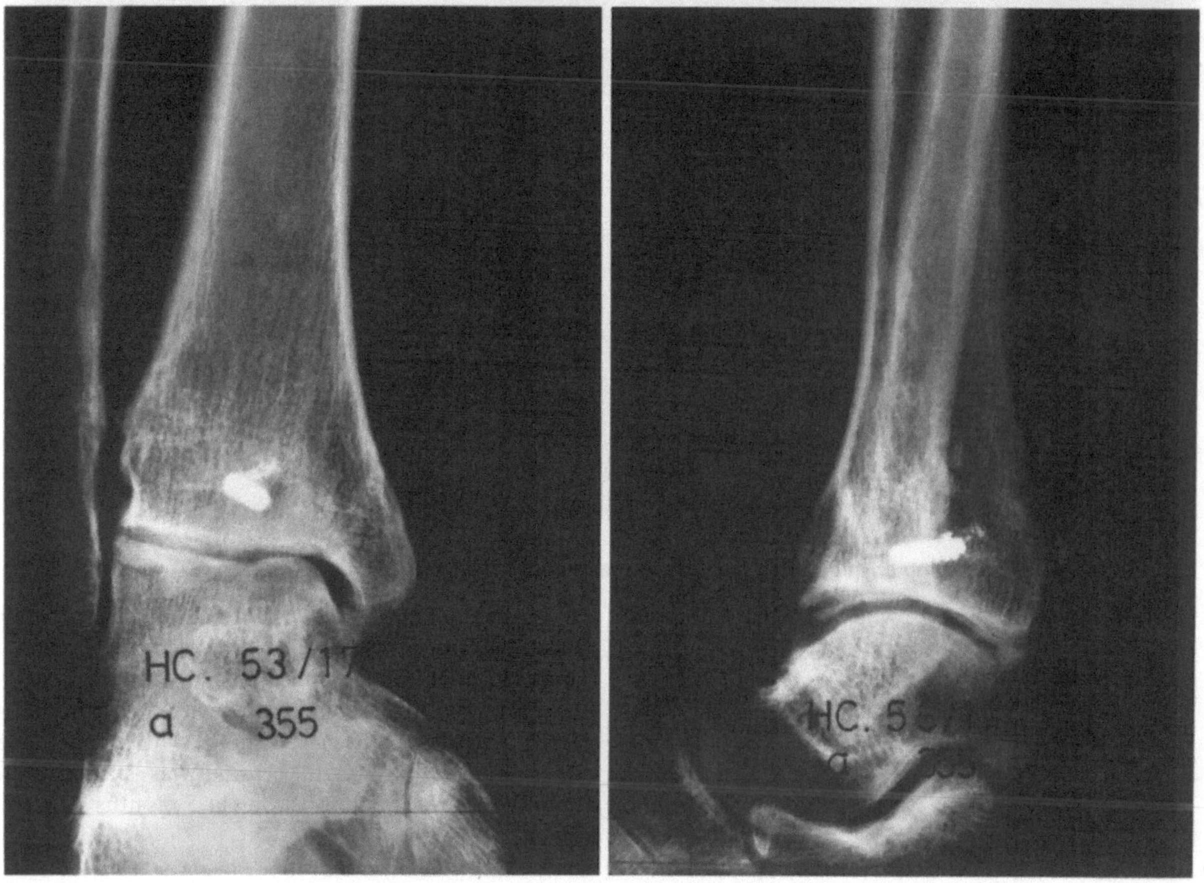

c

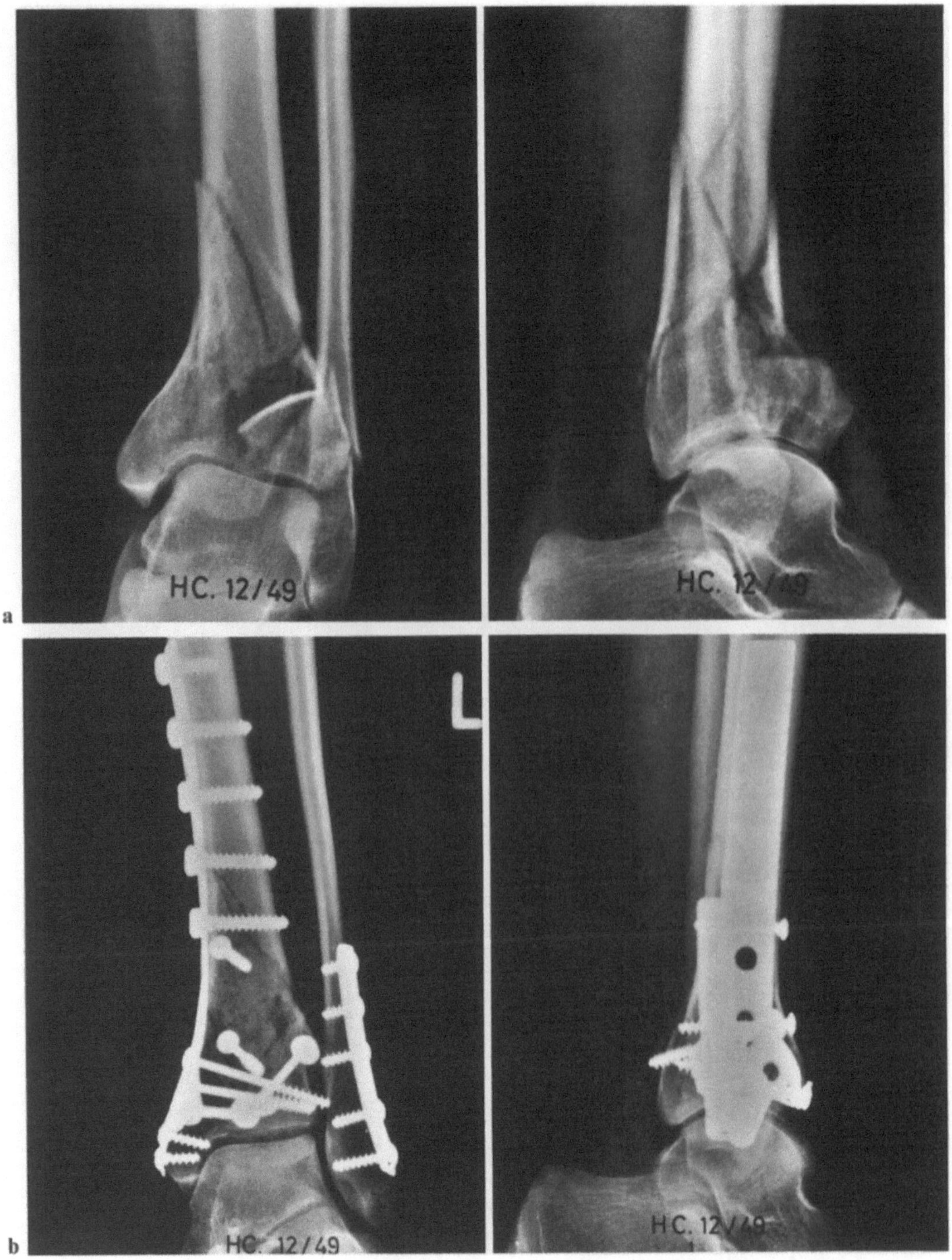

a

b

Fig. 193a–e. Clinical example: tibial pilon fracture extending into the shaft

Heidi B., 41-year-old housewife, fell while skiing on 1/30/73

a Complex tibial pilon fracture extending far up onto the shaft. Primary treatment consisted of traction and elevation

b Internal fixation was performed on 2/1/73 after swelling had subsided. The tibia was fixed with a long cloverleaf plate applied medially and with separate screws. Defects were grafted with iliac cancellous bone. Patient was discharged home with a removable U splint. Partial weight bearing was started at 4 months and full weight bearing at 5 months

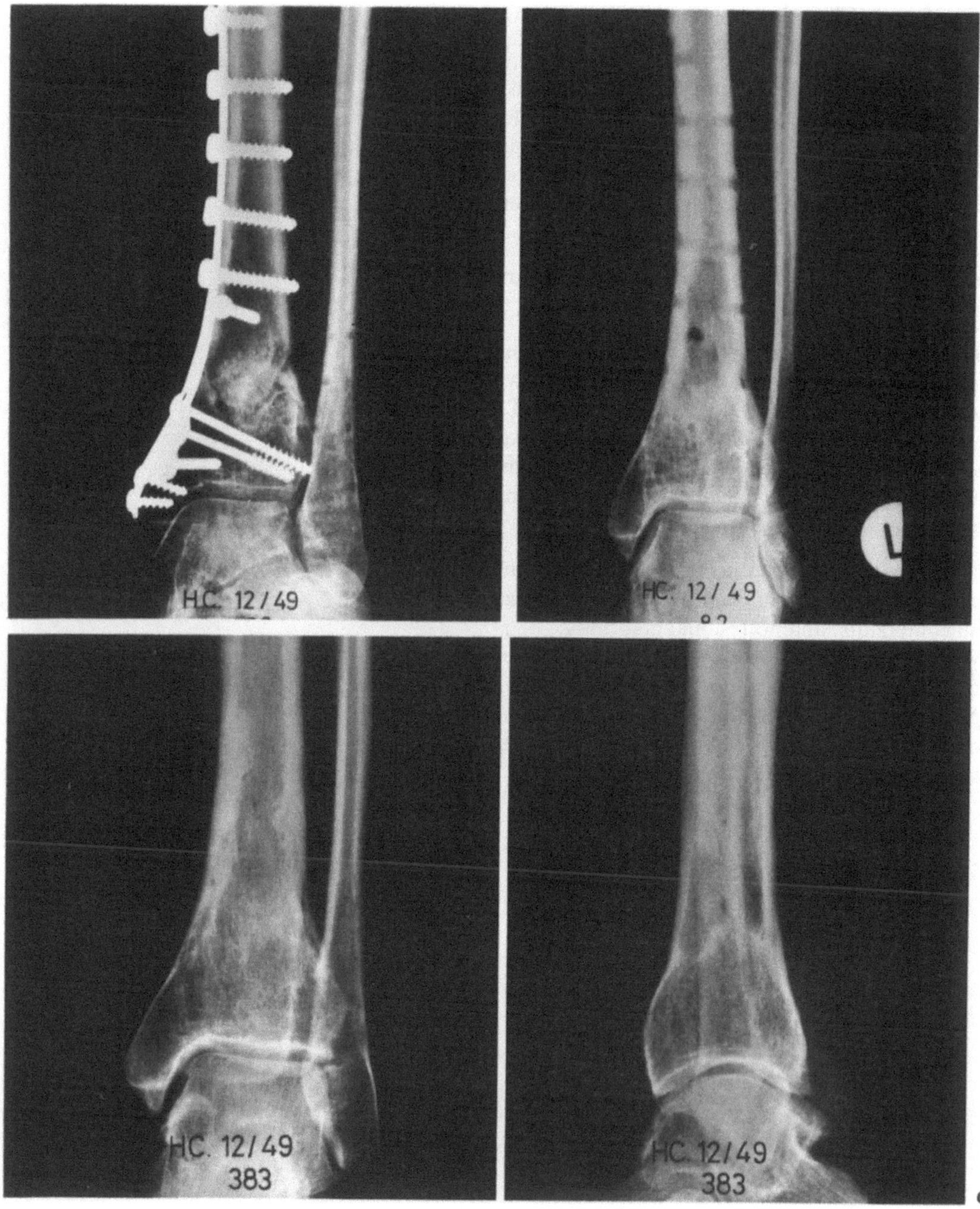

c d e

c The lateral implants were removed at 5 months. The bony structure was still irregular at that time

d On follow-up at $1^1/_2$ years, the rest of the implants were removed. Patient had no complaints, full motion, and no muscular atrophy

e Seven years after the injury, the patient claimed to have slight pain when first walking or standing, but she was athletically sound. X-rays showed moderate osteoarthritis

Fig. 194a–c. Clinical example: corrective osteotomy for a malunited fracture of the distal tibia

Brigitte H., 16-year-old trade school student, sustained a supramalleolar fracture of the tibia in a skiing accident in February, 1971. Primary treatment consisted of traction and cast immobilization. Increasing deformity ensued, and patient was referred to us at 3 months after the injury

a Delayed malunion in position of 16° varus and 20° posterior angulation

b Corrective osteotomy was performed through a medial approach. Iliac cancellous bone graft was interposed and the site fixed with a cloverleaf plate attached medially. The limb was not put in plaster. By 8 weeks the osteotomy was solid, and full motion was achieved. Full weight bearing was commenced at 10 weeks

c Follow-up at 10 months, prior to implant removal, confirmed fracture union. Patient had full function, no complaints, and no residual deformity.
When contacted at 9 years, the patient, who lives far away, stated that she had absolutely no complaints. The X-rays sent to us (not suitable for reproduction) showed no osteoarthritic changes in the ankle joint

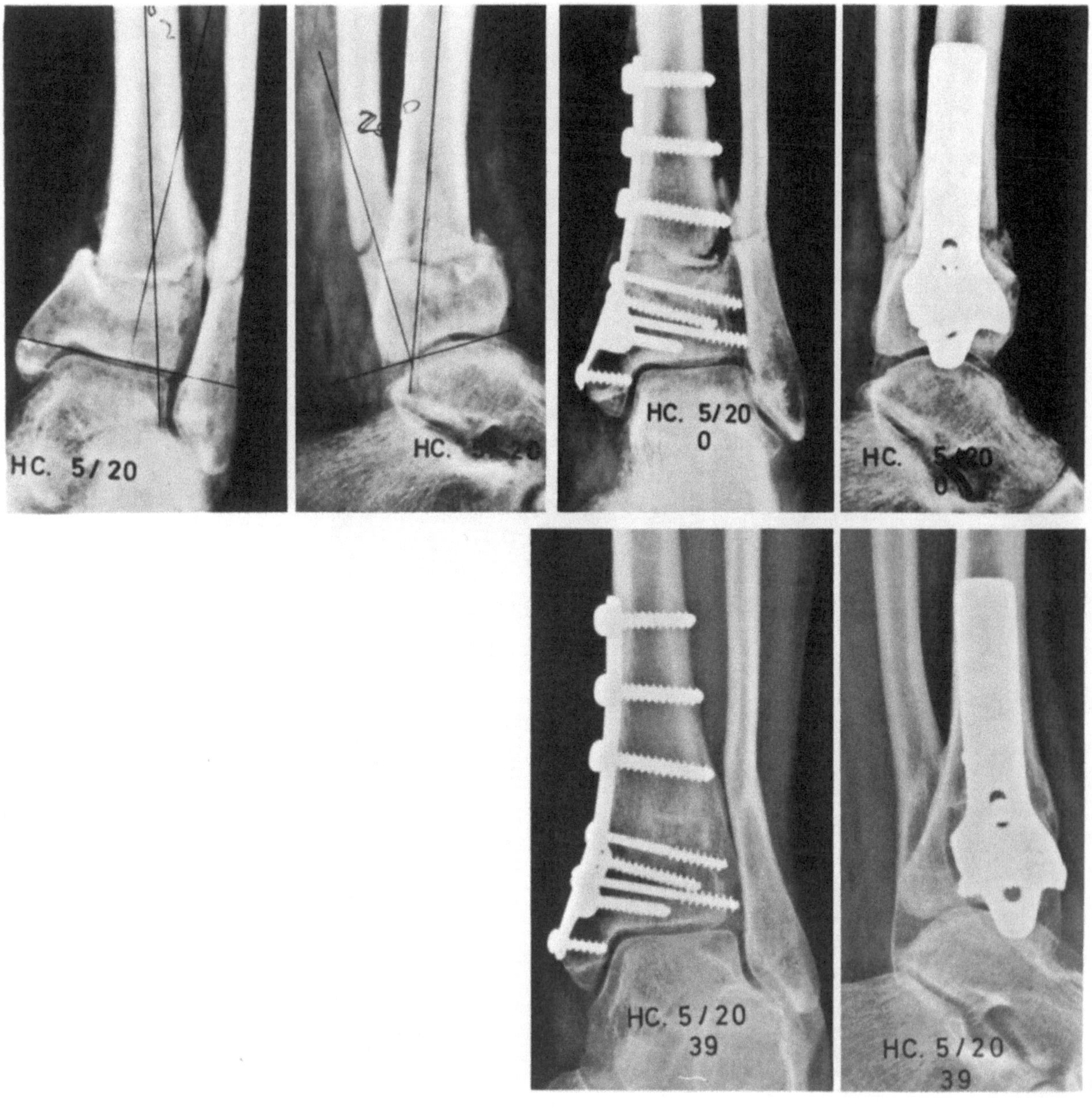

a b c

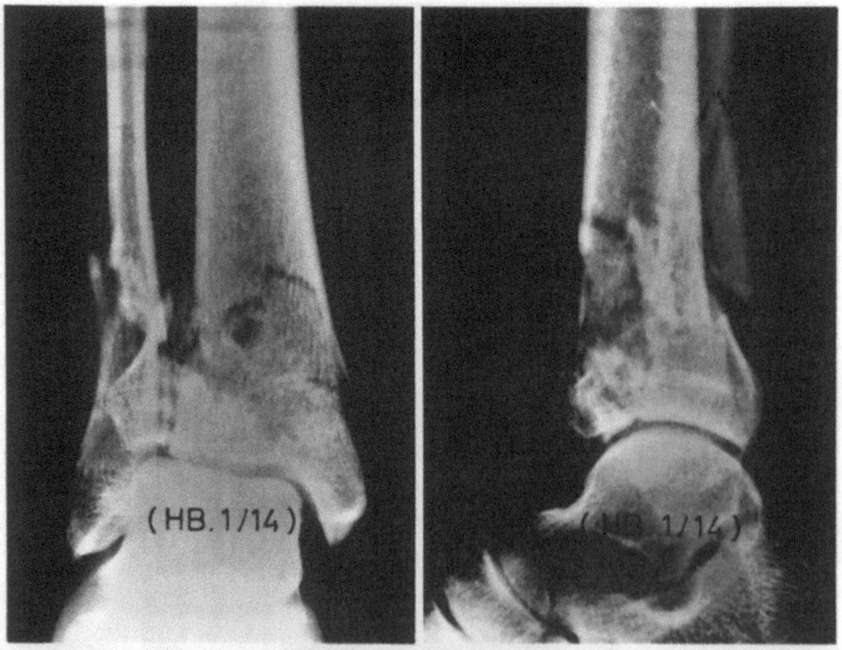

a

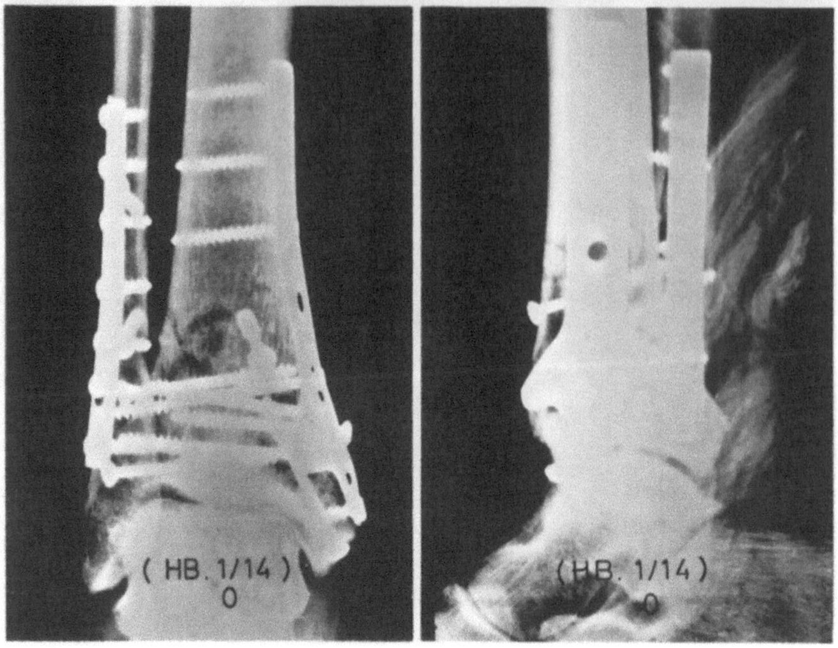

b

Fig. 195a–m. Clinical example: revisionary internal fixation of bilateral pilon fractures because of delayed union

Andre M., 39-year-old mechanic, fell while skiing on 1/3/84. Emergency internal fixation of bilateral pilon fractures was performed in a local hospital.

Postinjury films: right = **a**, left = **g**. Both fractures were type C2.

Postfixation films (fibular plates, cloverleaf plates, cancellous bone grafts on both sides): right = **b**, left = **h**.

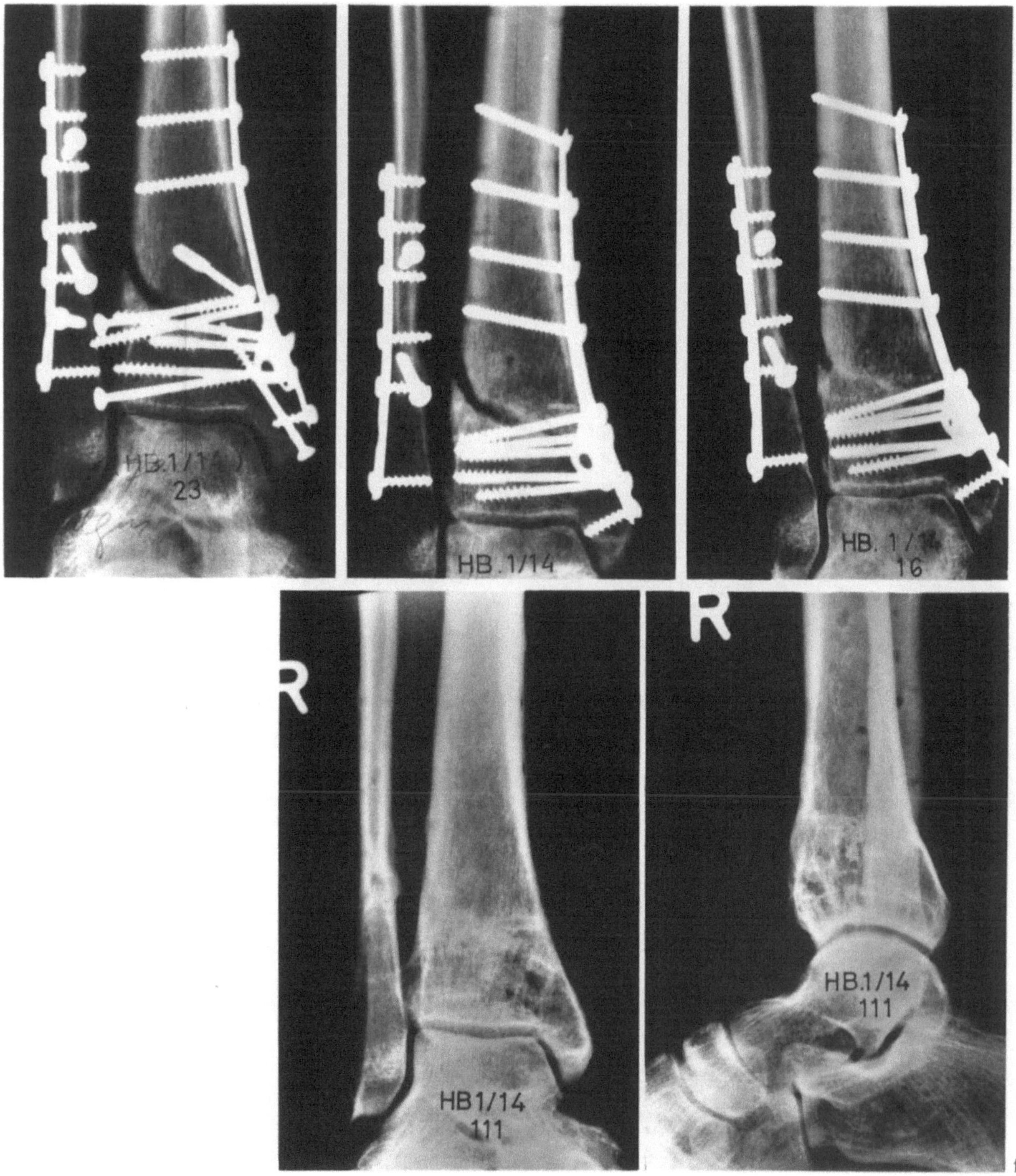

c, d

e

f

Delayed union of both fractures was confirmed at $5^1/_2$ months: right = **c**, left = **i**. Marked valgus deformity.

Both internal fixations were revised on 7/12/84 through the original incisions: The implants were removed, deformity was corrected, new iliac cancellous grafts were applied, and each tibia was stabilized with two different-length cloverleaf plates applied one over the other and compressed proximally with the tension device. Postoperative films: right = **d**, left = **k**.

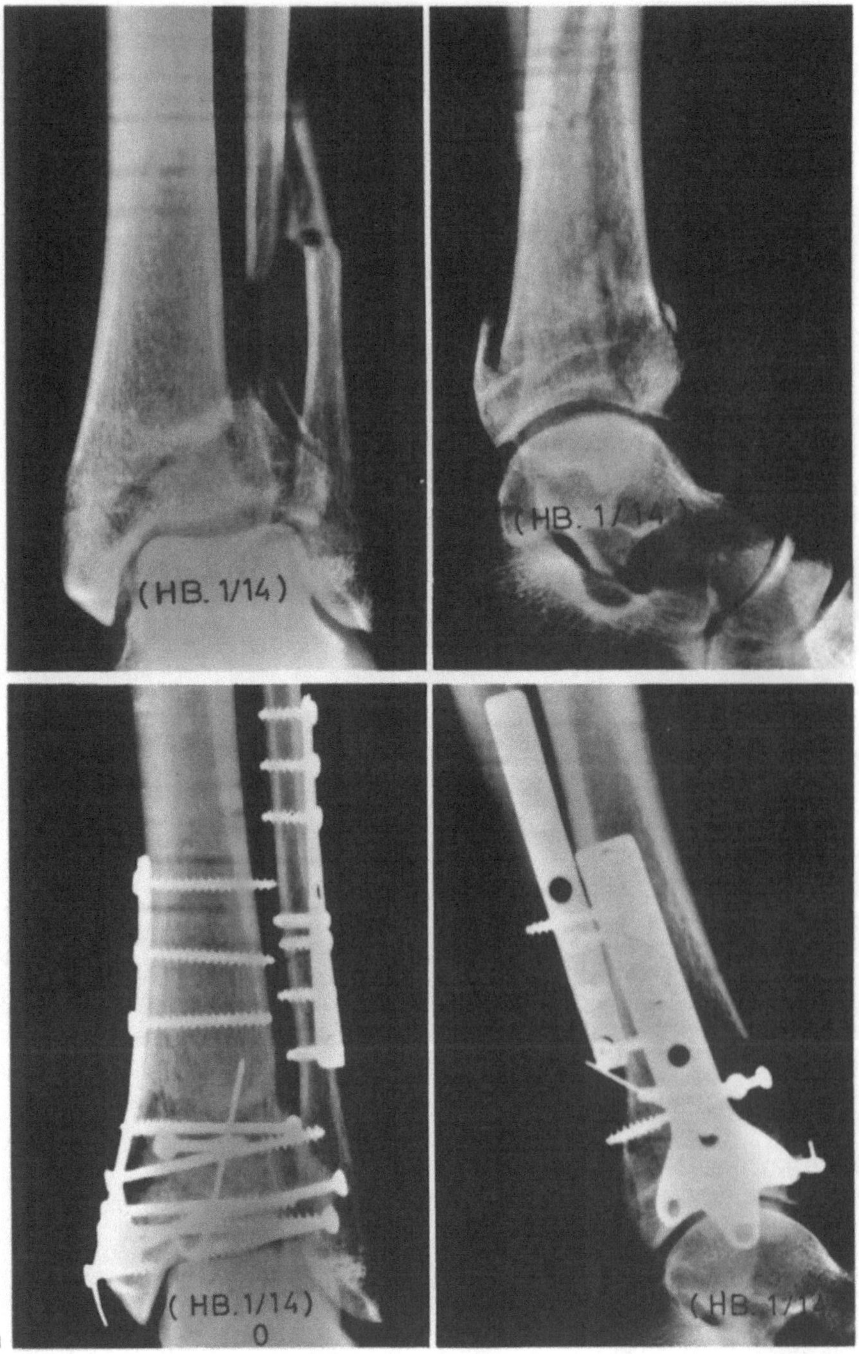

g

h

Fig. 195 (cont.)

The limbs were mobilized early, and swimming exercises were commenced after wound healing. Walking calipers were worn from the 3rd week.

At 12 weeks the patient was ambulating and bearing full weight. Radiographs: right = **e**, left = **l**. Patient had regained 50% work fitness by 6 months and 100% by 14 months. The implants were removed elsewhere at $1^1/_2$ years.

Follow-up at 2 years on 9/3/86: The right ankle (**f**) was painless and had full motion. The left ankle (**m**) was slightly painful during walks on uneven terrain, but walking distance was unlimited. That ankle showed a 15° loss of dorsiflexion and mild osteoarthritic changes.

Subtalar joint motion was limited by about 50% on both sides. No circulatory or trophic problems were evident, and there was no edema. The patient is not drawing disability.

i, k

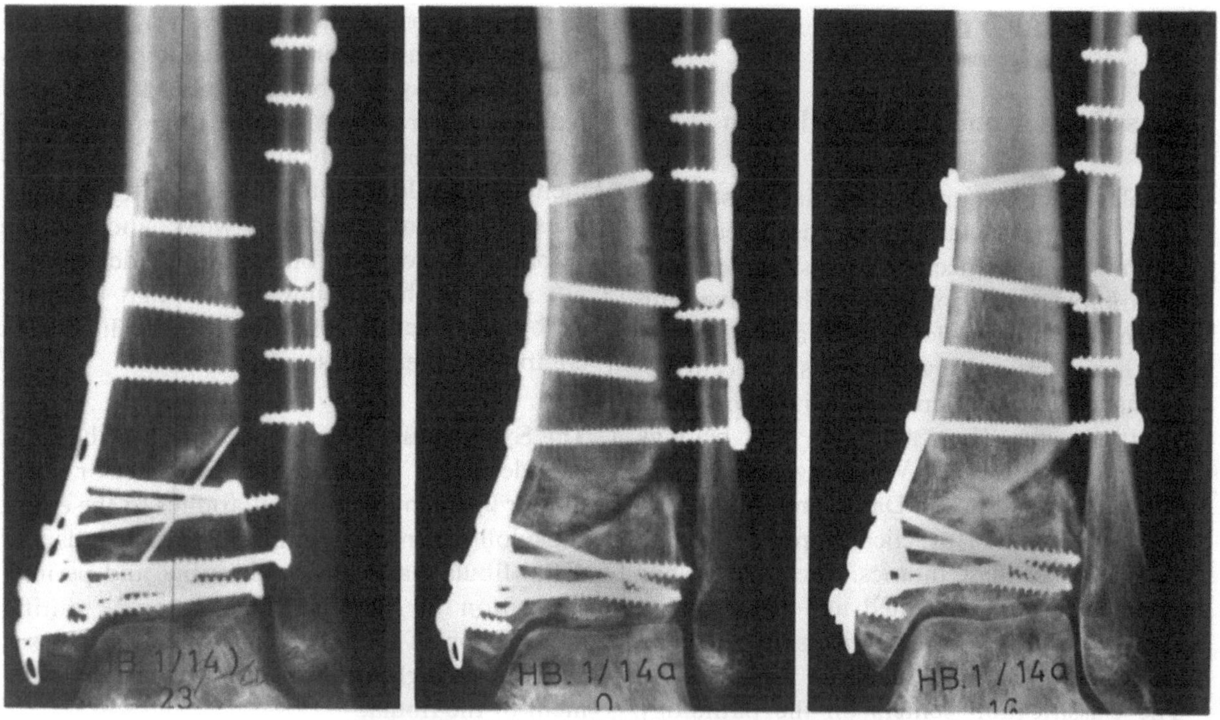

l

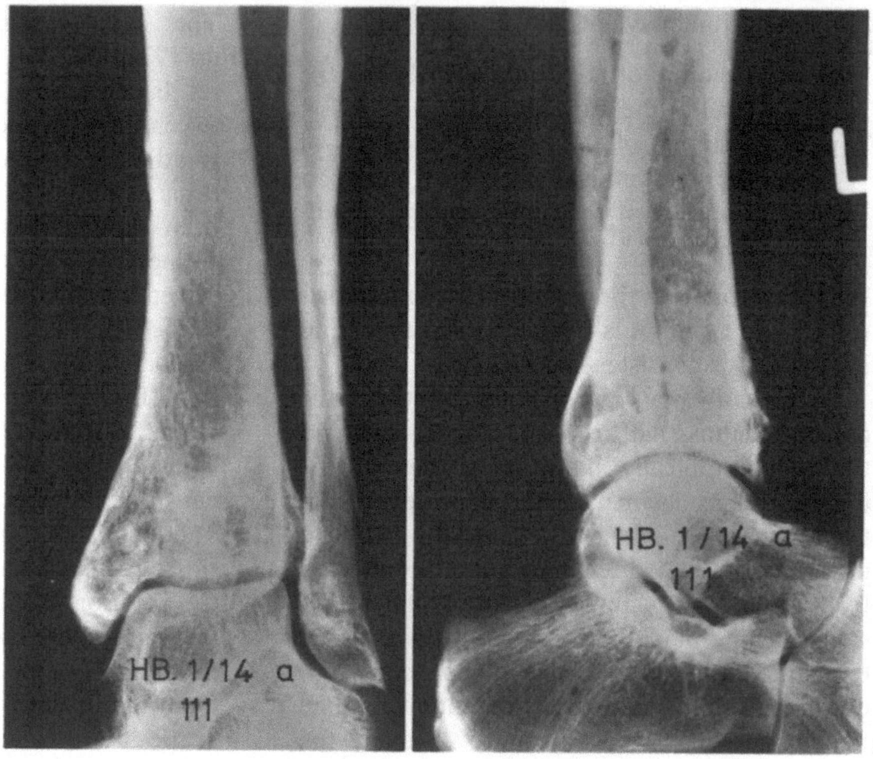

m

Fig. 195 (cont.)

B. Malleolar Fractures

1. Classification and Patient Selection

Malleolar fractures are among the most common of human skeletal injuries. They occur with a minimum of violence and are associated with a remarkable variety of lesions. They have long been an object of etiologic, clinical, and therapeutic investigation. Developments in recent decades have led to an increasing reliance on operative treatment. The credit for this belongs mainly to Weber and Willenegger, who expanded on the ideas of Danis and Bonnin to develop a clear and practical approach to the classification of these injuries. Their system has become widely implemented and has made it possible to establish basic, universally accepted rules of operative technique.

The classification centers on the pathology of the tibiofibular syndesmosis (Fig. 196):

Type A: Fracture of the fibula at or below the level of the joint space
Type B: Fracture of the fibula at the level of the syndesmosis
Type C: Fracture of the fibula above the syndesmosis

In type A fractures the tibiofibular syndesmosis is intact, in type B it is frequently ruptured, and in type C it is consistently ruptured.

We must draw a strict distinction between the osseous lesions that are visible on X-rays and the radiographically invisible injuries of the joint cartilage, ligaments, and capsule. A portion of these lesions may be clinically manifest or presumed, but often they must be inferred from the overall picture. Certainly, bilateral lesions on one plane and lesions on two planes (circumferential) are much more common than one might think, and it is prudent to assume that unilateral lesions are rare. Besides the classic types listed above, variants are possible, and anomalous forms are not uncommon. These cannot be described here in detail.

The main technical concern at operation is to obtain an anatomically exact and stable reconstruction of the fibula, as this lays the groundwork for postoperative functional exercises.

The most crucial factor, however, is the stability of the ankle mortise. This may not be satisfactory unless the fibula, stabilized by internal fixation and returned to the fibular notch of the tibia, is held elastically in place by its ligaments. It should be noted that the anterior tibiofibular ligament is relatively weak, and that the stability of the tibiofibular joint is determined not so much by the integrity of that ligament as by the overall condition of the ligaments comprising the syndesmosis.

The Syndesmosis. Many surgeons use the term "syndesmosis" to mean only the anterior tibiofibular ligament. Actually it applies to the entire capsuloligamentous complex which binds the distal fibula elastically to the tibia and permits separation of the tibiofibular mortise during dorsiflexion of the foot–a movement also associated with slight rotation and upward displacement of the fibula.

The syndesmosis consists of four parts (Fig. 197):

- At its center is a triangular sheet passing between the tibia and fibula. It is situated directly adjacent to the synovial recess and functions as both a buffer and a stabilizer. It has been shown to contain fat and collagenous connective tissue fibers. This structure has received little attention since it was first described by Fick in 1904. Most fractures are associated with a tearing of this sheet, and small fibular fragments sometimes remain adherent to it and create obstacles to reduction.
- The anterior and posterior tibiofibular (syndesmotic) ligaments. Both ligaments run obliquely superiorly and medially, the posterior ligament being thicker and broader than the anterior. Ruptures and avulsion fractures involving these ligaments are extremely common.
- Continuous with the syndesmosis proximally is the interosseous membrane, an important stabilizer. Superimposition of cross-sectional films of the diaphysis and epiphysis confirms the central location of this structure. The membrane is the site of origin for the extensor hallucis, digitorum longus, and tibialis anterior muscles anteriorly, and for the peroneus, flexor hallucis, flexor digitorum longus, and tibialis posterior muscles posteriorly.

The interosseous membrane always ruptures at its tibial insertion, but its tears are never isolated and are invariably combined with tears of one or both tibiofibular ligaments.

Ligamentous and membrane tears unaccompanied by a fracture have been described in sports-related injuries. Arthrograms usually are necessary for preoperative diagnosis.

Malleolar fractures are often associated with tearing of the interosseous membrane, and this can occur at any level. Complete rupture of the membrane is most common in the high type C fracture (Maisonneuve fracture).This injury destroys the ligamentous stability of the ankle joint. Similar ruptures are seen in approximately 30% of malleolar fractures in general and may produce overt instability.

In describing the techniques for the operative treatment of these injuries, we shall place particular emphasis on the use of small implants. We shall also discuss techniques of ligament repair and reinforcement, as these are often crucial to a successful reconstruction.

For practical reasons we shall consider internal fixations and ligament repairs separately for the lateral and medial sides.

2. Internal Fixations and Ligament Repairs on the Lateral Side

a) Surface Anatomy and Structure of the Distal Fibula (Fig. 197)

It is important to consider the shape and structure of the distal fibula if we are to use skeletal fixation effectively in that area. The lateral aspect of the bone is best suited for plating owing to the absence of muscular insertions.

Near the ankle joint the fibula expands and acquires a double curvature, to which implants must be suitably adapted. The bony structure also changes in that area from hard cortex to softer cancellous bone.

There is a lateral ridge several centimeters above the ankle joint which widens proximally and causes the lateral surface of the fibula to face posteriorly. Lateral plates must be twisted accordingly to avoid malrotation. It will be noted that screws in the upper part of the plate point obliquely forward, toward the tibia. This is advantageous in cases where a transfixion screw must be placed through a fibular plate.

The cross-section of the fibula is roughly oval-shaped at the level of the ankle joint. This is favorable for posterior plating, as the broader AP dimension provides a better hold for screws than the narrower lateral dimension. Moreover, this placement avoids the necessity of drilling toward and possibly injuring the syndesmosis and talus.Posterior implants also acquire a better softtissue coverage. This technique requires the use of special surgical approaches, however.

b) Positioning

The *standard position* for most operations on the malleoli and "posterior malleolus" of the tibia is with the lower leg elevated on a padded rest and the knee moderately flexed. The opposite leg is level with the table top.In this way the foot can be rotated laterally or medially by pressing on either side of the knee, and the posterior aspects of the lateral and medial malleoli can be alternately brought into view (Fig. 199a). The rotational position of the foot can be increased if necessary by placing a wedge-shaped cushion beneath the buttock.

Special positions should be considered preoperatively for the treatment of posterior malleolar fractures through the lateral or posteromedial approach.

- For a strictly lateral internal fixation that does not require a medial incision, the patient may be positioned on his side with the knee slightly flexed (Fig. 199b).
- In some circumstances the approach to a posterior marginal fragment from the posteromedial side can be aided by crossing the injured foot over the healthy leg during the operation. This makes it easier to insert screws from the posteromedial aspect, adjacent to the Achilles tendon. For this maneuver a wedge-shaped cushion is placed beneath the buttock on the corresponding side (Fig. 199 c).

c) Lateral Approaches

Skin incisions at joint level should not be placed directly over the protruding malleoli, where the soft-tissue envelope is thin and vulnerable. This is not a concern farther proximally.

To obtain sufficient exposure, one may find it necessary to curve the ends of the incisions slightly. It is better in terms of circulation to lengthen incisions than terminate them in actual curves.

We prefer a slightly oblique skin incision that starts above and behind the fibula, crosses it proximal to the mortise, and passes forward and distally, parallel to the fibula (Fig. 200a). This incision, which is extended as needed, must give exposure of the fibular fracture, the anterior tibiofibular ligament, the distal interosseous membrane, the tubercle of Tillaux-Chaput and adjacent tibial surface, as well as the anterior talofibular and calcaneofibular ligaments and the retinaculum of the peroneal tendons.

By extending the incision proximally and curving it back to the Achilles tendon (sparing its peritenon), a flap can be formed that gives excellent access to the posterior malleolus behind the peroneal tendons.

A type A fracture can be approached through a longitudinal incision placed anterior to the malleolus.

The posterior surface of the fibula is optimally exposed through a longitudinal incision placed behind the fibula, especially in cases where the lesions are strictly lateral and only a lateral operation is proposed.This incision gives good access for exposing and fixing a posterior malleolar fracture. Exposure of the anterior tibiofibular ligament is somewhat more difficult and requires that the incision be extended distally and curved anteriorly at the end. With all anterior incisions, care is taken to spare the subcutaneous sensory branch of the superficial peroneal nerve, which supplies the lateral side of the dorsum of the foot (Fig. 200b). This branch should always be identified, as its injury causes permanent and troublesome sensory deficits. Neuromas can cause extremely refractory complaints. The nerve is about 1–1.5 mm in diameter and usually runs parallel to the anterior fibular border, although its course is highly variable. In most cases it emerges from the anterior tibialis compartment at a fairly high level, passing anteriorly into the subcutaneous tissue. But it may also arise from the peroneus compartment and cross the fibula. Duplication of the nerve is also possible.

Its topographic relations to the implants should be documented in order to avoid injury at the time of implant removal. Usually the removal is performed by a different, less experienced surgeon who will benefit from notes on the location of the nerve.

Exposure of the anterior tibiofibular ligament, distal interosseous membrane, tubercule of Chaput, and lateral tibial metaphysis requires division of the cruciform ligament. This does not cause any problems of which we are aware. The muscle bellies of the long digital extensors are then carefully retracted medially with a blunt retractor (Fig. 205a).

d) Fracture of the Distal Fibula Accompanying a Tibial Fracture

Most of these fractures are of the subordinate or "vassal" type. This means that internal fixation of the tibia will usually result in spontaneous reduction of the fibula, which then requires no further treatment (see Fig. 41b). Spontaneous reduction of the fibular fracture is considered evidence for correct axial alignment of the tibia. Shortening signifies valgus deformity of the tibia, distraction signifies varus (Fig. 198d), and diastasis signifies malrotation.

Spontaneous reduction is not guaranteed, however, and we have found operative stabilization of the distal fibula to be necessary in approximately 7% of tibial shaft fractures. This may occur in two situations:

- *Irreducible angular deformity* (Fig. 198a) of the distal fibular fragment after internal fixation of the tibia. This is most common with transverse tibial fractures. The angulated distal fragment can adversely affect the malleolar mortise. Open reduction is easily accomplished through a small longitudinal incision and can be secured with a short implant (Fig. 198b).
- *Instability of the ankle mortise* after internal fixation of the tibia. Here the fibular fracture is accompanied by tearing of the anterior tibiofibular ligament and possibly of the interosseous membrane. This laxity of the ankle joint is not clinically evident prior to internal fixation of the tibia, and so the mortise should

be examined after the tibial phase of the operation is completed. This may be done by palpation, but an image intensifier is more reliable. If instability is noted, the fibula must be fixed (and the ligamentous injury repaired) following the technique used for type C fractures (Fig. 198c).

e) Internal Fixation of the Fibula in Type C Fractures

Usually the fibula is stabilized with a neutralization plate, possibly combined with screw fixation. The one-third tubular plate has replaced medullary nailing of the fibula, which offers poor rotational stability and can further traumatize the bone.

After fixation of the fibula, repair of the anterior tibiofibular ligament is carried out. Reinforcing sutures also may be used (Fig. 206). Next the stability of the mortise is tested, giving special attention to posterior drawer mobility (Fig. 205c). If stability is inadequate, additional measures must be taken. These may involve placing an extra screw in a small posterior malleolar fragment (avulsion fracture of the posterior tibiofibular ligament or posterior margin of the fibular notch) or possibly the insertion of a transfixing screw.

Three special situations must be considered from the standpoint of internal fixation: comminuted fractures, high type C fractures, and conditions that warrant transfixion of the fibula to the tibia.

Comminuted Type C Fractures

These fractures are not uncommon and may present as butterfly fractures, segmental fractures, bilevel fractures, or fractures with bone loss, the latter usually occurring in proximity to the syndesmosis. The reduction must be anatomic, i.e., it must restore physiologic length, angular alignment, and rotation. The procedure is very difficult technically, and errors are common. Occasionally, provisional reduction of the fragments will require the use of cerclage wire in addition to small forceps. Long one-third tubular plates (8- to 12-hole) are excellent for definitive fixation and may be combined with separate screws.The plates must be accurately contoured by bending and twisting to prevent malrotation (Fig. 202 a). Primary cancellous grafting is recommended for sites of bone loss.

High Type C Fibular Fracture

We make a distinction between fibular shaft fractures and subcapital Maisonneuve fractures. The latter is associated with circumferential tearing of the ankle joint ligaments and a complete rupture of the interosseous membrane. In the absence of fibular shortening, the prognosis is considerably better than when there is shortening or dislocation of the fibular head (Fig. 196 C3).

Direct Internal Fixation. This is possible only up to about the middle of the fibular shaft. Farther proximally the fibula is deeply embedded in muscle. Exposure is difficult, and there is a high risk of peroneal nerve injury.

Indirect Stabilization (Fig. 201): In Maisonneuve fractures with shortening, the major problem is to restore the anatomic length of the fibula and return it to the center of the fibular notch. We recommend taking preoperative spot radiographs of the contralateral joint for comparison with the intraoperative film. The fixation is carried out in stages:

- Reduction of the fibula: A small hole is drilled in the lateral cortex of the distal fibula. A curved hook is inserted and the fibula pulled distally until it seats into the fibular notch of the tibia. The fibula is temporarily transfixed to the tibia with a 1.6-mm Kirschner wire drilled in horizontally.
- A spot film is taken of the ankle joint and compared with the bilateral preoperative films.
- The position of the fibula can also be assessed by noting the direction or coaptability of the fibers of the torn anterior tibiofibular ligament.
- The fibula is definitively stabilized with one or two transfixing screws placed 4–6 cm proximal to the ankle joint (3.5-mm cortex screws using three-point fixation, Fig. 203).

- Lateral ligament repairs should follow the technique illustrated in Fig. 206.
- Ankle joint motion is tested by passive dorsiflexion of the foot. The repaired ligamentous fibers should become tense without tearing as the foot is dorsiflexed.

Transfixing the Fibula to the Tibia

(Figs. 201, 202, 203)

The indications for a tibiofibular transfixing screw are quite limited, because the procedure is unphysiologic. We feel that there are only two situations which justify its use:

1) Residual instability (posterior drawer sign) following internal fixation of the fibula and ligament repairs. The cause is always a proximal tear of the interosseous membrane or a small, untreated fracture of the posterior malleolus.

2) The Maisonneuve fracture (type C subcapital fibular fracture), which precludes direct internal fixation of the fibula.

The transfixing screw must stabilize the syndesmosis without compressing it. That is why a cortex screw is used rather than a cancellous or malleolar screw. Both cortices of the fibula are threaded (i.e., a gliding hole is not prepared). The screws threads engage a total of three cortices–the lateral and medial cortex of the fibula and the lateral cortex of the tibia (three-point fixation). A 3.5-mm cortex screw placed in this way provides an elastic fixation that does not restrict movements of the ankle mortise and preserves the range of ankle motion (especially dorsiflexion of the foot) as well as fibular length. The screw need not engage the medial cortex of the tibia.

A transfixing screw can also be inserted through the hole of a previously attached plate: When residual instability is noted after internal fixation, a screw is removed from the plate at the appropriate site. A pilot hole is drilled into the lateral tibial cortex through the plate hole with a pointed 2.0-mm Kirschner wire, and it is enlarged with the 2.5-mm drill bit. Then the lateral tibial cortex is tapped and a long 3.5-mm cortex screw is inserted, engaging all three cortices and solidly transfixing the fibula to the tibia (Fig. 203). The usual screw length is 30–34 mm.

The transfixing screw may also be inserted separate from the plate. We do this mainly for the indirect stabilization of high, type C fibular fractures (Fig. 201 b). The technique is as follows: After fibular length has been restored and the fibula returned to its notch as described above, a 2.5-mm hole is drilled horizontally through the fibula 4–6 cm above the joint. The hole is directed about 30° anteriorly so that it will meet the lateral border of the tibia squarely (Fig. 203 a). This hole is started with a pointed 2-mm Kirschner wire and completed with a 2.5-mm drill bit. A bit used without a pilot hole might bend or break against the tibial surface if it did not meet the border squarely. Next the threads (3.5-mm cortex) are cut in the three drill holes, and a cortex screw of appropriate length is inserted. The lateral fibular cortex is not countersunk, as this would sacrifice some of the tapped portion of the hole. The screw head protrudes slightly and is easily located at the time of removal (Fig. 203 b,c).

After the transfixion is completed, the foot is passively dorsiflexed to confirm free motion in the ankle joint.

We have found early removal of the transfixing screw to be unnecessary. The screw does not exert a compressive effect, or interfere with ankle motion. If the screw is stressed by rotational movement of the fibula at an early stage, a small area of osteolysis may appear at its tip on X-rays, or the screw may break during mobilization. It is safe to leave the broken screw tip within the tibia during subsequent implant removal.

Transfixion with standard-size 4.5-mm cortex screws leads to stiffening of the syndesmosis. These screws are removed separately when fibrous healing is complete, i.e., no later than 8–10 weeks after the internal fixation.

f) Internal Fixation of the Fibula in Type B Fractures

Long oblique or spiral fractures can be fixed with small cortex screws or cancellous screws alone (Fig. 204 a). With multi-part fractures or a short fracture line, the screws should be supplemented by a contoured one-third tubular plate (Fig. 204 b). We usually apply this plate laterally, although posterior plating can give better stability in certain oblique fractures with a distal fragment that terminates posteriorly in a spike (Weber's "anti-gliding plate") (Fig. 204d). The proximal retinaculum of the peroneal tendons must be spared when a posterior plate is used.

In comminuted fractures, especially when osteoporosis exists, fixation is occasionally accomplished with multiple Kirschner wires inserted at varying angles. These may be interconnected and reinforced with a tension-band wire if desired. The oblique transfixion of the tibia and fibula produced by the Kirschner wires in the area of the syndesmosis is not detrimental, although care must be taken to avoid separation of the mortise. Fibular shortening is also a danger with this technique (Fig. 204e).

g) Internal Fixation of the Fibula in Type A Fractures

Most of these fractures are short oblique or transverse types. A straight plate or small T plate is sometimes appropriate, but most cases are managed with a tension-band loop applied over Kirschner wires (Fig. 204f).

h) Ligament Repairs about the Ankle Joint

The importance of the ligaments as stabilizers of malleolar fractures is often underestimated. The following ligamentous injuries may be encountered at operation:

Anterior Tibiofibular Ligament:
- Tibial avulsion with or without a small cortical fragment (at the "tubercle of Tillaux-Chaput")
- Midsubstance tear, often Z-shaped
- Fibular avulsion with or without a small cortical fragment

Posterior Tibiofibular Ligament:
Tears of this ligament are difficult to approach surgically, and little is known about their morphology. They may be identified in situ through an anterior approach if there are coexisting tears of the anterior tibiofibular ligament and interosseous membrane. In these cases the tibia and fibula can be separated by passing a spreader between them, and a fine instrument (elevator) can be introduced to probe the posterior ligamentous injury (Fig. 205b).

Interosseous Membrane:
- Avulsion at the tibial insertion. The extent of these tears is independent of the level of the fibular fracture. Tears of the interosseous membrane and anterior tibiofibular ligament can occur in the absence of a fibular fracture.

Distal Fibular Ligaments (Anterior and Posterior Talofibular Ligaments, Calcaneofibular Ligament):
- Fibular avulsion (frequent)
- Talar avulsion
- Midsubstance tear
- Posterior avulsion from the calcaneus; includes tearing of the inferior retinaculum of the peroneal tendons

Tears of the distal fibular ligaments are frequently combined with "isolated" fractures of the medial malleolus.

Deltoid Ligament:
- Tibial avulsion (frequent)
- Z-shaped avulsion
- Talar avulsion (rare)

Displacement and entrapment of the tibialis posterior tendon is possible in these tears.

A common objection to the operative treatment of these injuries is that suture repairs have insufficient tensile strength, cannot restore the anatomy of the torn ligament fibers, and interfere with their blood supply.

The only mechanically effective and biologically sound method of repairing a torn ligament is to reinsert it on an avulsed piece of bone. This restores the fascicular architecture of the fibers, reestablishes their physiologic tension, and preserves their blood supply. Avulsion fractures are the rule in children and are less common in adults (Figs. 204 c, 206 b).

The suture repair of torn ligaments–except for the powerful deltoid ligament–is merely a coaptation. It is performed with fine suture material and is an important prerequisite for ligament healing. But if mechanical strength is required, the coapting suture needs to be reinforced.

Transosseous reinforcement of the anterior tibiofibular ligament (Fig. 206):

- Channels are drilled in the tibia and fibula on both sides of the tear and are rounded with a curved hemostat. Heavy absorbable sutures are passed through the channels and tied under tension.

On the fibular side, the reinforcing suture can be anchored by passing it around a plate, wire loop, Kirschner wire, or other internal fixation material.

For years we have used only absorbable suture material (polyglycol or polyacetate) for reinforcing ligament repairs. This material protects the repair until the ligament fibers have regenerated, and it does not interfere with fine movements at the syndesmosis.

After completing the reinforcement, the surgeon tests its mechanical strength (elimination of drawer mobility) and also verifies free passive motion of the foot.

The reinforced repair permits active mobilization of the ankle joint as well as partial weight bearing, depending on the stability of the internal fixation.

Coexisting tears of the interosseous membrane heal completely without sequelae under the protection of a reinforced anterior tibiofibular ligament repair and do not require suturing. We have abandoned our earlier practice of repairing the interosseous membrane with transosseous sutures.

i) Fractures of the "Posterior Malleolus"

Approximately one-third of all malleolar fractures are accompanied by bony lesions of the posterior tibial margin. Most of these occur in the posterolateral quadrant, in the most delicate part of the joint.The rare posteromedial lesions of the tibia are discussed under the heading of medial malleolar fractures.

Five morphologically distinct types of posterolateral lesion are recognized (Fig. 207):

Articular Fragments:
Articular fragments are sheared off by pressure from the dislocating talus, which may be spontaneously or iatrogenically reduced by the time the postinjury radiograph is obtained.

Articular fragments account for approximately half of all posterior malleolar lesions.

- *Larger marginal fragments* involve a substantial portion of the articular surface of the tibia. Involvement of one-third or more of the joint line is apparent on the lateral spot film.
- *Smaller marginal fragments* involve a smaller area of the articular surface.

  Often it is difficult to estimate the size of the fragment. Postinjury radiographs usually are poorly centered in the presence of foot deformity, and dislocation of the talus can compound the difficulty of evaluation. Diagnosis can be aided by an AP view demonstrating the proximal, displaced tip of the fragment as a fine radiopaque line ("Gothic window sign"). Such fragments definitely involve the articular surface.
- *Marginal fragments with compression of the tibial articular surface.* Marginal compression occurs in approximately one-fourth of articular rim fractures but often cannot be appreciated on the initial radiograph. It magnifies the lesion of the tibial joint surface and can pose an obstacle to reduction.

Extra-articular Fragments:

- Small peripheral fragments outside the weight-bearing articular surface are common. Most represent avulsion fractures of the joint capsule. They do not cause traumatic arthritis.
- Small, flake-like avulsion fractures of the posterior tibiofibular ligament occur slightly proximal to the joint margin. They are relatively rare.

Patient Selection. Today it is generally acknowledged that fragments involving a portion of the articular surface should be anatomically reduced to establish a normal articular relation between the talus and tibia.It is equally important to stabilize the joint so that functional exercises can be performed.

Another argument is the necessity of seating the fibula securely in the fibular notch of the tibia. Marginal fragments form the posterior lip of the fibular notch and, when displaced, cannot retain the fibula within the notch (Fig. 207d). In doubtful cases fixation of a small marginal fragment is preferable to the use of an unphysiologic transfixing screw.

The main difficulty in patient selection is the estimation of fragment size. Another problem is the natural hesitancy of many surgeons to approach these deeply situated fracture elements.

Before the operation is begun, consideration must be given to the best patient position, or position change, for gaining access to the posterior malleolus (see above), and corresponding preparations must be made.

It is advantageous to perform the reduction and fixation under direct vision, as it is difficult to center X-ray apparatus properly for films or for image intensification fluoroscopy.

Indirect Screw Fixation from the Anterior Side (Fig. 208 a,b)

The fragment is exposed and reduced through a posteromedial incision, but the fixation screw is inserted from the anterior side. This technique is especially suitable for large fragments. After internal fixation of the fibula and repair of the lateral ligaments, a long, curved incision is made in front of or behind the medial malleolus (Fig. 200c).If there is a fracture of the medial malleolus, it is tended to first.

The tibialis posterior tendon sheath is incised longitudinally (Fig. 209a). With a large fragment, the sheath will contain a hematoma. A Hohmann retractor is passed along the posterior surface of the tibia and retracts the tendons and neurovascular bundle posteriorly.The medial edge of the posterior malleolar fragment should present immediately adjacent to the tendon sheath. The thick periosteum is incised to expose the tip of the fragment (Fig. 209 b).This will serve as the guide for obtaining an anatomic reduction. If a depressed area is found, it is reduced under vision with an impactor (Fig. 209c). With a hook, the fragment is pulled distally and brought into a normal position; it is temporarily held in place with a reduction forceps (Fig. 209d). A 1.6-mm Kirschner wire is drilled into the fragment from the anteromedial aspect of the tibia and serves as a guide for drilling two 2.5-mm holes into the fragment (Fig. 209e). The drill holes are skewed slightly, taking care to avoid any implants that have been previously placed in the medial malleolus. Two cancellous screws with washers are driven into the holes. Interfragmental compression is obtained by having at least one of the screw threads lie entirely within the posterior fragment (Fig. 208a).Experience has shown that a small amount of screw thread projecting posteriorly will not harm the soft tissues. With smaller fragments, the screw thread can be shortened with a special cutting forceps (Fig. 208b).

If there is doubt as to the accuracy of the reduction, a lateral spot film should be taken while the Kirschner wire is in place, but *before* the screws are inserted.

Some surgeons prefer to insert the screws through a small, separate anterolateral incision.

Weber's Technique of Anterolateral Screw Fixation (Fig. 211)

In this technique, reduction and fixation of the posterior malleolar fragment are done as an initial step *before* reduction of the fibula. The Weber technique is appropriate only in type B cases with a relatively mobile, oblique fibular fracture, which can be distracted to expose the fibular notch of the tibia. Traction on the tip of the fibula restores the posterolateral fragment to a congruent position, in which it can be temporarily held with a Kirschner wire inserted percutaneously from the posterior side. The fragment is then fixed indirectly with screws inserted from the anterolateral side.

Direct Screw Fixation (Fig. 208c,d)

This technique gives significantly better interfragmental compression, but the approach is more difficult, and suitable preparations for positioning must be made (Fig. 199). The screws may be introduced from the posterolateral or posteromedial side. We prefer the latter in cases where there is compression of the tibial articular surface.

Posterolateral Approach (Fig. 210)

The patient's foot is placed in medial rotation (either at the flexed knee or in lateral decubitus).

The surgeon performs the operation in a sitting position.

We recommend the standard incision lengthened by a curved posterior extension, or a vertical incision placed immediately behind the lateral malleolus (Fig. 200).

The posterior malleolus is approached between the peroneal tendons and the flexor hallucis longus tendon, which are held apart with blunt retractors. As before, the tip of the fragment is exposed by incision of the thick periosteum; it is fitted into place and held there with a Kirschner wire. Definitive fixation is obtained with one or two cancellous screws with washers inserted close to the joint from the posterior side.

When drilling, care is taken to avoid penetration of the ankle joint – a mishap that can easily occur because of the inclined position of the articular surface with the knee in flexion. As a precaution, we mark the joint space with a hypodermic needle or thin Kirschner wire inserted percutaneously from the anterior side (Fig. 210a).

Posteromedial Approach (Fig. 209f)

This approach is used mainly when there is compression of the tibial margin. The fragment is exposed as for an indirect screw fixation (Fig. 209a–d), but the approach is extended by curving the skin incision proximally toward the Achilles tendon. The area of compression is exposed by separating the fracture surfaces with a hook, Hohmann retractor, or small bone spreader. It is reduced with an impactor under vision, then reduction and temporary forceps fixation are carried out as described earlier for indirect screw fixation.

The screw holes are drilled from the posterior side, directly adjacent to the Achilles tendon, while the tendons and neurovascular bundle are retracted medially. This approach is deeper than the posterolateral, and it is more difficult to conserve the soft tissues. Later removal of the implants is not advised.

k) Anterolateral Tibial Fracture (of Tillaux-Chaput)

Fractures of the anterolateral tibial margin may be difficult to appreciate on radiographs. The fragments vary in size from tiny bony avulsions of the syndesmosis to larger wedge-shaped fragments. Stabilization is imperative because the fracture line extends into the syndesmosis, disrupting the integrity of the ankle mortise, and because the fragment is attached to the anterior tibiofibular ligament of the syndesmosis. Internal fixation is generally accomplished with a cancellous screw, possibly combined with a spiked metal or plastic washer (Fig. 206b). The incision is placed just anterior to the lateral malleolus, sparing the cutaneous branch of the superficial peroneal nerve, which takes an irregular course (Fig. 200a).

l) Peroneal Tendon Displacement

Traumatic anterior displacement of the peroneal tendons has become more prevalent in recent years. It may occur in isolation or it may accompany other ankle injuries such as malleolar fractures, ligamentous and Achilles tendon ruptures, etc. The lesion is easily missed clinically because of swelling, and its neglect can lead to significant disability that will eventually require surgical correction. The acute injury occurs in three forms (Fig. 212 a):

- Tearing of the superior retinaculum with avulsion of periosteum from the anterior fibula. The displaced tendons lie beneath a raised flap of periosteum, which is continuous with the retinaculum. After the tendons are reduced, the retinaculum can be fixed to the posterior fibular margin with a screw and spiked plastic washer. The periosteum is repaired with coapting sutures (Fig. 212 b).
- Avulsion fracture of the fibula. The fragment is anatomically reduced and fixed with small screws.
- Tear of the retinaculum at its insertion (relatively rare). Direct suture repair may not be possible because of swelling. The retinaculum is reconstructed with a free plantaris longus tendon graft or with a flap of periosteum based on the tip of the lateral malleolus. Recurrences are uncommon.

A long-standing peroneal tendon displacement can be managed with a *Kelly osteotomy*. In this procedure a piece of cancellous bone on the lateral malleolus is osteotomized, transposed posteriorly, and fixed with screws to create a ridge that opposes further tendon displacement (Fig. 212c). The retinaculum can also be reconstructed with a free plantaris tendon graft or a distally based strip of Achilles tendon. Transposition of the peroneal tendons beneath the calcaneofibular ligament by osteotomy of the tip of the lateral malleolus also has been described.

3. Internal Fixations on the Medial Side

Fractures of the medial malleolus and associated ligamentous injuries have less biomechanical significance than lateral injuries, and so less attention has been given to the technical aspects of internal fixations on the medial side.Nevertheless, this does not diminish the importance of accurately reducing and stabilizing these fractures. Consideration must be given to the doubly curved surface anatomy of the medial malleolus, and special attention must be given to compression injuries of the anterior portion of the joint surface and to posterior fractures involving the tendon canals.

In isolated medial fractures, it is important to consider the possibility of coexisting ligament tears. Ruptures of the anterior talofibular ligament and calcaneofibular ligament are most common and can be recognized only on functional films taken under anesthesia. Concomitant tears of the syndesmotic ligaments and interosseous membrane are also possible. Fixation of the medial fracture alone will not adequately stabilize the joint, and ligamentous tears about the distal end of the fibula should be identified and repaired whenever such lesions are presumed or confirmed.

The fracture is exposed through a slightly curved longitudinal incision placed anterior or posterior to the medial malleolus. This preserves lymphatic drainage (danger of lymphedema with transverse incisions) and also permits the incision to be extended as needed–especially proximally and posteriorly, as for indirect screw fixation of the posterior malleolus (Fig. 200c).

a) Tibial Shaft Fractures that Involve the Ankle Joint

It has been our experience that approximately 10% of spiral fractures of the tibia involve the ankle joint. Most fracture lines skirt the periphery of the medial malleolus. Sometimes the lines are too fine to be seen on X-rays and are not detected until operation. Often the fragments are unstable and, if displaced, must be accurately reduced. Experience has shown that reduction of the more proximal, main fracture is made easier by first reducing and fixing the intra-articular extension. This is especially true with posterior fracture lines.

Approach and Internal Fixation. The standard incision for tibial fractures is extended distally along the anterior border of the medial malleolus. It crosses the great saphenous vein, which may have to be divided between ligatures. The ankle joint is opened just anterior to the deltoid ligament at the border of the medial malleolus. Any blood in the joint is aspirated.The incision in the joint capsule is extended until the fracture line can be clearly visualized and reduced.

The fracture may be stabilized with the tibial plate itself, as long as the main fracture can be plated distally and there are no soft-tissue problems. When a DCP is used, the distal plate screw may be low enough to give simultaneous fixation of the malleolus when inserted parallel to the joint (i.e., obliquely through the plate as in Fig. 213a). Usually, however, distal fracture lines have to be stabilized by one or two small cancellous screws with washers inserted separately (Fig. 213b).

b) Oblique Fracture of the Medial Malleolus (Fig. 214)

This is the classic indication for internal fixation with two small cancellous screws. With a large malleolar fragment, the procedure is like that shown in Fig. 22: The fragment is temporarily fixed with Kirschner wires, which serve as guides.

Comminuted fractures are often managed by combining Kirschner wire fixation with a wire-loop tension band.

When the condition of the soft tissues is poor, it is sometimes helpful to insert a separate screw through a small stab incision.

c) Small Avulsion or Chip Fracture

This may involve only the anterior part of the malleolus. Very small fragments may become embedded in the stretched but unruptured deltoid ligament and must be "hunted" in the fibrous tissue. The fracture is stabilized with a screw or small tension band, depending on the fragment size (Fig. 214d). Associated ligamentous tears should also be repaired.

Weber has described a special technique for the indirect screw fixation of small medial malleolar fragments. This must precede internal fixation of the fibula, because it requires opening of the medial joint space, which in turn requires some amount of lateral mobility. The 2.7 mm screw is inserted proximally to distally after creating a gliding hole and a special recess for countersinking the head (Fig. 214 f).

d) Posterior Fractures (Fig. 214 e)

Shell-like fractures can extend far posteriorly and involve the articular surface of the tibia. Sometimes they occur directly adjacent to a fracture of the posterior malleolus. It is necessary to open the tibialis posterior tendon sheath and retract the soft tissues posteriorly in order to expose and accurately reduce this fracture. Following reduction and temporary fixation with a Kirschner wire, the screws are inserted such that their heads lie at the edges of the tendon canals and not within them. It is not necessary to suture the tendon sheath.

e) Adduction Fractures (Fig. 215)

These are vertical fractures with extension into the proximal medial cortex of the tibia. They are stabilized with two small, diverging cancellous screws with washers. Only one of the screws is placed parallel to the joint line.

The surgeon should watch for compression of the anteromedial tibial joint surface. Areas that are deep and densely impacted can make it difficult to approximate and reduce the fracture surfaces. There may also be areas of wider compression that are transitional to tibial pilon fractures. These lesions must be recognized and corrected before reduction is carried out. Any visible bone defect that is created should be obliterated with autogenous cancellous bone. A small amount of graft material is obtainable from the proximal, intact, non-weight-bearing portion of the tibial metaphysis (Fig. 215b). Screw fixation stabilizes this articular zone against secondary collapse.

4. Aftertreatment

Besides postoperative elevation, it has proved beneficial to immobilize the foot on a 90° splint after all internal fixations of the malleoli. This is necessary to prevent the equinus deformity that would otherwise result from the predominance of the plantar flexors. This fixation can be accomplished in various ways. Some surgeons use dorsal plaster splints, which are not very solid, while others prefer stirrup-like splints that encompass the sides of the foot and the anterior side of the lower leg. These give better immobilization but can place unwanted pressure on the sides of the foot.

Active exercises are performed from the splint on the first postoperative day (dorsiflexion of the foot and toes). Active rotational exercises are started after 3–4 days. At that time, if wound healing is satisfactory, the patient is mobilized from bed under the protection of a rigid elastic bandage. He may perform heel-to-toe rocking and start partial weight bearing according to the stability of the fixation (the weight-bearing schedule should be specified by the surgeon). Usually we allow the patient to place 10–15 kg of weight on the operated limb, measured with a step-on scale. Once the patient is comfortable on crutches, he may be discharged. Weight bearing is increased according to the designated schedule. Most patients progress to full weight bearing in 6–10 weeks, depending on the type of fracture. Some centers routinely place the limb in plaster to provide external protection once active ankle mobility has been achieved. Mobility is quickly regained after the cast is removed.

Usually the implants are removed at six months, although a one year interval is recommended for complex type C fractures of the fibula.

5. Secondary Operations after Malleolar Fractures

a) Late Internal Fixation

Deformities that do not respond to conservative treatment or develop secondarily require operative intervention. If instability exists or there is a soft, easily identifiable callus that can be removed, internal fixation may be carried out just as in a primary operation. Often this is still possible weeks or even months after the original injury.

b) Nonunions

Malleolar nonunions have become rare following primary operative treatment. They are more common after medial malleolar fractures that have been managed conservatively.Operative treatment consists of interfragmental compression with small cancellous screws and washers. These are combined with autogenous cancellous bone grafts if osteoporosis exists.

c) Osteotomy

Shortening of the lateral malleolus after nonoperative fracture treatment or after inadequate length restoration in complex fractures or fractures with bone loss is the most frequent indication for osteotomies about the ankle joint. A lengthening osteotomy of the fibula can be fixed very securely with a one-third tubular plate. Distraction of the osteotomy site can be obtained by using the articulated tension device on a plate attached to one side of the osteotomy (see Fig. 33d), making sure that rotational alignment is correct before tension is applied. Up to about 1 cm of lengthening can be obtained in this way.The lengthening defect is bridged with a block of corticocancellous bone. The medial tibial metaphysis of the same leg makes an excellent donor site.It has been recommended that skin strips be used to reconstruct the anterior tibiofibular ligament, but this is rarely necessary.

C. Fractures of the Talus

Talar fractures may be central or peripheral in location.Avulsion fractures of the lateral process and posterior process of the talus are indications for open reduction and internal fixation to restore joint stability. The same applies to larger osteochondral "flake fractures" of the superior surface of the talus. Treatment consists of screw fixation (Fig. 216). Small fragments can be reattached with fibrin adhesive or with fine, absorbable polyacetate sutures.

Central fractures of the talus (neck, trochlea) are susceptible to avascular necrosis, and emergency treatment is indicated when displacement exists. This can be difficult to evaluate on a standard lateral roentgenogram.

The fracture is exposed through a medial approach and fixed with small cancellous screws inserted obliquely in skewed fashion (Fig. 216b). Defects at the edges of fragments are repaired with autogenous cancellous bone. The patient must use a walking caliper for several months after surgery to relieve weight on the ankle joint.

D. Illustrative Case Reports and X-Rays

(Figs. 217-227)

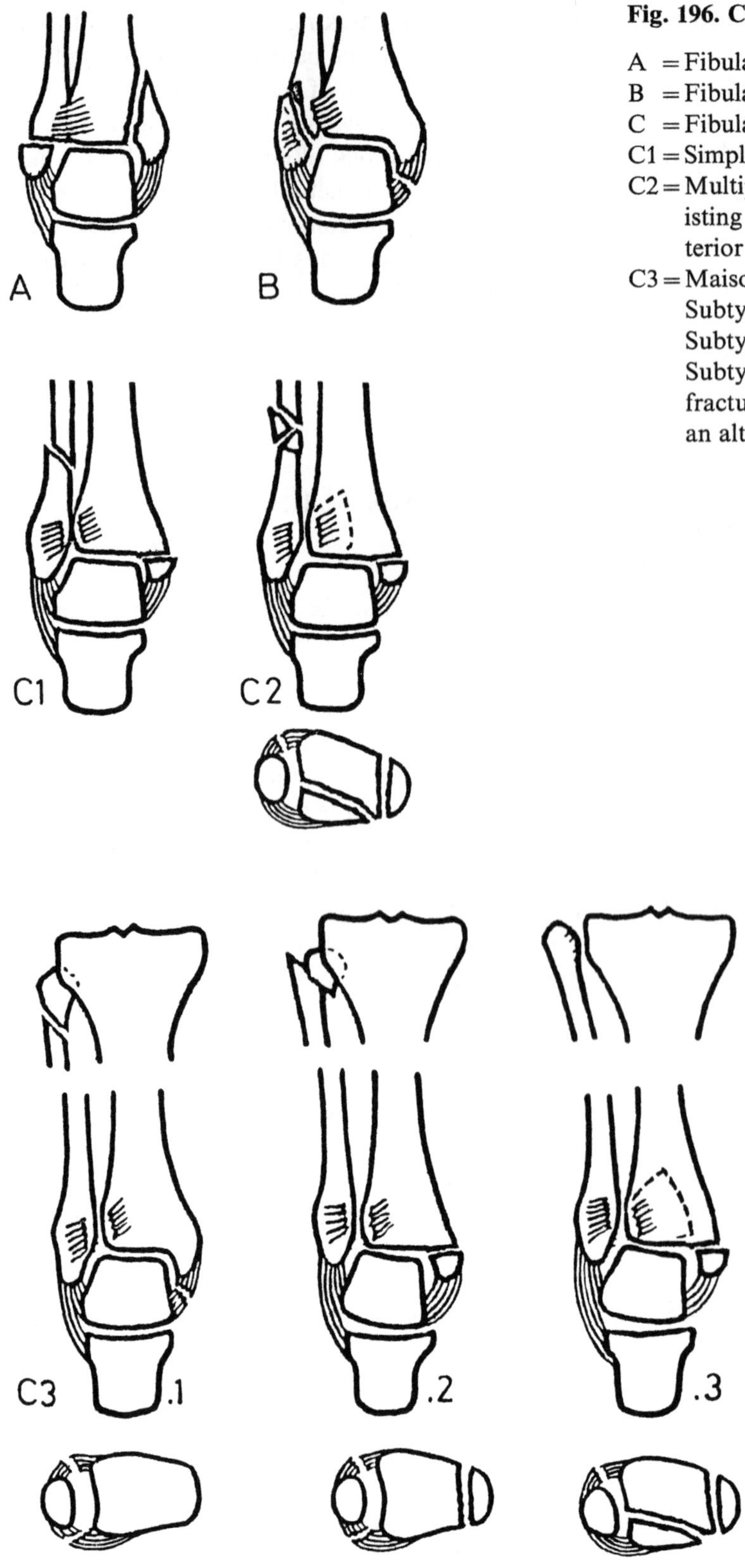

Fig. 196. Classification of malleolar fractures

A =Fibular fracture distal to the syndesmosis
B =Fibular fracture level with the syndesmosis
C =Fibular fracture proximal to the syndesmosis
C1 = Simple fibular fracture
C2 = Multiple fibular fracture (shown here with coexisting fractures of the medial malleolus and posterior malleolus)
C3 = Maisonneuve fracture
Subtype 1 = without shortening
Subtype 2 = with shortening
Subtype 3 = shortening plus posterior malleolar fracture (instead of a fracture the drawing shows an alternative: dislocation of the fibular head)

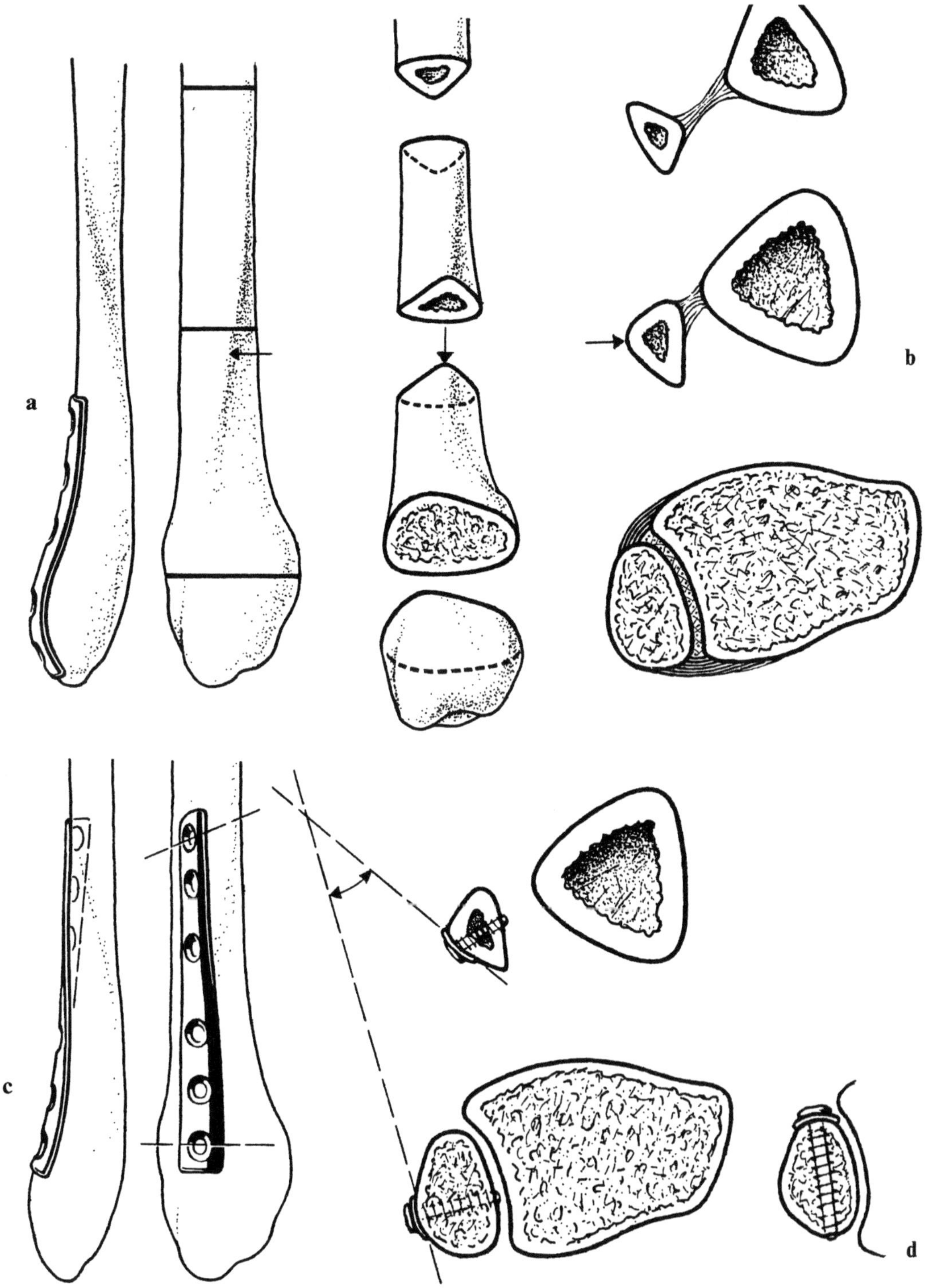

Fig. 197 a–d. Anatomy of the distal fibula

a Distal fibula viewed from the anterior side (with contoured one-third tubular plate) and laterally. Cross-sections at various levels show the changes in the morphology and bony structure of the fibula

b Comparative cross-sections of the fibula and tibia at various levels. Note the posterior rotation of the lateral aspect of the fibular shaft, the interosseous membrane, the fibrous syndesmotic sheet between the two bones at the most distal level (buffer and stabilizer), and the anterior and posterior syndesmotic (tibiofibular) ligaments

c The physiologic torsion of the fibula requires appropriate contouring of the one-third tubular plate (anterior, lateral, and cross-sectional views)

d Posterior plating: The wide cross-section provides a better hold for the screws, and the points do not endanger the talus or syndesmosis

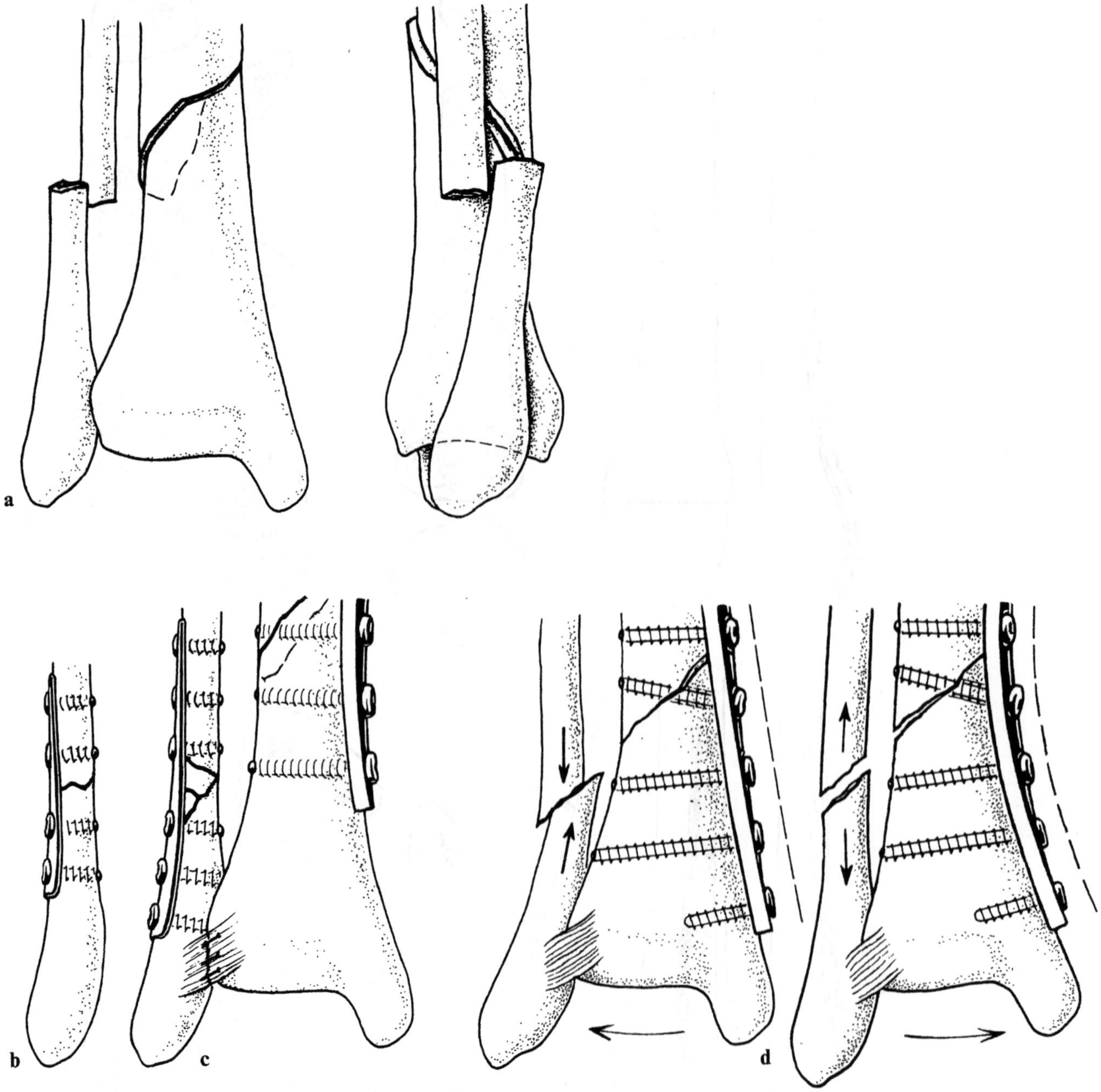

Fig. 198 a–d. Fracture of the distal fibula accompanying a tibial fracture

a Persistent, irreducible displacement of the distal fibula is possible even with internal fixation of the tibia. This disturbs the physiology of the malleolar mortise and is often combined with a tear of the anterior tibiofibular ligament

b A transverse fracture is openly reduced through a separate incision and fixed with a short one-third tubular plate

c A complex fracture and ruptured tibiofibular ligament are managed by a long one-third tubular plate and direct ligament repair

d The position of the fibular fracture reflects the accuracy of the tibial reduction: shortening signifies valgus, distraction signifies varus

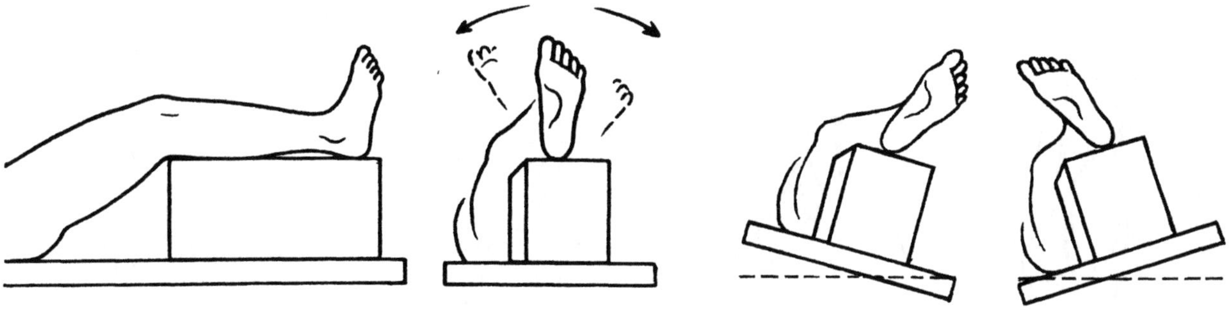

a

Fig. 199 a–d. **Positioning and repositioning for the internal fixation of malleolar fractures**

a Standard position: The lower leg is elevated with the knee moderately flexed. Lateral or medial access can be gained by rotating the knee and is improved by tilting the operating table slightly

b Lateral position for a pure lateral internal fixation; also allows access to the posterior malleolus through a posterolateral approach

c The leg is repositioned for screw fixation of the posterior malleolus through a posteromedial approach. The buttock is supported on a cushion, and the injured leg is flexed at the knee and crossed over the uninjured leg

d Posterolateral approach to the posterior malleolus with the lower leg upright. The surgeon operates from the cranial side of the patient, whose ipsilateral arm is flexed and held toward the opposite side

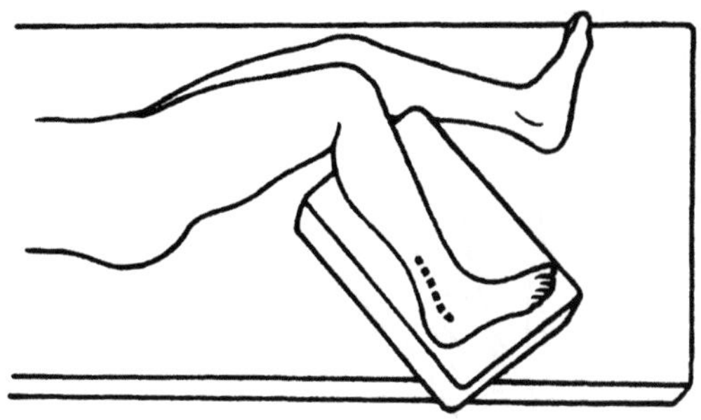

b

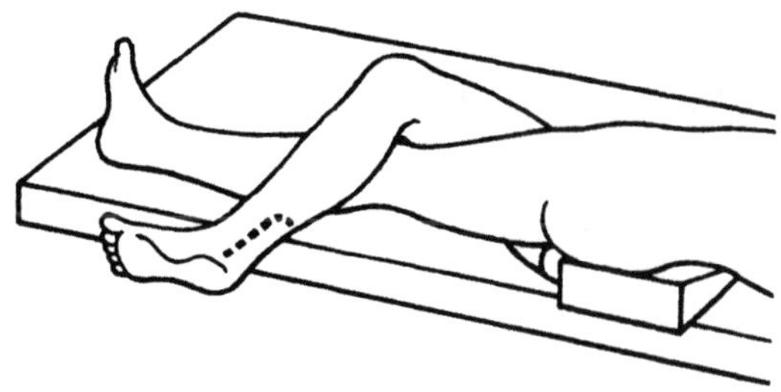

c

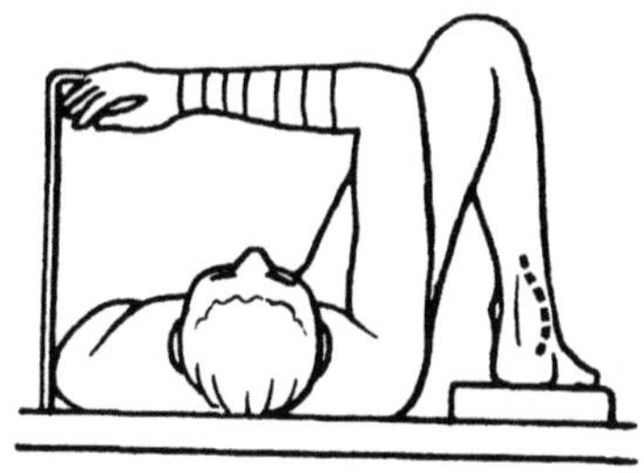

d

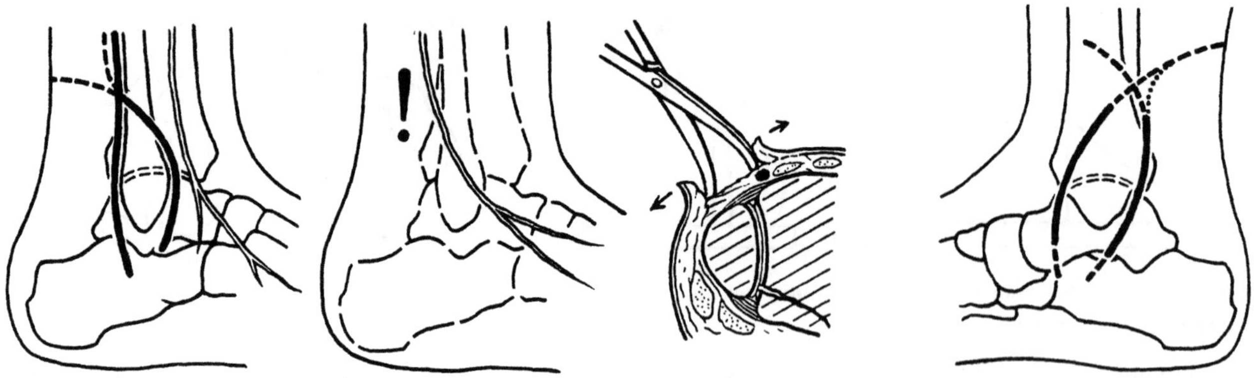

a b c

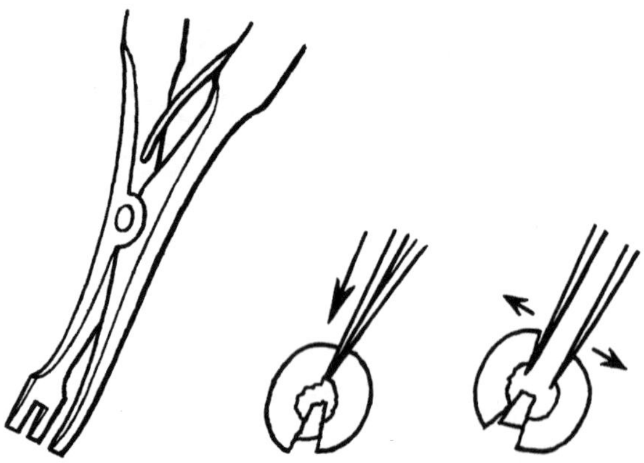

d

Fig. 200 a–d. Skin incisions for the open reduction and internal fixation of malleolar fractures, with extensions for exposing the posterior malleolus

a Standard lateral incisions around the tip of the lateral malleolus. The broken lines indicate possible extensions. The lateral dorsal cutaneous branch of the superficial peroneal nerve normally courses anterior to the lateral malleolus

b The nerve may also emerge from the peroneal tendon compartment and cross the lateral malleolus. Thus it must be identified during the dissection so that it can be protected. It is also vulnerable during later removal of the fixation material

c Standard incisions for exposing the medial malleolus and medial ligaments. The broken lines indicate possible extensions for exposing the posterior malleolus

d The small bone spreader is useful for separating fragments to aid deep reduction under vision

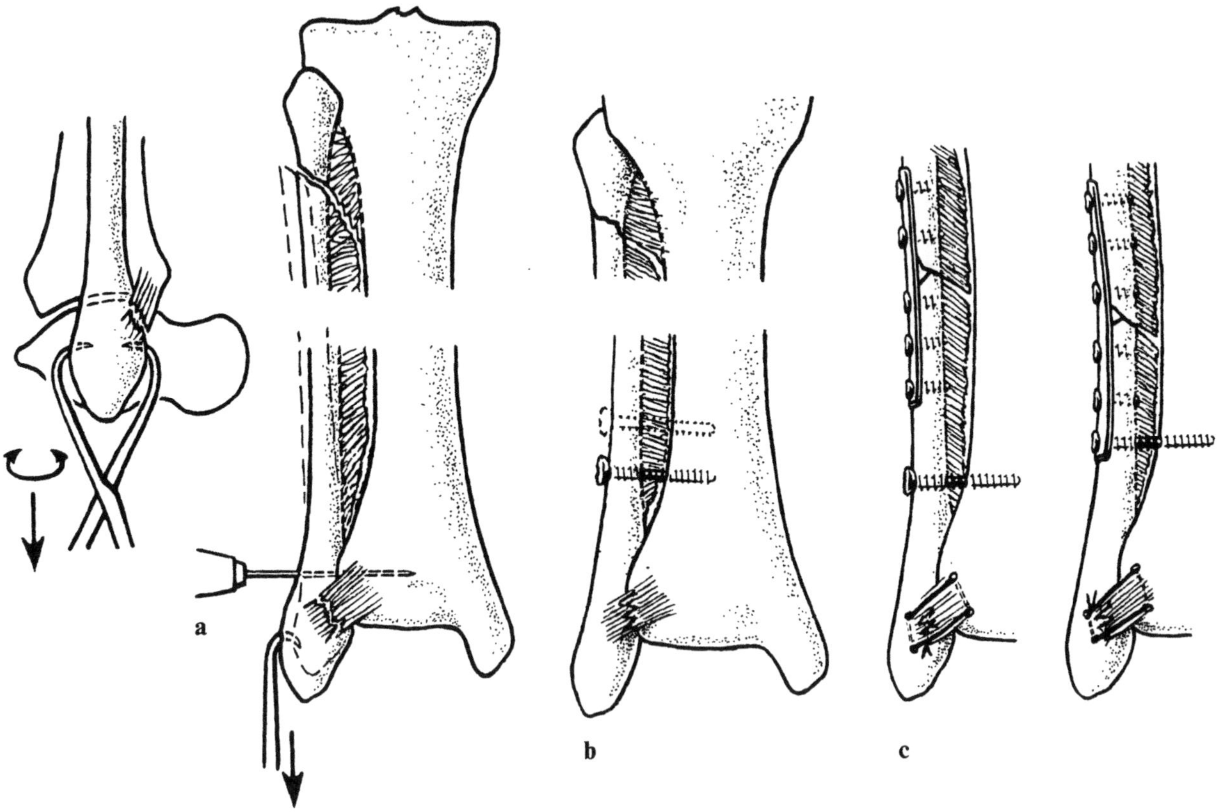

a b c

Fig. 201 a–c. Internal fixation and ligament repairs in type C fibular fractures

a In a Maisonneuve fracture with shortening, the fibula is returned to the fibular notch by applying distal traction with a forceps or curved hook. The torn anterior tibiofibular ligament serves as an indicator. The fracture is temporarily fixed with a transfixing Kirschner wire

b When reduction into the fibular notch is clinically and radiologically confirmed, a supramalleolar transfixing screw (3.5-mm) is inserted, and the ligament is repaired

c Reinforced internal fixation of type C fibular fracture with residual instability of the mortise: one-third tubular plate and a tibiofibular transfixing screw placed distal to the plate or through a plate hole to protect the ligament repair

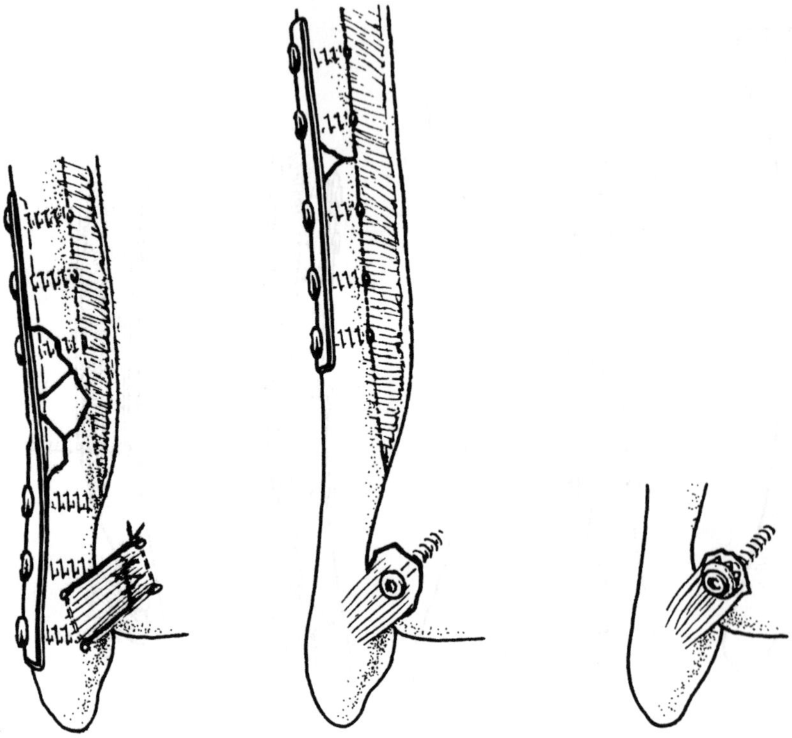

a

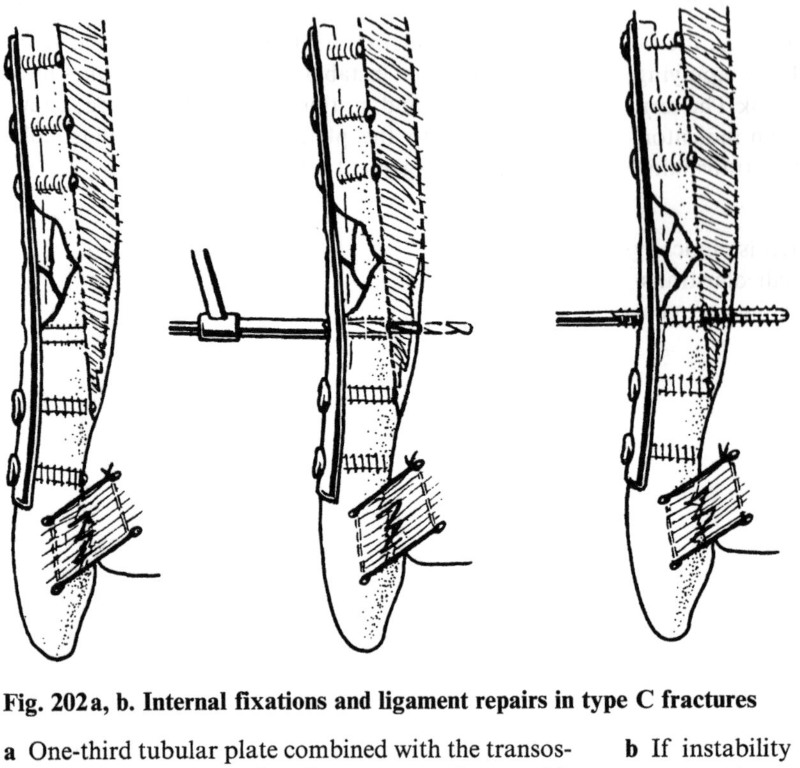

b

Fig. 202a, b. Internal fixations and ligament repairs in type C fractures

a One-third tubular plate combined with the transosseous reinforcement of a ligament repair or with screw fixation of an avulsed fragment to the tubercle of Tillaux-Chaput

b If instability persists despite the reinforced ligament repair, an ordinary plate screw may be replaced with a longer screw that transfixes the fibula to the tibia. The transfixing screw should be placed at least 4 cm proximal to the joint space

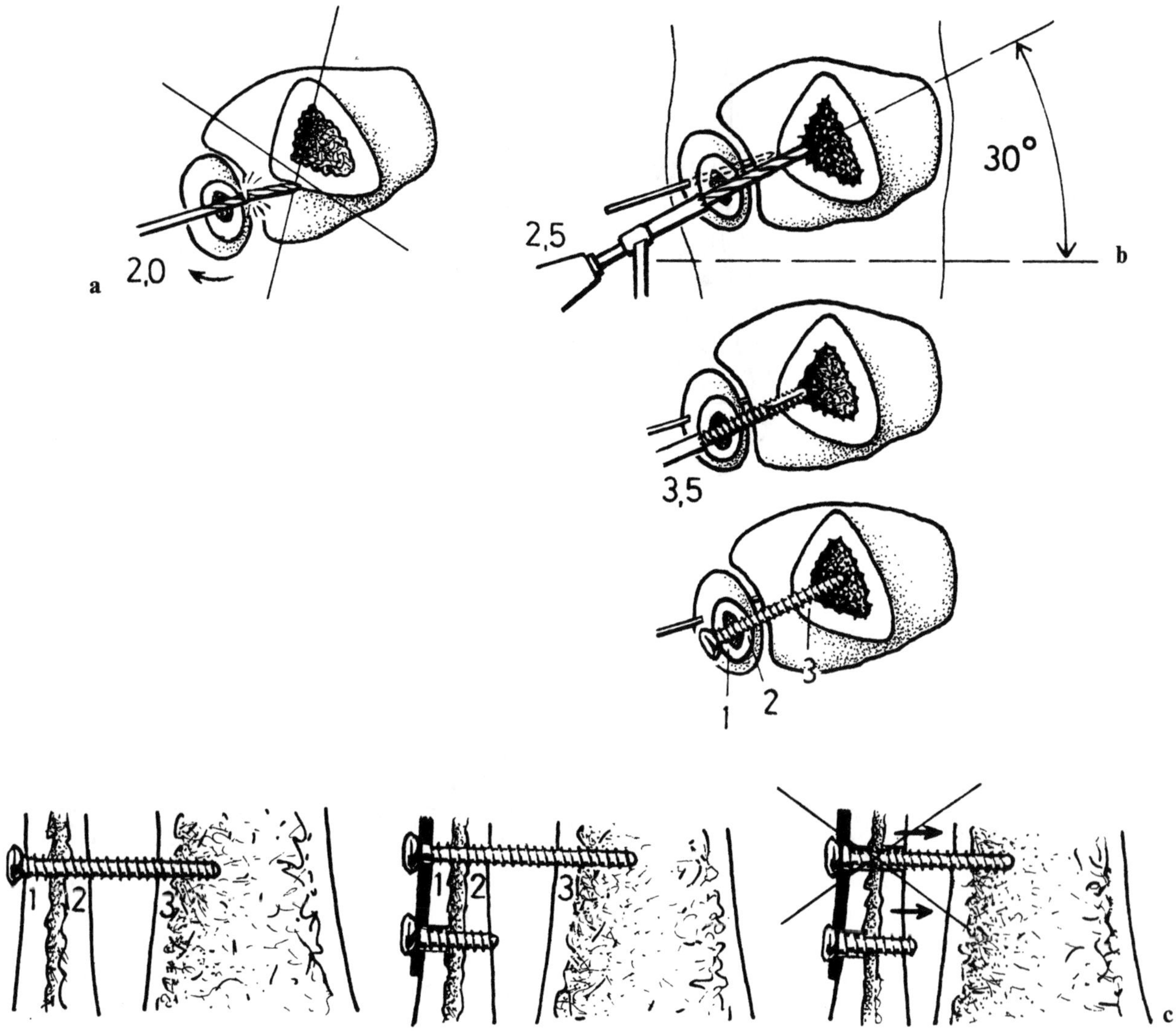

Fig. 203a–c. Technique of tibiofibular transfixion (cross-sectional and anterior views)

a If the screw hole were drilled directly through the fibula to the tibia, the drill bit might bent or break against the tibial cortex and rotate the fibula medially

b This is avoided by first transfixing the fibula to the tibia distally with a Kirschner wire. The three cortices (lateral and medial fibula, lateral tibia) are then perforated with the 2.5-mm bit. The cortices are tapped, and the screw is inserted; the head should project laterally somewhat. This arrangement prevents upward migration of the fibula without immobilizing the syndesmosis. The preliminary Kirschner wire is removed

c Tapping all three cortices (1, 2, 3) avoids tibiofibular compression by an unwanted lag-screw effect. A gliding hole is not made in the fibula

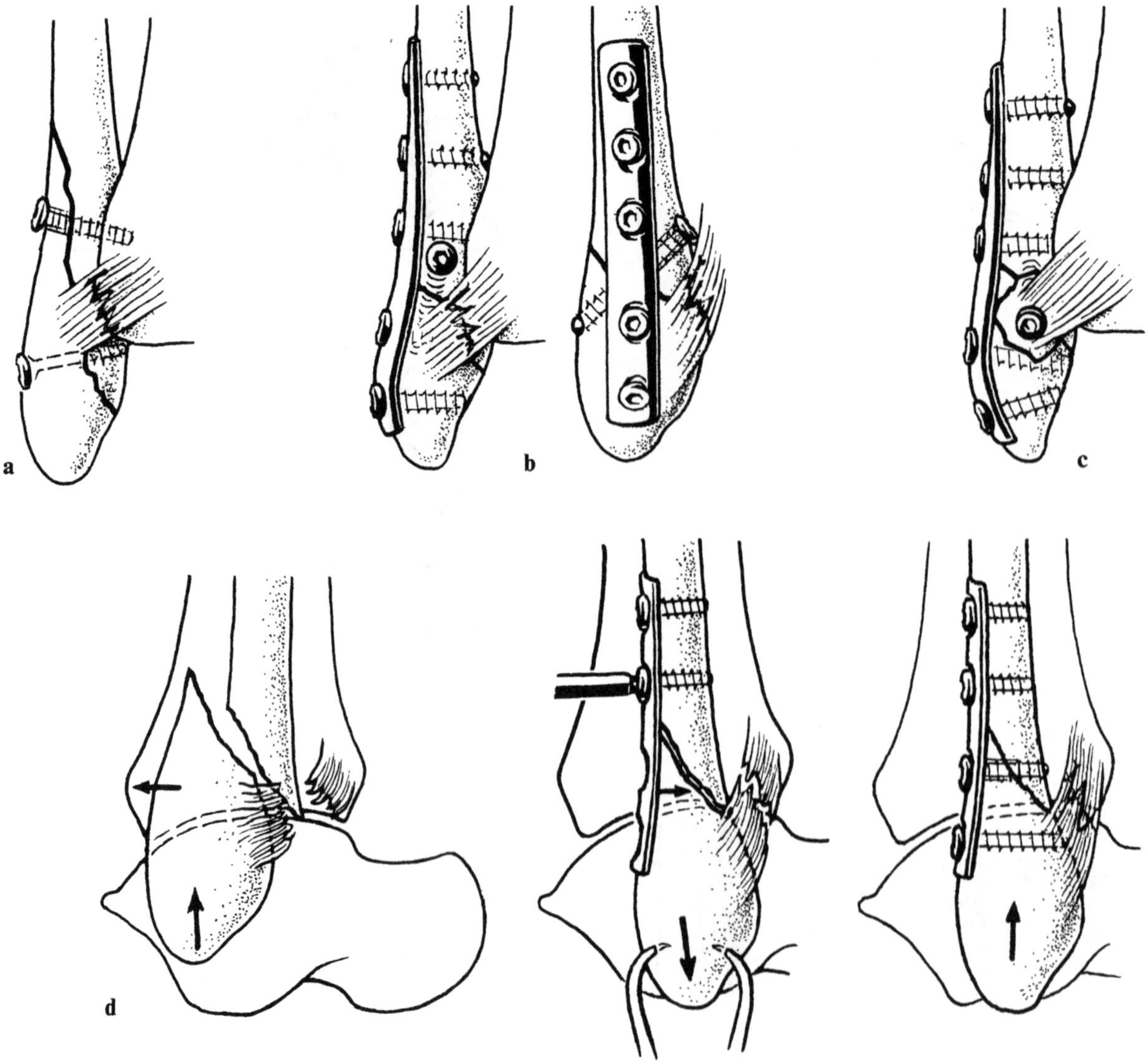

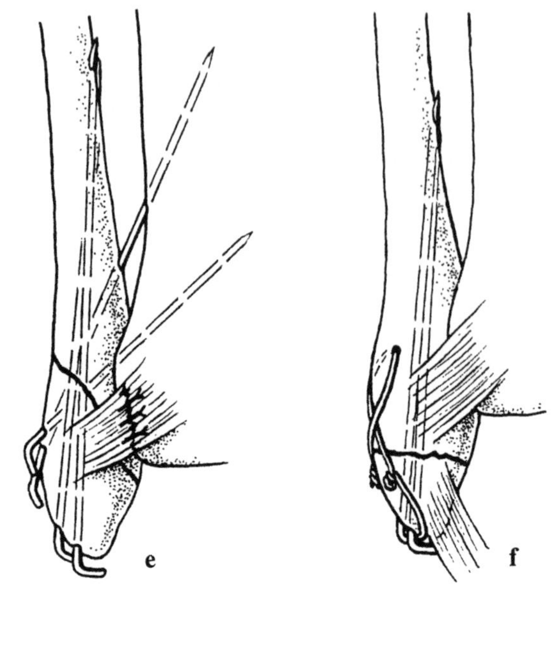

Fig. 204a–f. Internal fixations of the fibula in type B and type A fractures

a Screw fixation of a long oblique type B fracture with repair of the anterior tibiofibular ligament

b, c Screw fixation combined with a one-third tubular plate for a short oblique fracture (anterior and lateral views).The ligament is also repaired

d Weber anti-gliding plate: A one-third tubular plate is attached posteriorly above the fracture line before definitive reduction is performed. The fragments interlock when distal traction is released.The posterior plate may be shorter than a lateral plate

e Multiple Kirschner wires and oblique transfixion; may be combined with a tension-band wire if severe osteoporosis exists

f Tension-band fixation of a type A fracture

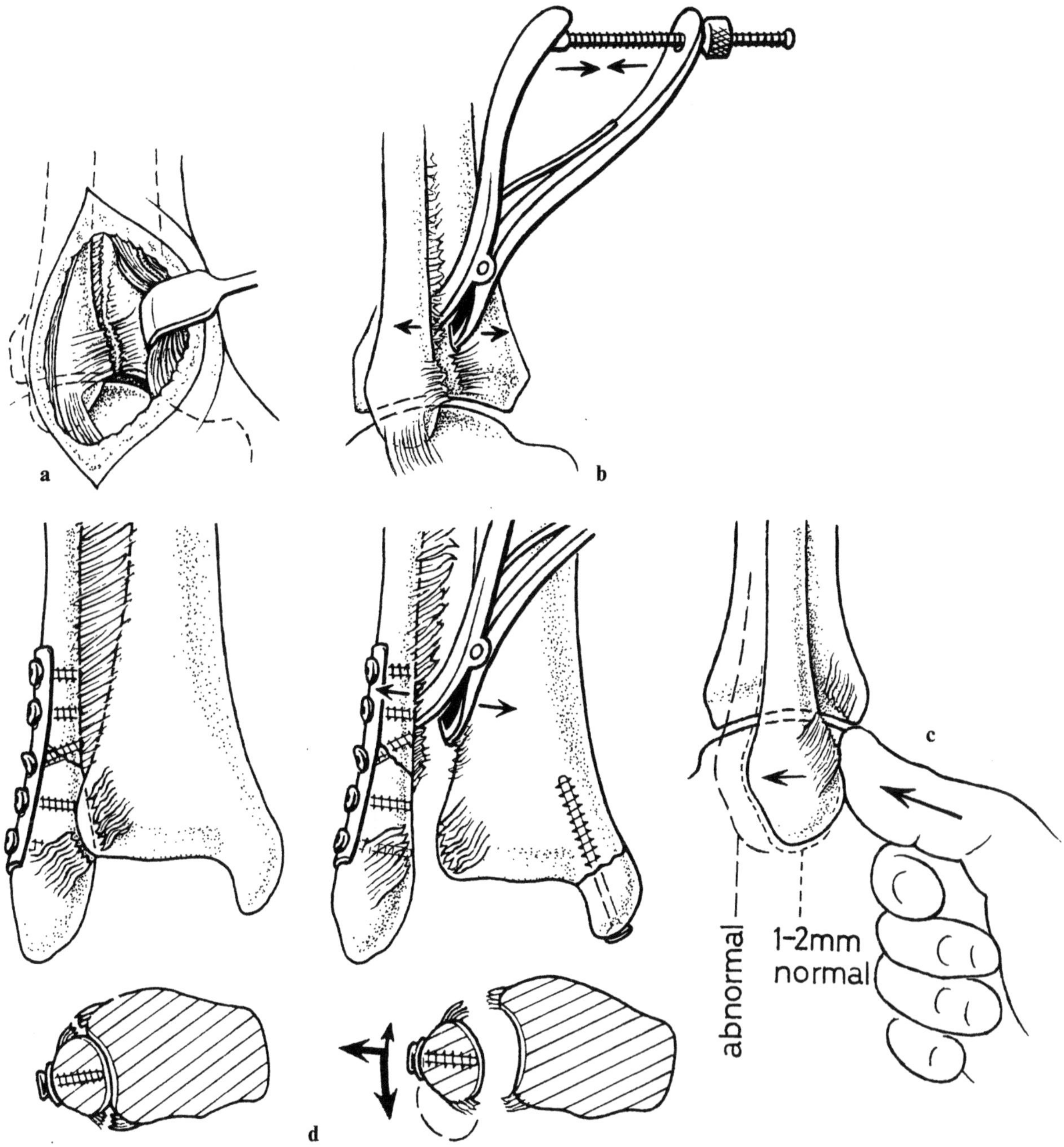

Fig. 205a–d. Assessing the stability of the ankle mortise

a The anterior tibiofibular ligament and distal interosseous membrane are exposed following division of the cruciform ligament, and the long extensors are retracted anteriorly

b With a torn interosseous membrane, the spreader is introduced between the tibia and fibula to expose the fibular notch. The posterior tibiofibular ligament can be probed with an elevator

c Abnormal motion in the ankle mortise is manifested by diastasis and especially by a posterior drawer sign. Anterior thumb pressure should elicit no more than 1–2 mm of movement

d The importance of interosseous membrane integrity for mortise stability: With an intact membrane, the internal fixation will hold the fibula elastically at the center of the notch; the ligament repair has no mechanical significance. With a ruptured membrane, diastasis and drawer mobility exist

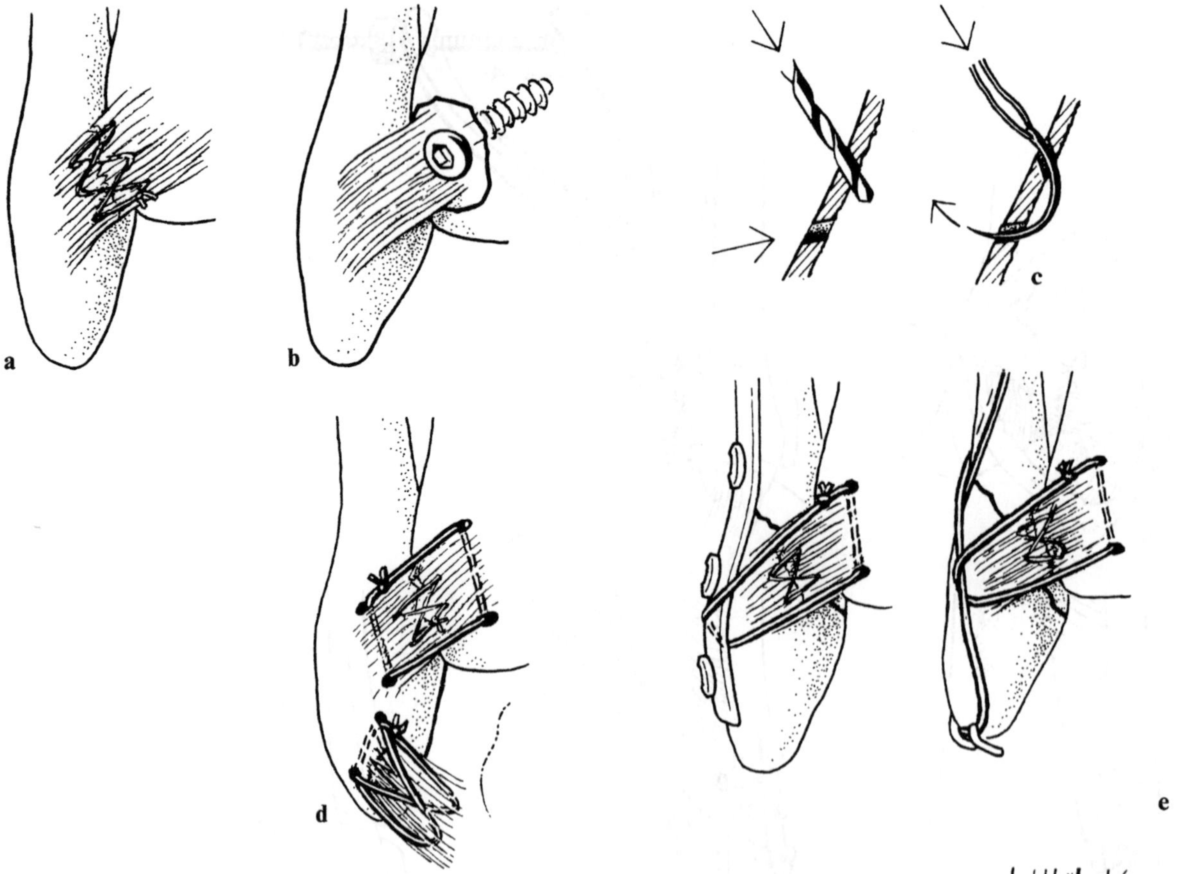

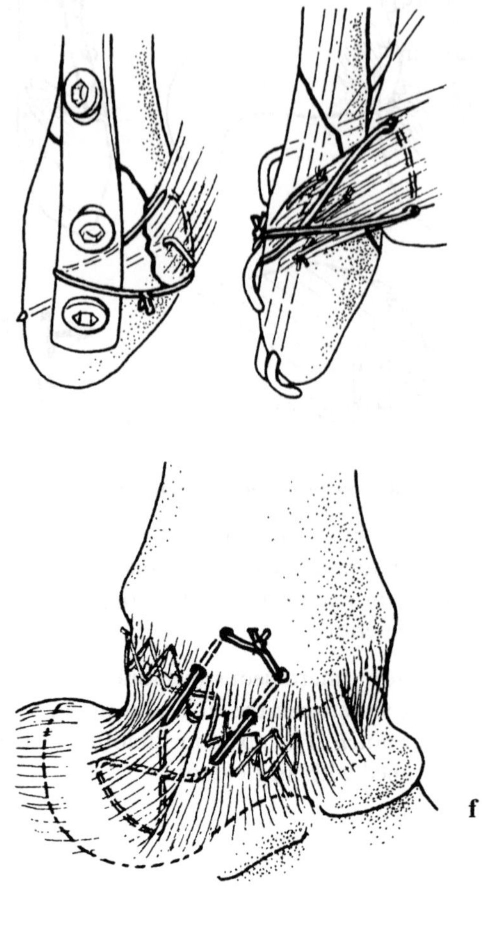

Fig. 206a–f. Technique of ligament repairs about the ankle joint

a Midsubstance tear repaired with an approximating suture (continuous suture of fine material)

b The reattachment of a bony ligament avulsion with a screw and washer is biomechanically ideal

c Drill holes are made for placing a transosseous reinforcing suture

d Transosseous reinforcement of a standard ligament repair with heavy, absorbable suture material

e The reinforcing suture may be anchored around a fibular implant

f Repair of the deltoid ligament: A central, transosseous supporting suture of heavy, absorbable material is applied, and the torn fibers are carefully reapproximated with a continuous suture

Fig. 207 a–e. Fractures of the posterior malleolus (classification)

Sagittal, posterior, and cross-sectional views

a Extra-articular avulsion fracture of the insertion of the posterior tibiofibular ligament

b Marginal avulsion (joint capsule) that does not involve the articular cartilage

c Large articular fragment

d Small articular fragment

e Small articular fragment with compression of the posterior margin of the tibial articular surface. This greatly compounds the severity of the articular lesion

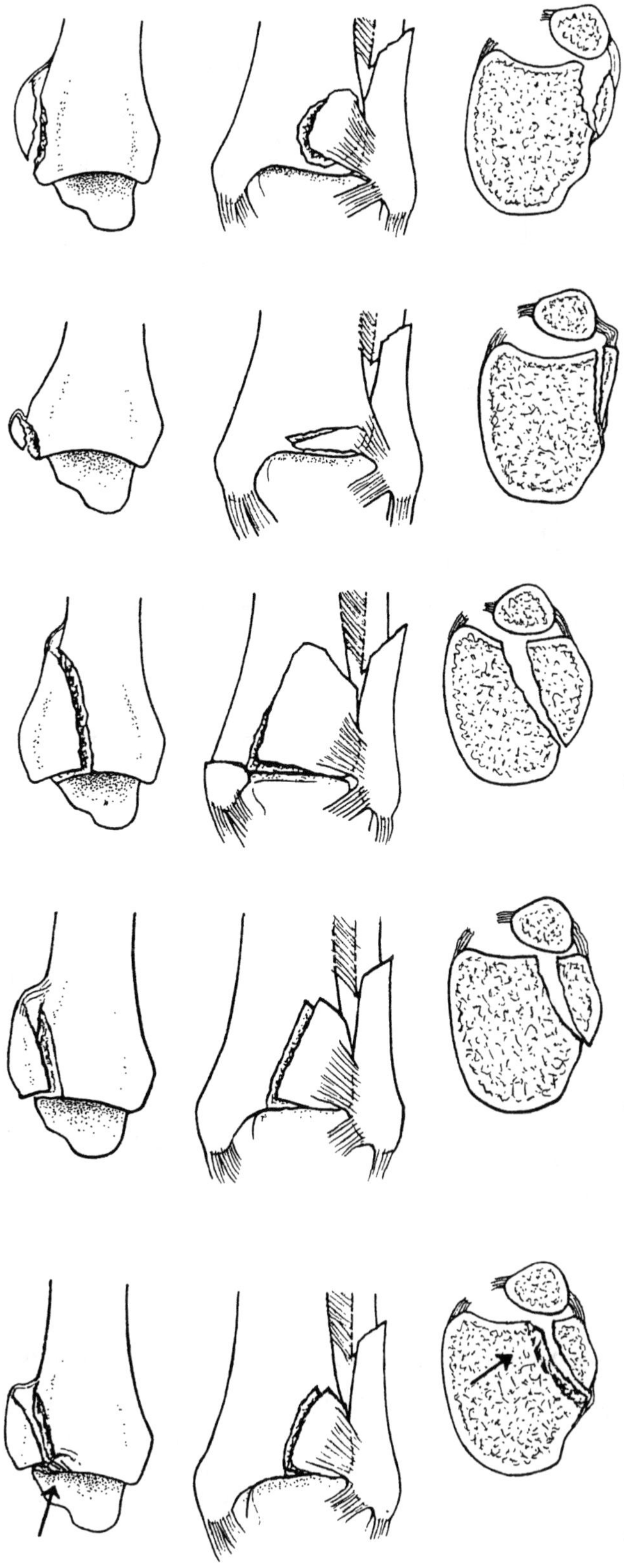

a

b

c

d

e

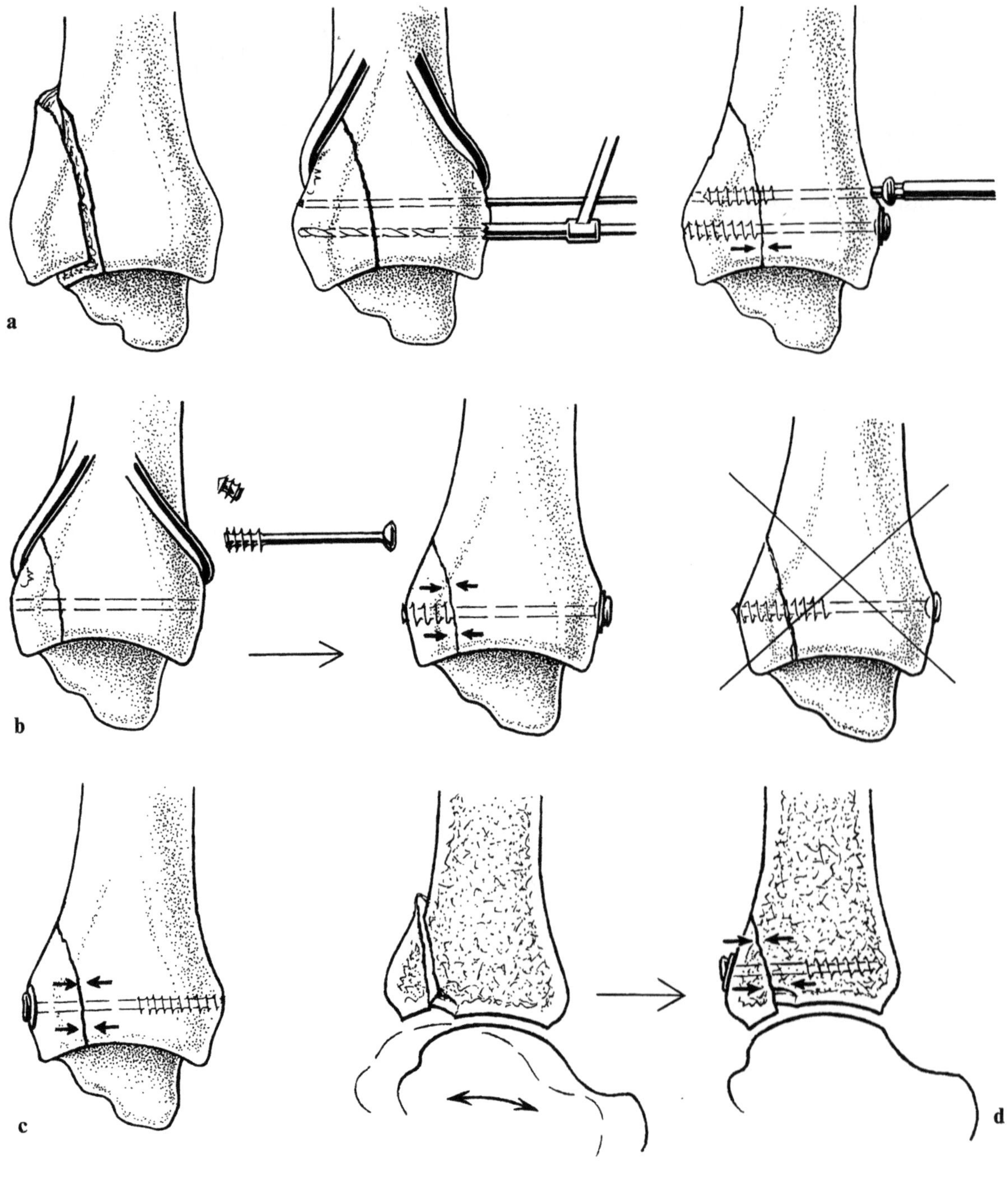

Fig. 208a–d. Principle of internal fixation of the posterior malleolus

a Indirect screw fixation from the anterior side following reduction and temporary fixation with a forceps and Kirschner guide wire. Definitive fixation is effected with two small cancellous screws and washers

b Indirect screw fixation of a smaller fragment using a cancellous screw with a shortened thread. The compressive effect is less than in **a**. If the thread were not shortened, the screw would not produce interfragmental compression

c Direct screw fixation of a small fragment from the posterior side using a 4.0-mm cancellous screw with washer. This provides optimum interfragmental compression

d Same technique is used for a small fragment with a depressed area. Sufficient screw pressure can reappose the posterior joint margin, preventing subluxation of the talus

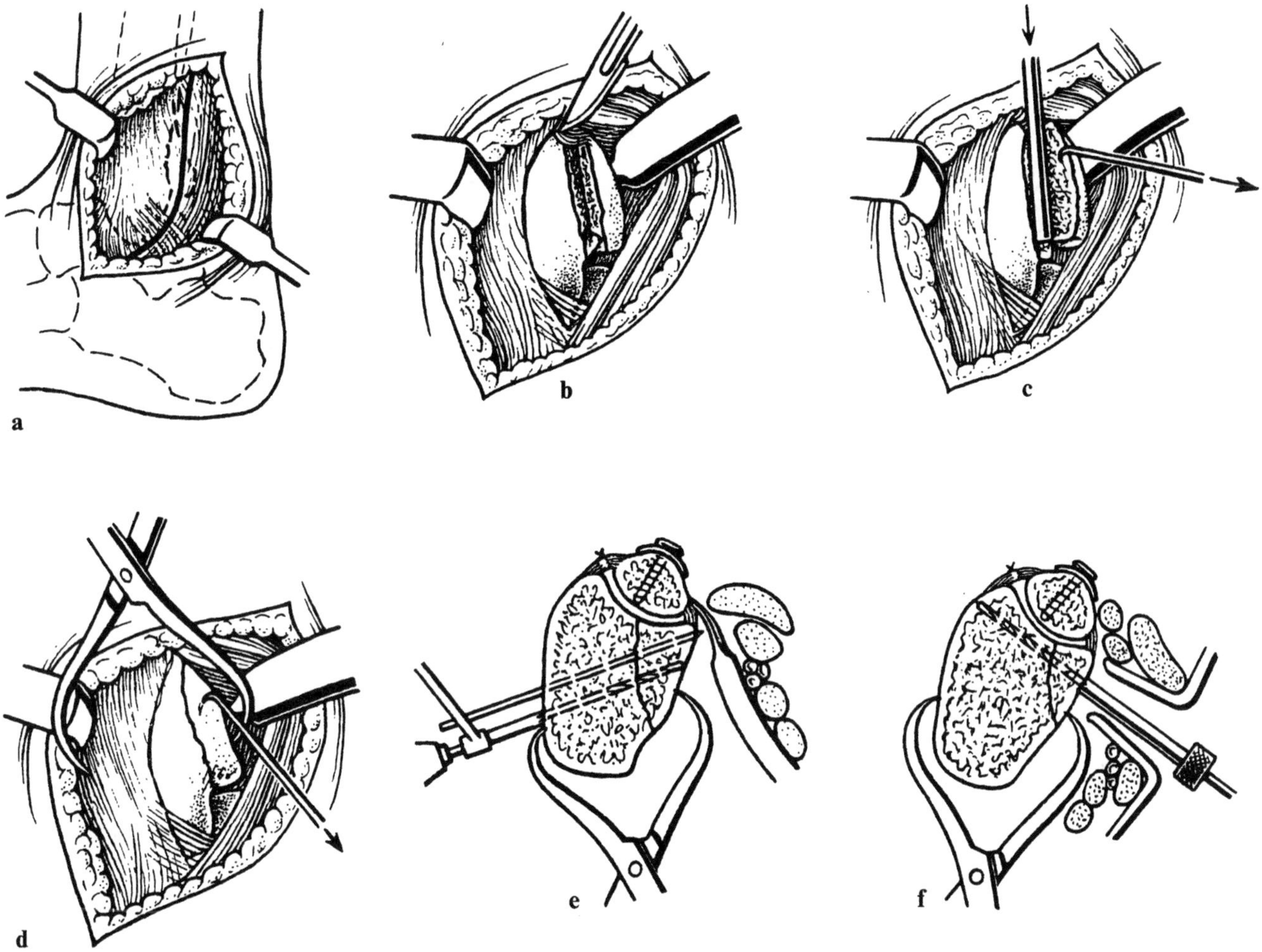

Fig. 209a–f. Technique of indirect screw fixation of the posterior malleolus through a posteromedial approach

a Incision of the tibialis posterior canal after extension of the skin incision as shown in Fig. 200

b The fragment is exposed, and the thick periosteum is incised at its tip so that the reduction can be assessed

c The fracture surfaces are separated, and a depressed area is reduced under vision with an impactor

d The fracture is reduced by distal traction and held in place with pointed forceps

e Cross-sectional view of the screw fixation: A 2.5-mm hole is drilled parallel to a Kirschner guide wire, and 4.0-mm cancellous screws are inserted

f For direct screw fixation from the posteromedial side, reduction is performed through the same approach, the Achilles tendon is retracted laterally, and the medial tendons and neurovascular bundle are retracted medially. The insert drill sleeve serves as a tissue protector while the fixation is carried out

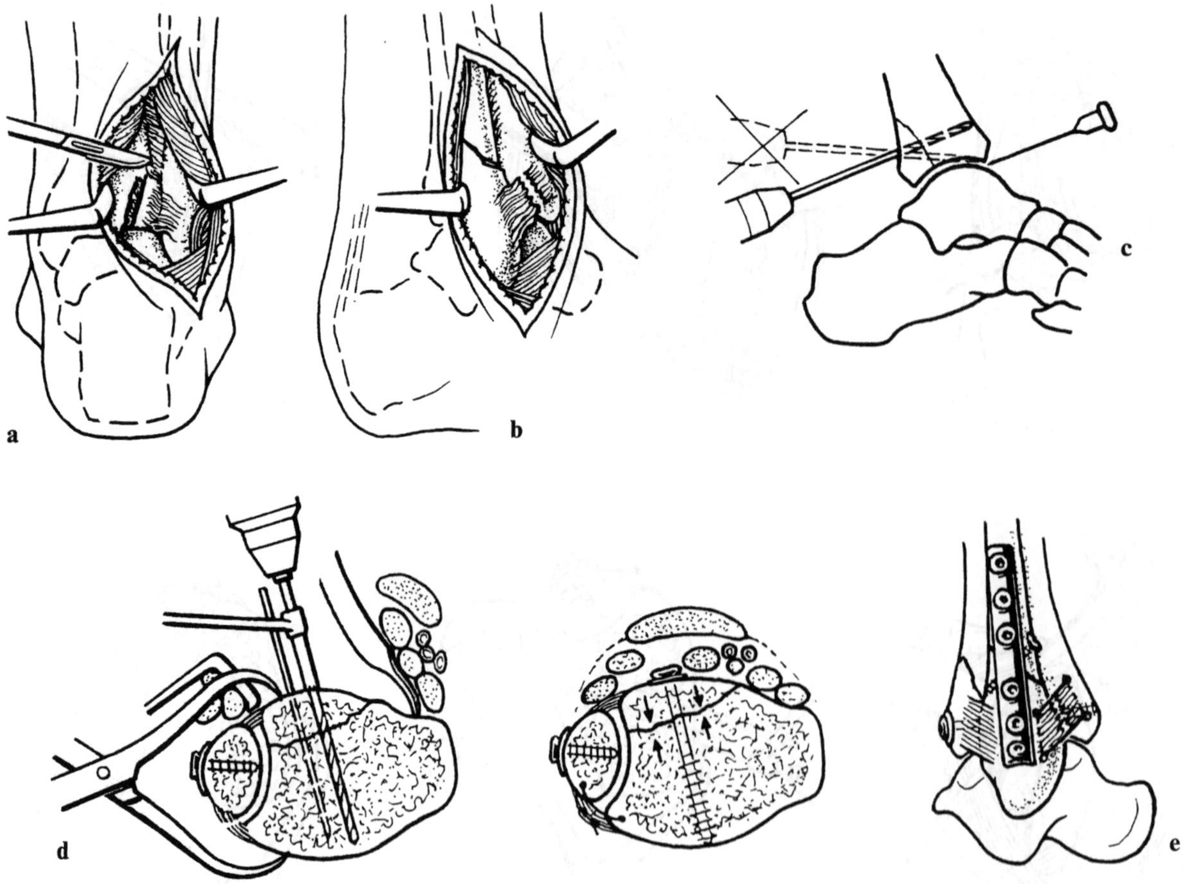

Fig. 210 a–e. Technique of direct screw fixation of a small fragment through the posterolateral approach

a The peroneal tendons are retracted laterally while the Achilles tendon, flexor tendons, and neurovascular bundle are retracted medially. The tip of the posterior malleolar fragment is exposed by incising the thick periosteum with a scalpel

b A fibular fracture and anterior ligament tear can be visualized through the same approach

c The anterior joint space is marked with a hypodermic needle or Kirschner wire to guide the drilling. Ankle joint injury must be avoided

d Cross-sectional view of the screw fixation: A forceps holds the fragment in reduction while the peroneal tendons are retracted laterally and the Achilles tendon, medial tendons, and neurovascular bundle are retracted medially. The screw is inserted parallel to a previously inserted Kirschner wire

e Cross-sectional and lateral views of the completed tibial fixation, with concomitant internal fixation of the fibula and transosseous reinforcement of the anterior ligament repair

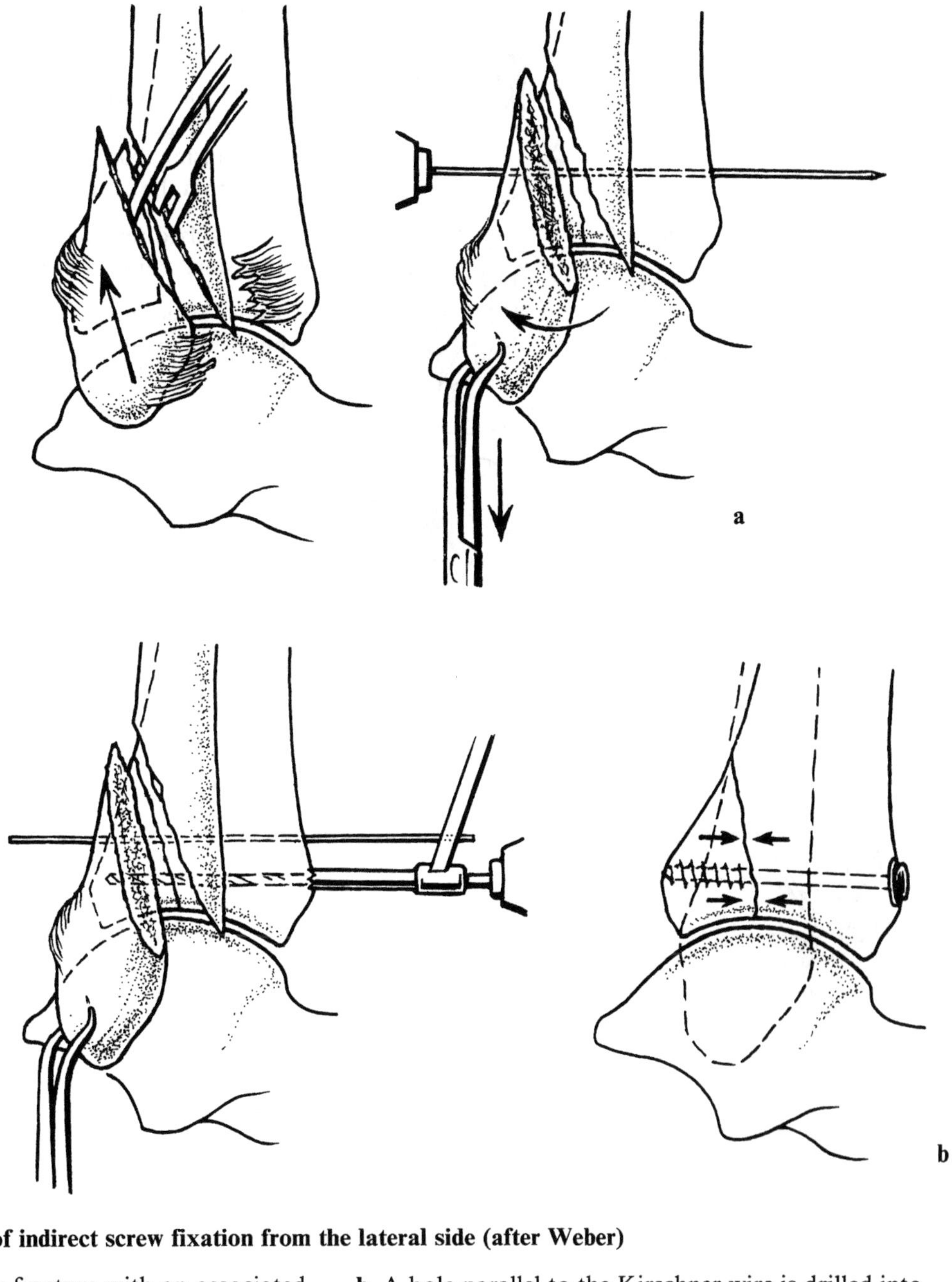

Fig. 211 a, b. Technique of indirect screw fixation from the lateral side (after Weber)

a Oblique type B fibular fracture with an associated fracture of the posterior malleolus. The fibular fracture is separated to expose the fibular notch. The tip of the fibula is pulled distally so that the posterior malleolus can be reduced under vision. It is temporarily fixed with a Kirschner wire drilled in percutaneously from the posterior side

b A hole parallel to the Kirschner wire is drilled into the fragment through a small anterolateral stab incision, and a cancellous screw is inserted

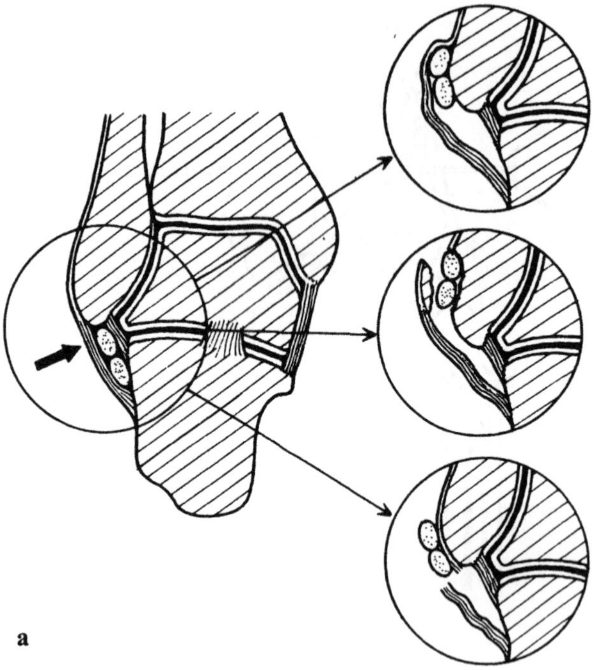

a

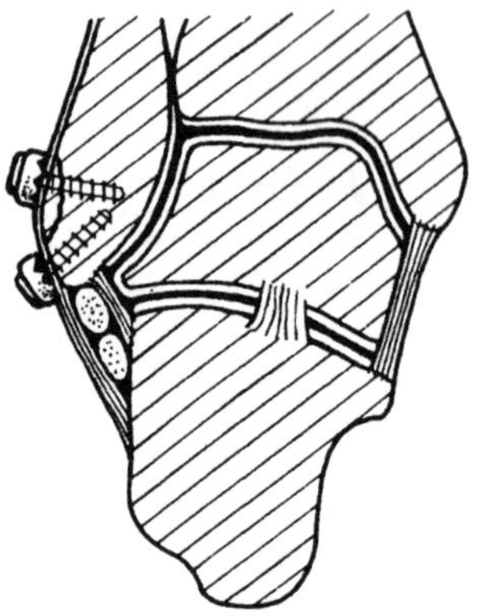

b

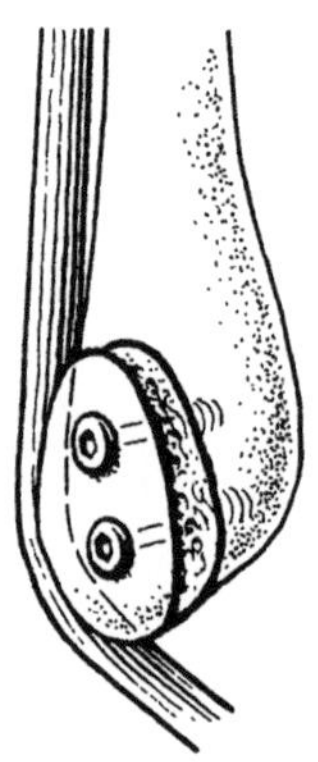

c

Fig. 212a–c. Treatment of peroneal tendon displacement

a Classification of the primary displacement: elevation of the periosteum with an intact retinaculum, bony avulsion from the fibula, avulsion of the retinaculum from the fibula

b The avulsed retinaculum or bone fragment is fixed with a small cortex screw and spiked plastic washer

c Kelly osteotomy of the lower fibula creates a groove that opposes tendon displacement. The osteotomy is fixed with two small cancellous screws

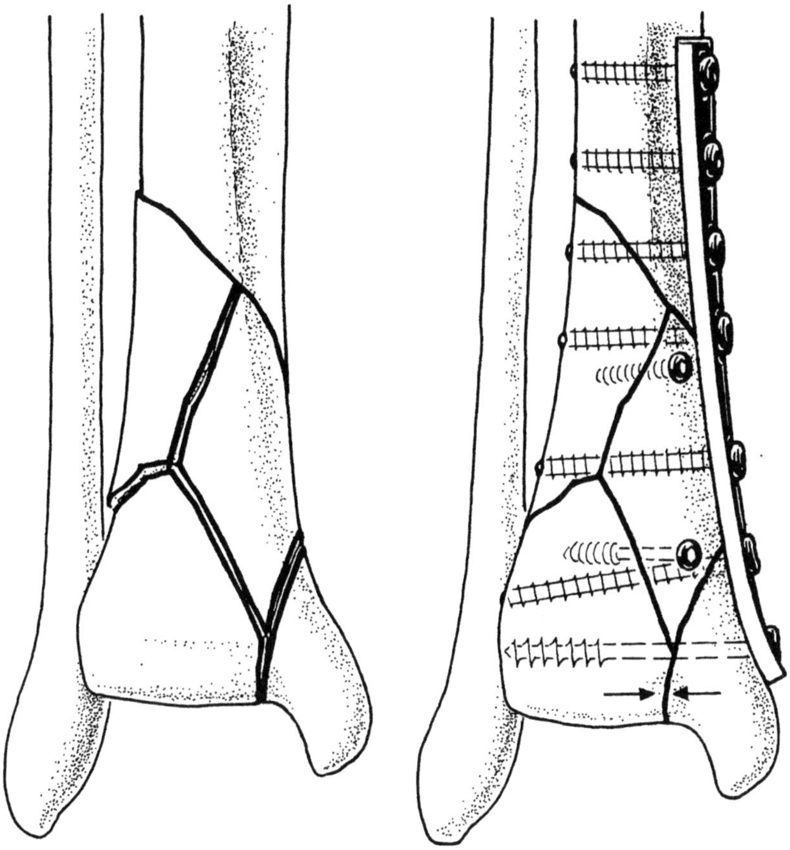

a

Fig. 213a, b. Internal fixation of a medial malleolar fracture accompanying a fracture of the tibial shaft

a The narrow DCP (fixed with 4.5-mm cortex screws and a 6.5-mm cancellous screw) overlaps the articular fragment. The distal cancellous screw inserted parallel to the joint line fixes and compresses the fracture

b The main tibial fracture and distal fracture line may be fixed independently, using small cancellous screws to fix the malleolus

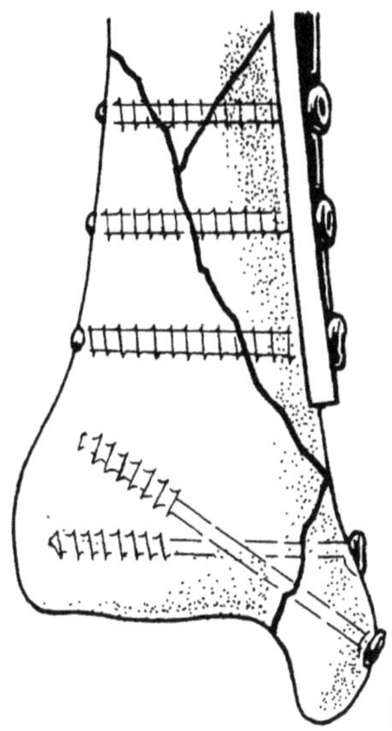

b

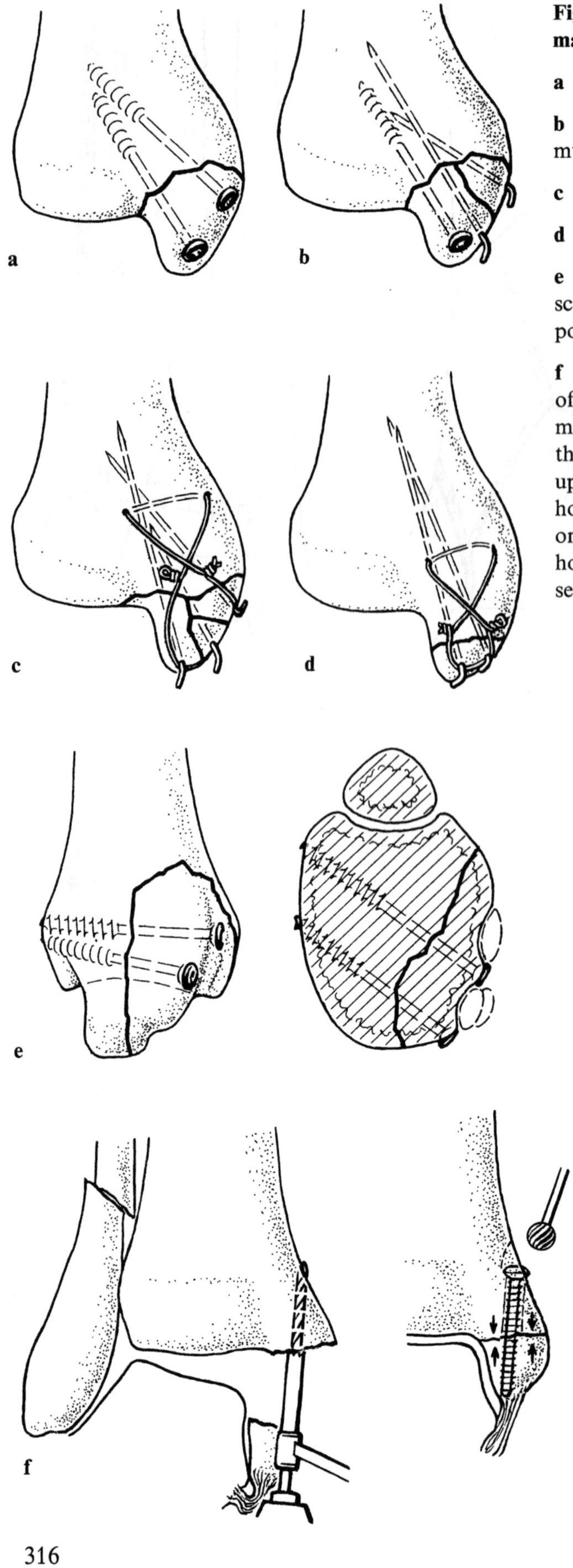

Fig. 214a–f. Typical internal fixations of the medial malleolus

a Screw fixation of a large anterior fragment

b Combined screw and Kirschner-wire fixation of multiple fragments

c Tension-band fixation of a comminuted fracture

d Tension-band fixation of a small avulsed fragment

e Screw fixation of a posteromedial fragment. The screws are inserted between the canals for the tibialis posterior and toe flexor tendons

f Weber's technique for the retrograde screw fixation of a very small fragment. The proximal tibial fragment is drilled before the fibula is reduced, so that the foot can be displaced laterally. The hole is drilled up through the fracture surface to serve as the gliding hole. A large countersink recess is cut with a gouge or spherical bur. The fracture is reduced, the thread hole is drilled and tapped, and a small screw is inserted in retrograde fashion

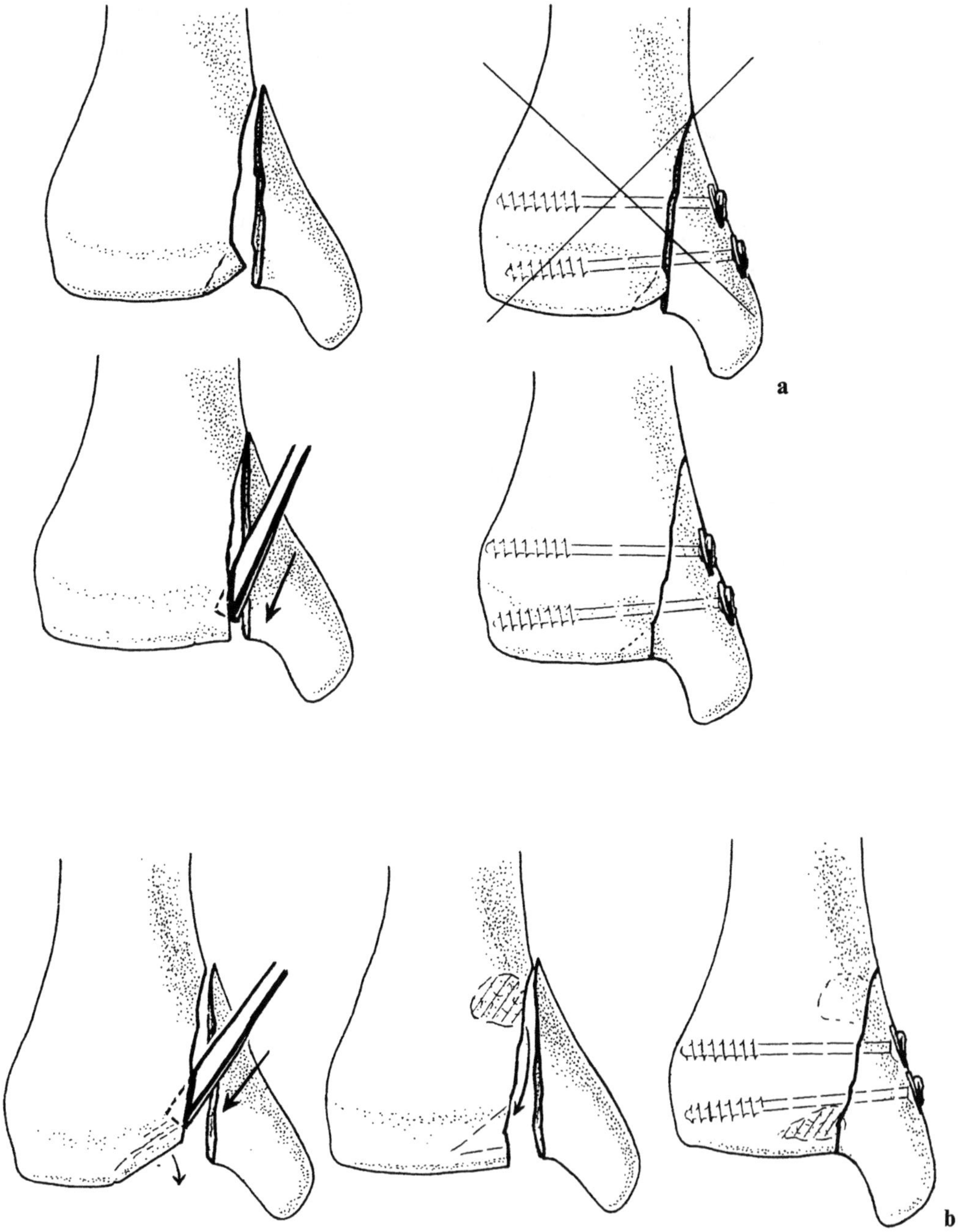

Fig. 215 a, b. Adduction fractures

a The small depressed area on the medial tibial articular margin must be elevated under vision before an anatomic reduction is possible

b Elevating a larger depressed segment creates a defect that must be packed with cancellous bone obtained locally

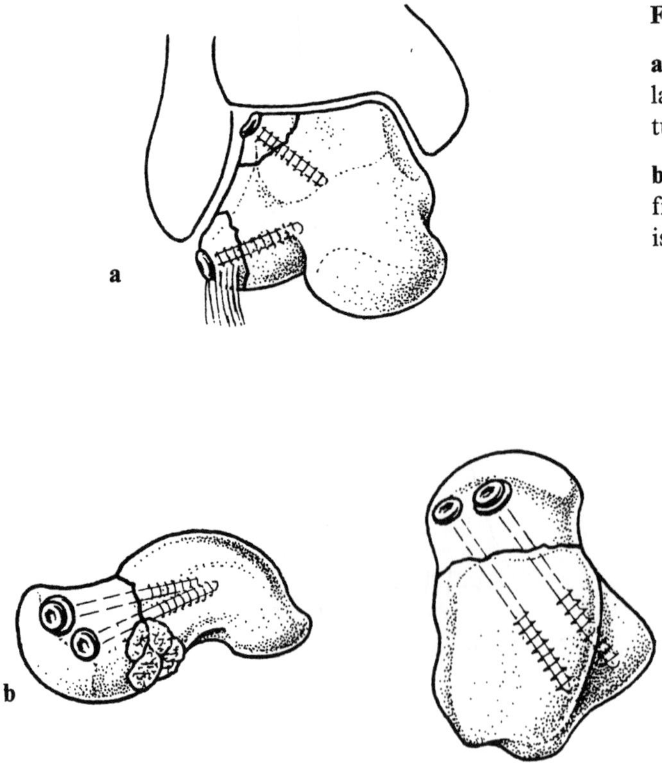

a

b

Fig. 216a, b. Internal fixation of fractures of the talus

a Screw fixation of peripheral talus fractures: articular shear fractures and a ligamentous avulsion fracture of the lateral process

b Screw fixation of the fractured neck of the talus from the anteromedial side. A distal defect, if present, is grafted with autogenous cancellous bone

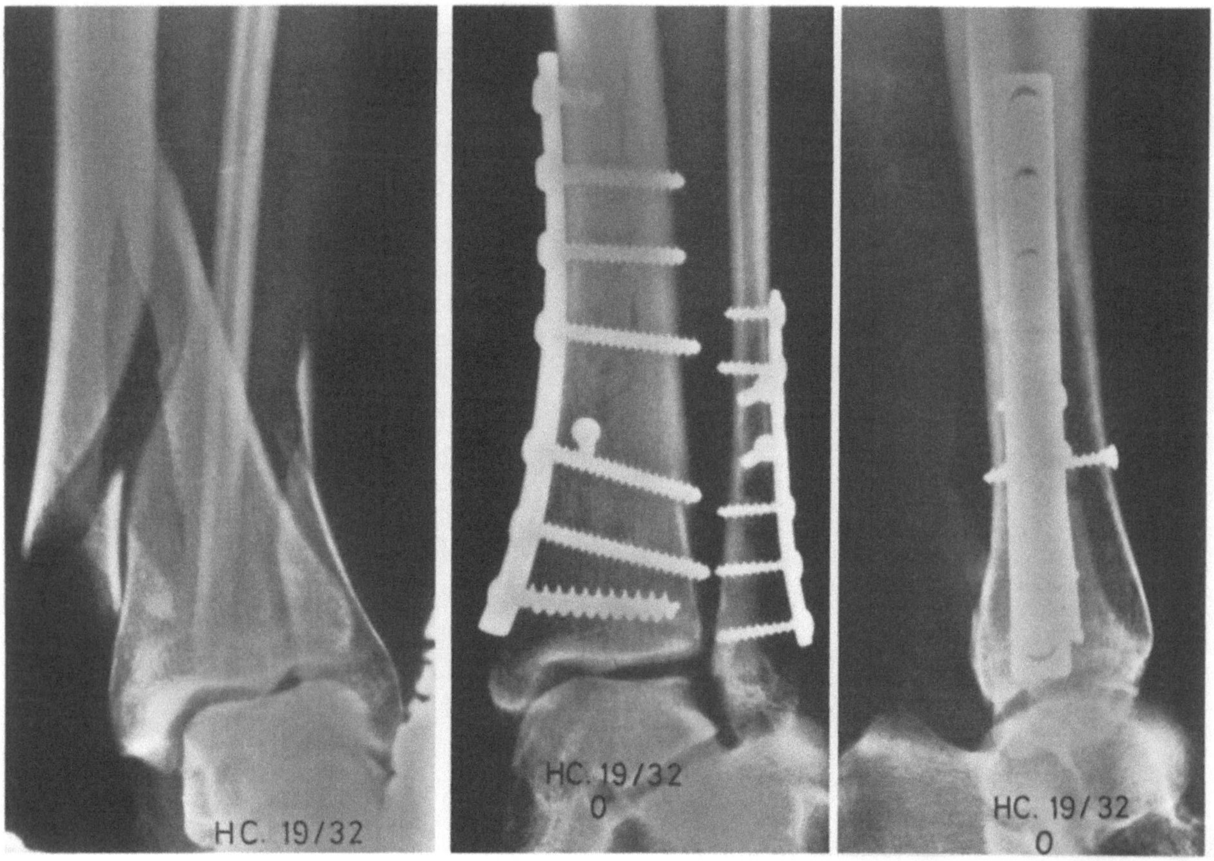

a b

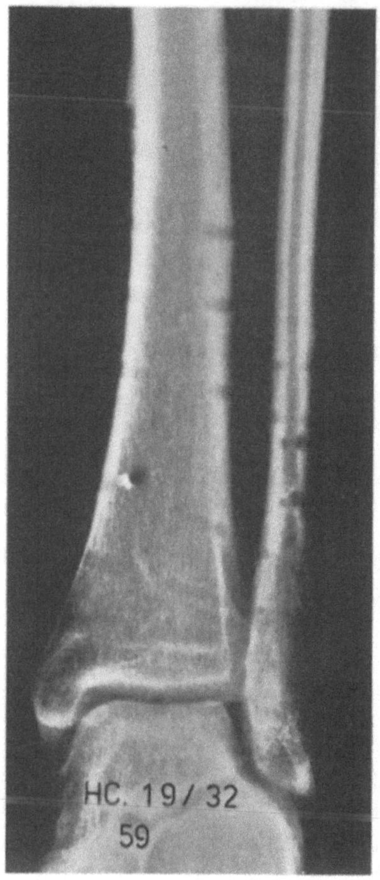

c

Fig. 217a–c. Clinical example: concomitant internal fixation of the distal fibula associated with a tibial fracture, fixation of small tibial fragments with small cortex screws

Christiane B., 45-year-old housewife, fell while skiing on 2/21/74

a Markedly displaced fracture of the distal tibia with butterfly fragments of the tibia and fibula

b The tibia was immediately stabilized with a 7-hole DCP placed just above the ankle joint.The posterior butterfly fragment (marked in **a**) was fixed with a 3.5-mm cortex screw.The fibula remained unstable within the mortise, so it was fixed with a 6-hole one-third tubular plate and two 3.5-mm cortex screws inserted through a second lateral incision
The postoperative course was uneventful, functional exercises were initiated, and full weight bearing was started at 4 months

c On follow-up and implant removal at 14 months, the patient had no complaints, full function, and slight muscular atrophy.Primary fracture union was confirmed

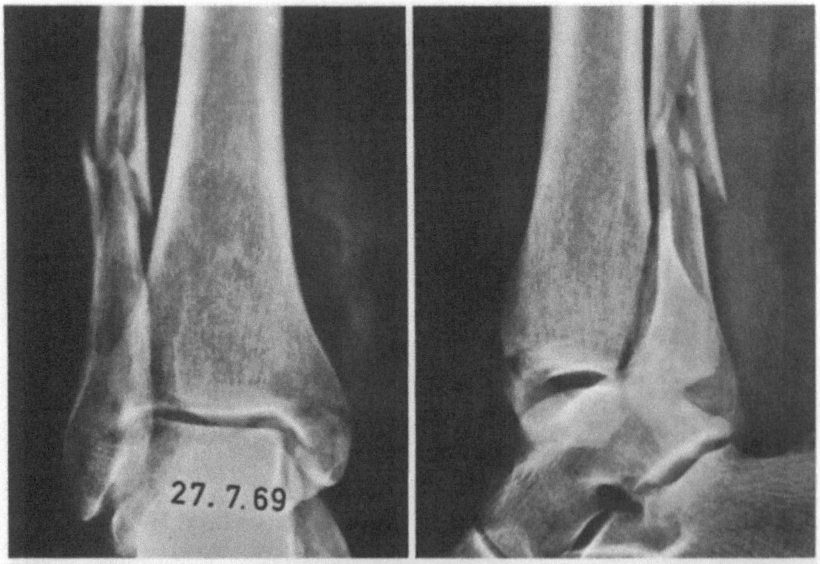

a

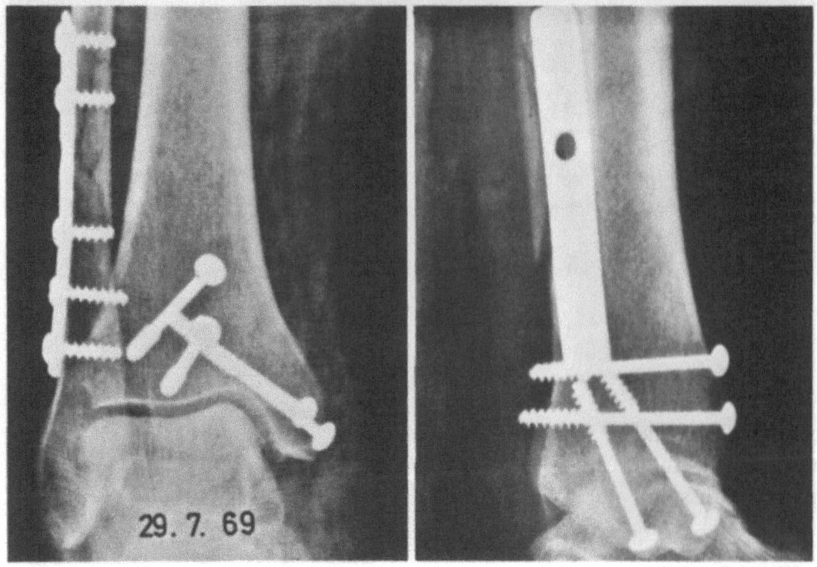

b

Fig. 218a–e. Clinical example: high type C fracture of the lateral malleolus with an associated fracture of the posterior malleolus

Betty H., 68-year-old housewife, fell on stairs on 7/27/69

a High type C fracture of the fibula with a butterfly fragment and a large posterior malleolar fragment

b The fibula was immediately stabilized with a 6-hole one-third tubular plate, and the lateral ligament was repaired. The oblique fracture of the medial malleolus was fixed with two small cancellous screws, and the posterior malleolus was fixed indirectly with two small cancellous screws inserted from the anterior side
Exercises were initiated from a removable splint. Patient was discharged home with a circular cast, which at 10 weeks was replaced with a walking cast. Full weight bearing was permitted at 12 weeks

c Implants were removed at 9 months. A zone of instability in the fibular fracture was missed at that time

d At 1 1/2 years the patient had full function and no complaints. Callus formation was noted at the level of the fibular fracture, with slight shortening

e When seen after 11 years on 7/7/80, the patient had no complaints, full function, and no muscular atrophy. Some thickening of the ankle joint was still apparent. X-rays showed no progression of osteoarthritis

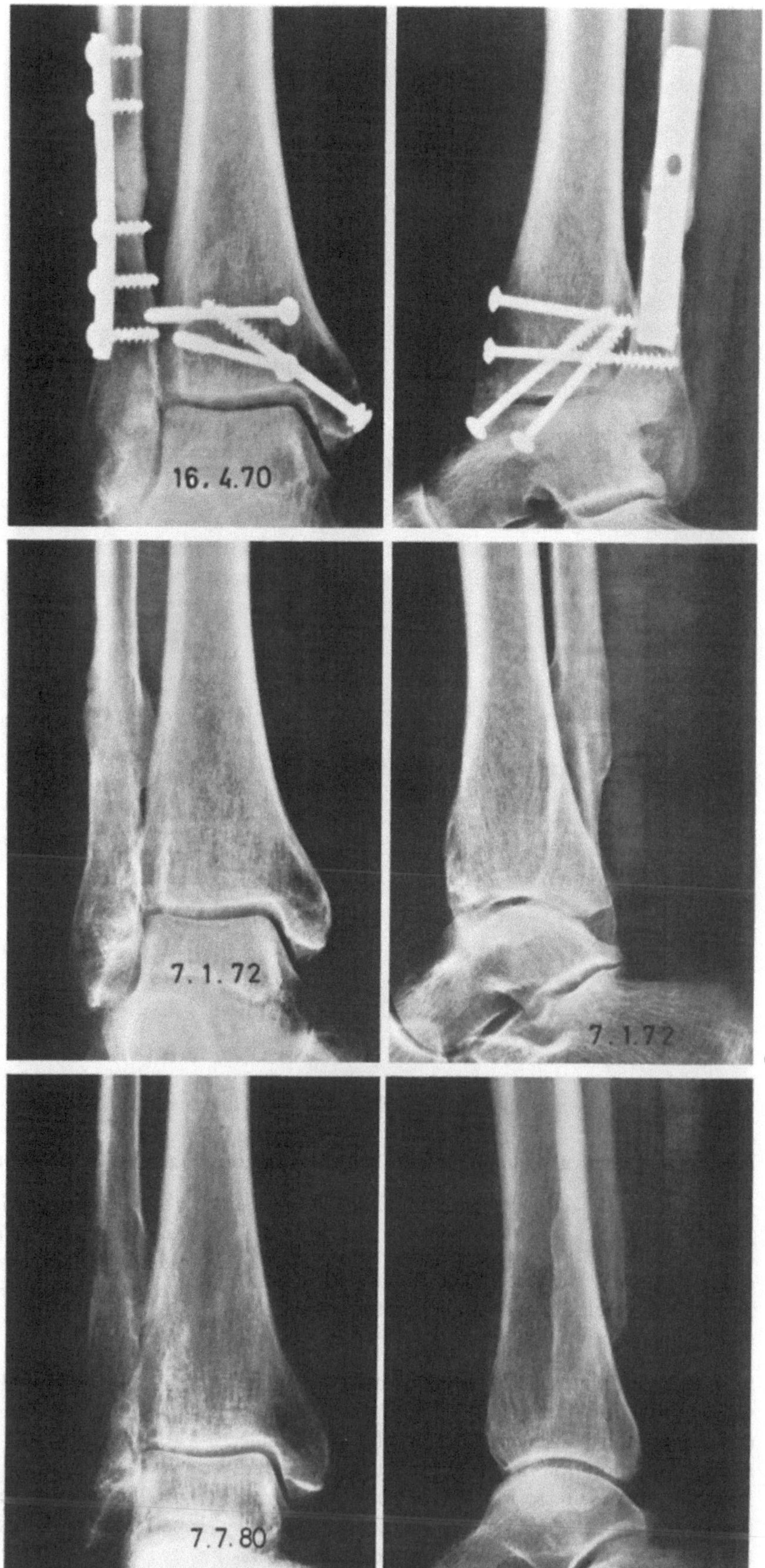

c

d

e

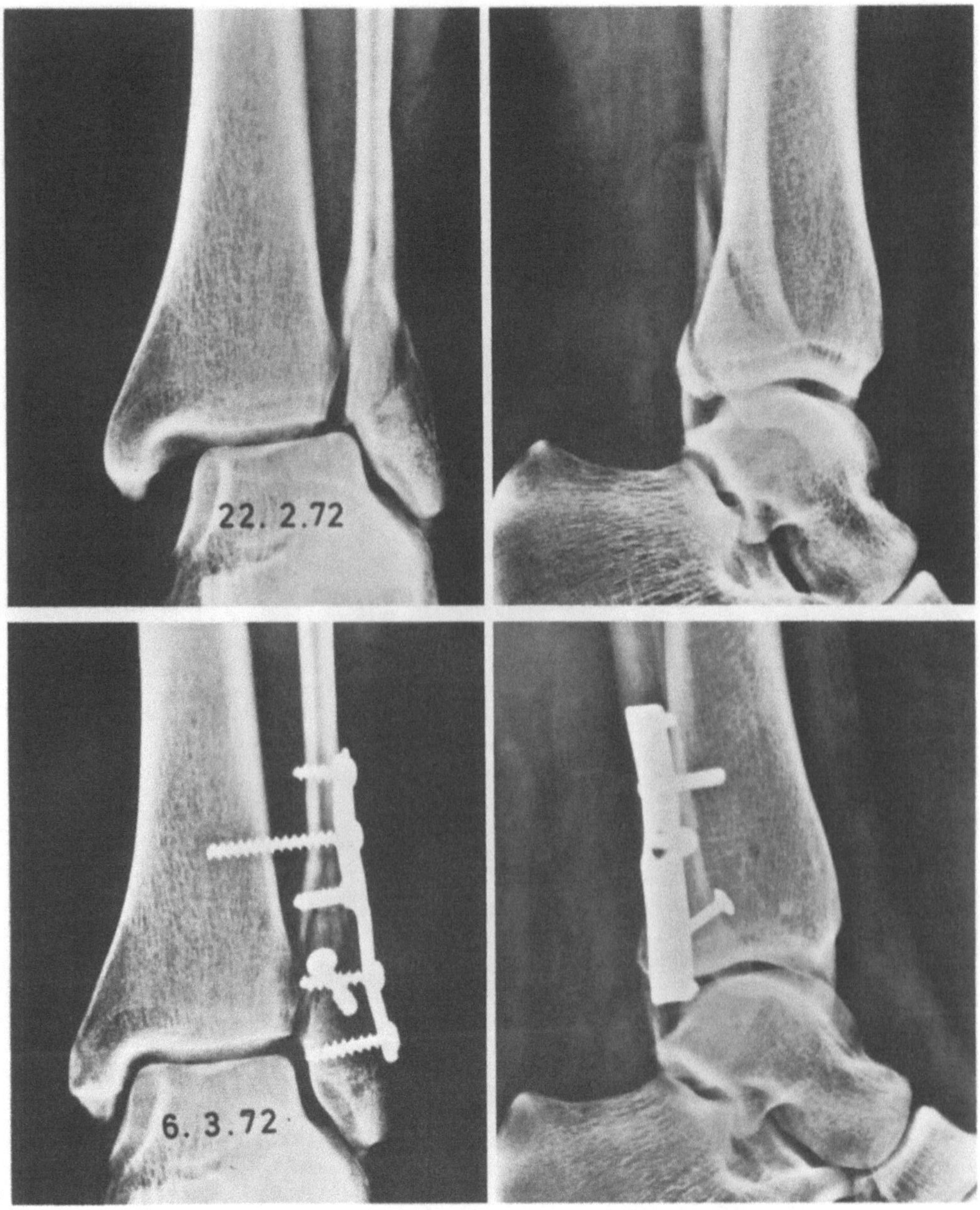

a

b

Fig. 219a–d. Clinical example: type C malleolar fracture managed by tibiofibular transfixion

Lotti K., 37-year-old housewife, fell while skiing on 2/22/72

a Type C spiral fracture of the fibula with a small posterior malleolar fragment and rupture of the medial ligaments

b At emergency internal fixation, the main fragments were fixed with screws and a neutralization plate (5-hole one-third tubular plate) on the lateral side, and the anterior tibiofibular ligament was repaired. Instability persisted, so the second plate screw from the top was replaced by a transfixing screw. Medially the deltoid ligament, avulsed from the tibia, was repaired with a transosseous suture

c The postoperative course was uncomplicated, and exercises were started from a removable splint. Patient was discharged with a plaster cast worn for 10 weeks, and full weight bearing was started at 12 weeks

On follow-up and implant removal at 33 weeks, the fractures were united. The patient had no complaints, full function, no muscular atrophy, and no osteoarthritis

d When seen 8 years later on 7/2/80, the patient still had no complaints or osteoarthritis

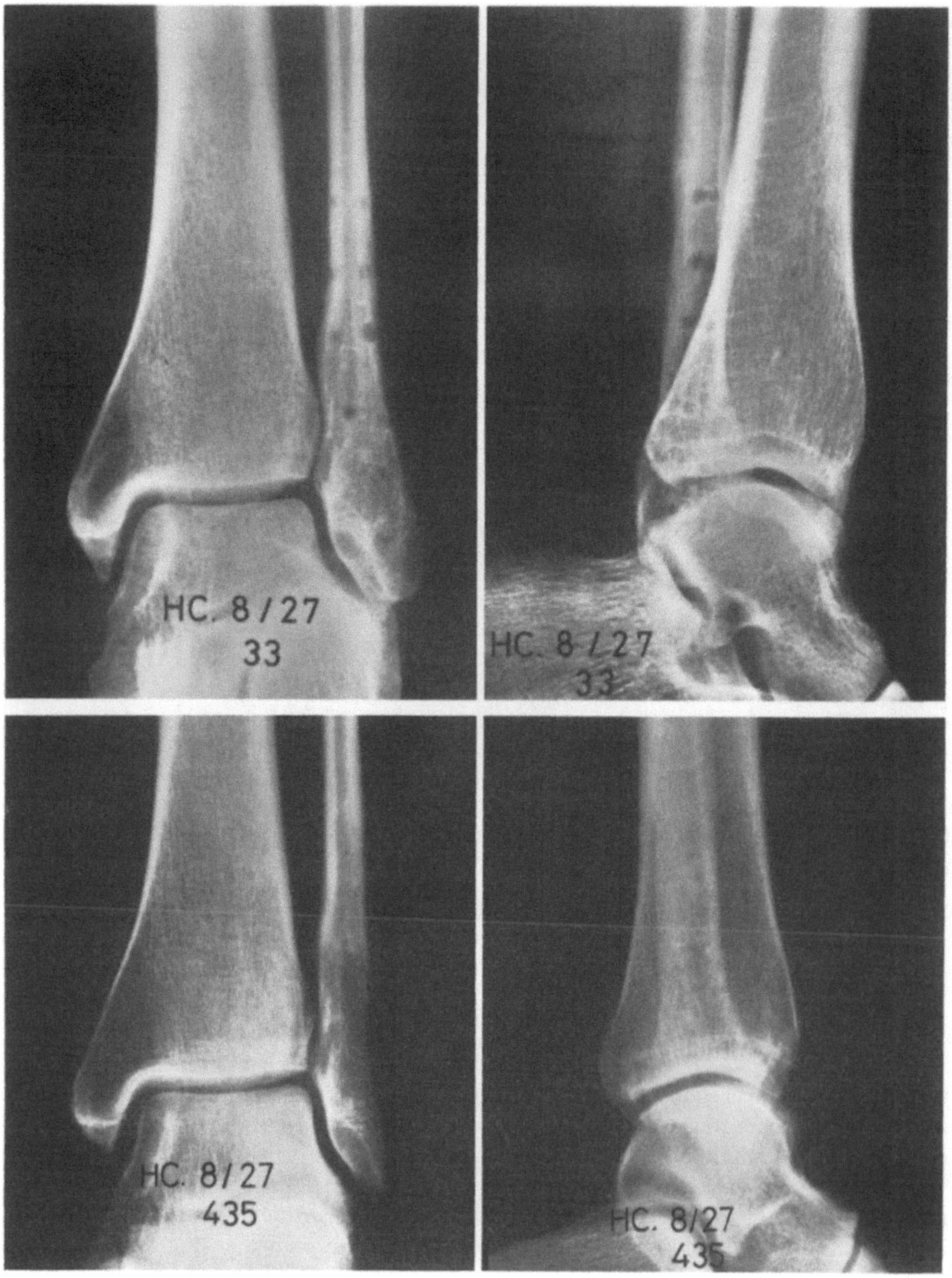

c

d

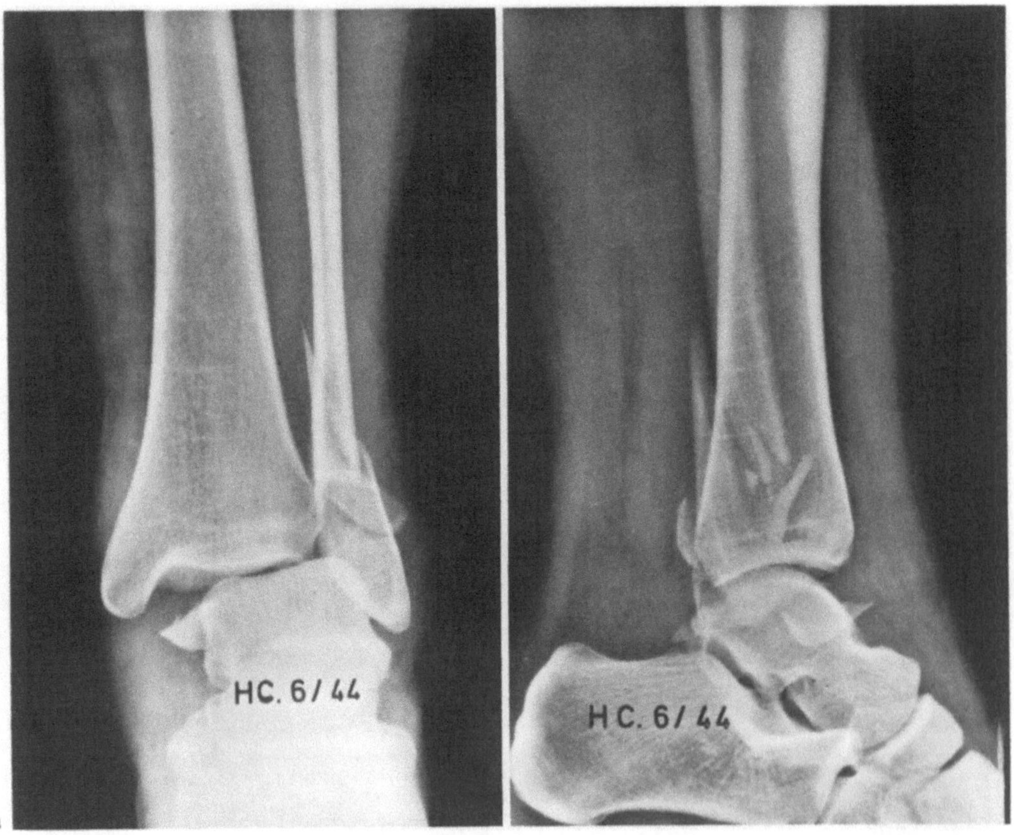

a

Fig. 220a–c. Clinical example: type C malleolar fracture with a small medial avulsion, fixed with a plate and tension band

Heidi H., 18-year-old gardener, fell while skiing on 12/29/71

a Type C comminuted fracture of the fibula with a small avulsion fracture of the medial malleolus and a small avulsion of the posterior malleolus

b At emergency operation the lateral fragment was screwed to the main fragments, and a neutralization plate (6-hole one-third tubular plate) was applied. The anterior tibiofibular ligament was repaired.The medial melleolus was fixed with Kirschner wires and a small tension band, and the joint capsule was sutured

The course was uncomplicated, and active exercises were performed from the splint. Patient was discharged with a circular cast, which was worn for 10 weeks. Implants were removed elsewhere at 8 months

c When examined 8 1/2 years later on 9/3/80, the patient had no complaints, full motion, and no muscular atrophy
X-rays showed slight irregularity of the tibial structure in the area of the syndesmosis and no osteoarthritic disease

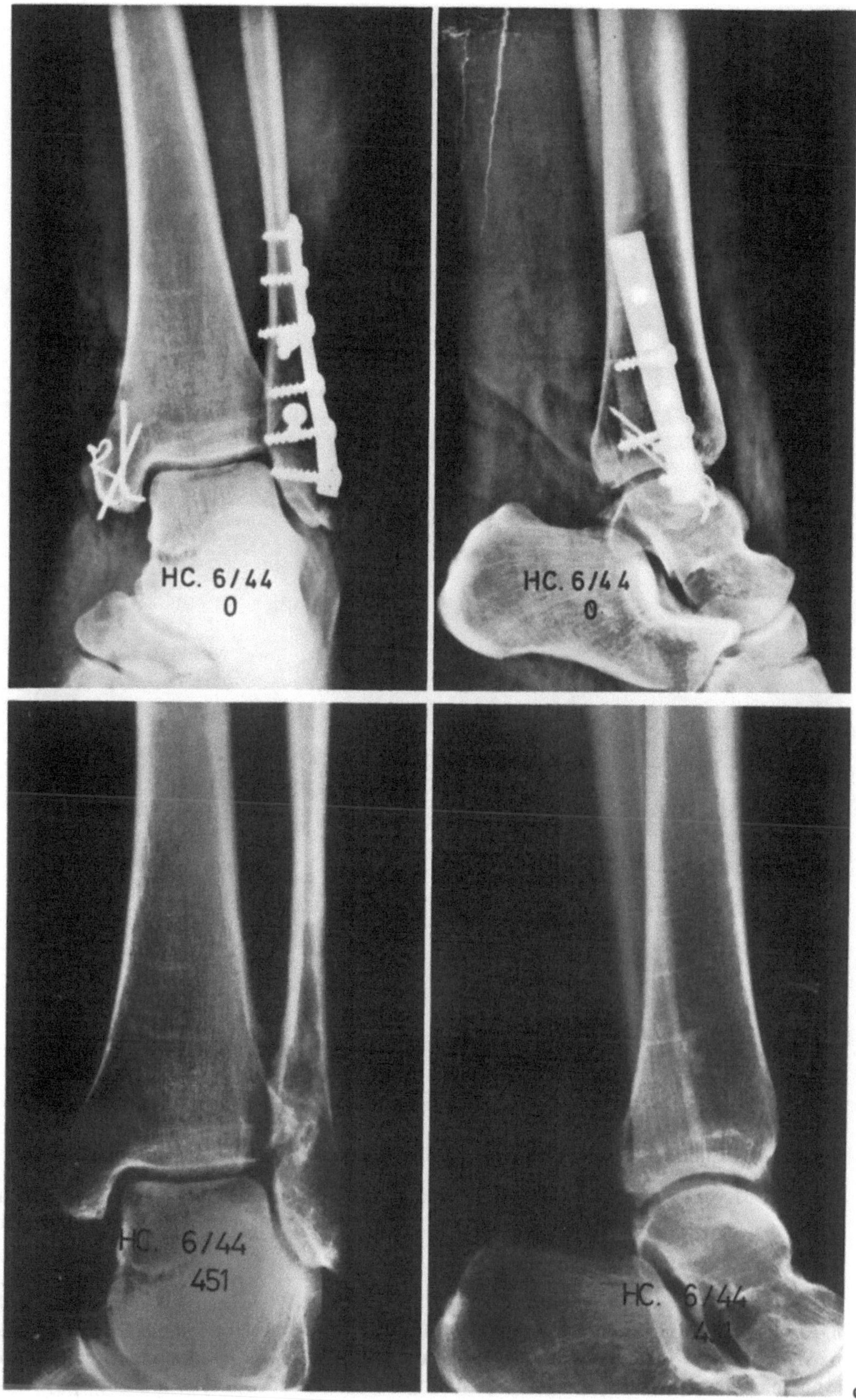

b

c

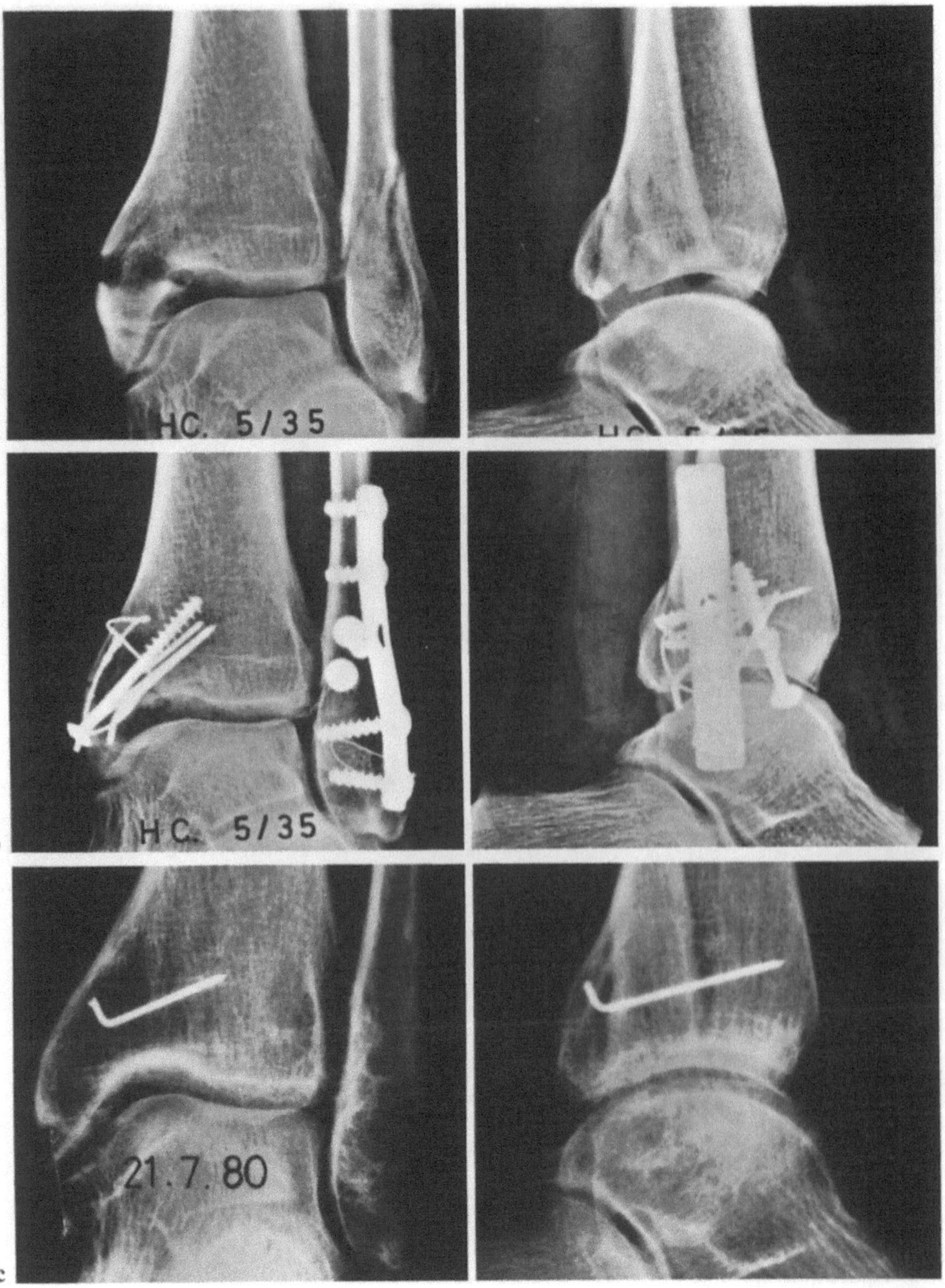

a

b

c

Fig. 221 a–c. Clinical example: type B bimalleolar fracture with posteromedial comminution

Ilse W., 51-year-old teacher, fell while skiing on 7/27/71

a Type B oblique fracture of the fibula with posteromedial comminution

b At emergency operation the fibular fracture was fixed with screws and a neutralization plate, and the syndesmosis was repaired (small avulsed fragment was fixed with a flexible wire). The medial fracture was managed by a combination of screws, Kirschner wires, and a wire tension band

The patient was discharged with a circular cast after an uneventful course. The implants were removed elsewhere after 1 year

c When seen 9 1/2 years later on 7/21/80, the patient was free of complaints and athletically fit. Examination disclosed a slight limitation of ankle joint motion; no muscular atrophy was present. X-rays showed one Kirschner wire left in the tibia; there was no evidence of osteoarthritis

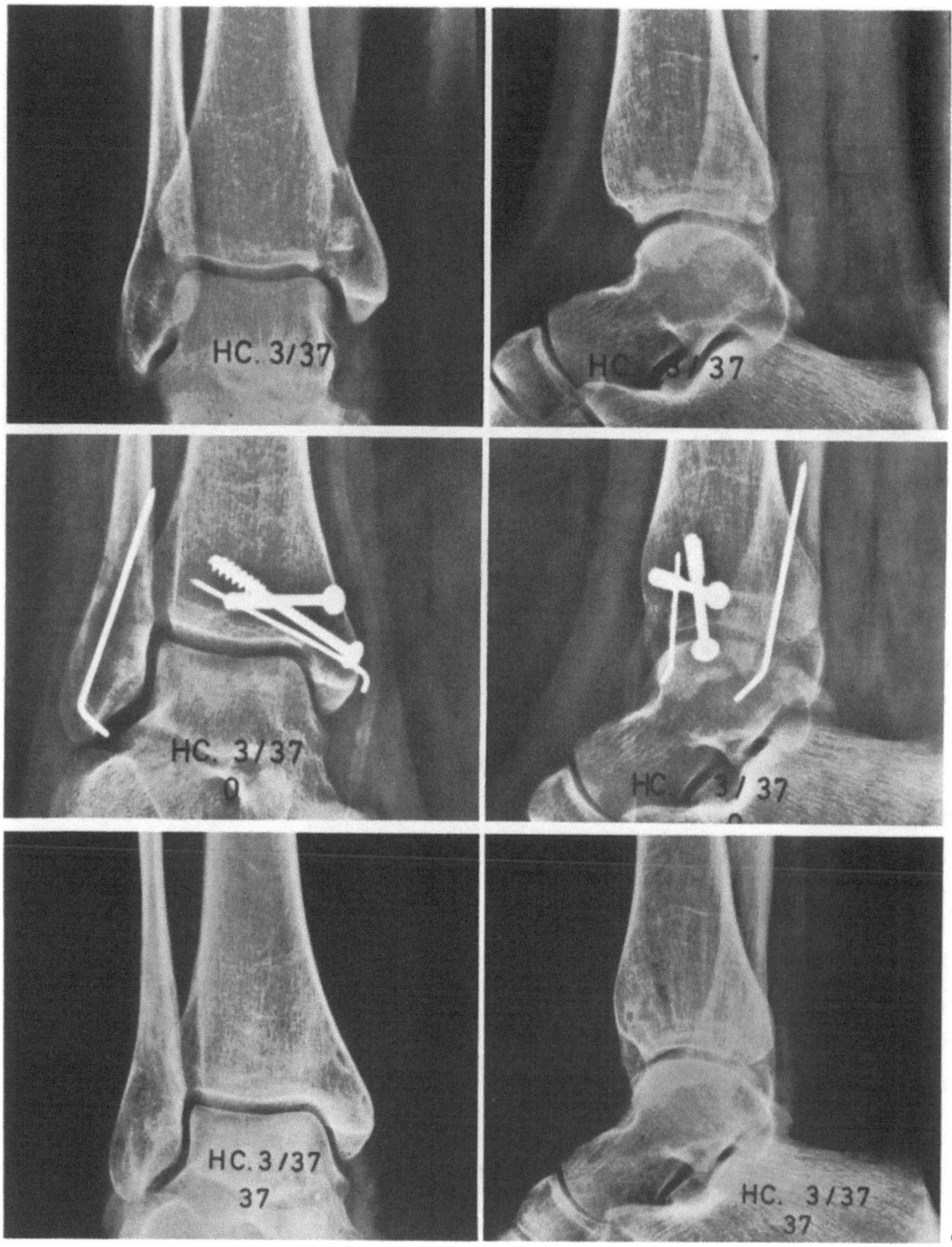

Fig. 222a–c. Clinical example: adduction fracture with compression of the joint surface

Brigitte K., 28-year-old housewife, had skiing accident on 3/12/71

a Adduction fracture of the medial malleolus. Interposition of a compressed articular fragment. Undisplaced fracture of the lateral malleolus, type A

b Emergency internal fixation: medially reduction and fixation with screws and a Kirschner wire. Laterally single Kirschner wire

A posterior plaster splint was later replaced with a circular cast. Full weight bearing at 12 weeks

c Implant removal after 8 months. Regular joint lines. Full mobility and no complaints
Nine years postinjury, on 7/20/80, we were informed that the patient was completely asymptomatic and had full motion

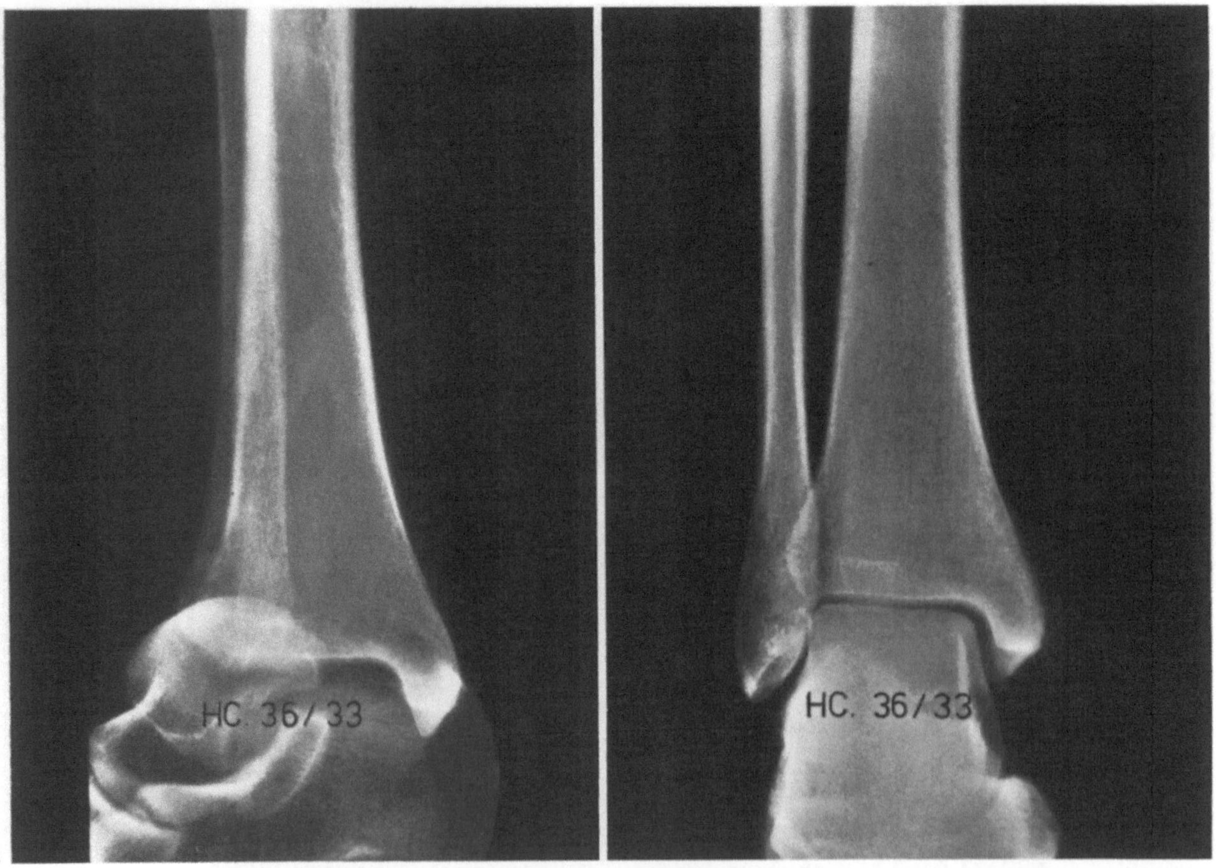

a

Fig. 223 a–c. Clinical example: internal fixation of a Maisonneuve fracture with 3.5-mm cortex screws

Edith R., 34-year-old housewife, fell while skiing on 3/13/77

a Maisonneuve's fracture-dislocation of the ankle joint with rupture of the deltoid ligament and a spiral fracture of the upper fibula. After immediate reduction of the dislocation, no further joint pathology was seen

b At emergency operation the tibiofibular ligaments and the anterior and posterior talofibular ligaments were found to be ruptured, and lateral and medial ligament repairs were carried out. The fibula was returned to its notch and indirectly stabilized with two transfixing screws inserted transversely above the syndesmosis, each screw gripping three cortices

After an uneventful course and early mobilization, the patient was discharged home with a circular cast, which was worn for 6 weeks. Full weight bearing was permitted at 12 weeks; the implants were removed elsewhere

c When seen at 3 1/2 years on 9/13/80, the patient had no complaints and was again active in skiing and tennis. She had symmetric ankle joint motion and a slight limitation of motion in the subtalar joint. No muscular atrophy was apparent. X-rays showed a uniform mortise with no osteoarthritis. A small osteophyte was visible on the anterior tibial margin

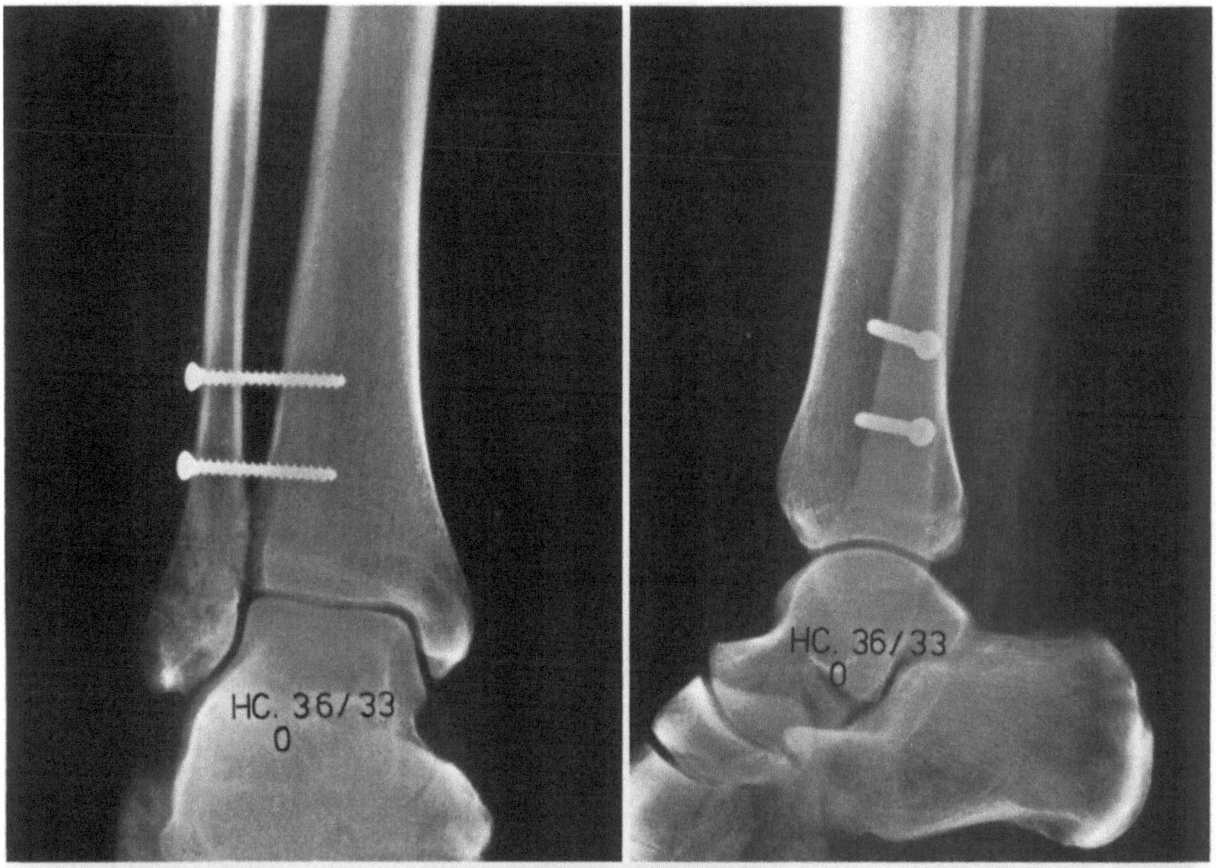

b

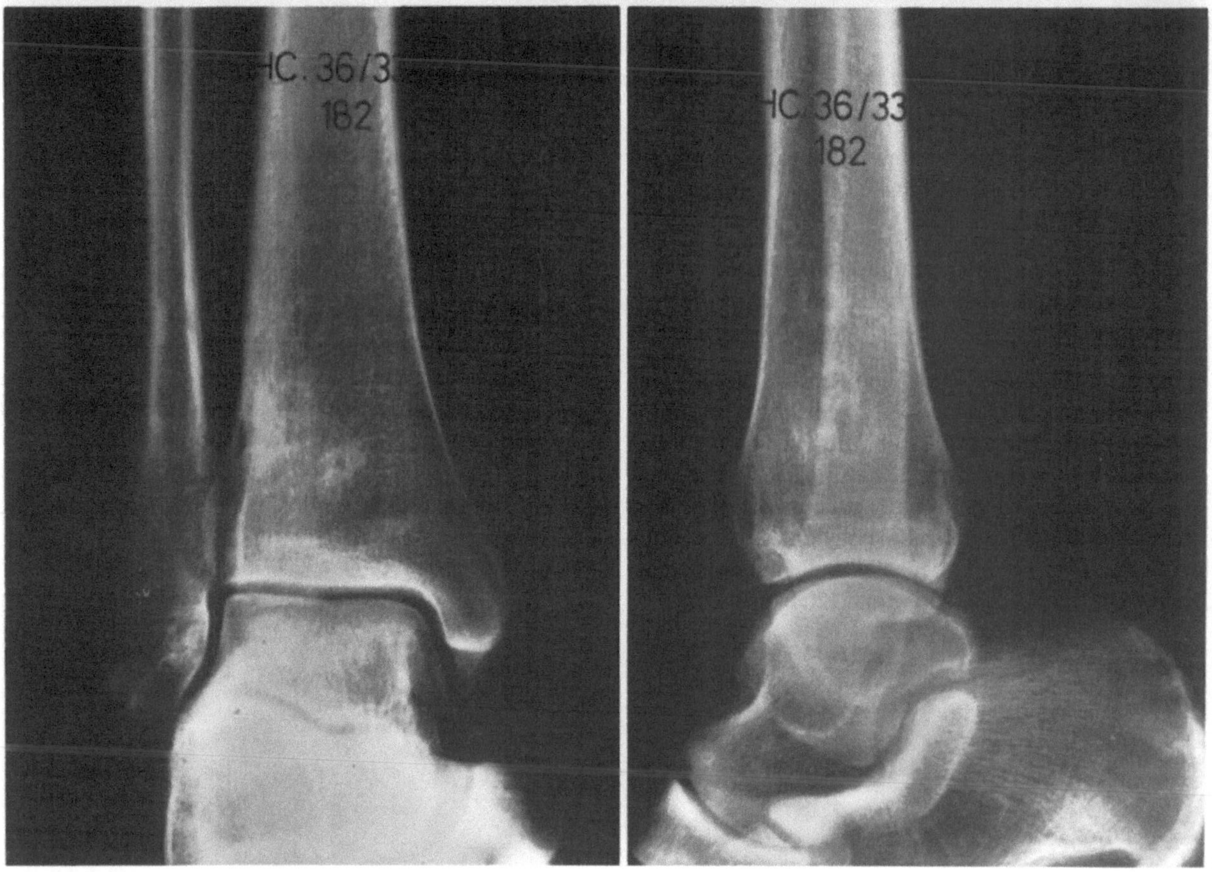

c

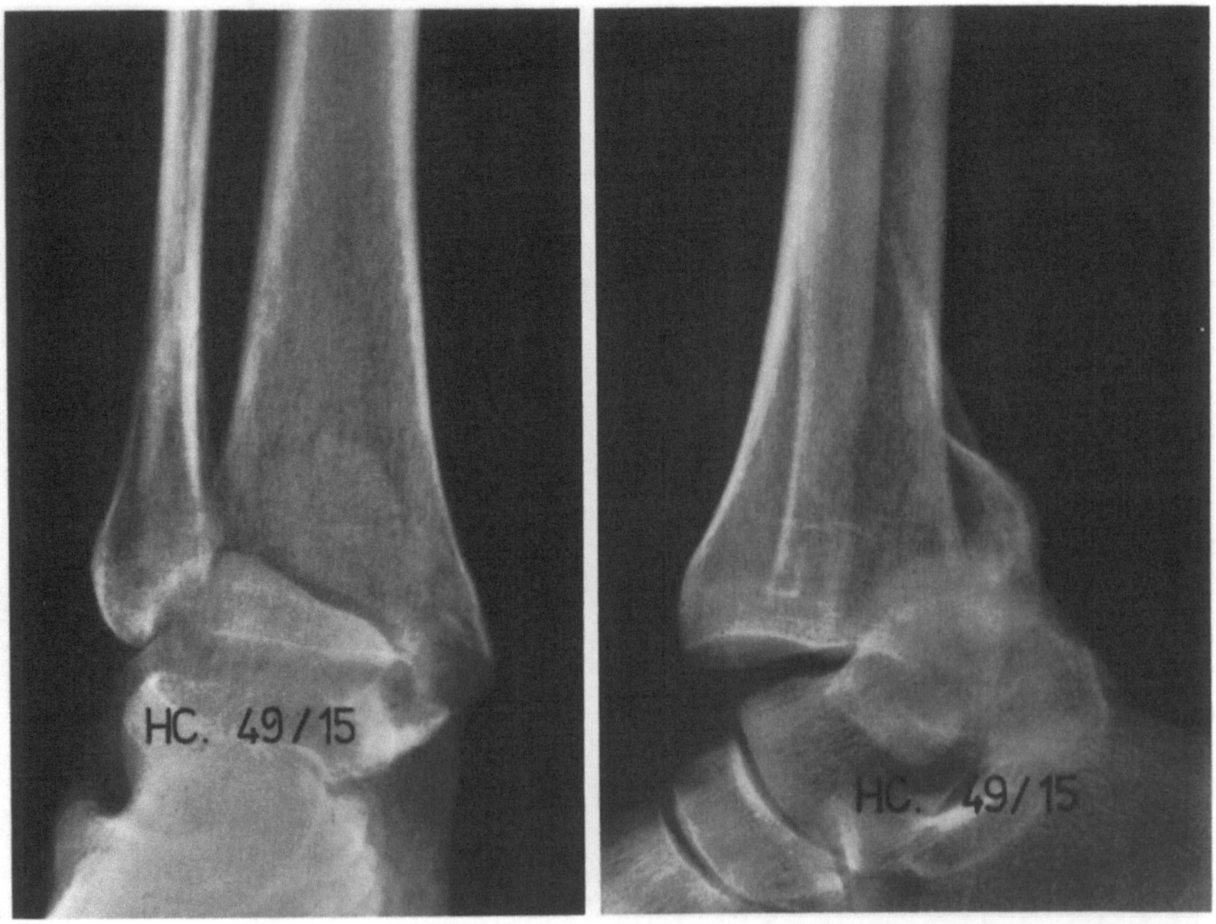

a

Fig. 224a–c. Clinical example: direct screw fixation of a small posterior malleolar fragment from the posterolateral side in a trimalleolar fracture

Paulina S., 58-year-old nun, fell during mountain walk on 8/17/79. Patient was unathletic and had mild diabetes mellitus

a Type B trimalleolar fracture-dislocation of the right ankle with a small displaced fracture of the posterior malleolus

b At emergency operation the lateral malleolus was fixed with an oblique lag screw and 6-hole one-third tubular plate. The anterior tibiofibular ligament was repaired with a transosseous suture.The lateral incision was extended proximally and posteriorly, and the posterior malleolus was fixed with two cancellous screws and washers. The medial malleolus was stabilized with a cancellous screw and Kirschner wire

Wound healing was uncomplicated, and active exercises were started. The patient was discharged with a below-knee cast, which was removed at 6 weeks to permit non-weight-bearing ankle exercises. Walking-pool exercises were started at 10 weeks, and full weight bearing at 12 weeks. Rehabilitation was prolonged by moderate trophic disturbances
The implants were removed after 10 months. There was still some limitation of ankle and subtalar joint motion, with regression of osteoporosis

c At 5 years the patient had no complaints, and the ankle was free of osteoarthritis

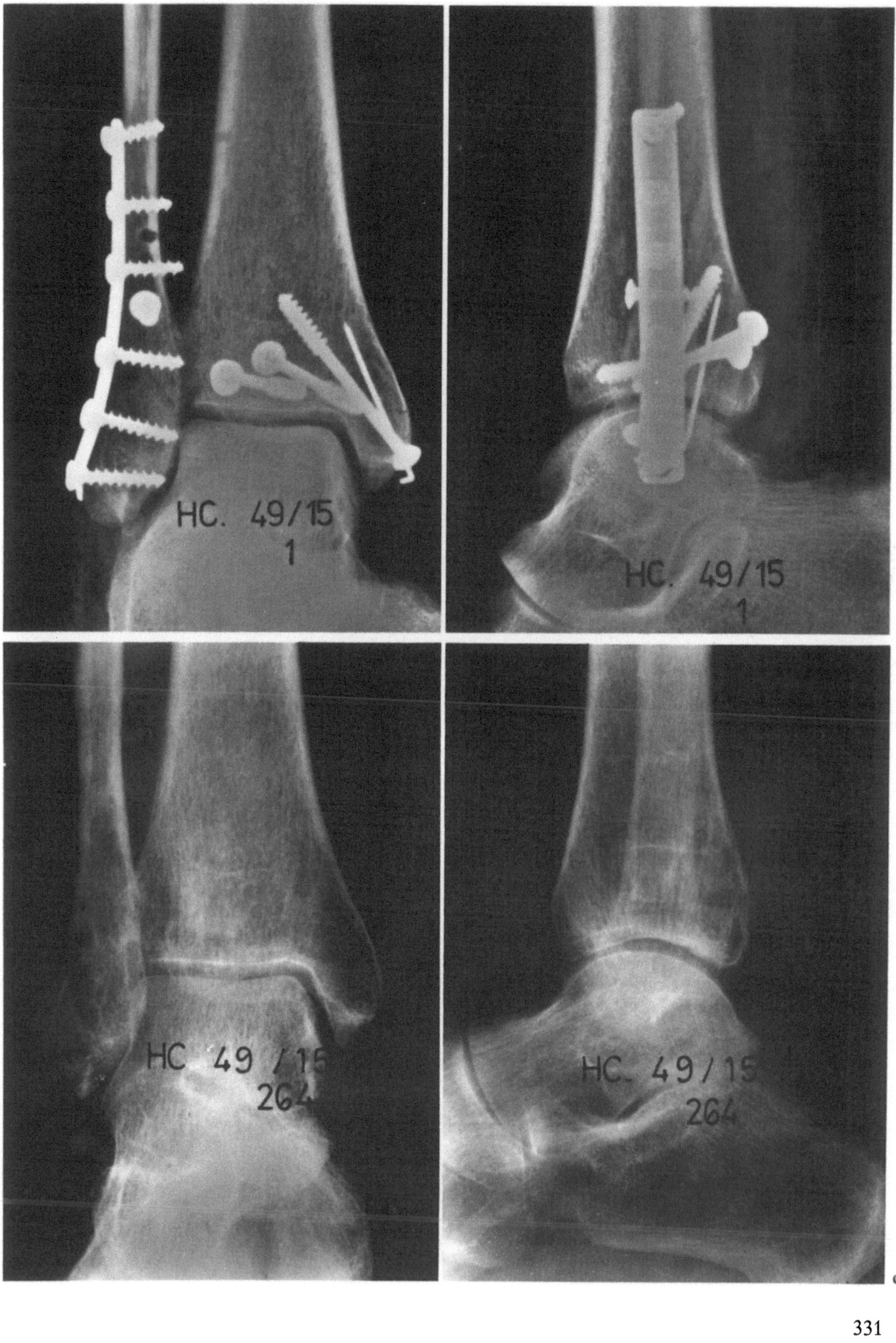

b

c

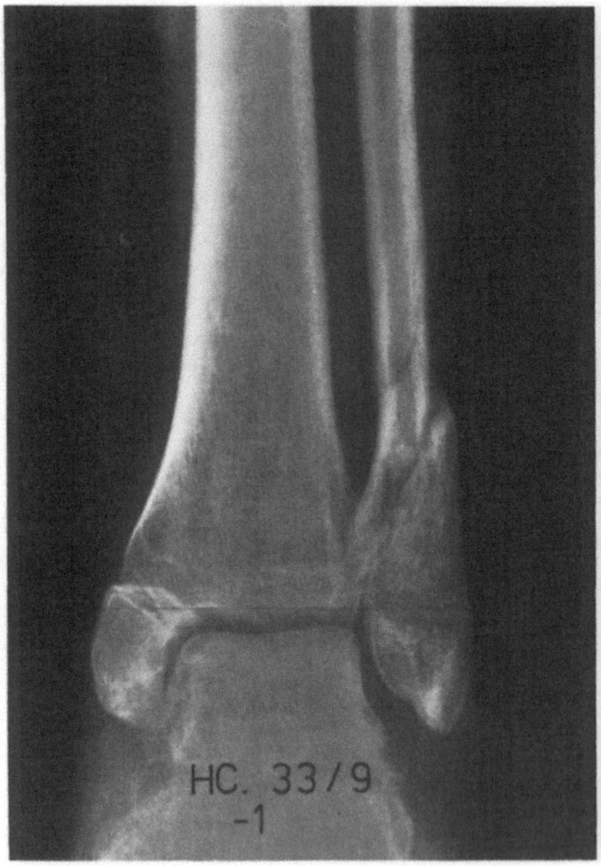

a

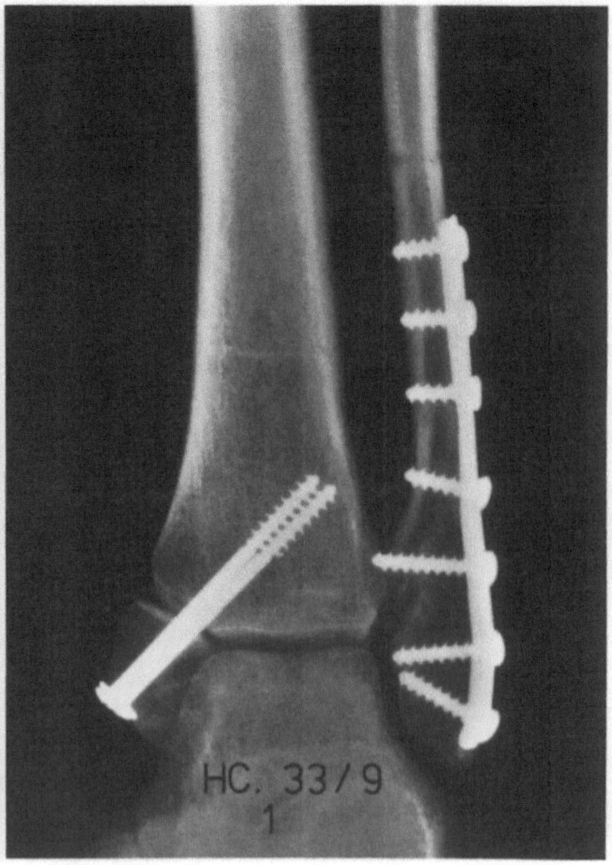

b

Fig. 225a–f. Clinical example: nonunion of the malleoli

Nesa C., 48-year-old housewife, struck from behind by a car, sustaining a bimalleolar fracture of the left ankle and a wound on the back of the lower leg. She was treated elsewhere with a plaster cast for 8 weeks

a Four months postinjury the patient presented with a nonunion of the lateral malleolus with 6-mm shortening and a nonunion of the medial malleolus with corresponding valgus deformity

b Internal fixation was performed on 10/19/76. Fibular length was restored and the lateral malleolus fixed with a 7-hole one-third tubular plate. The medial malleolus was fixed with two small cancellous screws with washers

After an uncomplicated course and primary exercises, the ankle was immobilized in a circular cast for 8 weeks

c The fibular nonunion consolidated, but the nonunion of the medial malleolus persisted

d At reoperation on 10/14/77 the lateral plate was removed, and one of the small cancellous screws on the medial side was replaced by a large, 6.5-mm cancellous screw with washer

e The medial nonunion consolidated

f When seen 3 1/2 years after implant removal, the patient had no complaints, full motion, 0.5-cm atrophy of the calf muscles, slight swelling in the malleolar area, and no osteoarthritis

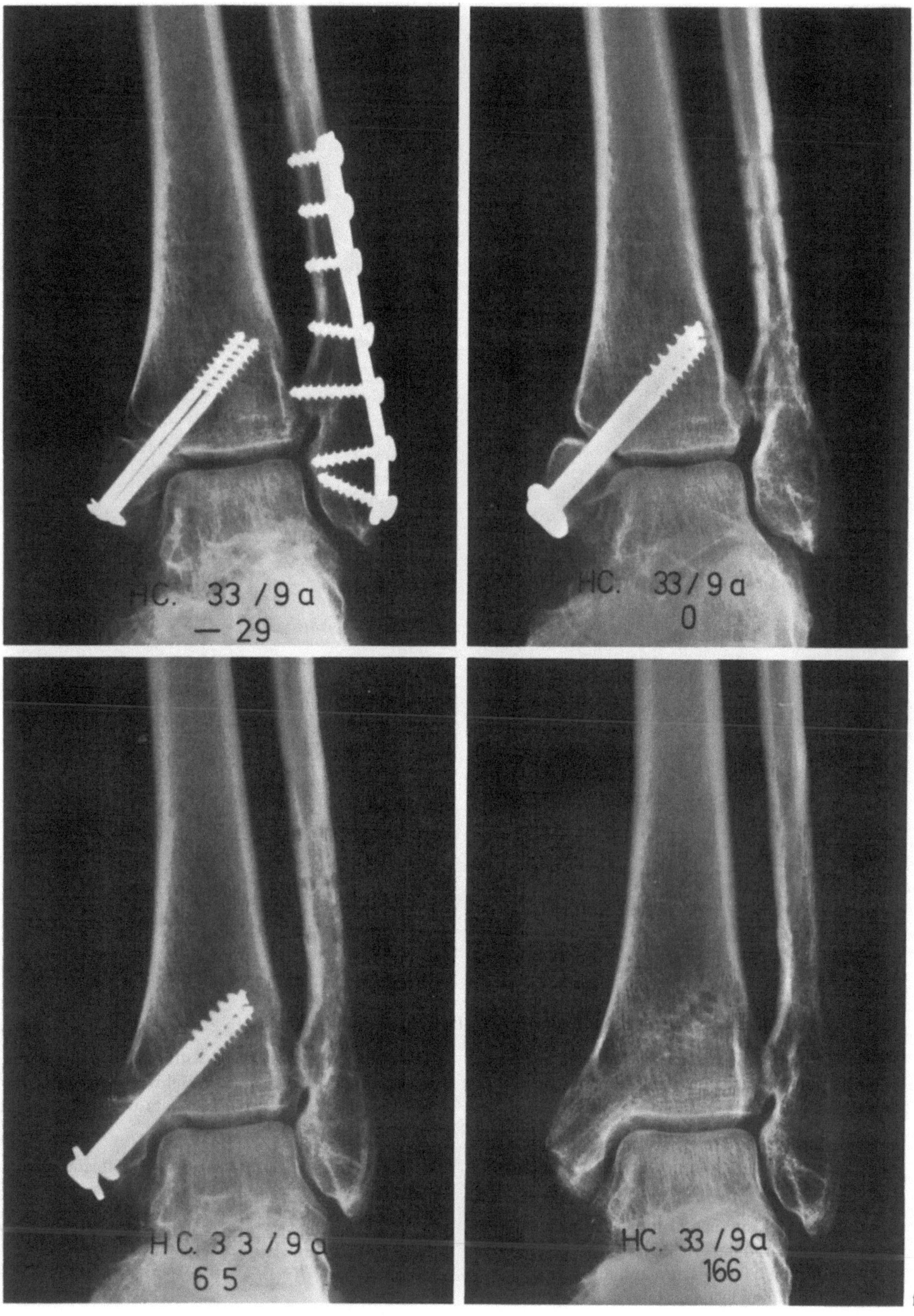

c d e f

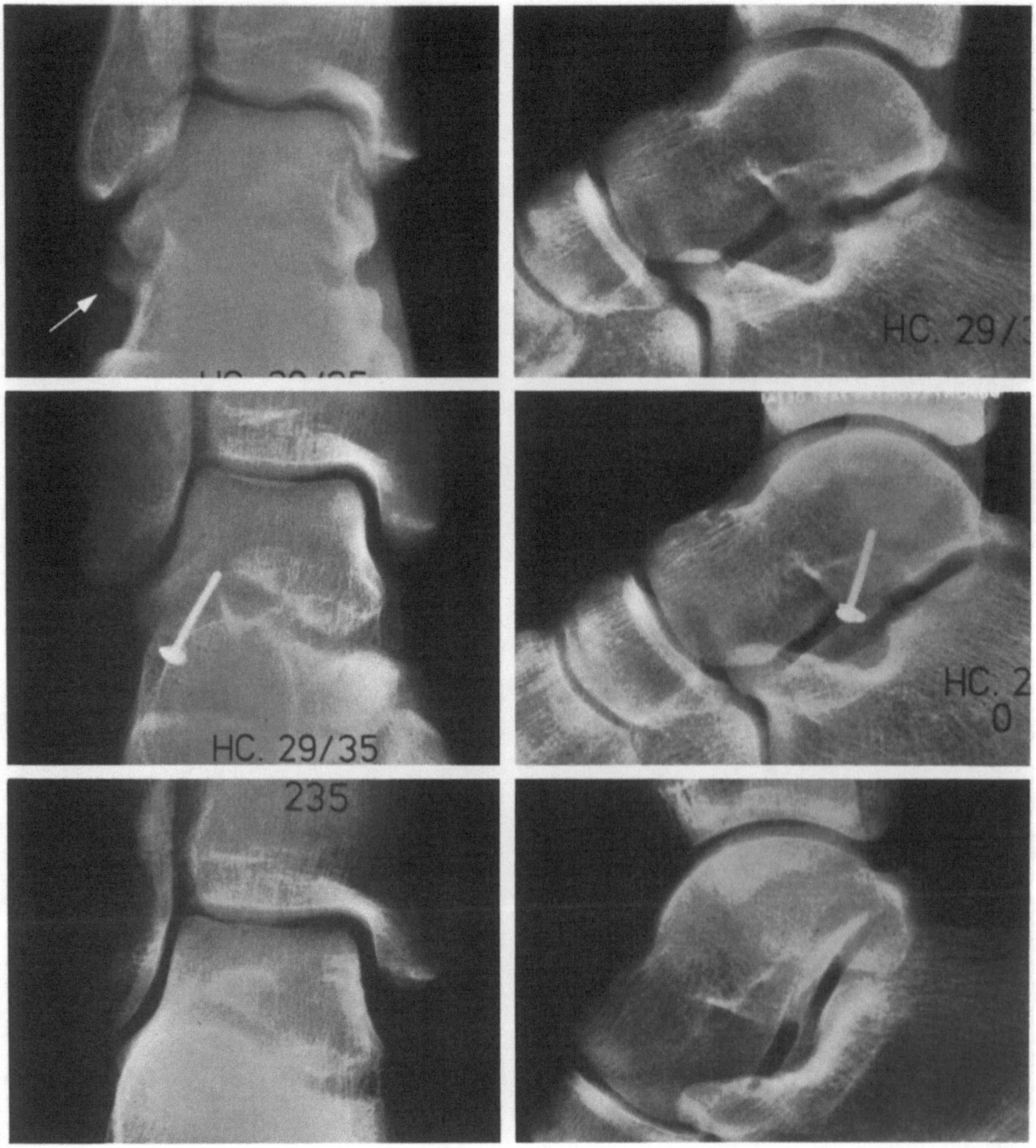

a
b
c

Fig. 226a–c. Clinical example: avulsion fracture of the lateral process of the talus

Silvio C., 21-year-old draftsman, fell while skiing on 1/10/76, noticed tenderness and swelling below the lateral malleolus

a The avulsion fracture of the lateral process of the talus(*arrow*) is difficult to appreciate on the X-rays. It signifies a ligament rupture in the subtalar joint

b At emergency internal fixation, the hemarthrosis was evacuated, and the avulsed fragment was reduced and fixed with a 2.0-mm screw and improvised washer.The surrounding ligament tears were repaired

The patient was discharged with a plaster splint after an uncomplicated course. Weight bearing was commenced at 10 weeks; the implants were removed at 9 months

c When seen at 4 1/2 years on 7/22/80, the patient had no complaints, full function, a linear scar, and no muscular atrophy. X-rays showed no osteoarthritis and a small calcification at the back of the talus

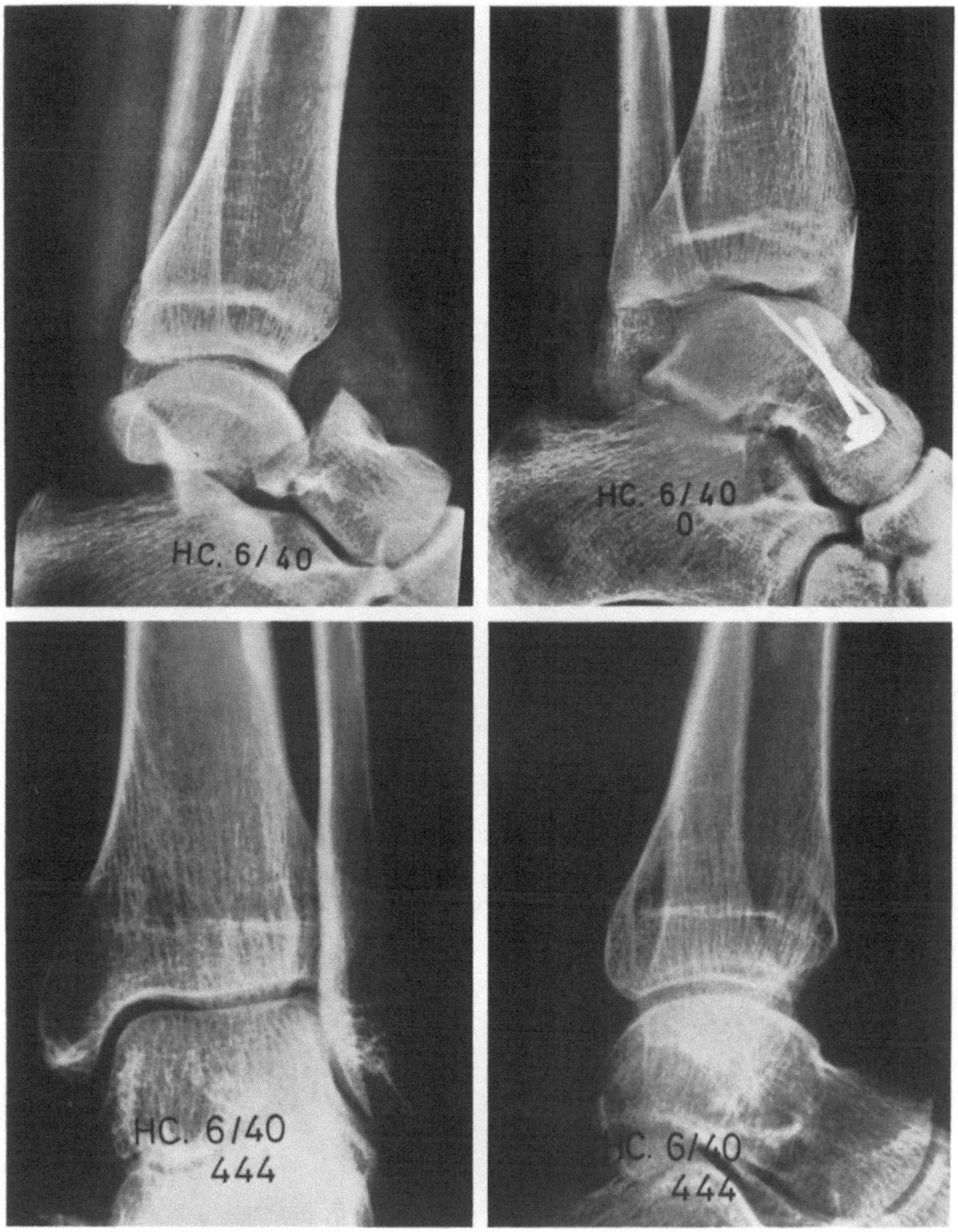

a b c

Fig. 227 a–c. Clinical example: fracture-dislocation of the talus managed by screw fixation

Daniel S., 18-year-old apprentice, fell while skiing on 12/19/71

a Fracture-dislocation of the neck of the talus. Closed reduction was unsuccessful

b The fracture was exposed through a medial incision, accurately reduced, and temporarily fixed with two Kirschner wires, one of which was replaced with a small cancellous screw (for interfragmental compression); the other was left in place

The postoperative course was uneventful, and a circular cast was worn for 4 weeks. Then a walking caliper was worn for 12 months

c When seen after 9 1/2 years on 7/7/80, the patient had no complaints, full function, a linear scar, no muscular atrophy, and normal X-rays

XVII. The Foot

1. Calcaneus

a) Avulsion fractures of the anterior process of the calcaneus are relatively rare. Because the calcaneofibular and interosseous ligaments insert on this process, open reduction and screw fixation are advised.

b) Beak fractures and avulsion fractures of the insertion of the Achilles tendon are fixed with a tension band, usually combined with Kirschner wires or cancellous screws. These injuries have conspicuous radiographic features. One should consider the possibility of coexisting malleolar fractures and peroneal tendon displacement.

c) Central Depressed Fractures

These are serious injuries of the calcaneus which destroy the subtalar joint. In the past, most of these fractures were managed conservatively. Treatment ranged from simple functional therapy to realignment by a pin drilled in from the tuberosity followed by cast immobilization in cases with a markedly decreased Böhler's angle. The results tended to be unfavorable, and many patients eventually developed a painful osteoarthritis that necessitated arthrodesis. Deformity, shortening, and disability of the foot were almost the rule.

Bèzes, building on the ideas of Judet, developed an open reconstructive technique for the treatment of central depressed fractures of the calcaneus. The late results of his technique were reviewed in a large patient series in 1980, and since then many ASIF surgeons have embraced the concept. The technical details of the procedure (approach, implants) have been modified somewhat in recent years. The original method will be described and illustrated below.

Objections to primary internal fixations of the calcaneus relate mainly to the risk of infection. In an area that already possesses a relatively poor vascular supply, compressive trauma and post-traumatic edema can compound the problem of circulatory compromise. Thus, we are faced with much the same problem (at a more distal level) as in the tibial pilon fracture, where it is often recommended that operative treatment be deferred until swelling has subsided.

The reduction should be anatomic.It should reconstitute the depressed posterior talocalcaneal joint and Böhler's angle, and it should eliminate widening and shortening. Stabilization with a lateral plate will enable the foot to be mobilized *without* the need for plaster fixation.

Opinions differ as to the need for cancellous bone grafting to fill the defect beneath the depressed segment. Bèzes considers bone grafting to be unnecessary.

The incidence of infection in Bèzes' series was 5%. This included two cases of osteitis with poor late results (following open fractures). Skin necroses (10%) tended to be superficial.

The late results are surprisingly good in terms of pain relief and ambulatory capacity, even in cases (about one-third) with restriction of subtalar joint motion.

Approach (Fig. 228 a,b)

With the patient on his side and the knee flexed, a gently curved skin incision is made between the apophysis of the fifth metatarsal and the lateral insertion of the Achilles tendon, running about one fingerwidth below the tip of the lateral malleolus. The incision is deepened with a scalpel down to the lateral cortex of the calcaneus, which will show varying degrees of comminution. The peroneal tendons, whose sheath is usually torn, are sharply mobilized and retracted proximally together with the sural nerve and small saphenous vein, which are identified but not dissected free. The calcaneofibular ligament is divided at its insertion. During this maneuver and the reduction that follows, care is taken to protect the retracted soft-tissue mass, which is susceptible to avascular necrosis.

At this point the surgeon should have a clear view of the posterior subtalar joint and the entire fracture site.

We have found that distraction with the small external fixator greatly aids the approach and facilitates temporary fixation after reduction of the articular fragments (Fig. 228 b).

Reduction and Fixation

The depressed articular segment may be up to 2 cm deep and solidly impacted. It is reduced by pulling the tuber calcanei posteriorly and distally with a large, sharp hook and elevating the impacted segment with a periosteal elevator.

Reduction of the joint and reconstitution of Böhler's angle will partially correct any widening that exists. The reduction is temporarily secured with Kirschner wires drilled horizontally and obliquely into the talus.

Definitive fixation is usually obtained with a one-third tubular plate (5- to 7-hole), which is appropriately twisted and contoured and applied beneath the peroneal tendons. The center of the plate is apposed to the comminuted area of the body of the calcaneus. The posterior end of the plate is near the proximal margin of the tuber, and the distal end is close to the anterior calcanean process (or the cuboid) (Fig. 228 c). The screws are inserted in a fanlike pattern, with the screw in the intact tuber directed medially and plantarly, and the distal screws directed proximomedially (Fig. 229). Centrally, small bridging cancellous screws grip the medial cortex of the calcaneus and the usually intact sustentaculum tali. We find that the preliminary insertion of Kirschner guide wires into the joint makes it easier to engage the distant sustentaculum with a screw. Tightening the central screws restores the anatomy of the calcaneus, even on the frontal plane. With severe lateral comminution, we recommend that the fixation be reinforced with a second, shorter plate applied more proximally (Fig. 228 d). Other authors prefer an H plate or radial T plate in this situation. If the fracture involves the anterior process of the calcaneus, a longer plate is selected and is anchored to the cuboid.

The operation is concluded by inserting a suction drain and closing the proximal soft tissues with fine cutaneous sutures. Often the presence of the implants will prevent reapproximation of the divided calcaneofibular ligament.

Aftertreatment

The extremity is elevated and immobilized on a plaster splint in standard fashion until wound healing is confirmed. Then active exercises are started, and the patient is allowed to stand with a supportive bandage. Rocking on the forefoot is recommended for ambulatory training. Full weight bearing is allowed when the fracture is solid, usually at about three months.

d) Open Fractures

These rare injuries are associated with a high risk of infection, and so internal fixation is not advised. The small external fixator has proved very effective in stabilizing these cases.

2. Tarsal Navicular

a) Fractures of the Body of the Navicular

These rare fractures can result from direct or indirect trauma. Especially with direct violence, first priority is placed on the treatment of the soft-tissue injuries. Displaced fractures generally require open reduction and internal fixation. If the fracture cannot be stabilized by screws alone, the cuneiforms can be incorporated into a plate fixation to create a temporary arthrodesis. When bone defects are found, one should not hesitate to perform a primary cancellous bone graft and especially to pack cancellous chips beneath depressed articular surfaces. The external fixator offers an alternative when soft-tissue conditions are precarious.

b) Fractures of the Navicular Tuberosity

These fractures are caused by eversion injuries that put extreme tension on the tibialis posterior tendon. But the majority show no significant displacement owing to the powerful capsuloligamentous attachments and the adjacent insertions of this tendon and therefore are amenable to closed treatment. When displacement is pronounced or union is delayed, screw and tension-band fixation should be considered and are preferable to later fragment excision in the event of nonunion.

c) Avulsion Fractures

Dorsal avulsion fractures are the most commonly observed navicular injury, and most can be treated conservatively. The same applies to fractures of the dorsal articular margin. Larger fragments can be anatomically reduced and fixed with a tension-band wire or with screws.

3. Cuneiforms and Cuboid

Fractures of the cuneiforms and cuboid are almost always caused by direct violence, which often is combined with dislocating injuries of the tarsometatarsal joint, comminution, and loss of height. To preserve the plantar vault, it is necessary to obtain anatomic realignment, fill any defect with cancellous bone, and apply rigid internal fixation (one-third tubular plate, T plate). A buttress plate applied to the lateral aspect of the cuboid can be placed across the calcaneocuboidal articulation and attached to the calcaneus (Fig. 237).The tarsometatarsal joint can be bridged in analogous fashion (Fig. 242). If soft-tissue conditions prohibit rigid internal fixation, external skeletal fixation may be applied. This permits the concurrent grafting of bone defects and provides free access to the soft tissues.

Full weight bearing on the foot is not possible until the fracture has consolidated and the joint-bridging plate has been removed or replaced.

4. Dislocations and Fracture-Dislocations

a) Transverse Tarsal Joint (Chopart's Joint)

The rare dislocations of the navicular, cuneiforms, and cuboid require anatomic reduction and rigid fixation. This can be done with Kirschner wires or by the internal fixation of these bones in the presence of bony avulsions or other accompanying fractures.

b) Tarsometatarsal Joint (Lisfranc's Joint)

The stabilizing "keystone" of the tarsometatarsal joint is the second metatarsal, whose base fits into a bony mortise formed by the medial and lateral cuneiforms and also has a strong ligamentous attachment to the lateral side of the medial cuneiform. In a Lisfranc dislocation, this powerful ligamentous attachment is responsible for the pathognomonic bony avulsion of the medial base of the second metatarsal. Especially when combined with other metatarsal fractures, Lisfranc dislocations are easily overlooked and can cause serious sequelae. It has proved helpful to supplement standard three-plane X-rays with CT scans so that joint congruity can be accurately assessed. With appropriate clinical findings, avulsions at the base of the second metacarpal and cuboid avulsions should always raise suspicion of tarsometatarsal instability or dislocation.

Most fresh dislocation injuries are amenable to closed reduction, whereas open reduction is generally indicated for older dislocations or fracture-dislocations. Diastasis between the medial and intermediate cuneiforms may signify interposition of the tibialis anterior tendon. If ischemia of the forefoot persists following a successful closed reduction, operative exposure of the dorsalis pedis artery and posterior tibial artery is mandatory. The reduction is stabilized with transarticular Kirschner wires. Intra-articular fractures require an anatomic reduction. A plate that temporarily spans the tarsometatarsal joint, combined with the cancellous grafting of significant bone defects, provides a rigid, stable fixation (Fig. 241). Comparable fixation is not obtainable with Kirschner wires reinforced by external immobilization.

When the tarsometatarsal joint is incorporated into the internal fixation, the plate must be removed or repositioned early, generally at about two months, to avoid serious damage to the joint cartilage. Weight is kept off the foot until removal of the transarticular plate to ensure that the implant will not fracture or dislodge.

The tarsometatarsal joint cannot tolerate deformities relating to inadequate reduction. Late degenerative changes necessitating arthrodesis will result.

5. Fractures of the Metatarsal Shaft and Neck

a) Indications

The rigid internal fixation of forefoot fractures is opening up new treatment options which avoid many of the disadvantages of conservative therapy. The early postoperative mobilization made possible by internal fixation is the best way to avoid or minimize the dystrophic sequelae that are so commonly observed in the foot. With consolidation of the fracture, the foot as a whole is healed and rehabilitated.

The normal adult plantar vault derives largely from the shape of the individual skeletal parts and from the congruity and intact capsuloligamentous structures of the various articulations. Active stabilizers play a less important role. Dorsal and especially plantar malunions of metatarsal fractures cause changes in the stresses on the forefoot that cannot be compensated. Besides the important *first and fifth rays*, the *second ray* of the foot performs a key function during walking. Owing to the rigid support of the second metatarsal in the area of the tarsometatarsal joint, the greatest stresses during the push-off phase of gait are transmitted through the head of the second metatarsal. Even minor plantar deformities of the second ray and to a lesser extent of the third ray result in loss of the normal transverse arch and cause unphysiologic stresses to act on the central forefoot (Fig. 231).

Thus, displaced metatarsal fractures that are not amenable to closed reduction, or whose reduction cannot be held in plaster, are an indication for open reduction and internal fixation.It is important to obtain an essentially anatomic reduction with regard to dorsoplantar deformity and to preserve normal metatarsal length, especially in the first, second, and fifth rays. The tolerance to lateral deformities is better in terms of late sequelae.

In certain situations–open fractures, fractures in multiple trauma patients, local fractures amenable to treatment without a cast–rigid internal fixation of the first and fifth rays in particular offers significant advantages, even for minimally displaced fractures of the shaft or neck.

In multiple fractures, reduction and fixation of the first and fifth rays often is sufficient to correct deformities of the central rays and thus enable early functional exercises to be performed without additional internal fixation of the central rays.

In contrast to the hand, dorsal plating of the forefoot is biomechanically unfavorable and does not create an effective tension band. Greater stability can be achieved by lateral plating of the first and fifth rays. Even so, it is necessary to keep weight off the injured foot for several weeks until the fracture is solid.

b) Operative Technique

Fractures caused by a sprain or indirect trauma are amenable to primary operative treatment on the day of the injury. With a fracture caused by severe, direct violence, greater caution is advised. If significant swelling is present and the viability of the integument is questionable, operative treatment should be delayed until soft-tissue swelling has subsided and should be combined with any skin grafts that are needed to secure coverage of bradytrophic tissues (tendons) and implants.

The special conditions of blood flow in the foot demand the use of atraumatic surgical technique ("hand surgery on the foot"). As in the hand, the first and fifth rays are exposed through longitudinal dorsomedial (first ray) or dorsolateral incisions (fifth ray) placed so that the scars will not be irritated by footwear. The central rays are best exposed through longitudinal incisions that have a slight Z- or S-shaped curvature (Fig. 230a). Severe circulatory impairment and troublesome scar neuromas are avoided by sparing the dorsalis pedis artery (between the first and second ray) and the superficial branches of the peroneal nerve. Three or more distal metatarsals (multiple neck fractures) can be exposed through one transverse incision, as in the hand (Fig. 230b). However, care is taken to spare the longitudinal blood vessels and nerve branches so that circulatory compromise and neuroma problems can be avoided.

The *first metatarsal* is most commonly fractured in the midshaft area. In accordance with the relatively large dimensions of the first ray, contoured one-third tubular plates, small T plates (distally), and radial plates (proximally) are the implants of choice for internal fixation. From a biomechanical standpoint, it is better to plate the bone medially than dorsally (Fig. 233a). Wedge-type fractures with extension into the tarsometatarsal joint generally can be fixed with screws alone (3.5/4.0-mm or 2.7-mm). When the plantar bony buttress is deficient due to bone loss, the primary application of cancellous bone grafts will significantly accelerate healing (Fig. 233b).

Displaced transverse, oblique, or comminuted fractures of the shaft or neck of the *fifth metatarsal* are fixed with small T and L plates or quarter tubular plates (Fig. 233a). The 2.7-mm DCP offers added stability for shaft fractures. Pure spiral fractures with shortening can be rigidly fixed with 2.7- or 2.0-mm screws in suitable cases. A concomitant fracture of the fourth ray usually does not require additional fixation after the fifth ray has been stabilized (see Fig. 41).

Fractures of the *three central metatarsals* that do not involve the marginal rays rarely justify internal fixation with plates or screws. If there is displacement that cannot be reduced by closed methods, open reduction and *medullary Kirschner wire fixation* offers a simple and elegant operative technique (Fig. 234). The fractured end of the distal fragment is lifted out of the wound, and a heavy Kirschner wire, pointed at both ends, is drilled through the medullary canal of the distal fragment until the point emerges through the plantar skin. The fracture is reduced, and the wire is drilled back proximally into the base of the metatarsal. The projecting end of the wire is bent over and is not buried beneath the skin. The foot is immobilized in a well-padded plaster splint until removal of the wire at 5–6 weeks. Further treatment consists in partial non-weight bearing or use of a below-knee walking cast for another 2–3 weeks.

c) Aftertreatment

Aftertreatment following rigid internal fixation consists of functional exercises. Immediately after surgery a plaster U splint is worn until wound healing is confirmed; the splint is removed for intervals of active physiotherapy. Non-weight bearing is maintained until the fracture is solid, which takes 5–8 weeks in uncomplicated cases. Heel-to-toe rocking with 10–15 kg of floor pressure can be performed by most patients and is highly beneficial in terms of trophism and blood flow.

6. Fractures of the Fifth Metatarsal

a) Fractures of the Tuberosity and Base

These are the most common fractures of the foot. The usual mechanism of injury is forced plantar flexion and inversion of the forefoot. Reflex contracture of the peroneus brevis muscle avulses the tuberosity from the base of the fifth metatarsal. Torsion of the forefoot also exerts an indirect tensile force on the tuberosity through the lateral extensions of the plantar aponeurosis. Because the same mechanism of injury (supination and inversion) causes damage to the anterolateral ankle joint, the entire lateral (fibular) chain of lesions should be considered during diagnosis. A simultaneous direct blow to the lateral side of the foot, or excessive straining of that area, can result in more extensive fractures of the proximal fifth metatarsal with multiple fragments.

The biomechanical characteristics of the fracture depend on the course of the fracture relative to the fifth tarsometatarsal joint and the dynamic checkreins formed by the peroneus brevis tendon, the abductor digiti minimi, and the lateral slip of the plantar aponeurosis (Fig. 232a). When the fracture plane is roughly parallel to the plane of the tarsometatarsal joint, the dynamic checkrein action of the soft tissues on the intact proximal fragment produces compression on the dorsomedial side of the fracture. Thus, these fractures should heal well with conservative treatment, even if there is initial diastasis in the lateral part of the fracture (Fig. 232b). Internal fixation with screws or a tension band is indicated only in exceptional cases.

When the fracture plane is oriented roughly at right angles to the joint plane, as it is often the case in multi-part fractures, reduction is no longer aided by this natural, dynamic checkrein effect (Fig. 232c). Treated conservatively, displaced fractures of this type will often lead to incongruity of the fifth tarsometatarsal joint and nonunion. Consequently, these fractures justify internal fixation with a screw, tension band, or small L or quarter tubular plate (Fig. 232d,e).

b) Transverse Fracture of the Proximal Diaphysis (Jones Fracture) (Fig. 245)

A different mechanism of injury underlies the rare transverse fracture of the proximal diaphysis (metaphysis) of the fifth metatarsal, also known as *Jones fracture*. This type of fracture can occur in young, athletic individuals who may or may not recall a single precipitating event (fatigue fracture).In contrast to fatigue fractures of the shafts of the central metatarsals, conservative treatment of Jones fracture is associated with a high rate of refractures and nonunions. Especially when X-rays show signs of sclerosis about the fracture site, and the medullary cavities are visible, it is appropriate to perform rigid internal fixation with a laterally applied quarter tubular plate, L plate or T plate, possibly combined with cancellous bone grafting. The aftertreatment is like that for metatarsal shaft fractures, but the implants generally are left in place for a longer time (usually more than one year).

If X-rays do not show reactive changes, and a recent injury is presumed to be the cause of the fracture, conservative treatment generally will yield excellent results.

7. Fractures of the Big Toe (Fig. 233)

Displaced fractures of the proximal phalanx of the big toe are an indication for open reduction and rigid internal fixation, especially when there is incongruity of the metatarsophalangeal joint, or a condylar fracture has produced incongruity of the interphalangeal joint.A small T or L plate, quarter tubular plate or condylar plate may be used, depending on the fracture type.

8. Secondary Operations on the Forefoot

a) Nonunions

Delayed fracture unions and true nonunions are seen relatively frequently in the forefoot. The peculiar circulatory conditions and biomechanics of the foot, where bending loads act in both the dorsal and plantar directions, allow nonunions to develop in all the metatarsals and less frequently in the proximal phalanx of the big toe. Nonunions of the marginal rays almost invariably cause severe subjective complaints, and so the indication for internal fixation is definite. In the central rays, the need for internal fixation will depend upon subjective complaints.

Internal fixation may also be indicated for a persistent, painful apophysis at the base of the fifth metatarsal. We have already mentioned the special features of Jones fracture and the high incidence of delayed union, nonunion, and refracture with conservative therapy.

The operative technique and choice of implant are the same as in acute fractures.Given the unfavorable circulatory conditions and biomechanics of the forefoot, the application of cancellous bone chips (from the iliac crest) is an essential part of therapy. To obtain adequate stability, the tarsometatarsal joint can be temporarily immobilized with the internal fixation material without causing significant damage to the articular cartilage.

b) Arthrodeses

The main objective of treating a joint injury must be the reconstruction and preservation of the articular surfaces. However, when there is extensive damage to the transverse tarsal and tarsometatarsal articulations, primary arthrodesis with a corticocancellous iliac graft and rigid internal fixation can be very effective in shortening rehabilitation. Mild to severe degenerative joint changes may be expected to occur in up to one-third of patients with a Lisfranc dislocation. Treatment consists in arthrodesis of the affected joints.

Primary resection of the metatarsophalangeal joint of the big toe should be avoided if possible. If a painful secondary osteoarthritis develops, it can be managed by any of several techniques of resective arthroplasty. Implant arthroplasty with a silastic prosthesis has not become an established procedure in the foot.

Painful osteoarthritis of the interphalangeal joint of the big toe is treated by retrograde fusion of the joint with a screw (Fig. 249).

9. Illustrative Case Reports and X-Rays

(Figs. 235–249)

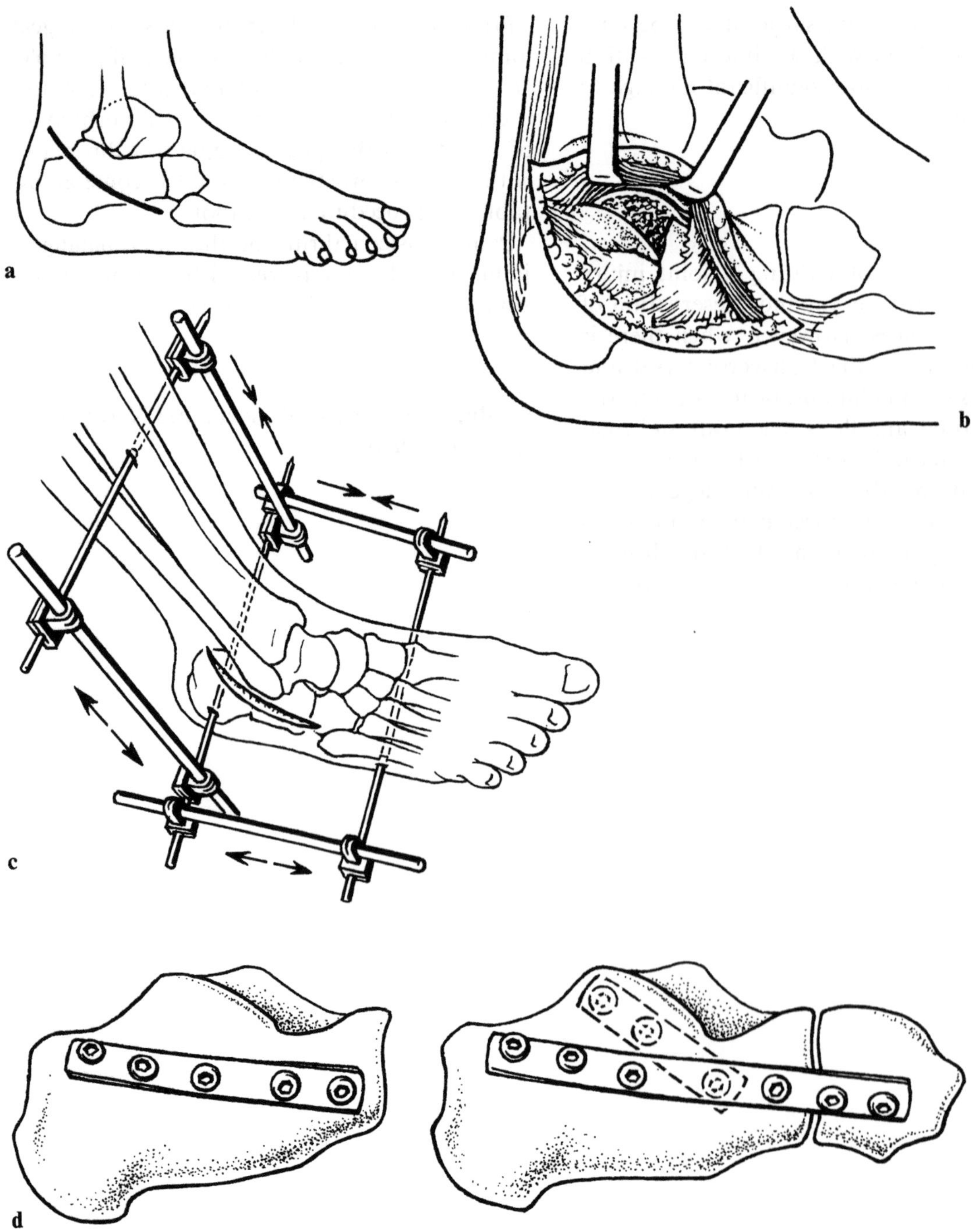

Fig. 228a–d. Internal fixation of a central depressed fracture of the calcaneus: approach and implant placement

a The skin is incised from the base of the 5th metatarsal to the distal end of the Achilles tendon

b The depression is exposed by elevating the peroneal tendons along with the sural nerve and vein

c The small external fixator is a useful aid to reduction and temporary fixation. Lateral distraction improves visualization of the fracture and facilitates reduction and temporary stabilization of the reduced articular fragments

d Position of the one-third tubular plate on the lateral calcaneus, with and without attachment to the cuboid (Y configuration with second, short plate for periarticular compression)

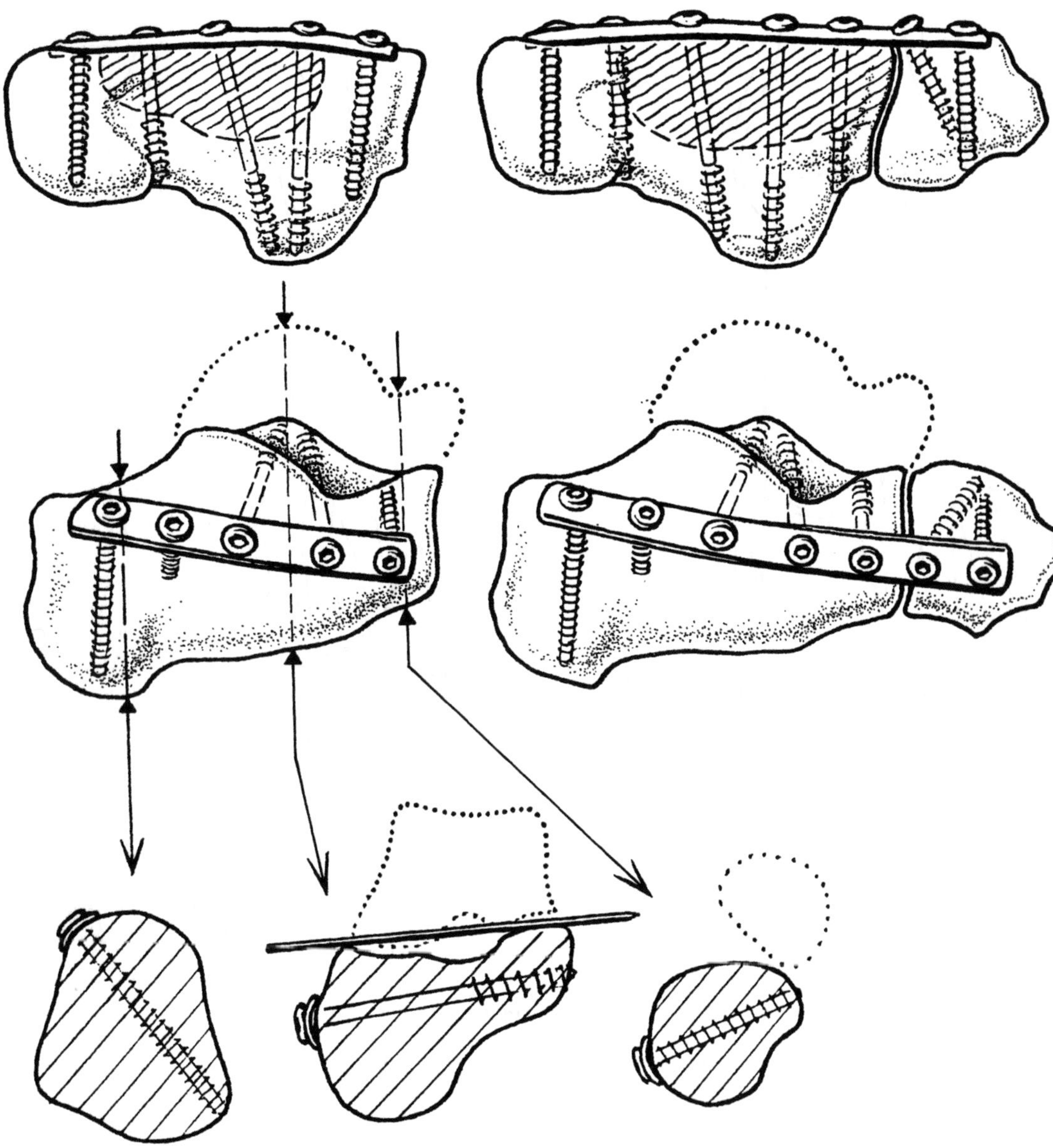

a

b

c

Fig. 229 a–c. Internal fixation of a central depressed fracture of the calcaneus: insertion of the plate screws

a Top view:
- Shaded areas: probable areas of comminution and depression
- Unshaded areas: normally intact areas that can hold a screw (tuber, sustentaculum tali, anterior process, cuboid)

b Lateral view with fanlike screw pattern

c Frontal cross-sections at the level of individual screws, from proximal (left) to distal (right). The screw for the sustentaculum tali is driven in parallel to a Kirschner guide wire inserted into the joint

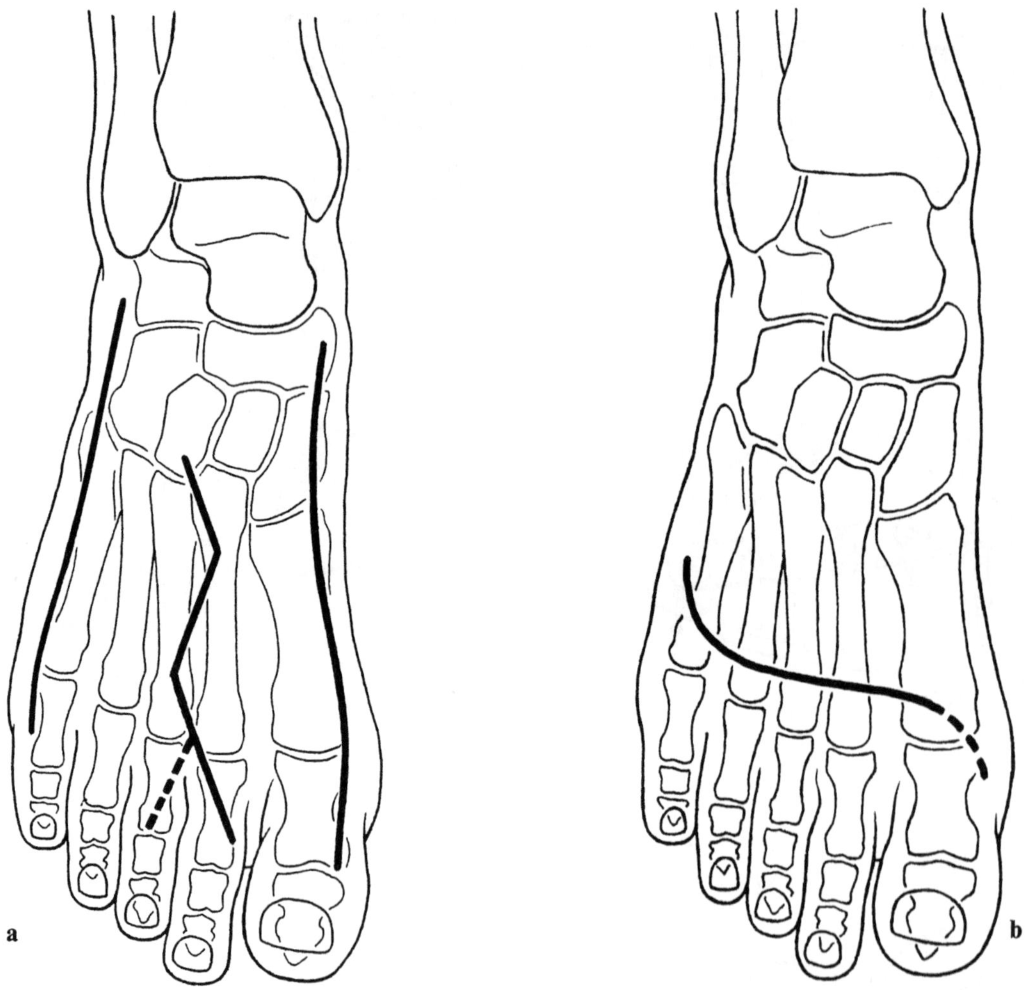

Fig. 230a, b. Skin incisions for internal fixations of the metatarsus and forefoot

a Longitudinal incisions for exposing the base and shaft of the metatarsals and the metatarsophalangeal joint of the big toe

b Transverse incision for operations on the distal forefoot (for multiple fractures of the distal metatarsals). Nerves and blood vessels coursing longitudinally must be protected in this approach

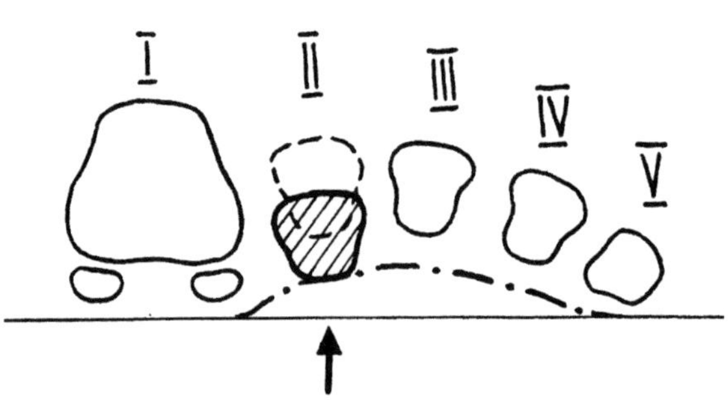

Fig. 231. The transverse arch with a displaced metatarsal fracture

Plantar angulation of the fragment causes excessive loading of the forefoot

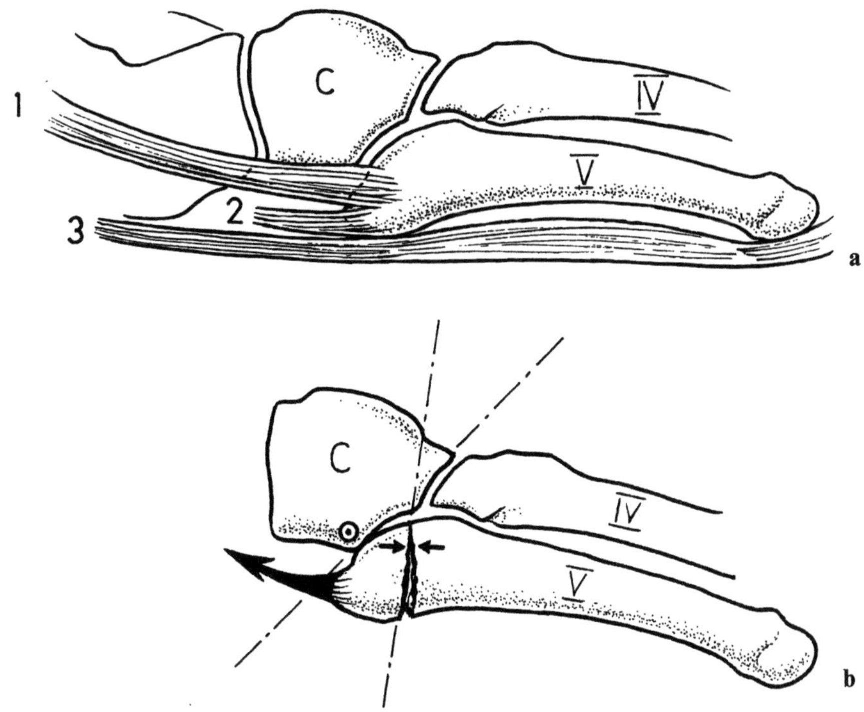

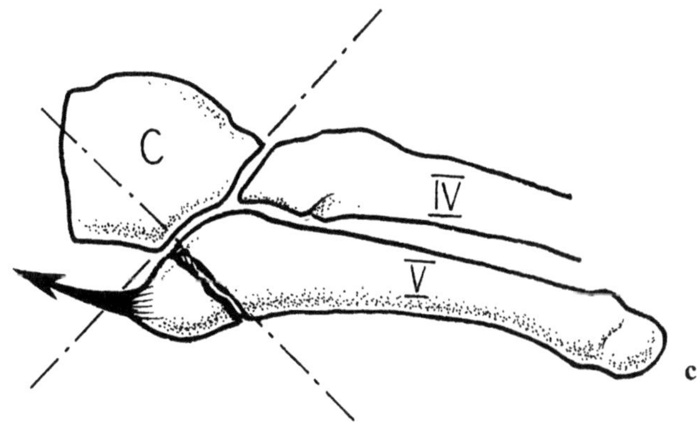

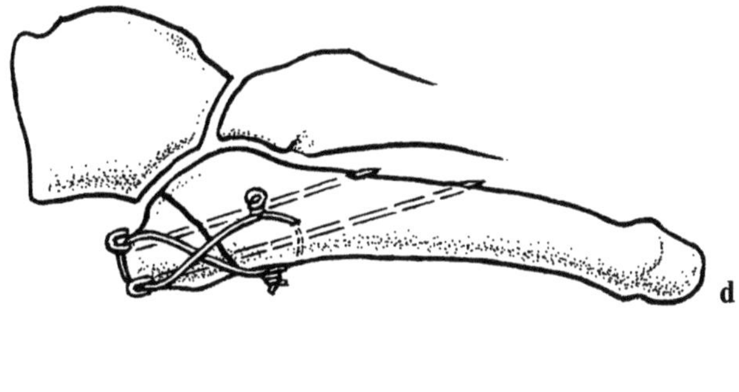

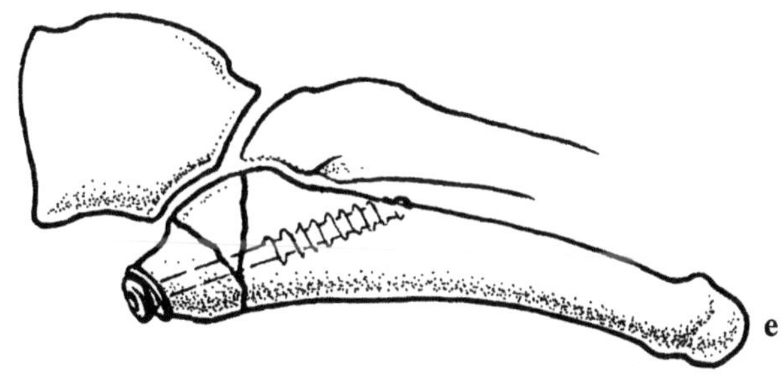

Fig. 232 a–e. Fractures of the tuberosity and base of the fifth metatarsal

a Biomechanics: The dynamic checkreins of the tuberosity and 5th metatarsal:
1 – Peroneus brevis tendon
2 – Lateral slip of the plantar aponeurosis
3 – Insertion of abductor digiti minimi on the tuberosity

b Here the fracture plane is "parallel" to the plane of the 5th tarsometatarsal joint. The dorsomedial part of the fracture is compressed by tendon traction. The plantar base of the cuboid (*ring*) is the fulcrum for this action

c Here the fracture plane is "perpendicular" to the plane of the 5th tarsometatarsal joint.The fracture surfaces separate

d Tension-band fixation of a small proximal fragment

e Screw fixation of a larger basal fragment that has internal fracture lines

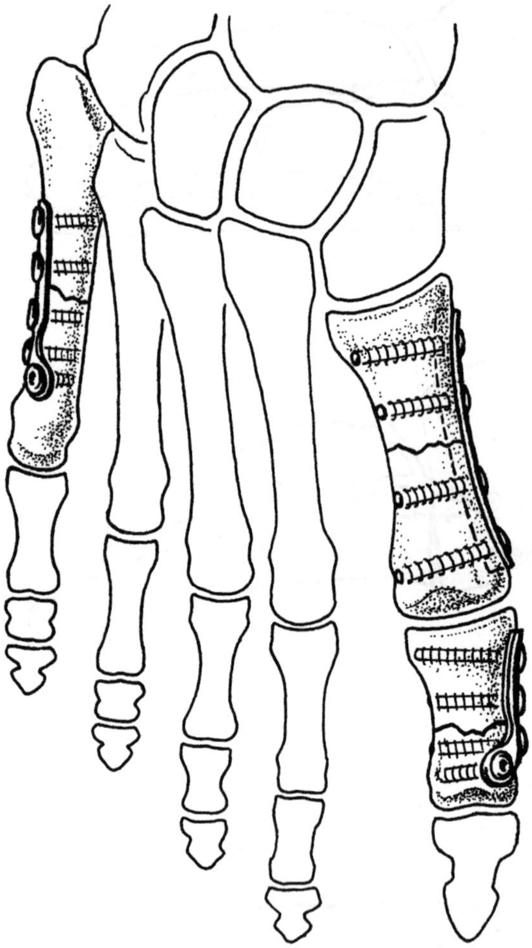

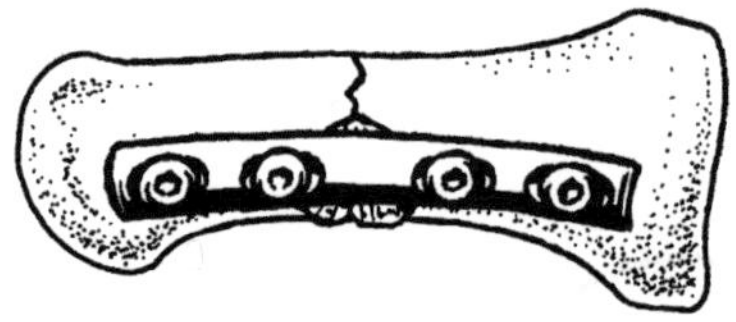

Fig. 233a, b. Typical plate fixations of the forefoot

a The 1st and 5th metatarsals are fixed with small plates attached to the tension side of the bones, shifted slightly toward the plantar surface (one-third tubular plate, radial T plate, finger L plate, mini L plate)

b Cancellous bone grafting of a comminuted area on the plantar side of the 1st metatarsal

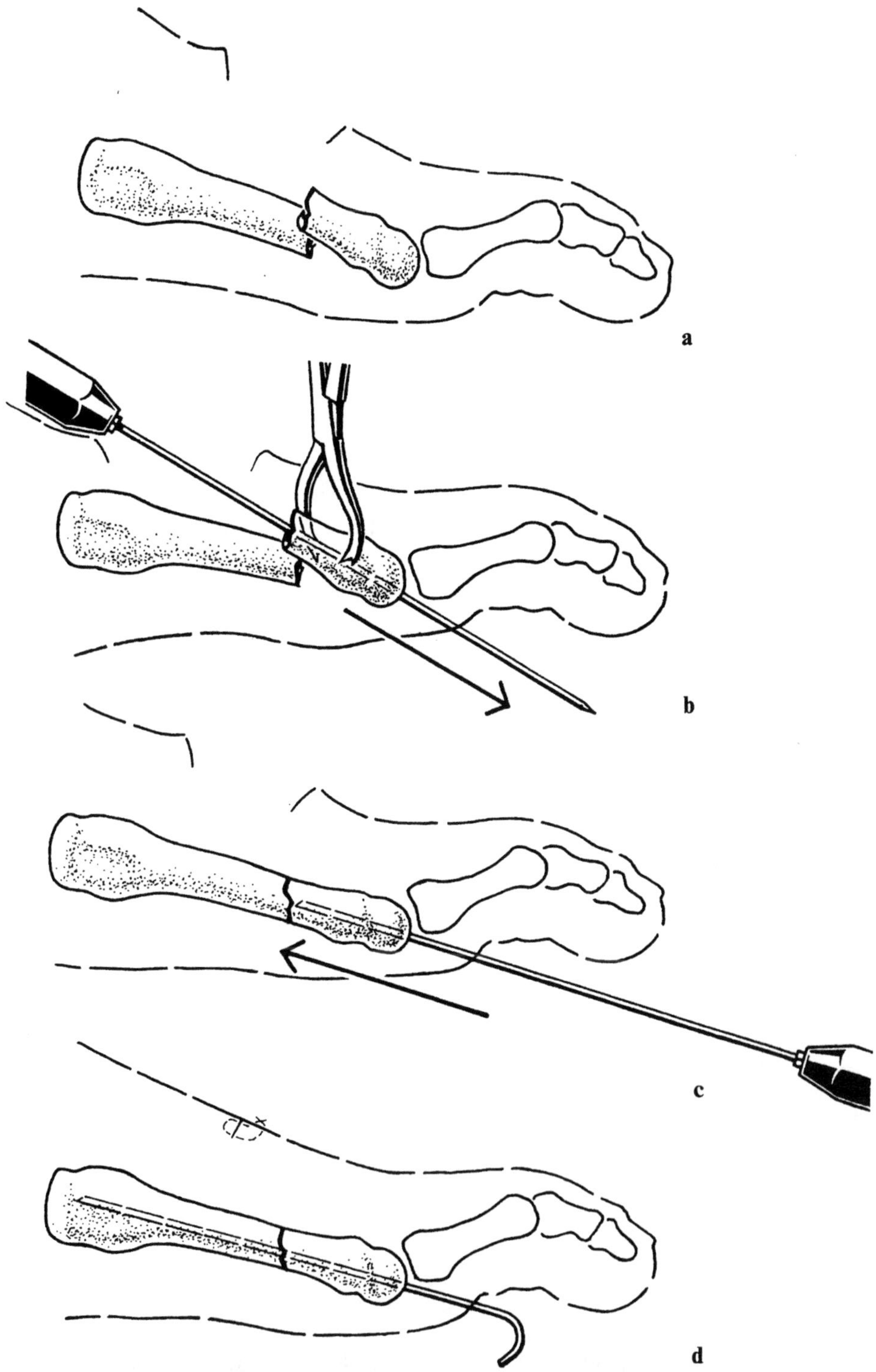

Fig. 234a–d. Open medullary Kirschner wire fixation of the second through fourth metatarsals

a Initial situation and approach

b From the dorsal incision, the Kirschner wire is drilled into the distal fragment and out through the plantar skin

c The fracture is openly reduced, and the wire is drilled back into the medullary cavity of the proximal fragment

d The end of the wire is not buried beneath the skin

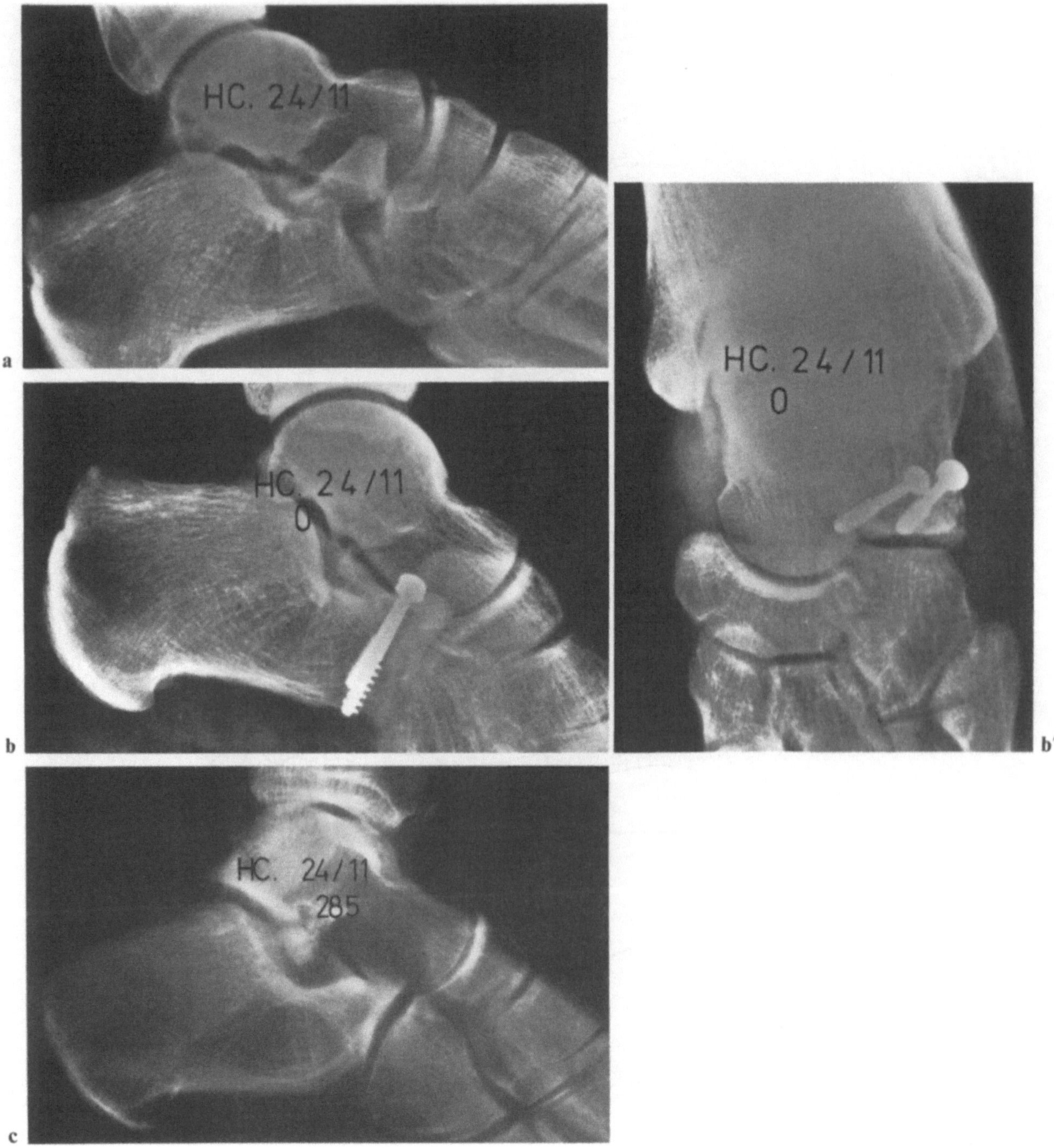

Fig. 235 a–c. Clinical example: avulsion fracture of the anterolateral calcaneus

Hans-Ulrich B., 21-year-old retail employee, fell while skiing on 1/3/75

a Avulsion fracture of the anterolateral margin of the calcaneus with subluxation of the transverse tarsal joint, also a small avulsion fracture of the lateral process of the talus

b At emergency internal fixation, the calcaneus was fixed with two small cancellous screws. A small comminuted zone was found below the avulsed fragment After an uneventful course, the patient was discharged with a circular cast worn for 12 weeks. The screws were removed elsewhere after 1 year

c At follow-up on 7/14/80, the patient had no complaints, full function, and a slightly pigmented scar. X-rays showed sclerosis of the lateral process of the talus and no osteoarthritis

Fig. 236a–c. Clinical example: tension-band fixation of a bony avulsion of the Achilles tendon

Eva-Maria G., 42-year-old housewife, fell while skiing on 2/1/79

a Bony avulsion of the Achilles tendon from the tuber calcanei

b The fragment was openly reduced and fixed with two small cancellous screws, washers, and a double tension-band wire loop
After an uncomplicated course and primary wound healing, the patient was discharged with a below-knee cast that held the foot in plantar flexion. A walking cast was applied at 4 weeks and removed at 8 weeks

c After 13 months the patient, who lives abroad, wrote that she was fully rehabilitated and athletically sound. The implants were removed at 8 months
Follow-up radiographs at 33 weeks confirmed fracture union

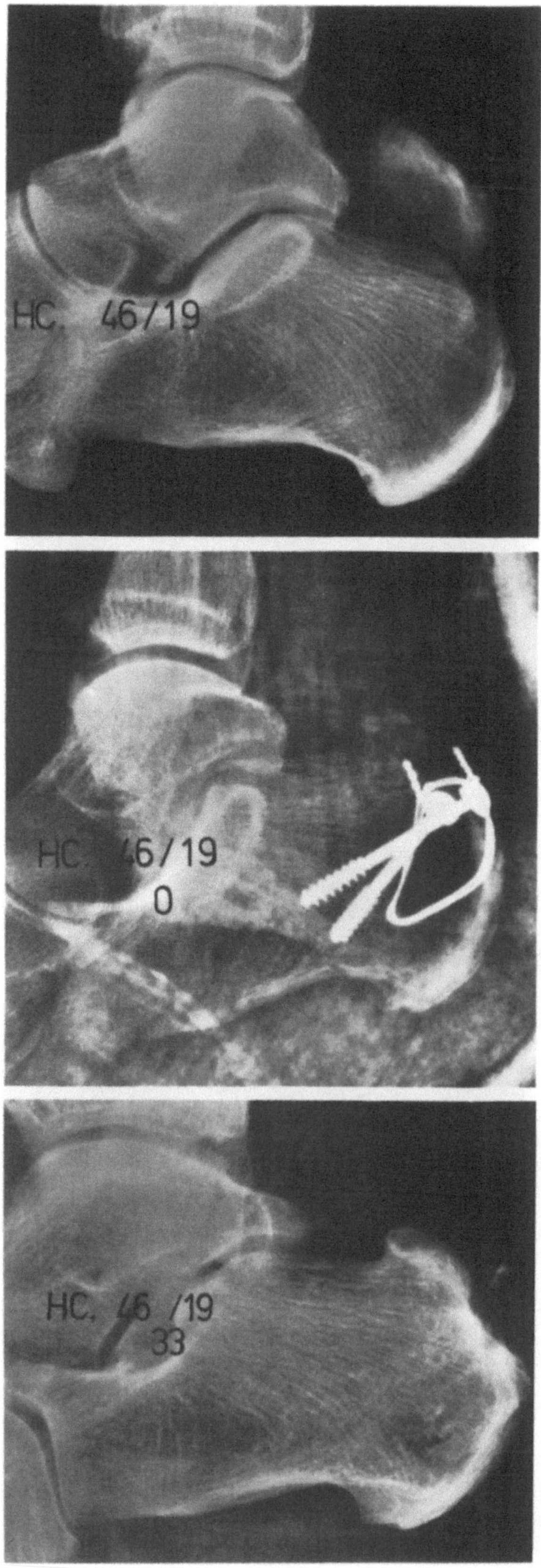

a b c

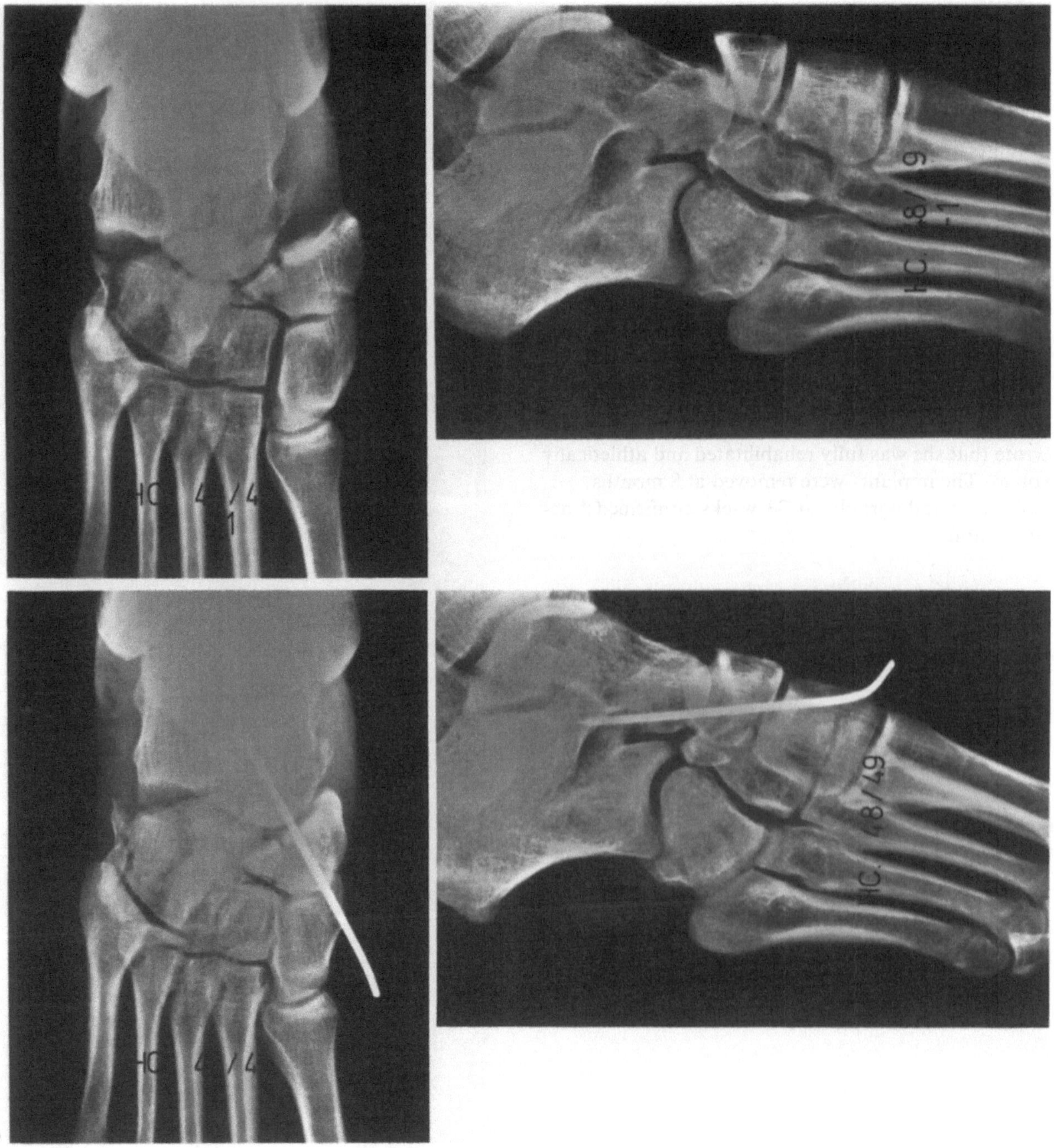

a

b

Fig. 237a–e. Clinical example: fracture-dislocation of the transverse tarsal joint

Verena F., 18-year-old hotel work trainee, fell while playing badminton on 7/11/79. Her dislocation was reduced and fixed in plaster by the family physician. Patient was hospitalized on day 9

a Dislocation of the transverse talar joint with compression fractures of the navicular and cuboid

b Closed reduction was performed under general anesthesia, and a percutaneous Kirschner wire was inserted through the navicular in the falus. At that time a chip fracture and defect of the cuboid were appreciated more clearly on X-rays.Further treatment was deferred because of the poor condition of the soft tissues

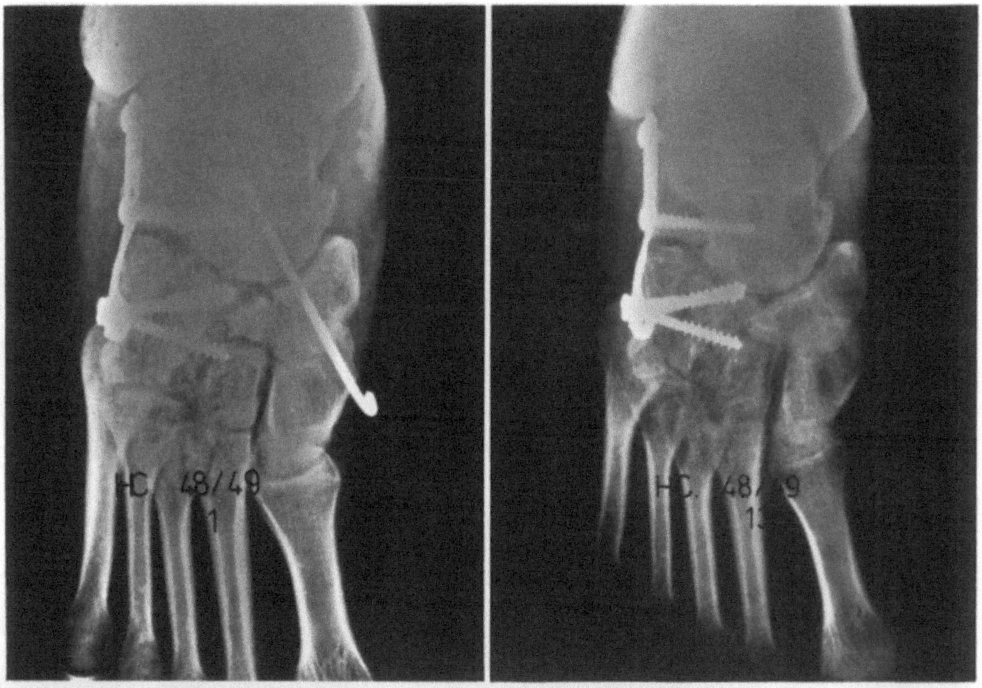

c

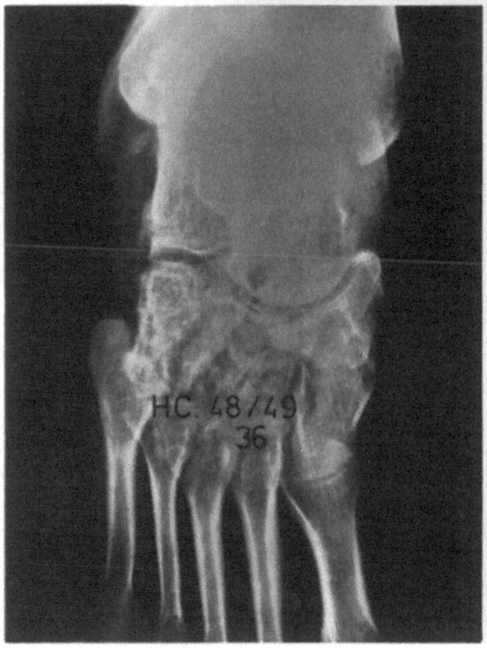

d

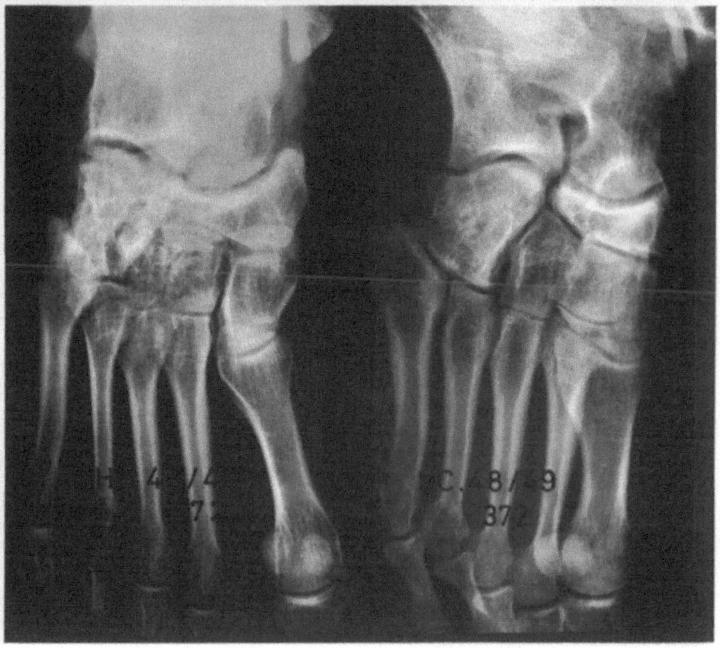

e

c Lateral internal fixation was performed one week later (8/1/79). The cuboid was openly reduced and realigned and the defect grafted with autogenous iliac cancellous bone. A buttress T plate was attached to the intact distal part of the cuboid and to the calcaneus. The lateral Kirschner wire was buried beneath the skin

Early exercises were performed, and the patient was discharged with a plaster splint. The Kirschner wire was removed 4 weeks later because of local irritation. Full weight bearing was started at 10 weeks

d The implants were removed at 8 months. Patient had full function except for a slight limitation of supination, no muscular atrophy, and a linear scar. The fractures were united with congruent joint lines

e When seen at 7 years on 9/15/86, the patient had no complaints, full function, and no osteoarthritis. A longitudinal split in the cuboid was still visible on X-rays

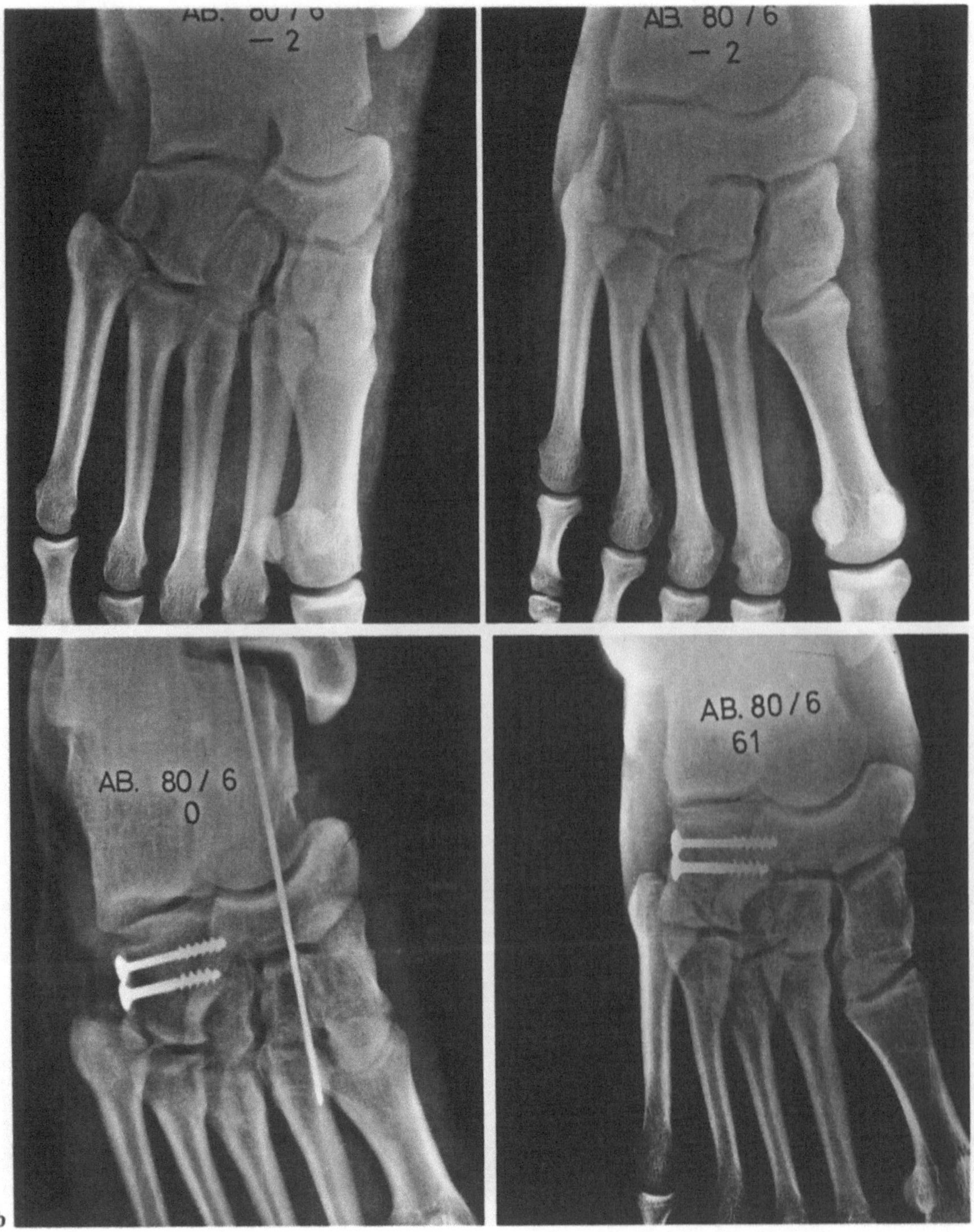

Fig. 238 a–c. Clinical example: lateral fracture-dislocation of the tarsometatarsal joint

Iris M., 16-year-old girl, fell on the right foot during gymnastic exercises on 3/13/74

a Basal fractures of the 2nd through 5th metatarsals with an avulsion from the base of the 2nd metatarsal– typical of tarsometatarsal dislocation. Chip fracture of the cuboid

b Internal fixation was performed at 2 weeks through 2 longitudinal incisions. The 2nd metatarsal was reduced and fixed with a Kirschner wire, and the ligament was repaired. The cuboid fracture was fixed with screws

A non-weight-bearing cast was worn for 7 weeks, then the Kirschner wire was removed and progressive weight bearing commenced

c At 11 months the patient had no complaints and a full range of foot motion. The screws were left in place

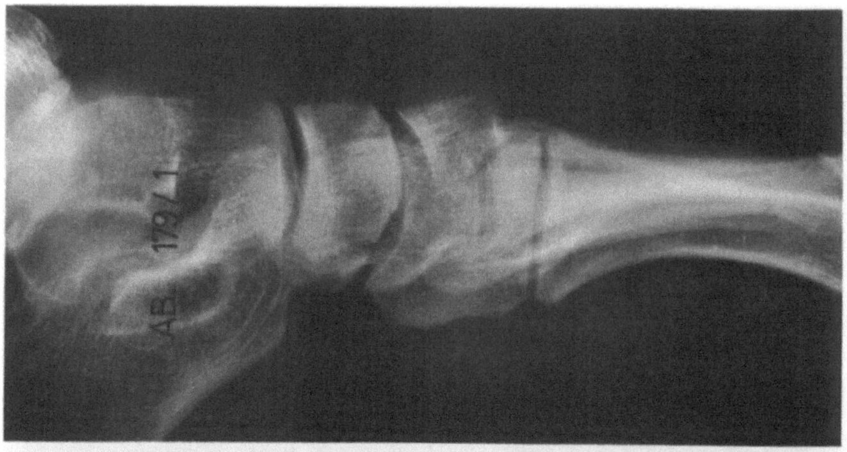

a

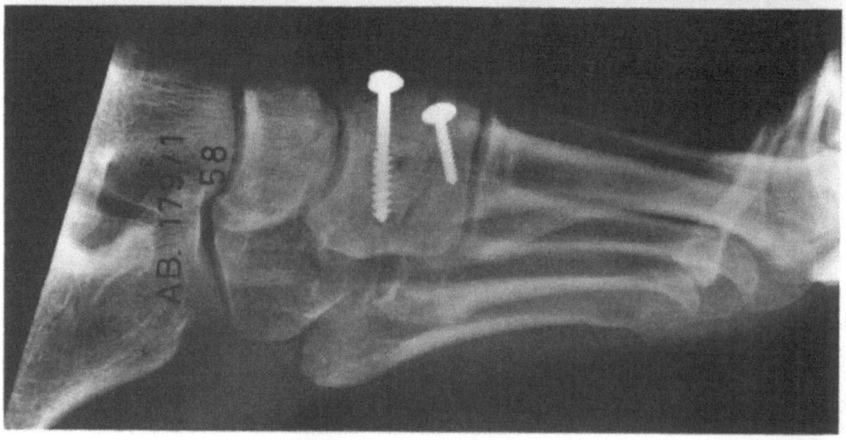

b

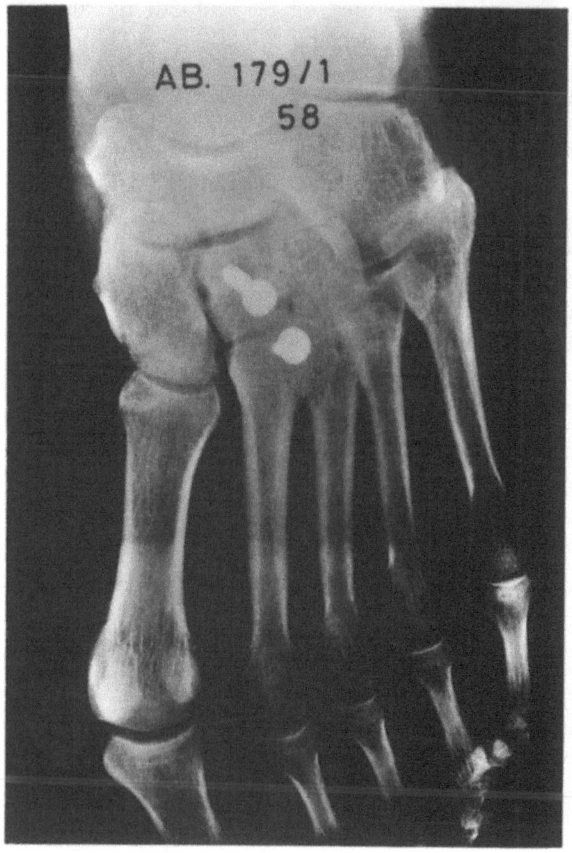

c

Fig. 239 a–c. Clinical example: central fracture-dislocation of the tarsometatarsal joint

Roland D., 49-year-old sales representative, injured in automobile accident (head-on collision) on 9/20/81

a Fracture of the base of the 2nd metatarsal with involvement of the intermediate cuneiform, which shows posterior displacement on the lateral X-ray

b Four days later the cuneiform fracture was fixed with a screw. A second screw was placed in the 2nd metatarsal because of persistent instability. The torn ligaments were sutured
After wound healing, a below-knee cast was worn for 4 weeks. Full weight bearing was started at 7 weeks

c At 1 year the patient had no complaints and a full range of foot motion. X-rays showed mild osteoarthritis. The screws were not removed

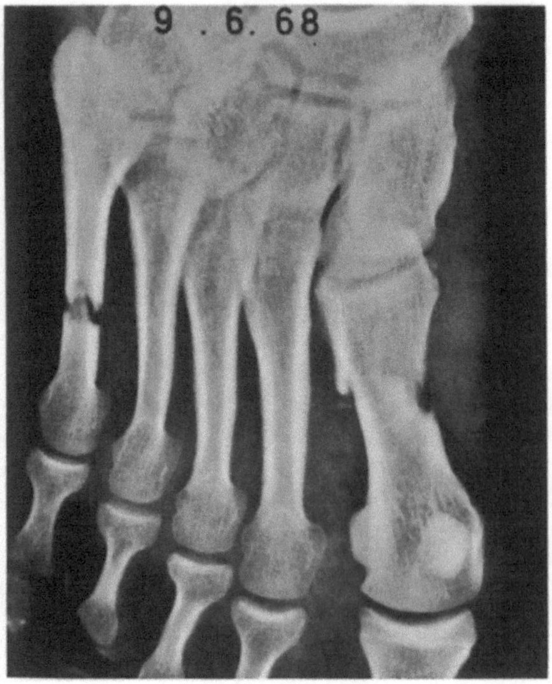

a

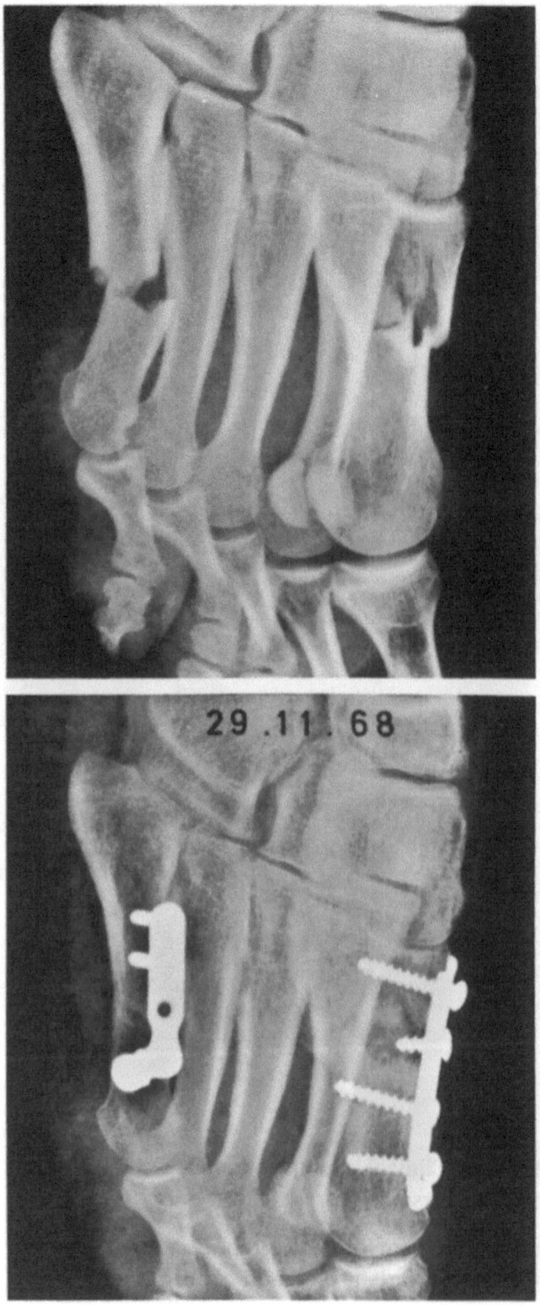

b

Fig. 240a–d. Clinical example: plate fixation of transverse fractures of the first and fifth metatarsals

Michele C., 32-year-old construction worker, caught foot in dredger bucket on 7/8/68

a Transverse fractures of 1st and 5th metatarsals with massive local swelling

b The limb was elevated, and internal fixation was performed at 11 days (7/19/68). The 5th metatarsal was fixed with an L plate, the 1st metatarsal with a one-third tubular plate. The central comminuted area was disregarded. The proximal plate screw was too short, and the second was placed in the comminuted area
There were no postoperative complications, and early exercises were performed without a cast. Patient was bearing full weight at 4 months and was back at work by 6 months

c The implants were removed at 8 months: no complaints, equivalent motion on both sides. X-rays showed primary union of the 5th metatarsal and delayed union of the 1st metatarsal

d When seen 12 years later on 7/12/80, the patient had no complaints and was fully active in his former work. He had full mobility, and no muscular atrophy, and a linear scar. X-rays showed osteoarthritic changes in the 1st tarsometatarsal joint

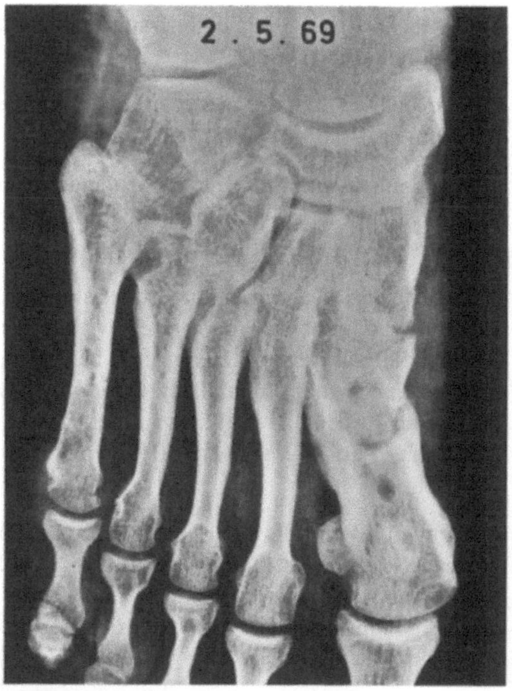

c

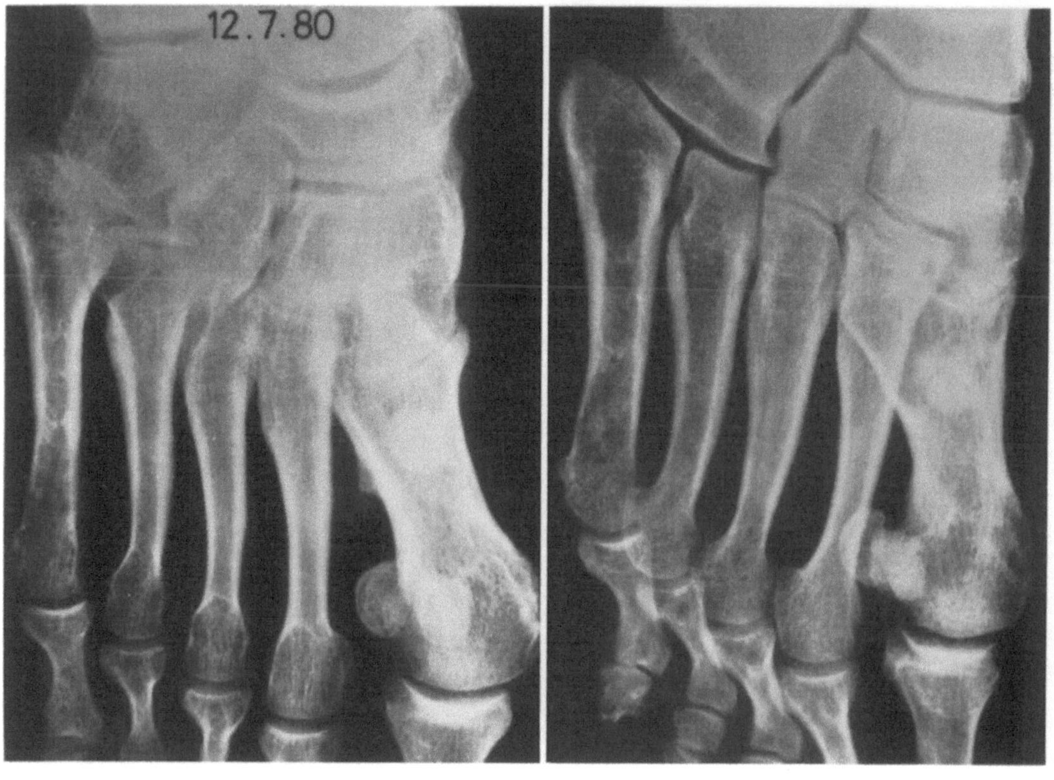

d

Fig. 241 a–c. Clinical example: fracture of the base of the first metatarsal

Domenico M., 28-year-old electrician, injured in a fall from scaffolding

a Proximal, comminuted, intra-articular fracture of the 1st metatarsal, subcapital fracture of the 2nd metatarsal (vassal fracture)

b Two weeks later primary arthrodesis of the 1st tarsometatarsal joint was performed with a one-third tubular plate and cancellous graft. The 2nd metatarsal was fixed with a medullary wire, which was removed at 4 weeks. A walking caliper was worn for 3 months. Patient regained 50% work fitness by 7 months

c X-ray at 13 months shows arthrodesis and fracture union. Treatment was concluded at 15 months. Patient was back at work and had no complaints. There was a 30% limitation of foot extension and inversion

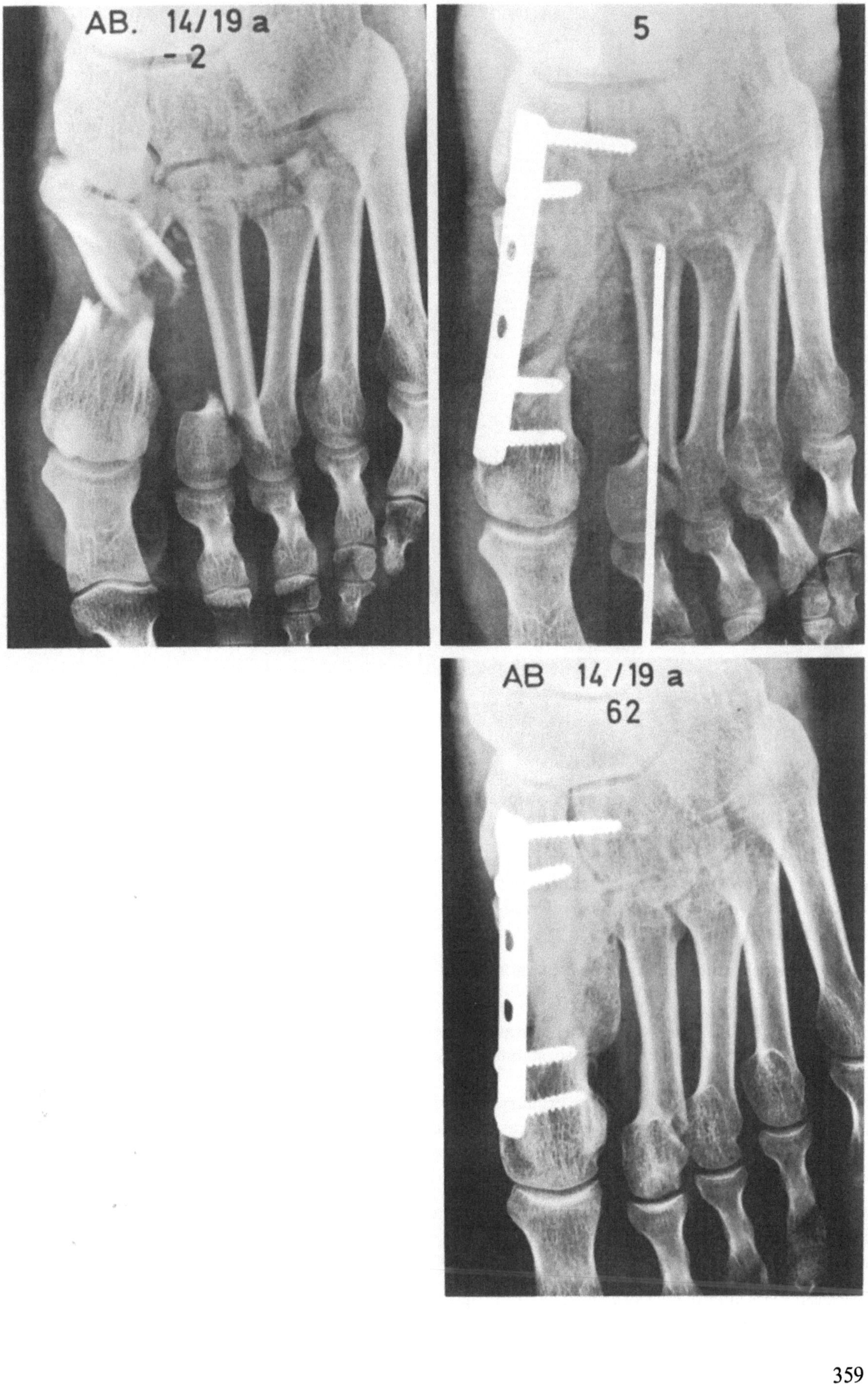

a b c

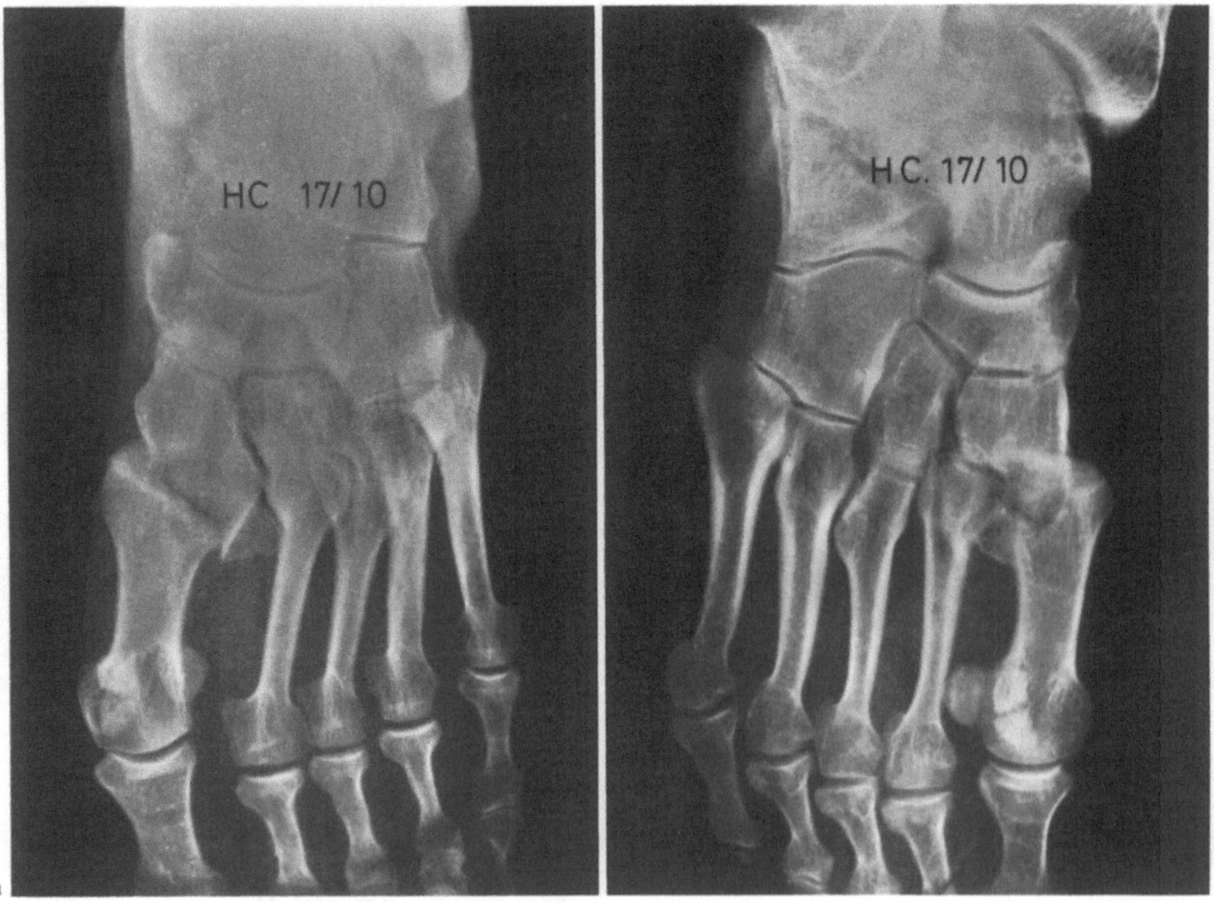

a

Fig. 242 a–d. Clinical example: fracture-dislocation of the base of the first metatarsal

Hermine H., 60-year-old factory worker, injured in a fall at work on 10/8/73. Injury was treated conservatively by the family doctor, who referred the patient for hospitalization at 6 days

a Fracture-dislocation of the base of the 1st metatarsal

b On 10/20/73 the base of the 1st metatarsal was fixed with a radius T plate that also stabilized the navicular
No complications arose, and after primary wound healing the patient was discharged with a walking cast because of a neurologic disease unrelated to the injury. The implants were removed at 7 months

c Union was confirmed at 13 months. The patient had minimal complaints, linear scars, and mild osteoarthritis

d Eleven years later there was no evidence of progression of the osteoarthritis

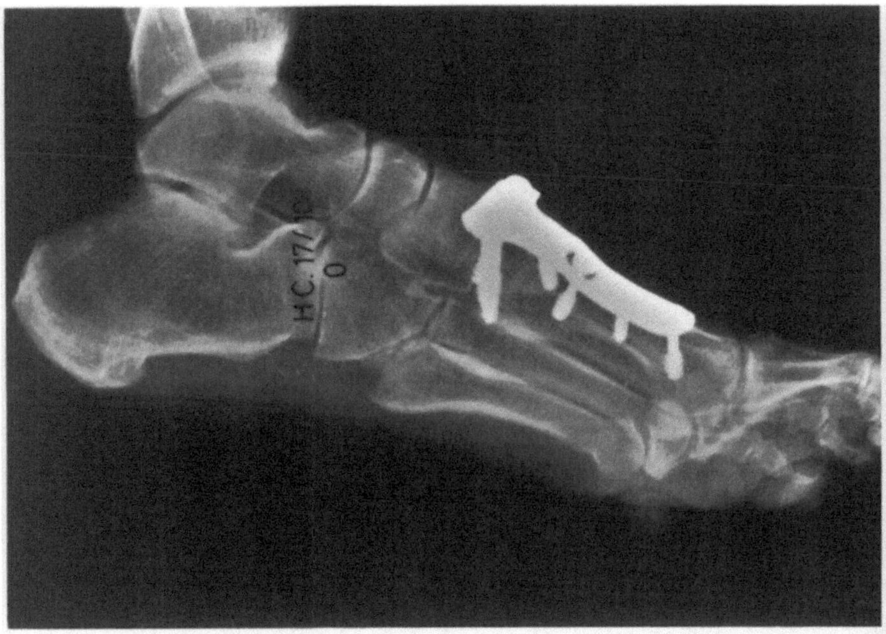

b

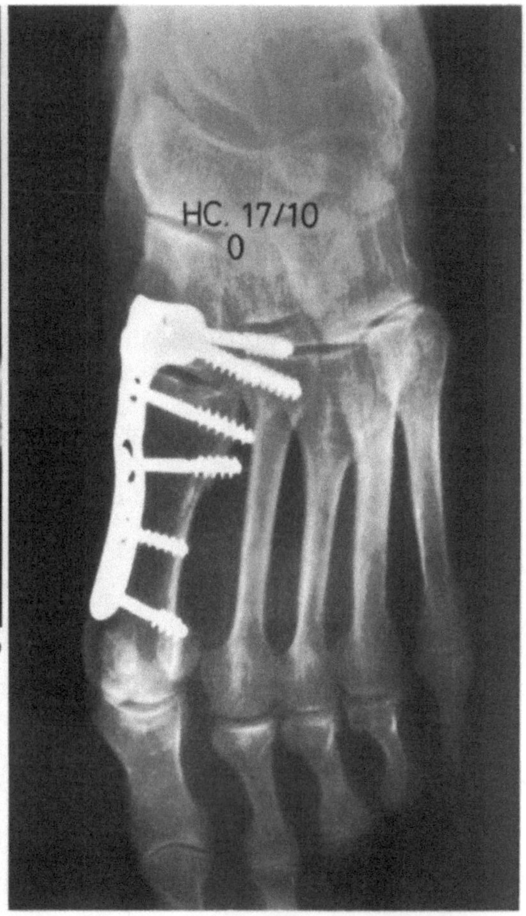

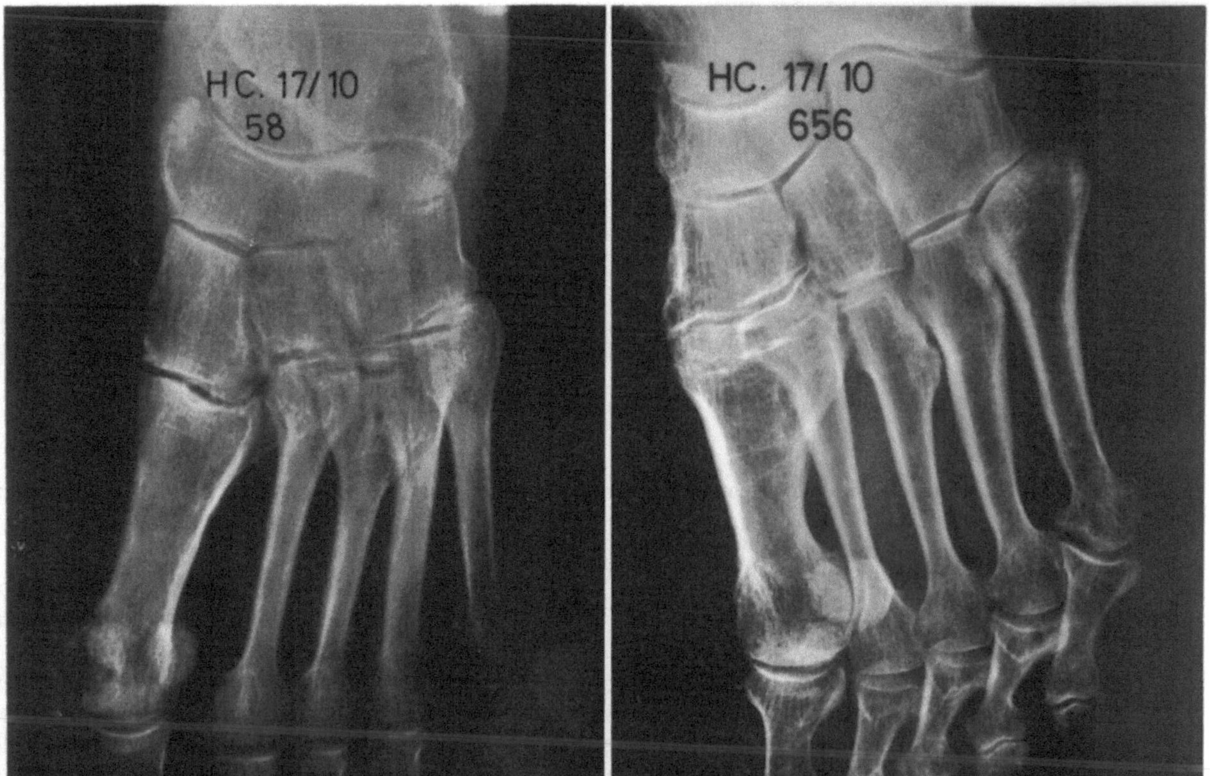

c, d

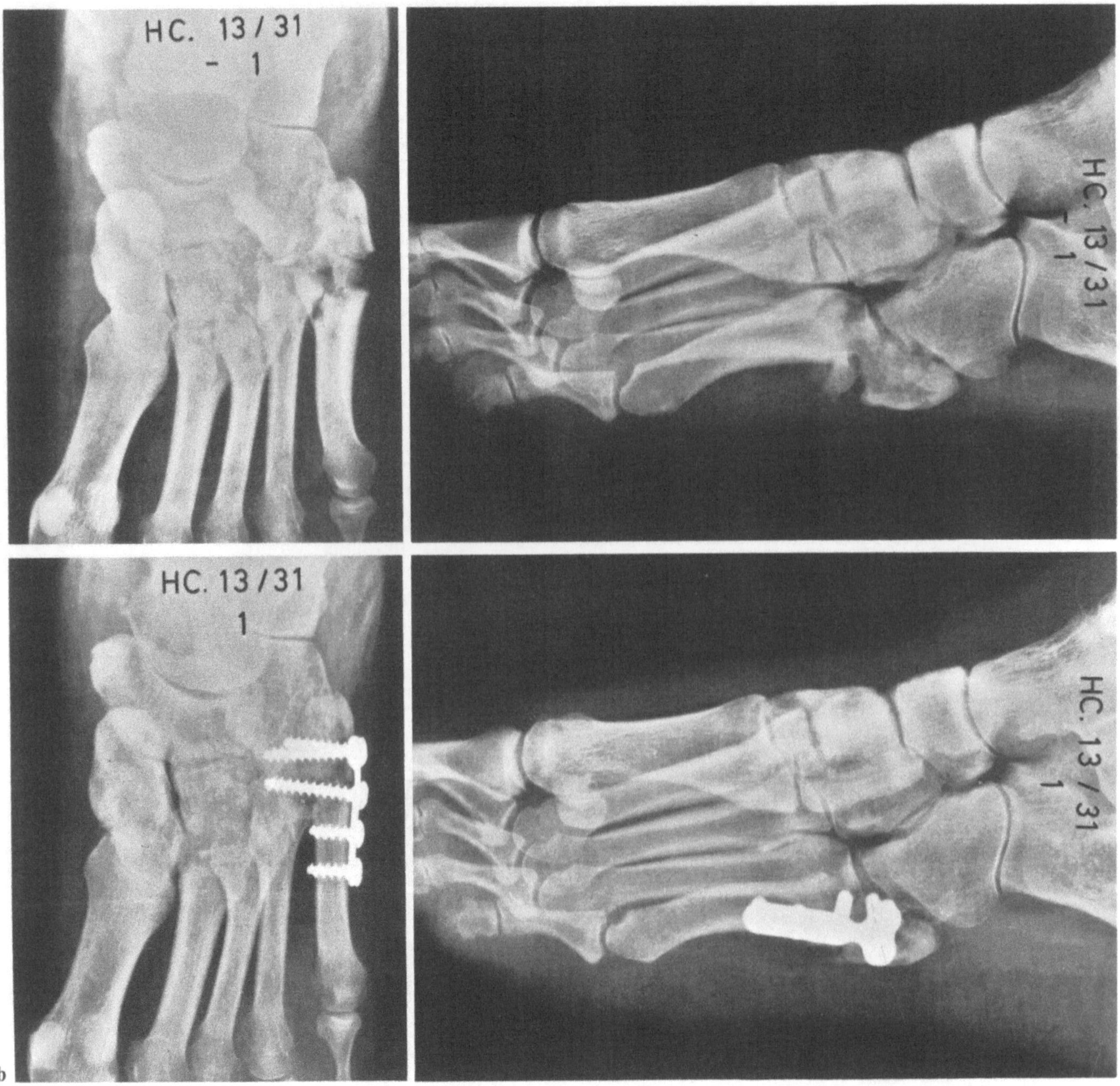

a

b

Fig. 243 a–d. Clinical example: secondary internal fixation of a comminuted fracture of the base of the fifth metatarsal

Agnes P., 53-year-old factory worker, caught left foot between forklift and wall on 1/4/73. Massive skin contusion

a Comminuted fracture of the base of the 5th metatarsal. Patient was treated at home with elevation and a plaster splint, and antibiotics were given for the skin wound. After 19 days she was hospitalized; closed reduction was unsuccessful

b Internal fixation was performed 5 weeks postinjury on 2/7/73 using a small T plate and iliac cancellous graft. Functional exercises were performed without a cast, and primary wound healing was achieved. Patient was discharged with a removable plaster splint, replaced with a walking cast at 7 weeks. Full weight bearing was possible at 18 weeks. Patient was fully rehabilitated for work at 34 weeks

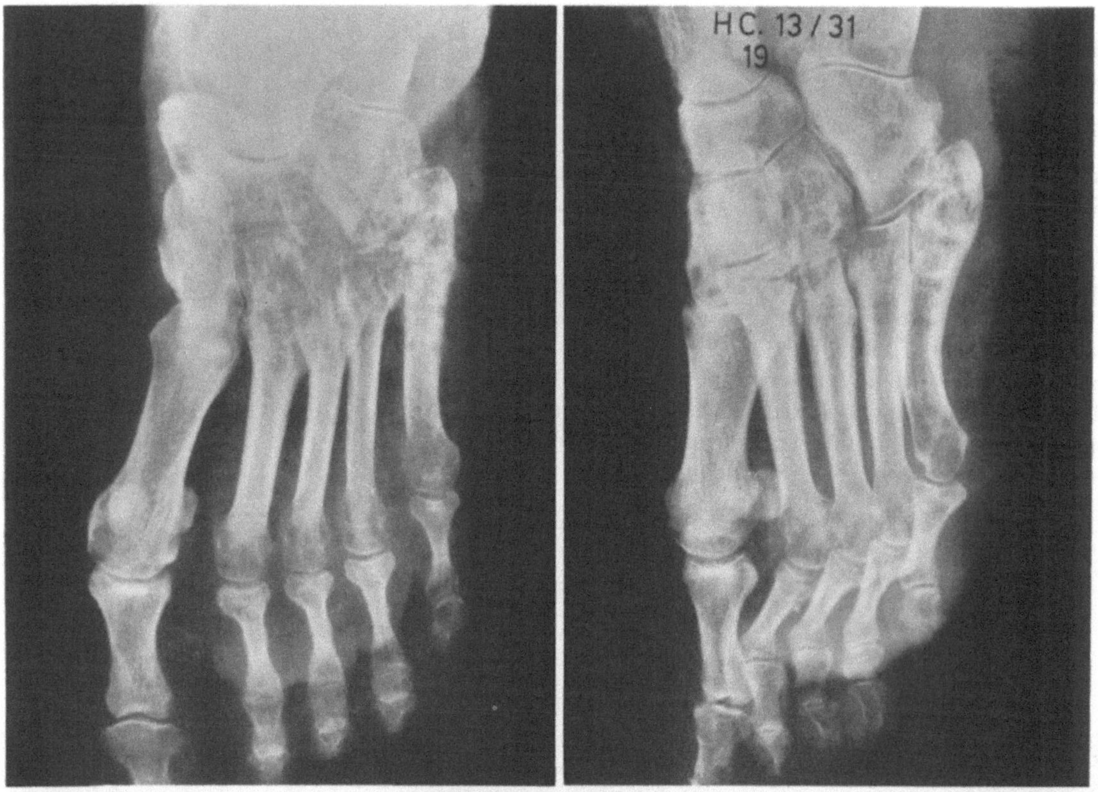

c

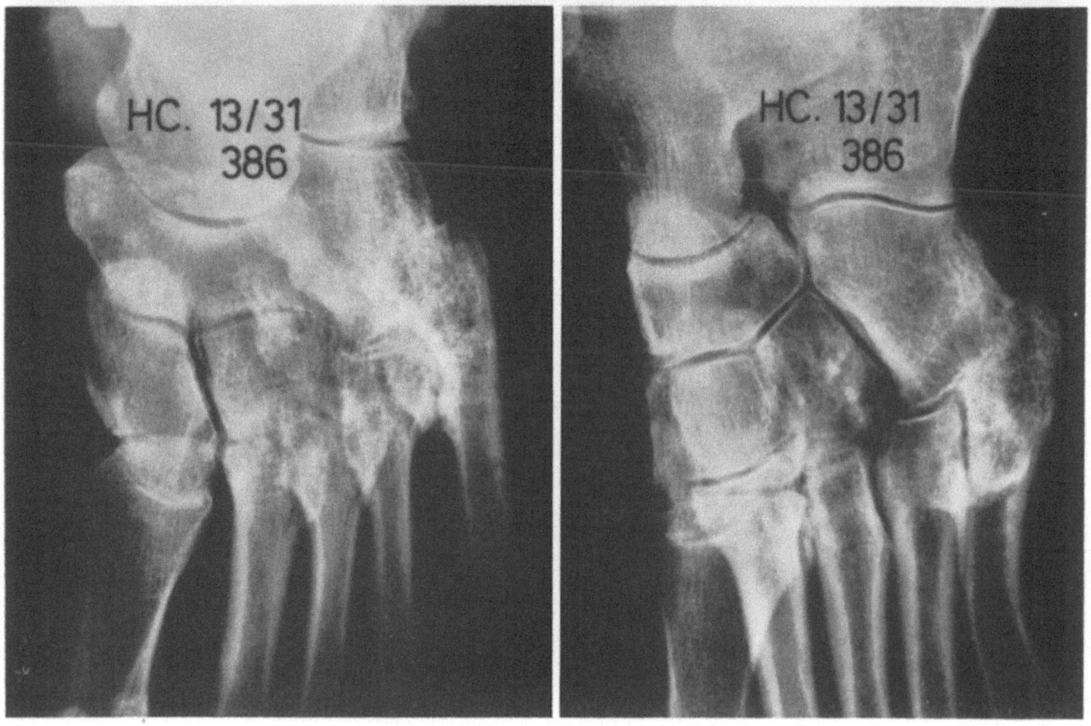

d

c The implants were removed at $4^1/_2$ months

d When seen at $7^1/_2$ years on 7/5/80, the patient had no complaints and was vocationally sound. She had normal ambulatory capacity, no muscular atrophy, and a linear scar. Ankylosis of the lateral tarsometatarsal joint was apparent

Fig. 244a–c. Clinical example: spiral fracture of the fifth metatarsal

Diane v.d.M., 39-year-old secretary, caught right small toe in a fall on stairs

a Very unstable spiral fracture of the shaft of the 5th metatarsal with a small area of proximal comminution

b Internal fixation was performed at 4 days with a mini screw and a quarter tubular plate placed toward the plantar side of the bone. Cancellous grafts from the distal tibial metaphysis were applied
The limb was not put in plaster, and heel-to-toe rocking exercises were initiated. Patient returned to work at 4 weeks and was bearing full weight at 7 weeks

c X-ray at 31 weeks after removal of the implants. The cancellous graft is now clearly visible.

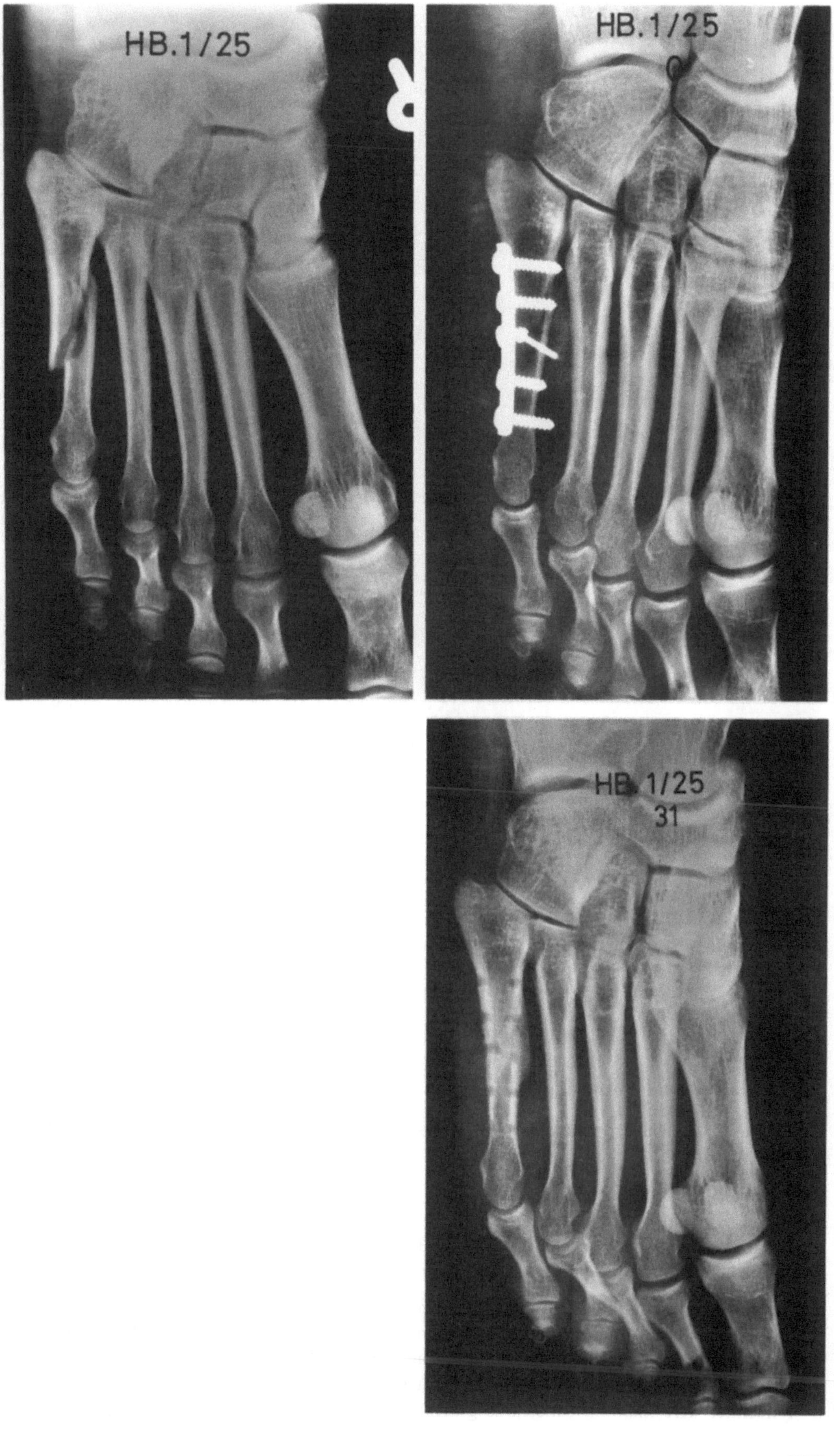

a b c

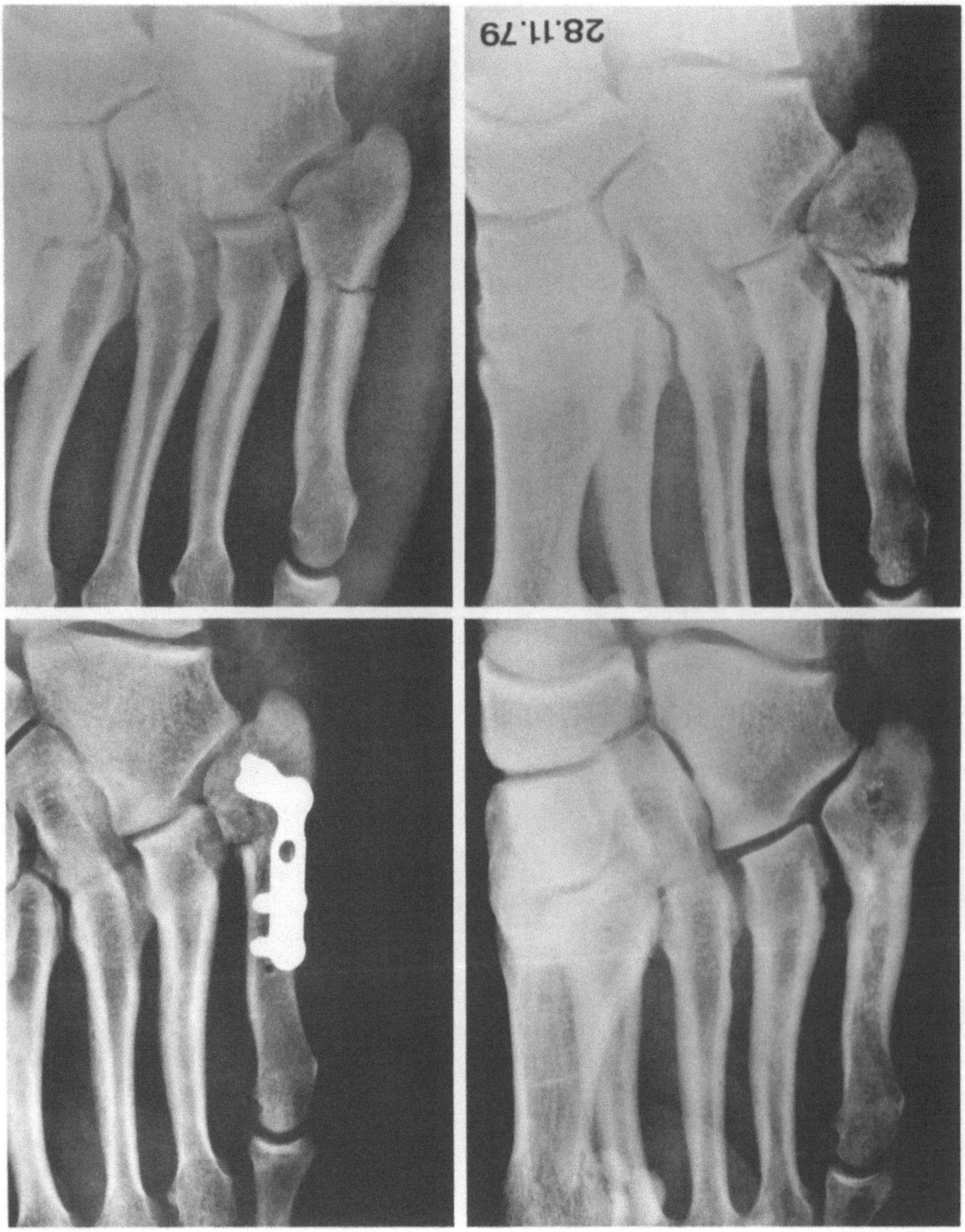

a b c d

Fig. 245 a–h. Clinical example: bilateral stress fractures of the proximal shaft of the fifth metatarsal (Jones fracture)

Refractures, treatment, course
Georg A., 19-year-old unatheletic patient, sprained the *left* foot while playing soccer on 12/19/78. Patient had prior history of mild load-dependent pain

a Undisplaced transverse fracture of the proximal 5th metatarsal (Jones fracture) united in $3^1/_2$ months with conservative treatment. The bone refractured 7 weeks later in a skiing accident and was treated by Kirschner-wire fixation, cancellous grafting, and cast immobilization. The fracture became clinically and radiologically solid (not documented)

b Twelve months after the initial injury, a second refracture was diagnosed following a mild sprain

c The fracture was fixed with an L plate and grafted with cancellous chips. It consolidated, and the plate was removed at 15 months

d When seen on 1/20/83, $3^1/_4$ years after the second refracture, the patient had no complaints

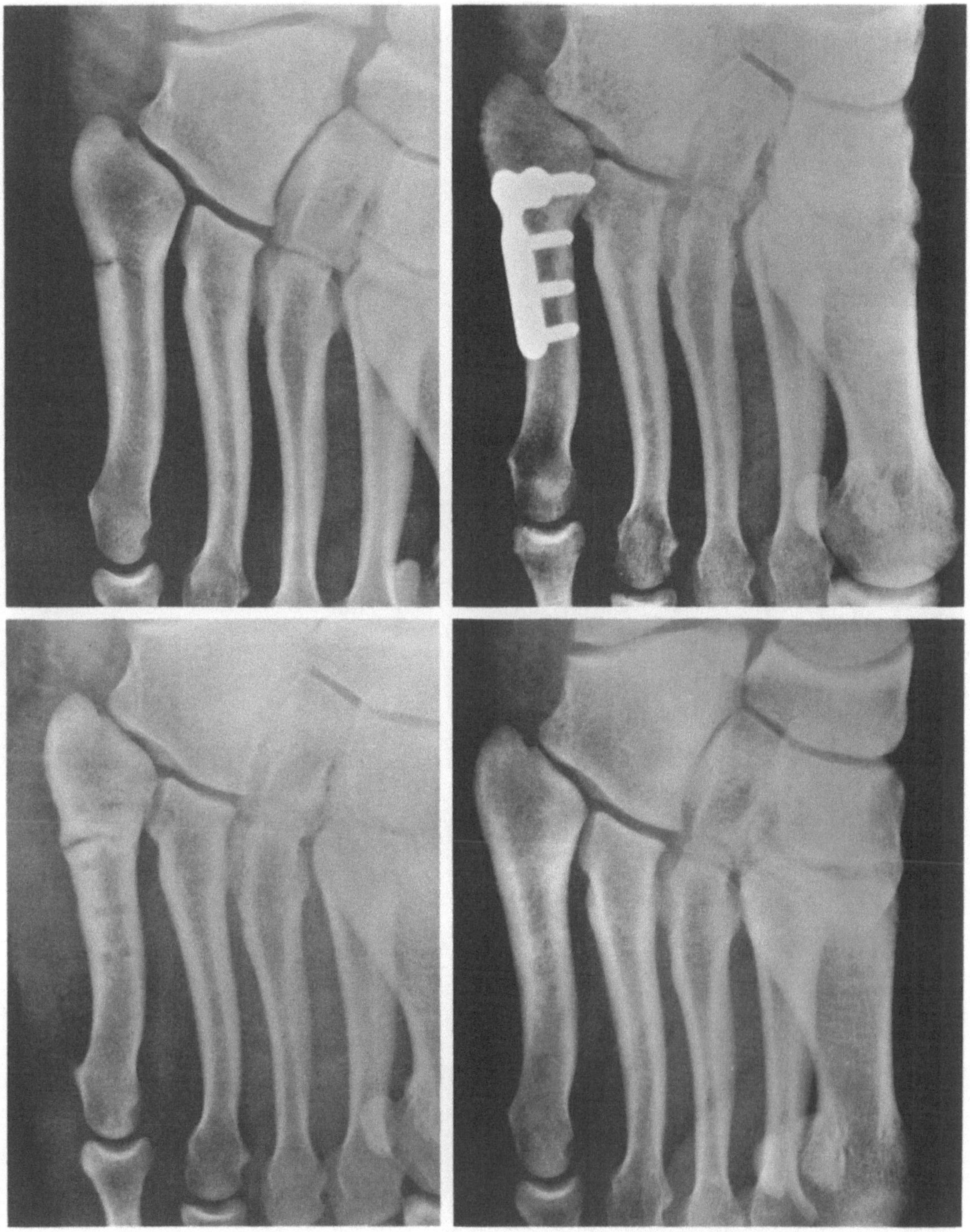

e f

g h

e Patient sprained his *right* foot during gymnastic exercises on 6/28/80, $1^1/_2$ years after injuring the *left* foot, sustaining a mirror-image Jones fracture on the right side. Primary internal fixation with cancellous grafting was performed

f Seven weeks after internal fixation, the fracture was united. The plate was removed at 9 months

g Refracture occurred 1 month after plate removal. The patient declined reoperation, and the foot was placed in a walking cast for 2 months

h When seen on 1/20/83, $1^3/_4$ years after the first refracture, the patient had no complaints, and all fractures were solid (Radiographs courtesy of Dr. H.P. Kundert, Zurich)

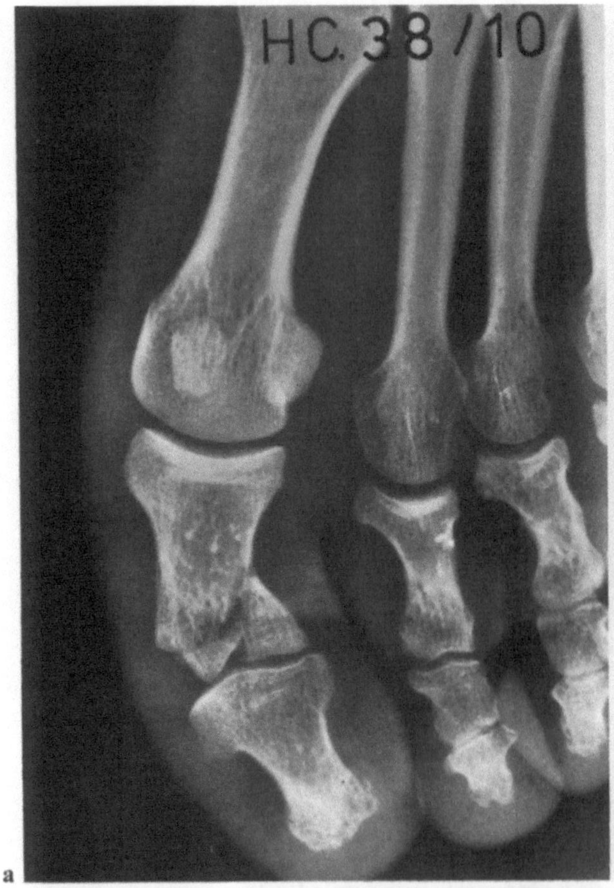

a

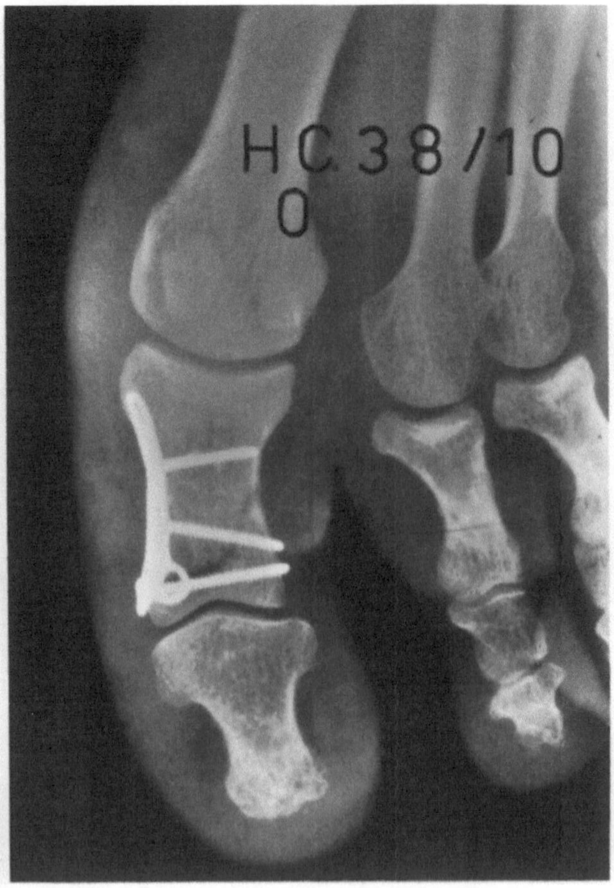

b

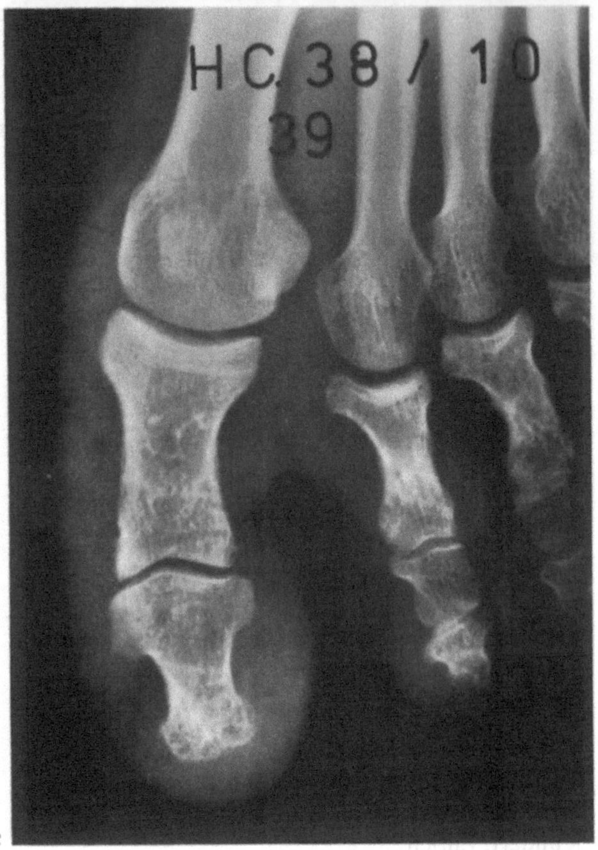

c

Fig. 246a–c. Clinical example: bicondylar fracture of the proximal phalanx of the big toe

Esther M., 27-year-old unskilled worker, fell on stairs on 7/28/77

a Bicondylar fracture of the proximal phalanx of the left big toe, moderate local swelling

b Internal fixation with a mini T plate the next day The postoperative course was uncomplicated, and functional exercises were performed. Patient was discharged with a walking cast, which was removed at 6 weeks for full weight bearing. Full rehabilitation was achieved by 10 weeks

c On follow-up and implant removal at 9 months, the patient had no complaints. Motion of the distal phalanx of the big toe was markedly restricted. X-rays confirmed fracture union and absence of osteoarthritic disease

Fig. 247 a–d. Clinical example: nonunion of the base of the fifth metatarsal

Santolo A., 36-year-old construction worker, struck the lateral side of the foot on a stone. He did not seek treatment despite constant, moderate pain

a Nonunion of the base of the fifth metatarsal was diagnosed at 8 months

b The site was compressed with a small cancellous screw and without a bone graft
A circular cast was worn for 3 months, and the nonunion became solid

c At 10 months the patient had full function and mild weather-dependent complaints. The nonunion was consolidated

d The screw was removed at 17 months (the threaded part broke off and was left behind). The patient left the country and was lost to further follow-up

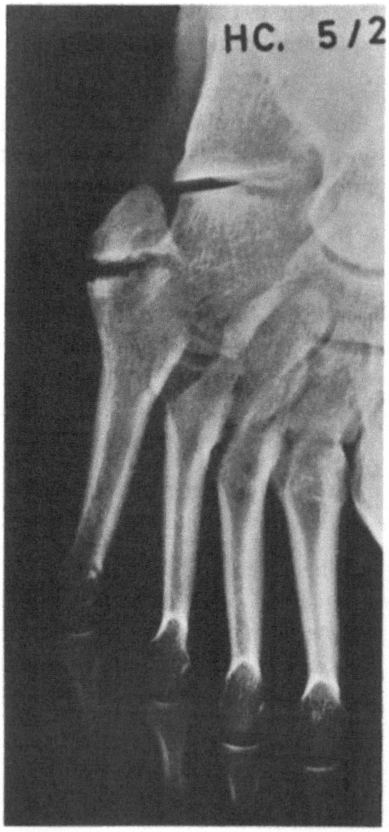

a

c

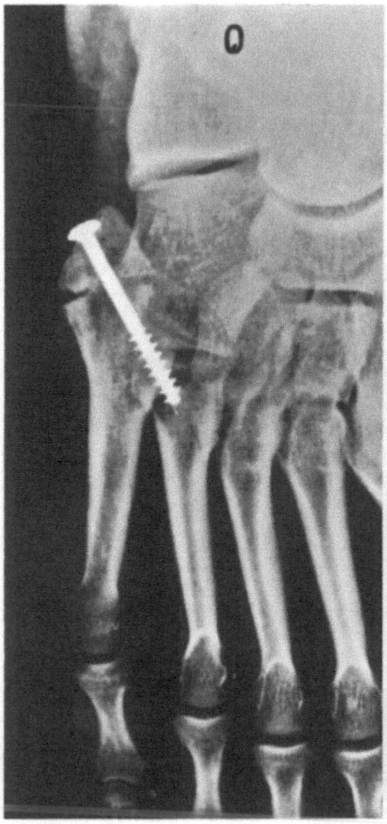

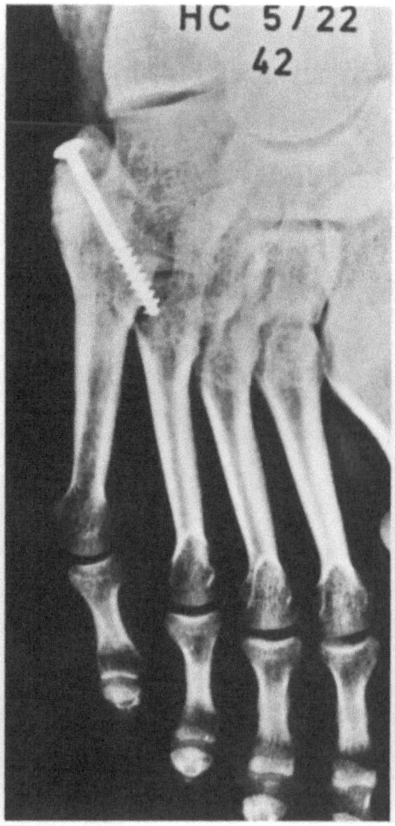

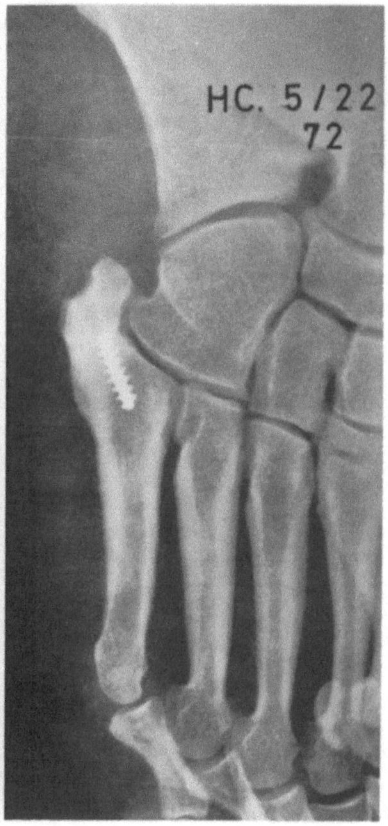

d

Fig. 248 a–d. Clinical example: delayed union of a distal fracture of the fifth metatarsal

Dante S., 47-year-old interior decorator, fell from a ladder on 7/29/70, sustaining a minimally displaced spiral fracture of the neck of the 5th metatarsal. The limb was placed in a walking cast

a By 8 weeks the fracture had not united, and there was increasing peripheral osteoporosis

b Internal fixation was performed on 9/23/70 using an autogenous iliac corticocancellous dowel graft stabilized with a small L plate and screws. Full weight bearing was commenced at 12 weeks. The implants were removed at 5 months

c At 9 months the patient had no complaints and full function. Moderate osteoporosis was still present

d When seen a decade later on 7/14/80, the patient complained of slight localized pain, most likely due to intervening primary chronic rheumatoid arthritis. Patient had full function, no muscular atrophy, and normal X-rays

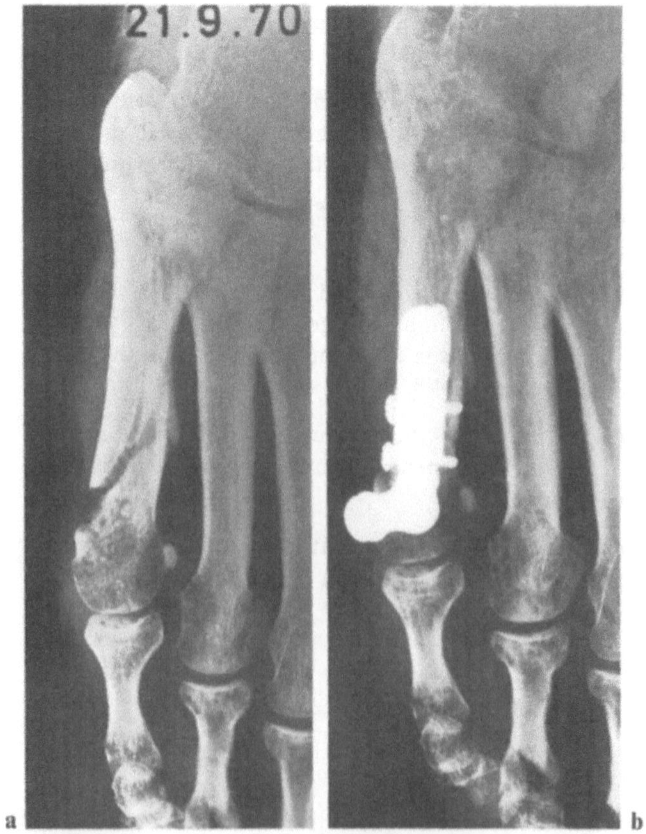

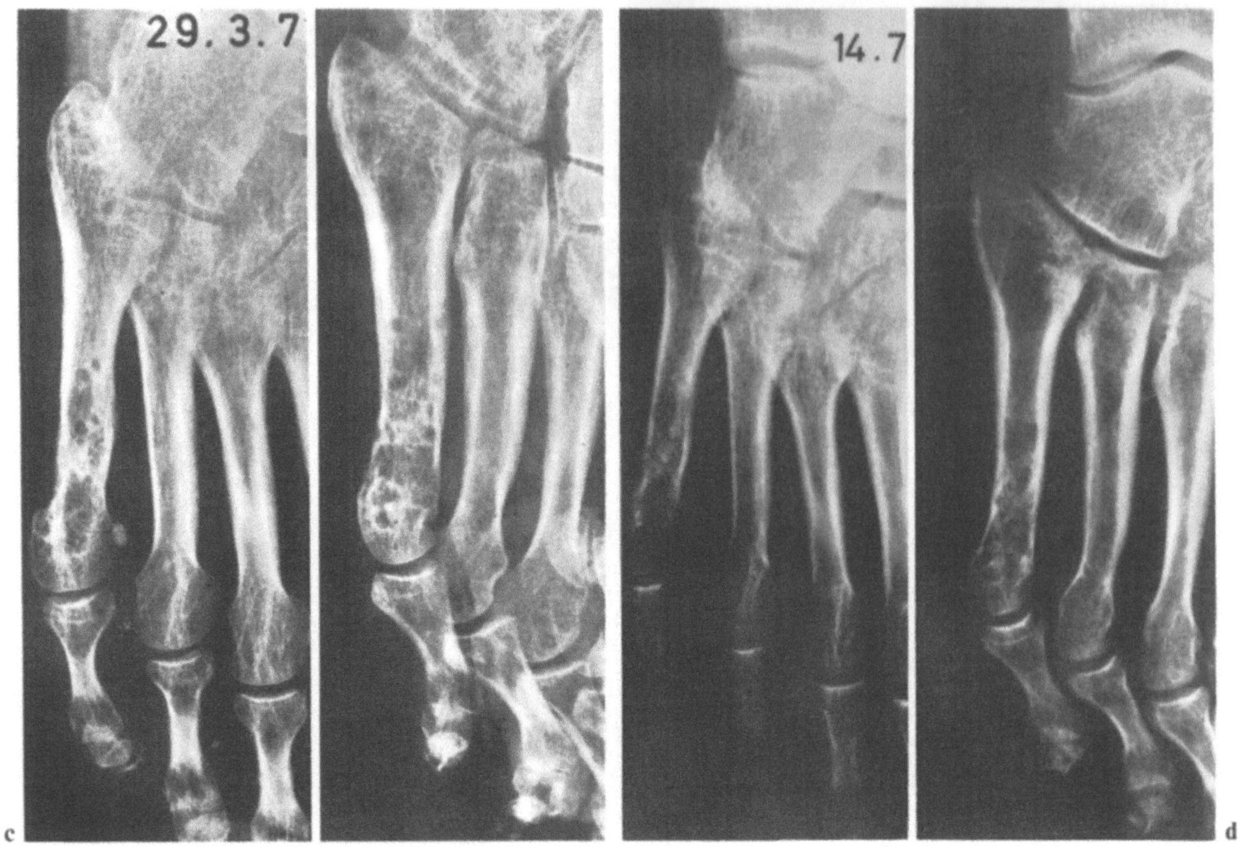

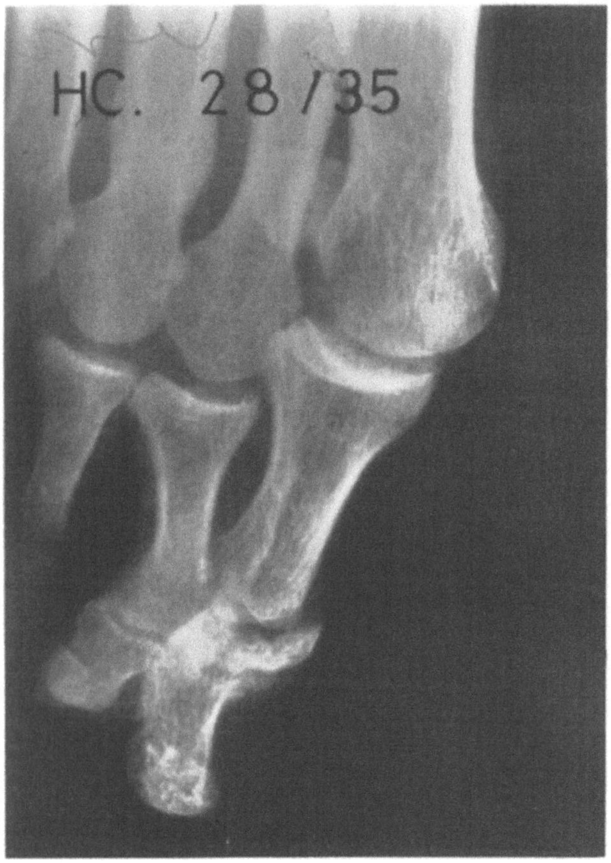

a

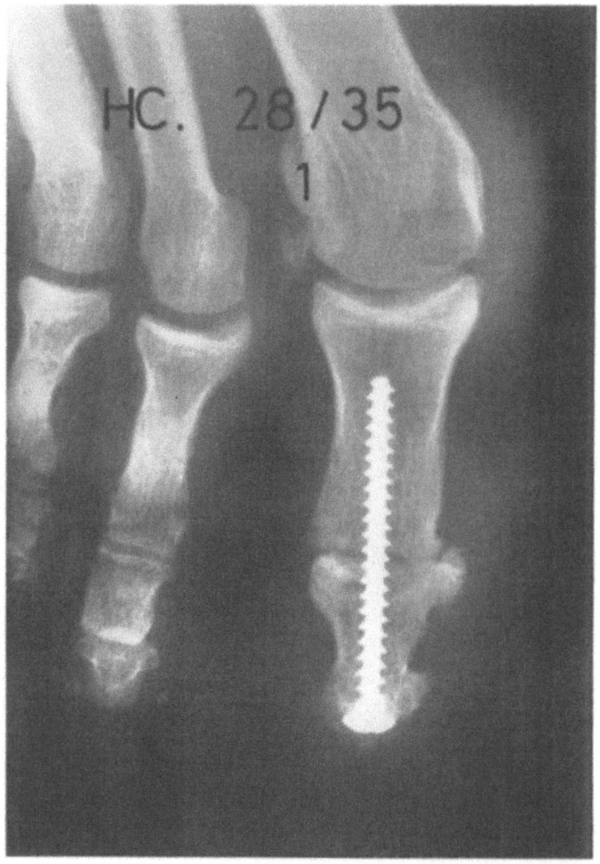

b

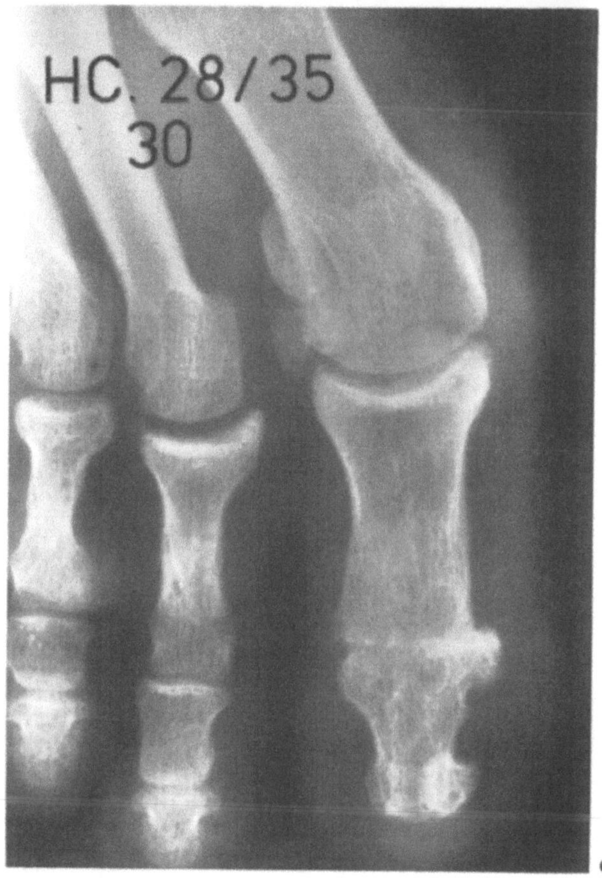

c

Fig. 249 a–c. Clinical example: screw arthrodesis of the interphalangeal joint of the big toe

Jose Juis D., 27-year-old construction worker, sustained impacted intra-articular fracture of the distal phalanx of the right big toe and a fracture of the 3rd metatarsal shaft while playing soccer in July, 1975. The interphalangeal joint of the big toe was painful

a Traumatic arthritis of the interphalangeal joint of the big toe

b Standard retrograde arthrodesis of the joint was performed on 10/31/75 with a 3.5-mm cortex screw The course was umcomplicated, primary wound healing was achieved, and functional exercises were performed. Patient was fully rehabilitated by 8 weeks

c The screw was removed at 7 months; the arthrodesis was solid

XVIII. Special Indications

Besides the classic and less frequent indications for use of the SFS, there are two areas of application that merit special discussion: 1) internal fixations in children and 2) rheumatoid surgery, which has assumed growing importance in recent years.

1. Internal Fixations in Children

The indications for internal fixations in the pediatric skeleton are rare and include open fractures, certain irreducible or unstable shaft fractures, and ligamentous avulsion fractures, which include epicondylar avulsions. The foremost indications, however, are epiphyseal plate fractures and traumatic separations of the epiphysis (Figs. 252–258).

Because the danger of post-traumatic ankylosis in children is negligible, external fixation may be used without concern, and internal fixation assumes more the character of an accurate open reduction. Nevertheless, it is still important to consider the biomechanical relationship between the implant and the bone. Of course, the small implants of the SFS are ideally suited for use in children. The plates most commonly used are the one-third tubular plates for the forearm and tibia. Lately the DCP for 3.5-mm screws is also being used with greater frequency in pediatric patients. Growth disturbance is avoided by making sure that the screws do not violate epiphyseal and apophyseal lines. Also, screws are frequently used with washers so that the screw heads will not sink into the cortical bone, which is still quite soft in children.

Because callus masses tend to form quickly around metallic implants in children, it is advisable to remove the implants early, as this may be very difficult later on. Another problem is the tendency of transverse fractures in children to stimulate longitudinal growth–a tendency that is enhanced by internal fixation.This could well influence patient selection for internal fixations of the lower extremity in the pediatric group.

2. Use of the SFS in Rheumatoid Surgery

The main role of metallic implants in rheumatoid surgery is for arthrodesis, following the techniques described in the General Section. The brittle and delicate bones of the rheumatoid patient frequently require the use of special, thin implants. On the other hand, the risk of infection in these patients is quite low, even after prolonged cortisone therapy, and scar formation is remarkably good. As in the pediatric skeleton, the SFS offers various means of stabilization with little or no external support–a circumstance that reduces discomfort and allows for rapid functional loading.

3. Illustrative Case Reports and X-Rays

(Figs. 253–258)

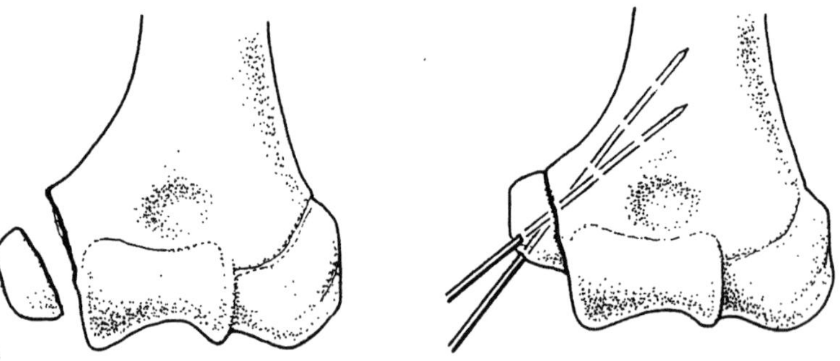

a

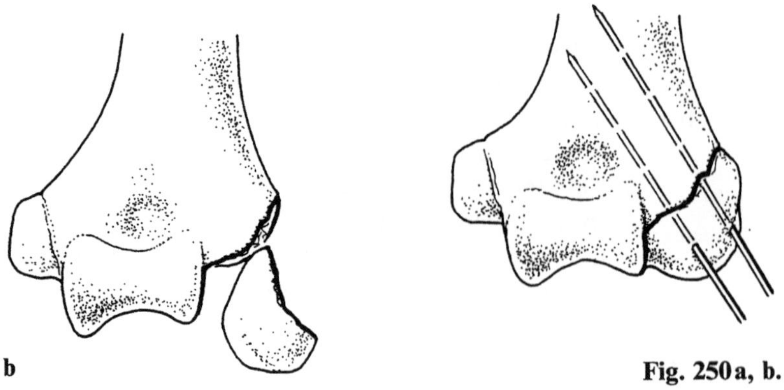

b

Fig. 250a, b. Internal fixation of pediatric elbow fractures

a Condylar and epicondylar fractures are fixed with Kirschner wires. The ulnar nerve is exposed and protected

b An irreducible radial neck fracture in children may be fixed with Kirschner wires drilled in obliquely from the distal side. This must be reinforced with external plaster. The wires may be removed at 4 weeks

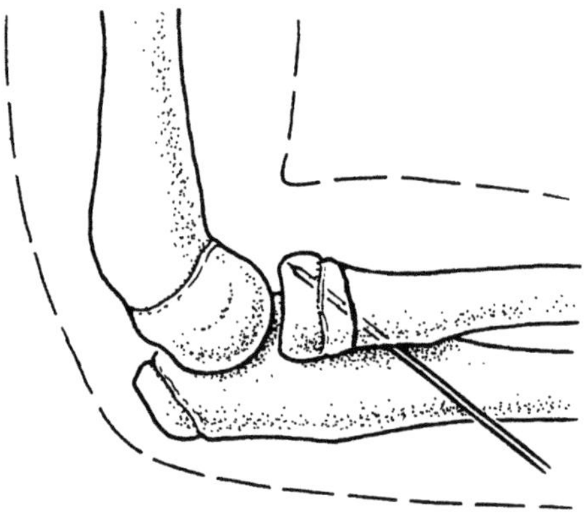

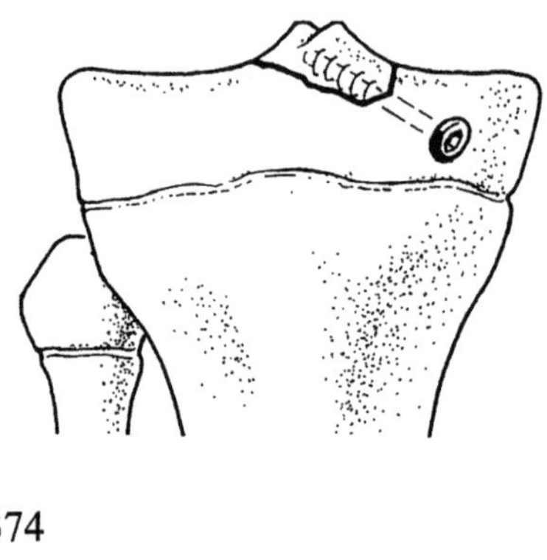

Fig. 251. Avulsion of the intercondylar eminence in children. The fixation screw does not cross the epihyseal growth plate

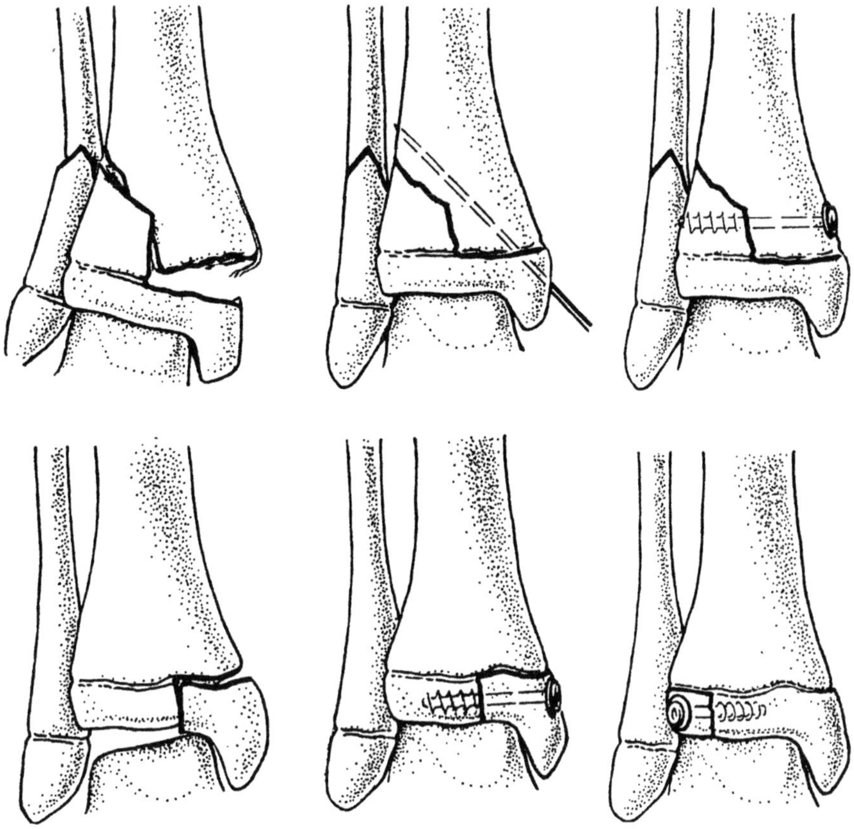

Fig. 252. Internal fixation of injuries of the distal tibial epiphysis

Examples fo screw fixations of epiphyseal injuries as alternatives to open reduction and fixation with Kirschner wires

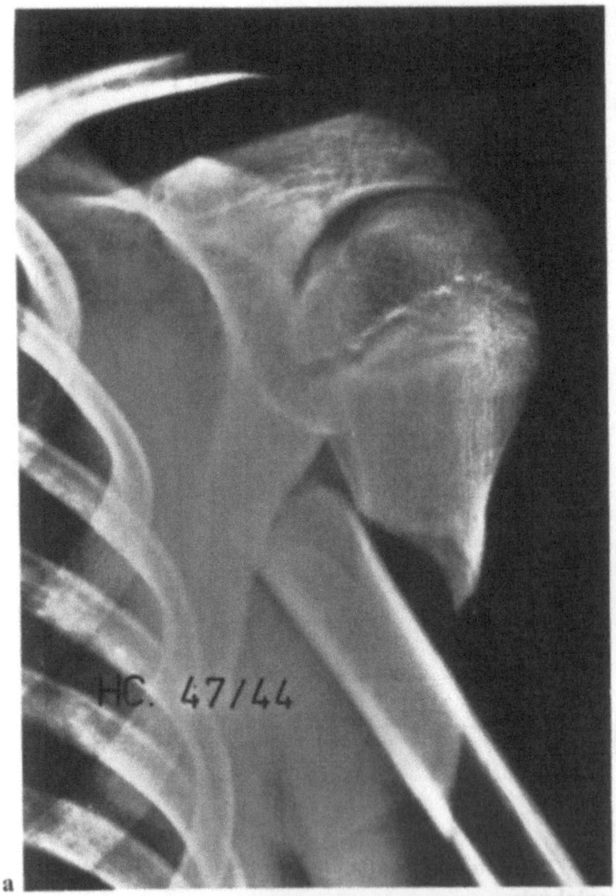

a

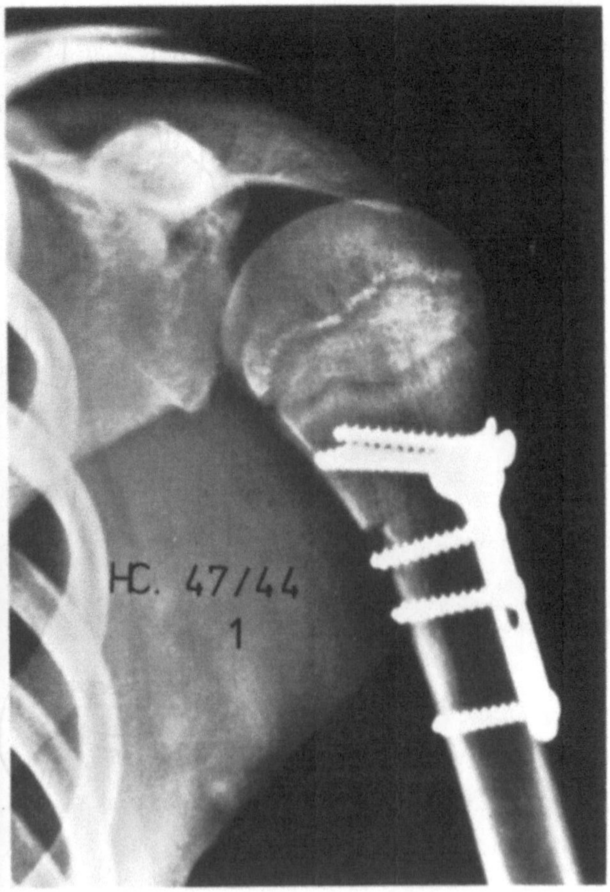

b

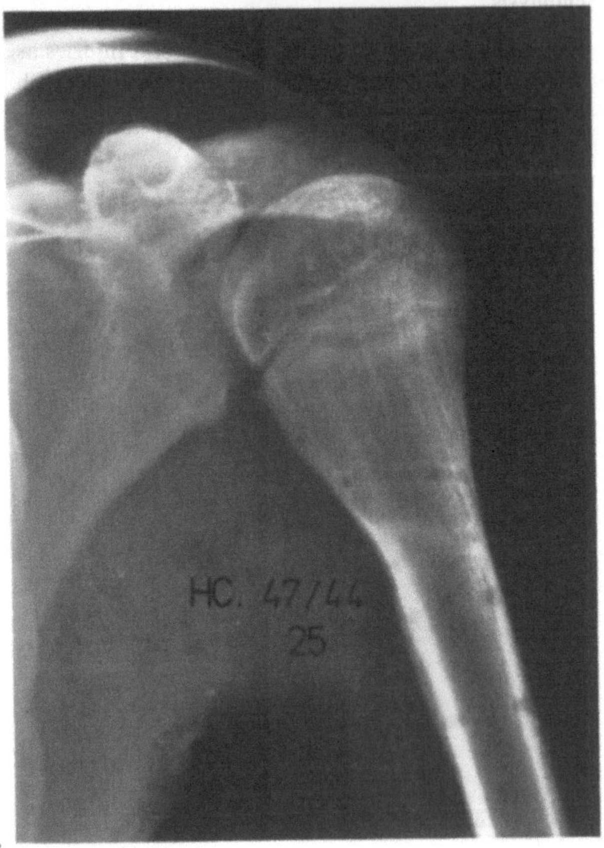

c

Fig. 253 a–c. Clinical example: unstable fracture of the proximal humerus in a child

Werner F., 14-year-old schoolboy, fell while skiing on 4/21/79

a Very unstable and markedly displaced fracture of the proximal humeral shaft. The interposed biceps tendon precluded a closed reduction

b Internal fixation with a small T plate was performed on 4/24/79. No complications arose, and the arm was mobilized. Full use was regained at 6 weeks

c On follow-up and implant removal at 6 months, the patient had no complaints, full function, and no muscular atrophy

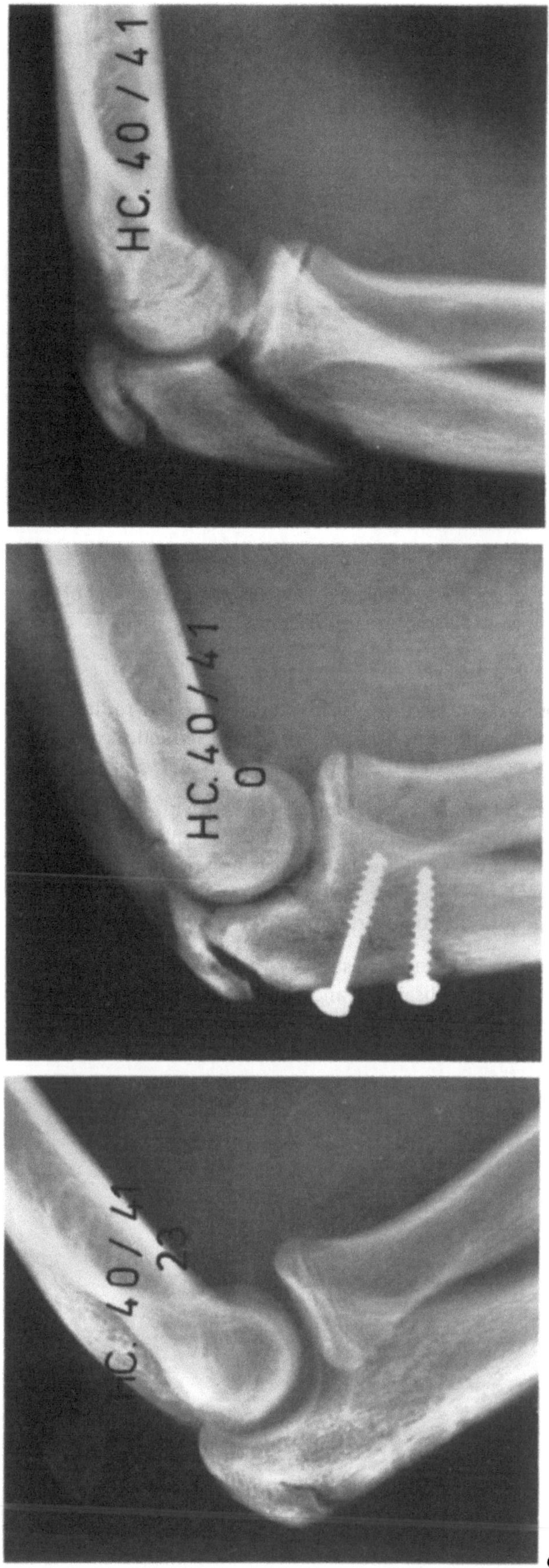

a

b

c

Fig. 254 a–c. Clinical example: screw fixation of a pediatric oblique olecranon fracture

Bernhard J., 15-year-old schoolboy, injured in collision while skiing

a Displaced oblique olecranon fracture outside the epiphyseal line

b Emergency internal fixation was performed with two screws and washers
After an uncomplicated course, the patient was discharged with a circular cast worn for 4 weeks. Full use was regained at 6 weeks

c The screws were removed at 5 months. Patient had no complaints, full function, and linear scars. The fracture was solid

a

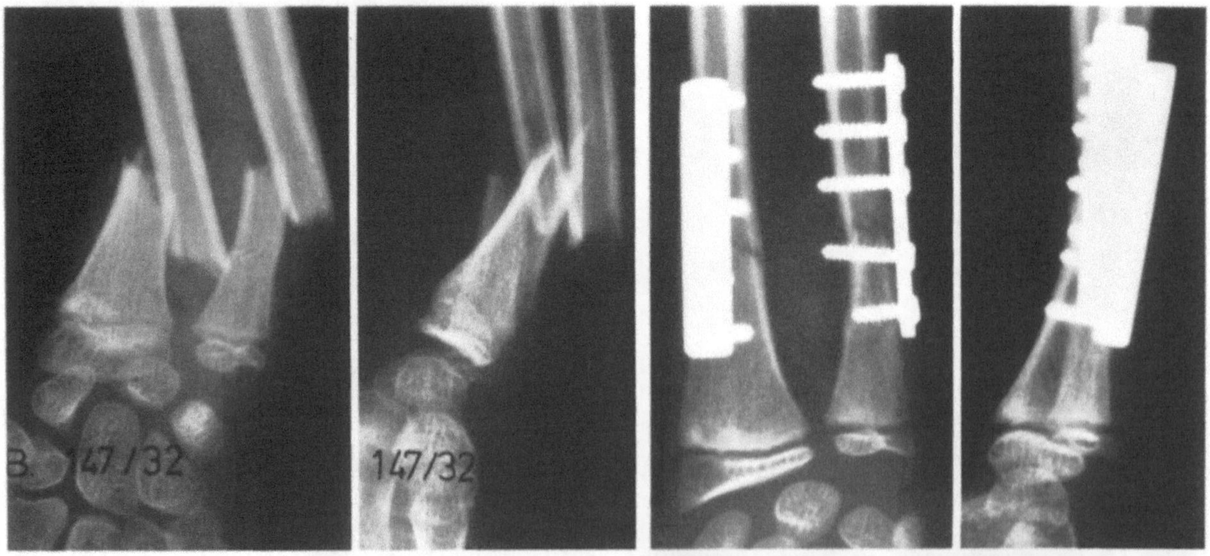

b

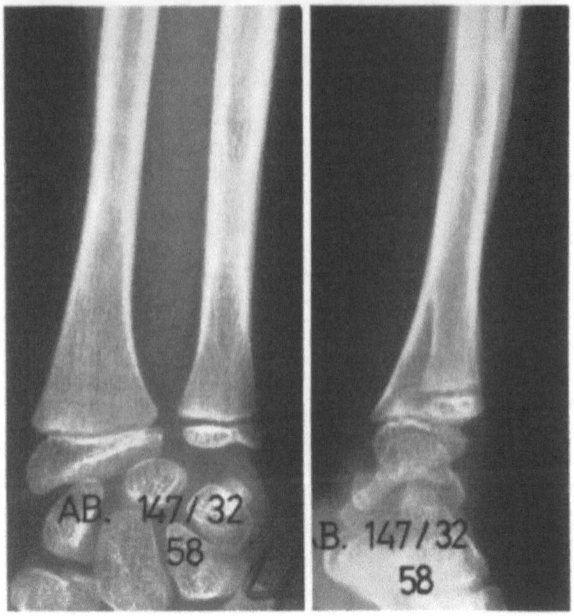

c

Fig. 255a–c. Clinical example: plate fixation of an open pediatric forearm fracture

B.G., 10-year-old schoolboy

a Fractures of the distal third of the left radius and ulna with skin perforation. Closed reduction was unsuccessful due to interposed soft tissue

b Internal fixation was performed with two 2.7-mm DCPs. A removable plaster wrist splint was worn for 4 weeks. Patient resumed apparatus gynmastics at 2 months. The plates were removed at 4 months as an outpatient procedure

c At 13 months postinjury the patient had no complaints or disability and equivalent strength and motion in both arms. There was no length discrepancy in the forearms

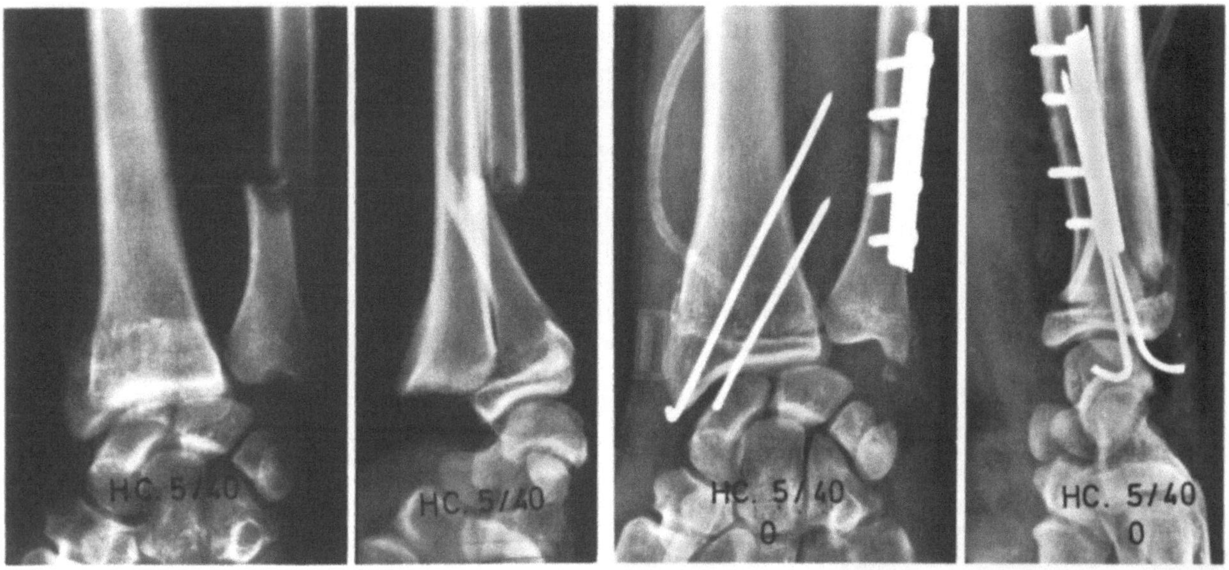

a b

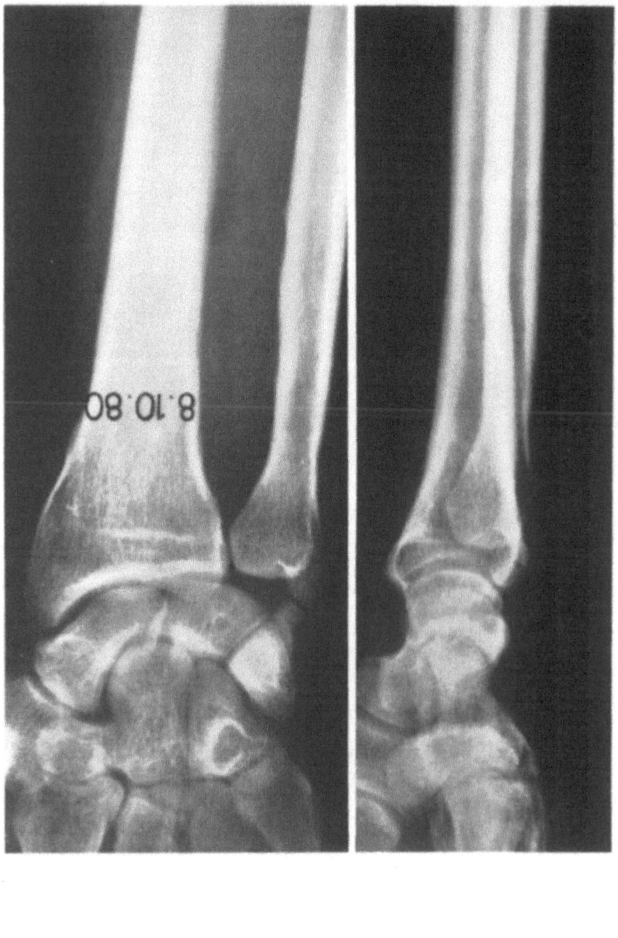

c

Fig. 256a–c. Clinical example: displaced fracture-separation of the distal radial epiphysis

Hansjorg B., 16-year-old schoolboy, fell from a fence onto the left hand on 8/18/71

a Aitken type I fracture-separation of the distal radial epiphysis with a fracture of the distal ulnar shaft. Closed reduction was unsuccessful

b At emergency operation the radius was openly reduced and stabilized with two parallel Kirschner wires; the ulna was fixed with a one-third tubular plate
Patient was discharged with a plaster splint after an uncomplicated postoperative course. The radial Kirschner wires were removed through a stab incision at 4 weeks, and the ulnar plate at 4 months

c When seen 9 years later on 10/8/80, the patient had no complaints, full function, and linear scars
X-rays showed regular joint contours and a nonunion of the avulsed ulnar styloid. Slight cortical irregularities were noted on the distal ulnar shaft

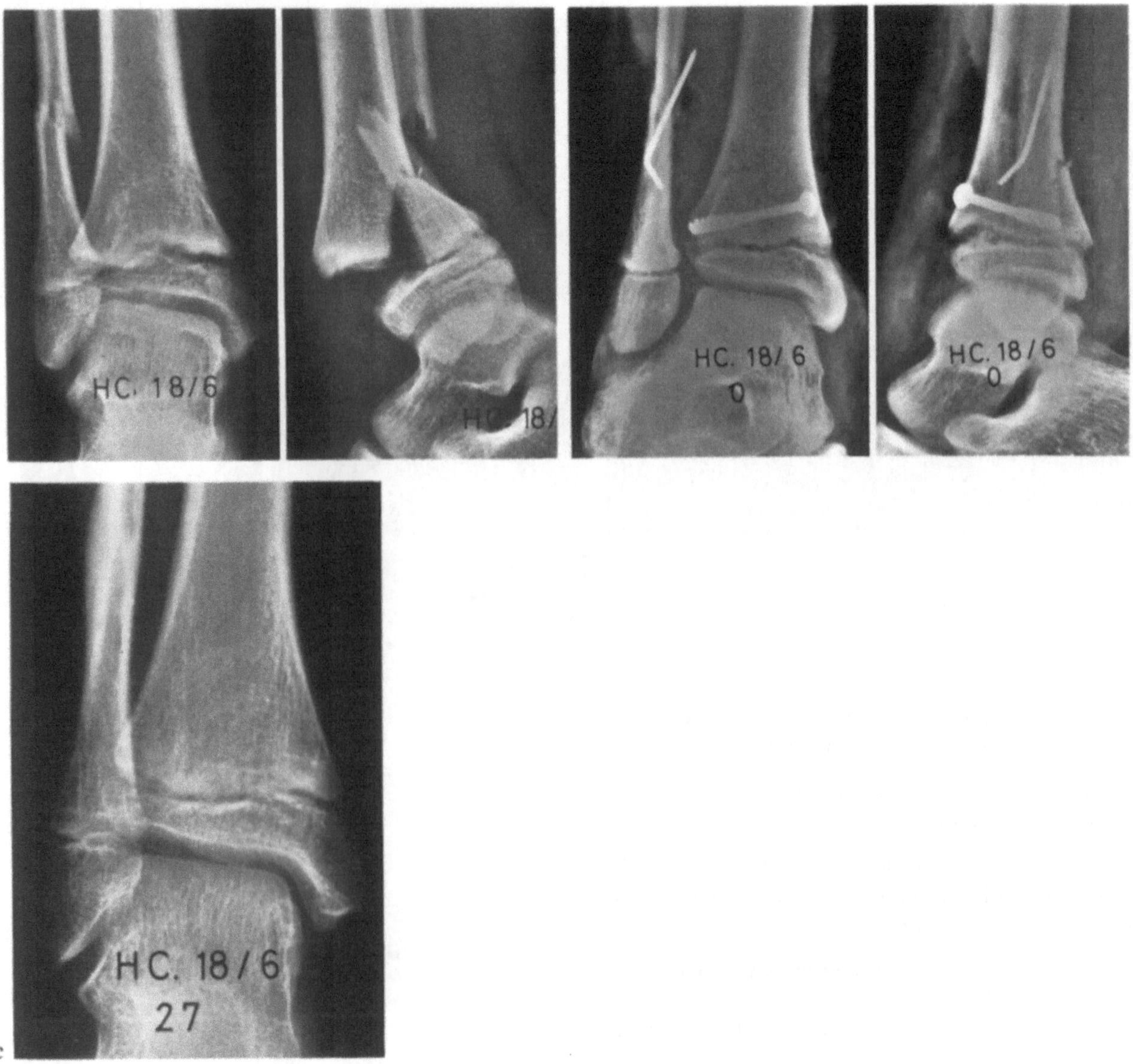

a b c

Fig. 257 a–c. Clinical example: fracture-separation of the distal tibial epiphysis

Thomas S., 11-year-old schoolboy, fell while skiing on 12/27/73

a Aitken type I fracture-separation of the right distal tibial epiphysis with a concomitant fracture of the distal fibula. Closed reduction was unsuccessful

b At emergency operation, medial interposed tissues were cleared, and the epiphysis was fixed with small cancellous lag screws. The irreducible fibular fracture was openly reduced and fixed with an oblique Kirschner wire

Patient was discharged home with a circular cast after an uneventful course. The implants were removed elsewhere at 6 weeks

c An X-ray sent to us $4^1/_2$ months later showed perfect fracture union with a regular epiphyseal line. In October of 1980, more than 6 years after the injury, the parents reported that their son, then 17, was growing normally and was athletically active

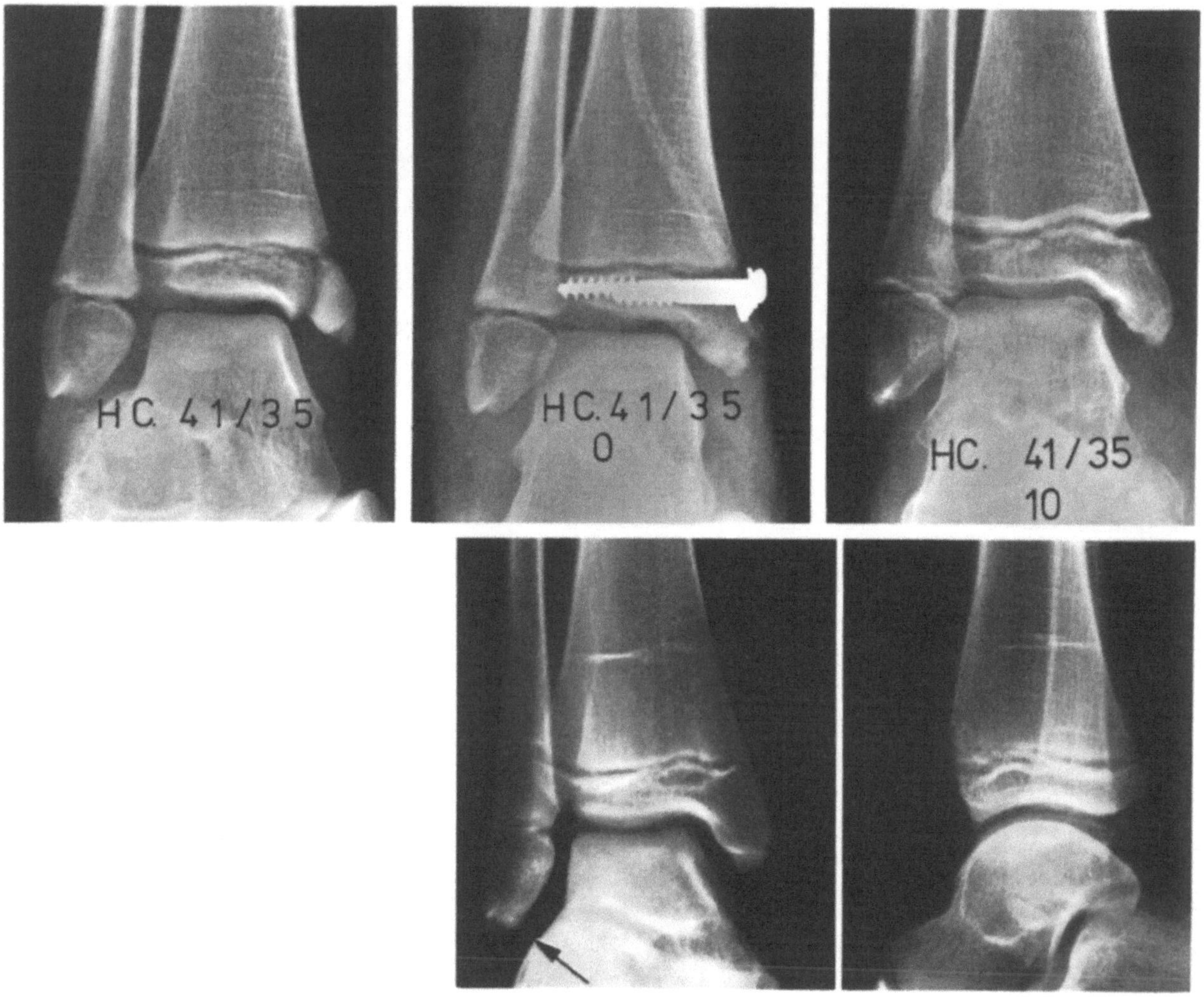

Fig. 258 a–c. Clinical example: fracture of the distal tibial epiphysis

Dagmar K., 8-year-old child, struck by a bicycle on 3/4/78

a Aitken type II epiphyseal fracture of the medial malleolus of the right tibia

b Emergency internal fixation was performed with two parallel cancellous screws and washers, and a circular cast was applied. Full weight-bearing was permitted at 6 weeks. The screws were removed at 8 weeks

c When seen at $2^1/_2$ years on 9/9/80, the patient had no complaints, full function, and a widened scar. There was partial fusion of the medial part of the epiphyseal line. No angular deformity was present. A tiny avulsed fragment at the tip of the fibula had developed into a large osteophyte

References

General Section

Breuing KH, Gotzen V (1986) Biomechanische Untersuchungen zur Haltekraft der neuen 3,5-mm-Corticalisschraube. Hefte Unfallheilkunde 181: 40–46

Heim U, Damur-Thür F (1977) Spongiosa aus dem Tibiakopf als autologes Transplantationsmaterial. Arch Orthop Unfallchir 89:211

Jakob RP (1982) Der kleine Fixateur externe. AO-Bulletin

Kilbourne B, Paul EG (1958) The use of small bone screws in the treatment of metacarpal, metatarsal and phalangeal fractures. J Bone Joint Surg 40-A:375

Müller ME (1966) Treatment of non-unions by compression. Clin Orthop 43:83–92

Müller ME, Allgöwer M, Willenegger H (1963) Technik der operativen Frakturenbehandlung. Springer, Berlin Heidelberg New York

Müller ME, Allgöwer M, Schneider R, Willenegger H (1979) Manual of internal fixation. 2nd edn. Springer, Berlin Heidelberg New York

Müller ME, Allgöwer M, Schneider R, Willenegger H (1977) Manual der Osteosynthese, 2. Aufl. Springer, Berlin Heidelberg New York

Pauwels F (1965) Gesammelte Abhandlungen zur funktionellen Anatomie des Bewegungsapparates. Springer, Berlin Heidelberg New York

Perren SM, Allgöwer M (1976) Biomechanik der Frakturheilung nach Osteosynthesen. Nova Acta Leopold 44, 223:61–84

Perren SM, Huggler A, Russenberger M, Allgöwer M, Mathys R, Schenk RK, Willenegger H, Müller ME (1969) The reaction of cortical bone to compression. Acta Orthop Scand [Suppl] 125:19

Rittmann WW, Matter P (1977) Die offene Fraktur. Beurteilung, operative Behandlung und Resultate. Huber, Bern Stuttgart Wien

Schweiberer L (1976) Theoretisch-experimentelle Grundlagen der autologen Spongiosatransplantation im Infekt. Unfallheilkunde 79:151

Séquin F, Texhammar R (1980) Das AO-Instrumentarium. Springer, Berlin Heidelberg New York

Weber BG, Cech O (1976) Pseudarthrosis. Pathophysiology, Biomechanics, Therapy, Results. Huber, Bern Stuttgart Wien

Chapter IX. The Shoulder Girdle

Bronz G, Heim D, Pusterla C, Heim U (1981) Die stabile Clavicula-Osteosynthese. Unfallheilkunde 84:319

Fischer W, Poigenfürst J, Reiler T (1987) Die Verplattung der frischen Schlüsselbeinfraktur. Erfahrungen an 60 Operationen. Unfallchirurgie (in press)

Jäger M, Breitner S (1984) Therapiebezogene Klassifikation der lateralen Klavikulafraktur. Unfallheilkunde 87:467

Knofler EW (1978) Ein Beitrag zur operativen Behandlung des Schulterblatthalsbruches. Beitr Orthop Traumatol 25:54–56

Koch F (1971) Die Claviculapseudarthrose; ihre Entstehung und Behandlung. Monatschr Unfallheilkd 74:330

Matzen PF (1978) Indikation der operativen Therapie bei Frakturen und Luxationen im Schulterbereich. Beitr Orthop Traumatol 25:44–52

Poigenfürst J, Orthner E, Hofmann J (1987) Technik und Ergebnisse der coraco-claviculären Verschraubung bei frischen Acromioclavicularzerreissungen. Acta Chir Austriaca 1:11–16

Rüedi T, von Hochstetter AHC, Schlumpf R (1984) Operative Zugänge der Osteosynthese. Springer, Berlin Heidelberg New York Tokyo

Steffelaar H, Heim U (1974) Sekundäre Plattenosteosynthese an der Clavicula. Arch Orthop Unfallchir 79:75

Thelen E (1976) Acromioclavicular-Sprengungen – Ergebnisse nach operativer und konservativer Versorgung in 162 Fällen. Unfallheilkunde 79:417–422

Tscherne H (1976) Konservative und operative Therapie der Schulterblattbrüche. Hefte Unfallheilkd 126:52

Wilkins RM, Johnston RM (1983) Ununited fractures of the clavicula. J Bone Joint Surg 65A:773

Chapter X. The Elbow

Beaufils Ph, Audren JL, Lortat-Jacob A, Benoit Y, Perreau M, Ramadier YO (1983) Traumatismes complexes de l'extrémité supérieure des deux os de l'avant-bras. Rev Chir Orthop 69:303

Beck E (1974) Osteosynthese von Speichenköpfchenbrüchen. Aktuel Chir 9:23–28

Burri C (1978) Die Behandlung schwerster Ellbogengelenksverletzungen. Aktuel Traumatolo 8:127

Essex-Lopresti P (1951) Fractures of the Radial Head with distal Radio-Ulnar Dislocation. J Bone Joint Surg 33-B:244

Halls AA, Travill A (1964) Transmission of pressures across the elbow joint. Anat Rec 150:243

Heim U, Trüb HJ (1978) Erfahrungen mit der primären Osteosynthese von Radiusköpfchenfrakturen. Helv Chir Acta 45:63

Labitzke R, Kehr H, Rehn J (1972) Zur Behandlung von Olecranon-Frakturen und Olecranon-Pseudarthrosen. Arch Orthop Unfallchir 74:247

Mason MB (1954) Some Observations on Fractures of the Head of the Radius with a Review of One Hundred Cases. Brit J Surg 42:123

Morrey BF (1985) The elbow and its disorders. W.B. Saunders, Philadelphia

Morscher E (1973) Posttraumatische Fehlstellungen und Pseudarthrosen am Ellbogen beim Erwachsenen. Hefte Unfallheilkd 114:76–84

Mumenthaler M (1961) Die Ulnarisparesen. Thieme, Stuttgart

Tscherne H (1973) Luxationsfrakturen im Ellbogenbereich. Hefte Unfallheilkd 114:59

Chapter XI. Forearm

Galeazzi R (1935) Über ein besonderes Syndrom bei Verletzungen im Bereich der Unterarmknochen. Arch Orthop Unfallchir 35:557

Schweiberer L, Hertel P (1974) Die Ergebnisse nach operativer Behandlung von 48 frischen Monteggia-Verletzungen. Aktuel Traumatol 4:147

Chapter XII. The Wrist and Carpus

Brennwald J, Pfeiffer KM (1980) Radiusfrakturen loco classico. Ther Umsch 37:743–746

Brunner R, Regazzoni P, Pfeiffer KM (1985) Distale, intraartikuläre Radiusfrakturen: Indikation für den Fixateur externe. Helv Chir Acta 52:861–864

Fernandez DL (1982) Correction of posttraumatic wrist deformity in adults by osteotomy, bone-grafting and internal fixation. J Bone Joint Surg 64-A:1164–1178

Fernandez DL, Jakob RP, Büchler U (1983) External fixation of the wrist. Current indications and technique. Ann Chir Gynaec 72:298–302

Gasser H (1965) Delayed union and pseudarthrosis of the carpal navicular: Treatment by compression screw osteosynthesis. J Bone Joint Surg 47-A:249

Heim U (1979) Die operative Behandlung der gelenknahen Speichenbrüche des Erwachsenen. Hefte Unfallheilkd 82:15–22

Herbert TJ, Fisher WE (1984) Management of the Fractured Scaphoid using a new Bone Screw. J bone Joint Surg 66-B:114–123

Jakob RP (1982) Der kleine Fixateur externe. AO-Bulletin, Bern

Lauber P, Pfeiffer KM (1984) Offene Osteosynthese distaler Radiusfrakturen. Unfallheilkunde 87:185–195

Matti H (1936) Technik und Resultate meiner Pseudarthroseoperation. Zentralbl Chir 63:1442

Müller J (1978) Ergebnisse verschiedener Operationsmethoden bei Kahnbeinpseudarthrosen der Hand. Unfallheilkunde 80:345–352

Pfeiffer KM (1972) Zur Frage der primären Schraubenosteosynthese von Navikularefrakturen. Helv Chir Acta 39:111–122

Pfeiffer KM (1978) Perilunäre, transskaphoidale, transkapitale, transstyloidale Handgelenks-Luxationsfraktur. Operative Rekonstruktion. Handchirurgie 10:39–40

Pfeiffer KM, Meine J, Linder P (1975) Radiusfrakturen loco classico. Ther Umsch 32:788–799

Pfeiffer KM, Lauber P (1984) Was leistet die stabile Osteosynthese am distalen Radius? Handchir Mikrochir Plast Chir 16:80–82

Russe O (1960) Nachuntersuchungsergebnisse von 22 Fällen operierter, veralteter Brüche und Pseudarthrosen des Kahnbeines der Hand. Z Orthop 39:5

Segmüller G (1973) Operative Stabilisierung am Handskelett. Huber, Bern Stuttgart Wien

Trojan E (1955) Die operative Behandlung des veralteten Kahnbeinbruches der Hand. Verh Dtsch Orthop Ges 43:160

Wagner HE, Jakob RP (1985) Operative Behandlung der distalen Radiusfraktur mit Fixateur externe. Unfallchirurg 88:473–480

Wilhelm K (1983) Radius-Korrekturoperationen. Indikation und Ergebnisse. Fortschr Med 101:299–302

Chapter XIII. The Hand

Angehrn R (1980) Resultate der operativen Knochenbruchbehandlung am Handskelett. Analyse von 570 Fällen der AO-Dokumentation. Inauguraldissertation, Basel

Ansorge D (1980) Die Leistungsfähigkeit der Zuggurtungsosteosynthese am Handskelett. Zentralbl Chir 105:468–474
Asche G (1981) Stabilisierungsmöglichkeiten einer intraartikulären Trümmerfraktur des ersten Mittelhandknochens mit dem Mini-Fixateur externe. Handchirurgie 13:247–249
Asche G, Burny F (1982) Indikation für die Anwendung des Mini-Fixateur externe. Eine statistische Analyse. Aktuel Traumatol 12:103–110
Bauer J, Andrasina J, Lesko J, Tomas D (1980) Vergleich der konservativ und operativ versorgten Bennett'schen Frakturen. Hefte Unfallheilkd 141:103–105
Belsky MR, Eaton RG, Lane LB (1984) Closed reduction and internal fixation of proximal phalangeal fractures. J Hand Surg (Am) 9:725–729
Berger A, Meissl G, Walzer L (1980) Probleme der Knochenbruchbehandlung in der Replantationschirurgie. Handchirurgie 12:247–248
Black D, Mann RJ, Constine R, Daniels AU (1985) Comparison of internal fixation techniques in metacarpal fractures. J Hand Surg (Am) 10:466–472
Bouchon Y, Merle M, Foucher G, Michon J (1982) Les cals vicieux des métacarpiens et des phalanges. Résultats du traitement chirurgical. Rév Chir Orthop 68:549–555
Brennwald J (1980) Die Osteosynthese als Grundlage der mikrochirurgischen Replantation. In: Osteosynthese und Endoprothese. Schweiz. Naturforschende Gesellschaft, Jahrbuch 1980/2:74–79
Büchler U, Fischer T (1987) Mini Condylar Plate for Hand Surgery. Orthop Clinic and Related Research, 214:53–58
Burri C, Rüedi T, Matter P, Pfeiffer KM, Pusterla C (1969) Stabile Osteosynthese: Frakturen im Handbereich. Aktuel Chir 4:305
Della Santa D, Chamay A, Blanco F, Marti MC (1985) Les fractures des métacarpiens longs. Résultats à long terme. Ann Chir Main 4:175–180
Dingels WR, Far E, Rolle J (1980) Osteosynthesen im Bereich der Hand. 168 Fälle von Einzel- und Kombinationsosteosynthesen. Handchirurgie 12:239–244
Durband MA (1969) Metacarpalfrakturen unter besonderer Berücksichtigung der therapeutischen Möglichkeiten aus neuester Sicht. Inauguraldissertation, Zürich
Duspiva W, Biemer E (1980) Knochenheilung in der Replantationschirurgie an der Hand. Z Plast Chir 4:84–89
Filipovic L, Hlaka M (1980) Operative Behandlung der Bennett-Brüche. Hefte Unfallheilkd 141:100–103
Foucher G, Merle M, Michon J (1977) Intérêt de l'ostéosynthèse dans la stabilisation des fractures du squelette métacarpo-phalangien. Ann Chir 31:1065–1069
Frère G, Massart P, Hoel G (1981) Trois cent dix ostéosynthèses de métacarpiens. Ann Chir 35:771–777
Fritz G (1980) Intraartikuläre Brüche an der Basis des 1. Mittelhandknochens (ohne Bennett). Hefte Unfallheilkd 141:96–99
Fyfe IS, Mason S (1979) The mechanical stability of internal fixation of fractured phalanges. Hand 11:50–54
Gedda KO, Moberg E (1953) Open reduction and osteosynthesis of socalled Bennett's fracture in the carpometacarpal joint of the thumb. Acta Orthop Scand 22:249
Gingrass RP, Fehring B, Matloub H (1980) Intraosseous wiring of complex hand fractures. Plast Reconstr Surg 66:383–394
Heim U (1969) Die Technik der operativen Behandlung der Metacarpalfrakturen. Helv Chir Acta 36:619
Heim U (1973) L'ostéosynthèse rigide dans le traitement des fractures de la base du premier métacarpien. Acta Orthop Belg 39:1073
Heim U, Pfeiffer KM, Meuli HC (1973) Resultate von 332 AO-Osteosynthesen des Handskeletts. Handchirurgie 5:71
Heim U, Osterwalder M (1977) Arthrodèse de l'interphalangienne distale (et de l'interphalangienne du pouce) par vissage. Ann Chir 31:291
Heiss J, Prokscha GW (1980) Zur Behandlung von basisnahen Frakturen des I. Mittelhandknochens: Technik, Spätergebnisse. Hefte Unfallheilkd 141:105–111
Hoffmann R, Buck-Gramcko D (1982) Osteosynthesis in digital replantation surgery. Ann Chir Gynaecol 71:14–18
Hunter JM, Cowen NJ (1970) Fifth metacarpal fractures in a compensation clinic population. J Bone Joint Surg 52-A:1159
Iselin M, Blanguernon S, Benoist D (1965) Fractures de la base du 1er métacarpien. Mém Acad Chir 82:771
Jupiter JB, Koniuch MP, Smith RJ (1985) The management of delayed union and non-union of the metacarpals and phalanges. J Hand Surg (Am) 10:457–466
Korisek G (1980) Korrekturosteotomien nach in Fehlstellung geheilten Fingerfrakturen. Hefte Unfallheilkd 141:176–179
Leach RE, Bolton PE (1968) Arthritis of the carpometacarpal joint of the thumb; results of arthrodesis. J Bone Joint Surg 50-A:1171
Lemberger U (1980) Langzeitergebnisse versorgter Bennett-Frakturen. Handchirurgie 12:245–246

Lister G (1978) Intraosseous wiring of the digital skeleton. J Hand Surg (Am) 3:427–435
Massengill JB, Alexander H, Parson JR, Schecter MJ (1979) Mechanical analysis of Kirschner wire fixation in a phalangeal model. J Hand Surg (Am) 4:351–356
McElfresh EC, Dobyns JH (1983) Intra-articular metacarpal head fractures. J Hand Surg (Am) 8:383–393
Merle M, Foucher G, Mole D, Michon J (1981) Résultats fonctionnels des fractures ostéosynthésées de la première phalange des doigts longs. Ann Chir 35:765–770
Meuli HC, Meyer V, Segmüller G (1978) Stabilization of bone in replantation surgery of the upper limb. Clin Orthop 133:179–183
Meyer-Clement M, Brüser P, Bönninghoff N (1984) Dexon-Cerclagen am Handskelett. Handchir Mikrochir Plast Chir 16:189–191
Meyer VE, Chiu DT, Beasley RW (1981) The place of internal skeletal fixation in surgery of the hand. Clin Plast Surg 8:51–64
Mitz V, Richard JC, Ohanna J, Vilain R (1981) Intérêt de l'ostéosynthèse par brochage transversal externe des fractures du 5e métacarpien. Rév Chir Orthop 67:571–576
Nonnenmacher J, Wagnon J, Mochel D, Issa JB (1981) Traitement des fractures de la base du premier métacarpien par mini-fixateur externe. A propos d'une série préliminaire de 14 cas. Acta Orthop Belg 47:399–405
Pannike A (1972) Osteosynthesen in der Handchirurgie. Springer, Berlin Heidelberg New York
Pfeiffer KM (1976) Fortschritte in der Osteosynthese von Handfrakturen. Handchirurgie 8:17–22
Pfeiffer KM, Nigst H (1970) Schraubenarthrodese von Fingergelenken. Handchirurgie 2:149–151
Poigenfürst J (1980) Bennett'sche Verrenkungsbrüche: operative Therapie. Hefte Unfallheilkd 141:93–95
Rehm KE, Ecke H, Schultheis KH (1983) Osteosyntheseverfahren in der Replantationschirurgie. Handchir Mikrochir Plast Chir 15:130–134
Renner A, Santha E, Manninger J (1979) Korrekturosteotomien nach in Fehlstellung verheilten Brüchen der Mittelhand- und Fingerknochen. Handchirurgie 11:213–218
Rolando S (1910) Fracture de la base du premier métacarpien et principalement sur une variété non encore décrite. Presse méd 18:303
Rudolph H, Klussendorf D, Dolle H (1980) Die Wahl des Osteosyntheseverfahrens bei Schaftfrakturen der Finger- und Mittelhandknochen. Hefte Unfallheilkd 141:53–57
Rupnik J (1980) Ergebnisse der Osteosynthese an Mittelhandknochen und Fingern. Hefte Unfallheilkd 141:78–84
Santha E (1980) Rotations-Korrekturosteotomien. Hefte Unfallheilkd 141:175–176
Schärli AF (1980) Osteosynthesen kindlicher Hand- und Fußfrakturen nach dem Zuggurtungsprinzip. Unfallchirurgie 6:24–27
Schottle H, Stier GB, Langendorff HU (1985) Ergebnisse der operativen Behandlung von Frakturen der Mittelhand und Finger. Unfallchirurgie 11:76–83
Schwarz N, Eber K (1980) Pseudarthrosen an Finger- und Mittelhandknochen. Hefte Unfallheilkd 141:180–188
Segmüller G (1973) Operative Stabilisierung am Handskelett. Huber, Bern Stuttgart Wien
Segmüller G (1981) Stabile Osteosynthese und autologer Knochenspan bei Defekt- und Trümmerfrakturen am Handskelett. Handchirurgie 13:209–211
Segmüller G, Schönenberger F (1971) Technik der Kompressionsarthrodese am Finger mittels Zugschraube. Handchirurgie 2:218
Simonetta C (1970) The use of AO plates in the hand. Hand 2:43
Stock A, Stock HJ (1983) Wert der Osteosynthese bei Handverletzungen. Beitr Orthop Traumatol 30:345–353
Suman RK (1983) Rigid fixation of metacarpal fractures. J Roy Coll Surg Edinb 28:51
Thomine JM, Bendjeddou MS, Gibon Y, Biga N (1981) Les fractures diaphysaires de la première phalange. Résultats du traitement. A propos de soixante-douze cas. Ann Chir 35:759–764
Titze A (1979) Indikationen zur Osteosynthese an der Hand und an den Fingern. Unfallchirurgie 5:146–149
Tubiana R (1981) A propos du traitement chirurgical des fractures des métacarpiens et des phalanges. Ann Chir 35:757–758
Vanik RK, Weber RC, Matloub HS, Sanger JR (1984) The comparative strengths of internal fixation techniques. J Hand Surg (Am) 9:216–221
Wagner M, Poigenfürst J (1980) Indikationen zur Osteosynthese bei Handverletzungen im Kindesalter. Z Kinderchir Grenzgeb 30:114–116
Winter I, Zilch H, Baudin BP (1981) Zur Problematik der Osteosynthese bei der peripheren Replantation. Handchirurgie 13:114–119

Chapter XIV. The Knee

Bandi W (1977) Die retropatellaren Kniegelenkschäden. Pathomechanik und pathologische Anatomie, Klinik und Therapie. Huber, Bern Stuttgart Wien

Ganz R (1976) Isolierte Knorpelabscherungen am Kniegelenk. Hefte Unfallheilkd 127:79

Smillie IS (1976) Treatment of osteochondritis dissecans. J Bone Joint Surg 39-B:248

Chapter XVI. The Ankle Joint

Bandi W (1970) Zur Mechanik der supramalleolären intraartikulären Schienbeinbrüche des Skifahrers. Kongressbericht 9. Int. Kongress für Skitraumatologie. Nebel-Verlag, Garmisch-Partenkirchen

Bonnin JG (1950) Injuries of the ankle. Heinemann, London

Burri C, Rüter A (1978) Verletzungen des oberen Sprunggelenkes. Hefte Unfallheilkd 131. Springer, Berlin Heidelberg New York

Danis R (1949) Théorie et pratique de l'ostéosynthèse. Masson, Paris

Decoulx P, Razemon JP, Rouselle Y (1961) Fractures du pilon tibial. Rev Chir Orthop 47:563

Destot E (1911) Traumatismes du pied et rayons X. Masson, Paris

Fick R (1904) Handbuch der Anatomie und Mechanik der Gelenke. G. Fischer-Verlag, Jena

Frick H (1978) Zur Entstehung Klinik, Diagnostik und Therapie der isolierten Verletzung der tibiofibularen Syndesmose. Unfallheilkunde 81:542

Gay R, Evrard J (1963) Les fractures récentes du pilon tibial chez l'adulte. Rev Chir Orthop 49:397

Heim D (1980) Die Peronealsehnenluxation. Inauguraldissertation, Basel

Heim U (1972) Le traitement chirurgical des fractures du pilon tibial. J Chir (Paris) 104:307

Heim U (1973) Indication et technique des sutures ligamentaires dans les fractures malléolaires. Rev Chir Orthop 59 [Suppl 1]:270

Heim U (1982) Indikation und Technik der Stabilisierung des hinteren Kantendreiecks nach Volkmann bei Malleolarfrakturen. Unfallheilkunde 85:388

Heim U (1983) Malleolarfrakturen. Unfallheilkunde 86:248

Heim U (1986) Arthrosehäufigkeit nach Osteosynthesen des Volkmannschen Dreiecks bei Malleolarfrakturen. Zeitschr Unfallchir Versicherungsmed Berufskrankh 79:99

Heim U, Näser M (1977) Fractures du pilon tibial. Résultats de 128 ostéosynthèses. Rev Chir Orthop 63:5

Kuner EH, Müller T, Lindenmaier HL (1978) Einteilung und Behandlung der Talusfrakturen. Hefte Unfallheilkd 131:197–211

Müller ME (1967) Posttraumatische Fehlstellungen an der unteren Extremität. Huber, Bern Stuttgart

Rüedi T (1978) Spätresultate nach operativer Behandlung der Gelenkbrüche am distalen Tibiaende. Unfallheilkunde 81:319–323

Rüedi T, Matter P, Allgöwer M (1968) Die intraartikulären Frakturen des distalen Unterschenkelendes. Helv Chir Acta 35:556

Weber BG (1972) Die Verletzungen des oberen Sprunggelenkes. 2. Aufl. Huber, Bern Stuttgart Wien

Weber BG (1971) Brüche von Knöcheln und Talus. Bewährtes und Neues in Diagnostik und Therapie. Langenbecks Arch Chir 355:421–425

Willenegger H (1961) Die Behandlung der Luxationsfrakturen des oberen Sprunggelenkes nach biomechanischen Gesichtspunkten. Helv Chir Acta 28:225

Willenegger H, Riede UH, Schenk R (1971) Gelenkmechanische Untersuchungen zum Problem der posttraumatischen Arthrosen im oberen Sprunggelenk. I. Die intraartikuläre Modellfraktur. Langenbecks Arch Klin Chir 328:258

Willenegger H, Riede UH, Schweizer G, Marti J (1973) Gelenkmechanische Untersuchungen zum Problem der posttraumatischen Arthrosen im oberen Sprunggelenk. III. Funktionell-morphometrische Analyse des Gelenkknorpels. Langenbecks Arch Klin Chir 333:91

Chapter XVII. The Foot

Bèzes H, Massart P, Fourquet J-P (1984) Die Osteosynthese der Kalkaneusimpressionsfraktur. Unfallheilkunde 87:363

Collis WJMF, Jayson MIV (1972) Measurement of pedal pressures. Ann of Rheumatic Dis 31:215–217

Giannestras NJ, Sammarco GJ (1975) Fractures and dislocations in the foot. In: Fractures, Volume 2, Rockwood CA and Green DP (Editors), 1400–1495. Lippincott, Philadelphia

Goossens M, De Stoop N (1983) Lisfranc's fracture-dislocations: etiology, radiology and result of treatment. A review of 20 cases. Clin Orthop 176:154–162

Hardcastle PH, Reschauer R, Kutscha-Lissberg E, Schoffmann W (1982) Injuries to the tarsometatarsal joint. Incidence, classification and treatment. J Bone Joint Surg 64-B:349–356

Heim U (1970) Die Behandlung von Frakturen der Metatarsalia und Zehen unter besonderer Berücksichtigung der Osteosynthese. Z Unfallmed Berufskr 63:305
Holzach P, Staubli A, Gerber B (1983) Die Behandlung der Basisfraktur des Os metatarsale V. Helv Chir Acta 50:69–72
Kavanaughj H, Brower TD, Mann RV (1978) The Jones'fracture revisited. J Bone Joint Surg 60-A:776–782
Kempf I, Touzard RC (1978) Les fractures du calcaneum. J Chir (Paris) 115:377–386
Kundert HP (1984) Beidseitige rezidivierende Streßfrakturen des proximalen Metatarsaleschaftes V (Jones' fracture). Chir Piede 8:125–129
Seitz WH jr, Grantham SA (1985) The Jones' fracture in the non-athlete. Foot-Ankle 6:97–100
Simmen BR, Dick W, Pfeiffer KM, Richard HP (1982) Behandlungstaktik bei Metatarsalfrakturen. Orthop Praxis 18:62–66
Tittel K, Schmidt P (1984) Die Fraktur der Basis des Metatarsale V – konservative oder operative Behandlung? Unfallchirurgie 10:207–210
Torg JS, Balduini FC, Zelko RR, Pavlov H, Peff TC, Das M (1984) Fractures of the base of the fifth metatarsal distal to the tuberosity. Classification and guidelines for non-surgical and surgical management. J Bone Joint Surg 66-A:209–214
Wiley JJ (1971) The mechanisme of tarsometatarsal joint injuries. J Bone Joint Surg 53-B, 474–482

Chapter XVIII. Special Indications

Schärli AF (1980) Osteosynthese kindlicher Hand- und Fußfrakturen nach dem Zuggurtungsprinzip. Unfallchirurgie 6:24–27
Stauffer UG (1978) Indications for operative treatment of fractures in childhood. Prog Pediatr Surg 12:187–208
Weber BG, Süssenbach F (1970) Epiphysenfugenverletzungen am distalen Unterschenkel. Huber, Bern Stuttgart Wien
Weber BG, Brunner C, Freuler F (1978) Die Frakturbehandlung bei Kindern und Jugendlichen. Springer, Berlin Heidelberg New York
Weber BG, Brunner C, Freuler F (1980) Treatment of fractures in children and adolescents. Springer, Berlin Heidelberg New York

Subject Index

ABC system for the classification 144f., 152, 261, 267, 286, 298
Acromioclavicular joint 86
Acromion 94, 95
Aftertreatment 69ff.
Agee – Technique for PIP fractures 208, 220
Allergy 74
Amputation (hand) 210f.
Ankle joint 261ff.
Annular ligament 110f., 120f.
Approaches
– Ankle fractures 264, 268, 311ff.
– Calcaneus 344
– Clavicula 90
– Elbow 115
– Foot 337
– Hand 180, 204, 212ff.
– Humerus, distal 115f.
– Malleolar fractures 264, 268, 311ff.
– Radial head 120
– Radius, distal 146, 154ff.
– Scaphoid 149, 156
– Scapula 94
– Tibia distal 264, 268
– Wrist 155ff.
Arthrodesis 78, 80
– CMC joint I 182, 190, 201
– DIP joint 209f., 223, 244f.
– Foot 343
– IP joint thumb 183, 203
– MP joint I 183, 189, 191, 202
– PIP joint 209f., 222, 243
– Temporary 218, 235, 243, 340, 344f.
– Toe 352ff., 359ff., 371
– Wrist 151, 160, 174, 176ff.
Articular fractures: see locations
Autogenous bone grafting 75
see also
– cancellous bone graft
– corticocancellous bone graft
Avulsion fractures: see locations
Axial interfragmental compression 31, 34ff., 42f., 54ff.

Bandi 262
Barton-fracture (reversed Barton) 145
Base of first metacarpal 180
Bending irons 13, 20ff., 49, 186
Bennett's fracture dislocation 180, 184ff., 192f., 201
Big toe 342, 368, 371
Bimalleolar fracture: see Malleolar fractures
Bone grafts: see
– cancellous or
– corticocancellous bone graft
Bonnin 286
Bridge graft 190, 201
Bridge plate 44f.
Buttress plate 31, 38, 45

Calcaneous 337, 344f., 350f.
Cancellous bone graft 31, 38, *75f.*, *77ff.*, 86, 102, 110, 120f., 132f., 146, 164, 176, 190, 195, 242, 260, 264, 271f., 280, 282ff., 297, 332, 339, 341, 348, 352f., 359, 362f., 364f., 366ff., 370
Cancellous screw 5, 15f., 18
Carpal bones 150
Carpal tunnel 147f.
Carpometacarpal joint 182
Cerclage wire 22
see also: Hemicerclage
Children 373
Chopart's joint 339, 352
Classification, ABC system 145, 152, 261, 267, 286, 298
Clavicle 85, 90, 92ff., 98ff., 104
Cloverleaf plate 9, 21, 106, 270f., 273, 278, 280, 282f.
Colles-fracture 145
Complex injuries (hand) 210f.
Condylar fractures
– Hand 199, 208, 238
– Humerus distal 107ff.
Condylar plate: see Minicondylar plate
Coracoid process 92ff., 100, 103
Coronoid process 112
Corrosion 73
Cortex screw: see Screw
Corticocancellous graft 44, *75*, *77ff.*, 118, 136, 148, 150f., 160, 170, 178, 190, 201, 252, 297, 343
Countersink 12, 33

Cuboid 252f., 339, 354
Cuneiform 339, 355
Cutting forceps 21, 23
Danis 286
DCP principle 31, 44
DC-Plate (DCP)
- 3,5 mm: 8, 20, 35, 55, 85f., 139, 151, 160, 274
- 2,7 mm: 9, 22, 149, 378
- 2,0 mm: 10, 23, 225
Delayed union 150, 282ff., 370
Deltoid ligament 291, 308
Depth gauge 12
Distal, see
- DIP joint
- Humerus
- Patella
- Radius
- Tibia
- Ulna
Distal interphalangeal joint (DIP) 206, 208, 221, 237ff.
Drainage 70
Drawer sign 307
Drill bits 11, 16
Drill guides, double 11, 16, 26, 28, 36

Elevation, postoperative 70
Elbow 107ff., 374
Epicondyles 107, 115, 120, 374
Epiphyseal injuries 375, 379f.
External fixator, small
- Applications 41, 45, 66f., 344
- Components 24
- Description 10
- Examples 166ff.
- Indications 40
- Technique 40
Extensor retinaculum 147, 149, 154

Fick 286
Fifth metatarsal 341f.
Flexor retinaculum 147, 156
Foot 337ff.
Forceps
- Compression forceps (mini) for plates 13, 56f., 191
- Cutting forceps 21, 23
- for bending and twisting miniplates 23, 61
- Reduction forceps 10f., 29f.
Forearm, see
- Radius
- Ulna
Fracture dislocation: see location

Galeazzi-fracture 139, 144
Gay and Evrard 261
Gedda-Moberg, Approach 180, 184
Glenoid rim 95, 103
Goyrand-Fracture 145
Graft: see
- Cancellous graft
- Corticocancellous graft
Guides, drill 11, 16, 26, 28, 36

H-Plate, mini 9, 40, 60, 150, 197, 200
Hand 179ff.
Hand chuck 22
Handle 13
Head of the Radius: see Radial head
Hemicerclage wiring 179, 209, 229
Hemostasis 69
Herbert 150
Humerus, distal 107ff., 114ff., 124ff.
Humerus, proximal 89, 96, 106

Incision: see Approaches
Instruments 10ff., 16f., 19ff., 26ff., 48f., 52, 56f., 302
Intercondylar eminence 248, 251, 256
Interfragmental compression 31, 34ff., 42f., 54ff.
Interfragmental lag screw in plate 54ff., 64
Interosseous membrane 110, 286f., 291, 307
Interosseous wire suture 179, 209, 229
Interphalangeal joint of the thumb (IP) 183, 203, 206, 208
Iselin - Technique for fractures of the base of the first metacarpal 180, 186

Jäger - Classification of the lateral clavicle fractures 92
Jones-Fractures 342, 366

Kirschner wire 22, 46, 49, 53, 59, 66, 70, 73, 116ff., 122, 145, 153, 169, 179, 186, *189ff.*, 210, 218ff., 222, 252, 270ff., 303, 306, 308, 310, 312f., 316, 345, 347, 349, 374f.
Knee joint 257

Lag screw
- Technique 31f., 42, 46ff., 63
- Problems 50f., 63
Length measurements of screws 48, 52
Ligaments
- annulare radii 110, 121
- avulsions, bony 182, 252, 291, 294, 306, 308
- collateral DIP 223
- collateral MP thumb 182, 188
- collateral PIP 206, 216
- collateral ulnar (elbow) 109, 119
- coracoclaviculare 86, 92f.
- deltoid 291, 308
- knee joint 248

- reinforcing suture 289, 308
- tibiofibular 286, 291 f., 306 f., 308
Lisfranc's joint 339, 354 f.
Lunate 149, 172, 178

Machine, mini compressed, air 13, 25
Maisonneuve-Fractures 289, 303, 328
Malleolar fractures 286 ff., 301 ff.
- aftertreatment 296
- anterolateral tibial fracture (of Tillaux-Chaput) 294, 304, 308
- approaches 287, 293, 302, 311 f.,
- classification 286, 298
- ligament repair 291, 308
- Maisonneuve-fracture 289, 303, 305
- medial malleolus 295, 316 f.
- positioning 287, 301
- posterior malleolus 292 f., 309 ff.
- transfixing the fibula to the tibia 290, 303 ff.
- type A fracture 291, 306
- type B fracture 390, 306 f.
- type C fracture 289, 304 f.
Malunion: see Osteotomy
Marginal Fragments 292, 309 ff.
Mason – Classification for radial head fractures 109 f.
Matti and Russe – technique 150
Measurement, length 48, 52
Median nerve 147 f., 155 ff., 164
Metacarpal fractures 180 ff.
- approaches 180, 184, 204 f., 212
- complex injuries 210
- first ray (base) 180 f., 184 ff., 192 ff.
- first ray (distal) 182, 188, 197 ff.
- second through fifth ray 204 ff., 213, 217 f., 224 ff.
- secondary operations 182 f., 190 f., 201 ff., 209 f., 222 f., 240
Metacarpophalangeal joint (MP) 183, 205, 214, 230
Metatarsal fractures 340 ff.
- approaches 346
- fifth metatarsal 341, 347 f., 362 ff.
- Jones-fracture 342, 366 f.
- secondary operations 342, 369 f.
- shaft and neck fractures 340, 348 f., 356 ff.
Mini compression forceps 13, 56 f., 191
Mini condylar plate 9, 23, 39, 59, 209, 213, 217, 232
Mini H-Plate 9, 23, 40, 60, 150, 197, 200
Mine plate (straight and T) 9, 23, 188, 198, 208, 217, 231
Mini screw 7, 15 ff., 48 f., 111, 132, 134, 172, 199, 208, 217, 230 f., 233, 238
Moberg, Approach 180, 184
Monteggia-fracture 110, 134, 139 f.
Multiple fractures 38

Navicular bone
- Foot 338, 352
- Hand: see scaphoid
N. medianus: see Median nerve
N. radialis: see Radial nerve
Neutralization plate 31, 37, 44, 58
Nonunions 78 f., 90
- Clavicle 86, 90, 102
- Forefoot 342, 369
- Hand 209, 242
- Humerus distal 136 f.
- Malleoli 297, 332
- Olecranon 113
- Patella 249
- Radial head 109
- Radius distal 139, 148
- Scaphoid 150, 174 f.
- Tibia distal 280
- Ulna 140

Olecranon 112, 114, 116, 122, 130, 134, 377
Olecranon, osteotomy 108, 116, 129
Open fractures 40, 338
Osteoarthritis 236, 262, 276, 279, 284
Osteochondral fractures 249, 252, 257
Osteochondritis dissecans 249
Osteotomy 78 f.
- Clavicle 86
- Hand 183, 189, 209, 240 f.
- Humerus epicondyle 120
- Malleoli 297
- Olecranon 116
- Radius distal 170
- Tibia distal 273 f., 280
- Tibial tuberosity 249, 258
- Ulna 148 f.

Patella 247 f., 250, 253 ff.
Percutaneous Kirschner wire fixation 145, 169, 179
Perilunar transscaphoid fracture dislocation 149, 171 f.
Peroneal tendon displacement 294, 314
Phalangeal fractures
- approaches 205, 215
- articular: see
- distal interphalangeal joint (DIP)
- metacarpophalangeal joint (MP)
- proximal interphalangeal joint (PIP)
- secondary operations 209, 222 f., 242 ff.
- shaft 48, 182, 188, 208, 210, 217, 231 ff., 236 ff.
Pilon tibial fracture 261, 267 ff., 275, 276 ff., 282 ff.
Plates 8 ff., 20 ff., 31, 35 ff., 43 ff., 54 ff., 64 f., 79 f. see also:
- Bridge plate
- Buttress plate
- Neutralization plate
- Tension band plate

Plates, dangers and problems 61f.
Plate stability 37, 65
Plate, tension band 43
Pliers 13, 20ff.
Posterior melleolar fragment: see Malleolar fractures
Posterior tibiofibular ligament 291
Postoperative treatment 70ff.
Prosthetic replacements (radial head)
- Radial head 112
- Trapezium 182
Proximal humerus: see Humerus proximal
Proximal interphalangeal joint (PIP) 205, 207f., 215f., 220, 235ff.
Pull-out wire fixation 221

de Quervain perilunar transscaphoid fracture dislocation 149, 171

Radial artery 147, 155f., 158, 183, 190
Radial head fractures 109ff., 114, 119ff., 131ff.
Radial neck fracture 111, 132, 374
Radial nerve 111, 120, 147ff., 155, 158, 190
Radial styloid 145f., 153, 155
Radiocarpal fracture dislocation 161
Radius distal
- Approach 146ff., 155ff.
- Classification 145f., 152
- External fixator 10, 24, 45, 66f., 139, 166ff.
- Kirschner wire 145, 153, 166f.
- Secondary operations 148f., 151, 170f.
- Plating 8f., 21, 146, 153f., 162ff.
- Technique 146ff.
Radius shaft 139ff.
Reconstruction plate 9, 20, 39, 87, 91, 99, 109
Reduction 69
Reduction forceps 10, 29f., 33
Refractures 139
Removal of implants 73
Retinaculum
- Extensor retinaculum 147, 149, 154f.
- Flexor retinaculum 147, 156
Reverse Barton fracture 145f., 162
Rheumatoid surgery 373
Rolando's fracture 181, 184, 187, 194f.,
Rüedi 263
Russe 150

Scaphoid (Navicular bone)
- Approach 149f.
- Delayed union 150
- Fracture 145, 172
- Fracture dislocation 145, 149, 171
- Nonunion 150, 174f.
- Screw technique 159
Scapholunar ligament 150
Scapula 87f., 94f., 104f.
Screws 5ff., 15ff., 46ff.
Screw arthrodesis 80, 203, 210, 222, 243ff.
Screw technique 31f., 34, 46ff.
Screwdrivers 12
Skin incisions: see Approaches
Small external fixator: see external fixator
Smith fracture 145
Stag-beetle forceps 11, 111
Swelling, posttraumatic 69, 263
Syndesmosis 286

T-Plate
- for 3,5 mm screws (Radius T-Plate) 8f., 21
- for 2,7 mm screws (metacarpal) 9f., 22
Talus 297, 319, 334f.
Taps 12
Tap sleeves 11, 26ff.
Tarsal joint, transverse (Chopart) 339, 352f.
Tarsal navicular 338, 352
Tarsometatarsal joint (Lisfranc) 339, 354f.
Techniques for internal fixation 31ff.
Tenolysis 73, 225
Tension band
- Arthrodesis 80, 190, 222
- Plate 43, 57, 64
- Principle 31, 43
- Wire technique 34, 53, 93, 95, 116, 122, 252, 306, 316, 347
Tension device 56, 122, 136, 273, 283
Termite forceps 10, 111
Thumb 182
Thumb reconstruction 183
Tibial tuberosity 248, 252, 258
Tibia distal (Pilon) 260ff.
- Approach 264, 268
- Classification 261, 267
- Tactics 263
- Technique 269ff., 275ff.
Tibial shaft 259f.
Tibiofibular ligaments 287, 291, 308
Tibiofibular transfixion 290, 303ff., 322, 328
Toe: see Big toe
Tourniquet 69, 107, 113, 263
Traction 263, 272, 278, 280
Transfer of finger rays 209
Transfixing the fibula to the tibia: see Tibiofibular transfixion
Transosseous pull-out wire 179, 188
Trapezium 150, 173, 193
Trapezium prosthetic replacement 182
Trochlea - reconstruction 108, 117f., 127
Tubular plate
- one-third tubular (for 3,5 mm screws) 8, 20, 54, 118, 122f., 128, 304, 306

– quarter tubular (for 2,7 mm screws) 9, 22, 191, 202, 213, 217

Ulna 113, 139ff., 143, 149
Ulnar head syndrom 149
Ulnar nerve 108, 114, 125, 129, 149

Vassal Rule 38, 65

Wagner 180, 186
Washers 8, 15, 33, 46, 52, 120, 236, 252, 254, 256, 304, 308, 310, 312, 314, 318, 331, 334
Weber 286, 293, 306, 313, 316
Wedge fractures 110, 119
Weight bearing 71
Willenegger 286
Wound closure 70
Wrist: see
– Radius distal
– Scaphoid

J. Glicenstein, J. Ohana,
C. Leclercq, Paris

Tumors of the Hand

1988. Approx. 130 figures. Approx. 290 pages.
ISBN 3-540-17439-7

This book deals with both benign and malignant tumors of the hand classified under the following headings: skin tumors, soft tissue tumors, bone tumors of the nail.

It analyses the different aspects of each of these tumors on a clinical, radiologic, pathologic, histologic and therapeutic level. The reader thereby has access to the most complete review to date on tumors of the hand, as well as on the most recent developments in therapy. There is a wealth of illustrative material, nearly all in color, together with an extensive bibliography.

This reference work will be of enormous value to the surgeons, actively involved in the fields of plastic surgery, dermatology and orthopaedics.

Springer-Verlag
Berlin Heidelberg New York
London Paris Tokyo

Springer

MIX
Papier aus verantwortungsvollen Quellen
Paper from responsible sources
FSC® C105338

If you have any concerns about our products,
you can contact us on
ProductSafety@springernature.com

In case Publisher is established outside the EU,
the EU authorized representative is:
Springer Nature Customer Service Center GmbH
Europaplatz 3, 69115 Heidelberg, Germany

Printed by Libri Plureos GmbH
in Hamburg, Germany